BUILDING
A MEDICAL VOCABULARY
with Spanish Translations

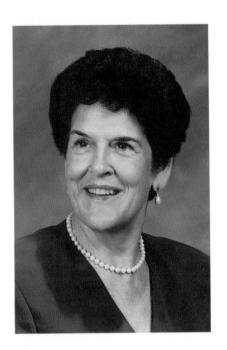

Peggy C. Leonard

BUILDING

A MEDICAL VOCABULARY

with Spanish Translations

PEGGY C. LEONARD, MT, MEd
St. Louis County, Missouri

FIFTH EDITION

SAUNDERS
An Imprint of Elsevier

SAUNDERS
An Imprint of Elsevier

The Curtis Center
Independence Square West
Philadelphia, Pennsylvania 19106

Editor-in-Chief: Andrew Allen
Executive Editor: Maureen Pfeifer
Senior Developmental Editor: Carolyn Kruse
Project Manager: Patricia Tannian
Project Specialist: Melissa Lastarria
Book Design Manager: Gail Morey Hudson
Cover Design: Teresa Breckwoldt
Cover Photo: PhotoDisc © 2001

Medicine is an ever-changing field. Standard safety precautions must be followed, but as new research and clinical experience broaden our knowledge, changes in treatment and drug therapy become necessary or appropriate. Readers of this text are advised to check the product information currently provided by the manufacturer of each drug to be administered to verify the recommended dose, the method and duration of administration, and the contraindications. It is the responsibility of the treating licensed prescriber, relying on experience and knowledge of the patient, to determine dosages and the best treatment for the patient. Neither the publisher nor the editor assumes any responsibility for any injury and/or damage to persons or property.

THE PUBLISHER

Library of Congress Cataloging-in-Publication Data

Leonard, Peggy C.
   Building a medical vocabulary / Peggy C. Leonard.–5th ed.
      p. ; cm
   Includes bibliographical references and index.
   ISBN 0-7216-8954-X
   1. Medicine—Terminology.   2. Human anatomy—Terminology.   3. English language—Glossaries, vocabularies, etc. I. Title
   [DNLM: 1. Terminology. W 15 L581b 2001]
   R123 .L46 2001
   610'.1'4—dc21   00-049690

BUILDING A MEDICAL VOCABULARY, Fifth Edition   ISBN 0–7216–8954–X

Copyright © 2001 by Harcourt Health Sciences

Copyright © 1997, 1993, 1988, 1983 by Saunders

Printed in China

Last digit is the print number: 9   8   7   6   5   4

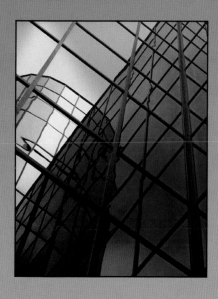

Reviewers

JACKIE T. ELLIS, MLT (ASCP)
Barnes Hospital
St. Louis, Missouri

GERTRUDE FRANGIPANI, RN, BS, MBA
Learning Tree University
Chatsworth, California

ROBERT L. GLADSON, EMT-D
Captain
Federal Fire Department
San Diego, California

DONNA GUIDOS, MA (Clinical Psych)
Diablo Valley College
Pleasant Hill, California

MARY RAHR, MS, RN, CMA-C
Northeast Wisconsin Technical College
Green Bay, Wisconsin

STEVEN J. THURLOW, BS, MS
Jackson Community College
Jackson, Michigan

In memory of my husband

Everette

who inspired those around him
to do more than they ever dreamed
and be better persons than they thought possible.

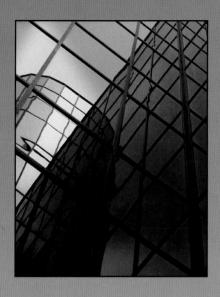

Acknowledgments

Several individuals have contributed to make the fifth edition of *Building a Medical Vocabulary* the best edition yet. Suggestions from instructors and students have been incorporated, as well as in-depth analyses by an outstanding group of reviewers.

The new pharmacological sections were made possible by James F. McCalpin, RPh, who spent many hours preparing material for each chapter. I am also indebted to the companies who have allowed use of illustrations that vividly enhance the written word and bring life to explanations of medical terms.

The production of this book would not be possible without the producers, editors, proofreaders, and all others whose expertise has produced a book that I know will be valuable to students in their search for understanding of the medical language.

Peggy Leonard, MT, MEd

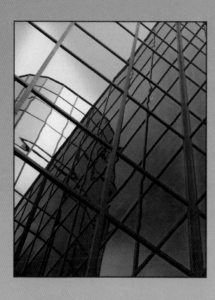

Preface

To the Student

Imagine being able to read and write medical words the first day you begin a terminology study! You will have this experience shortly after you begin studying *Building a Medical Vocabulary*.

FRAMES MAKE LEARNING EASY!

You will find that the material, though organized into frames, has the readability one expects of a textbook. It is important to study Chapters 1, 2, 3, and 4 in the order in which they are presented, since each chapter builds on the material learned in the previous chapter. Be sure to read all frames within a chapter.

YOU CAN WORK AT YOUR OWN PACE.

Some chapters will be shorter and some will be easier than others. You set the pace! It is important to write your answers in the blanks, since writing increases retention of the material. Be sure to work all review questions and check your answers with the solutions in the back of the book.

LISTING OF WORD PARTS WILL BE HELPFUL.

A listing of principal word parts is presented at the beginning of each chapter, beginning with Chapter 2. Most students use the list for review purposes, but others prefer to memorize the meanings before beginning the chapter. You may find that flashcards are helpful in either learning or reviewing.

DON'T BE INTIMIDATED BY LONG DRUG NAMES.

You are not expected to remember the names of drugs in the pharmacological sections; however, your instructor may expect you to remember the uses or effects of the drug classes. Since new drugs are introduced and other drugs are removed each year, it is important to consult current drug reference materials. Sources like the *Physician's Desk Reference* (PDR) and the *Nurse's Drug Reference* (NDR) provide continual updated materials.

HAVE FUN WITH THE PRACTICE DISK.

You will enjoy seeing how much you learned, and the disk is valuable in learning pronunciation.

THE APPENDIX MATERIAL IS A VALUABLE RESOURCE.

Become familiar with the appendices, which include a listing of all word parts and their meanings, a comprehensive glossary/index, Spanish translations, and a list of abbreviations.

To the Instructor

The fifth edition of *Building a Medical Vocabulary* is now even easier to use than previous editions! This easy-to-use interactive text was first published in 1983 to help students learn medical vocabulary, and instructors have depended on it for years. Although each profession and each specialty has its own particular terminology, much of the medical language is understood by all members of the health team. This shared vocabulary forms the foundation of this book.

THIS METHOD HAS INTRINSIC MOTIVATION!

A logical, step-by-step learning method is presented. **You will especially appreciate the new organization of chapter material in the fifth edition.** After learning the meaning of word parts and how they are combined, the student begins recognizing and writing new terms in the first chapter! Immediate involvement and feedback provide intrinsic motivation that is not found in other systems, and your students will have fun using this book. The challenge sections help the student distinguish and understand difficult concepts.

CHAPTERS 1 THROUGH 4 PROVIDE A FOUNDATION FOR CHAPTERS ABOUT THE BODY SYSTEMS.

It is important that students study Chapters 1 through 4 in the sequence in which they are presented. Students will learn many word parts, as well as concepts pertaining to body structure and body fluids, in this foundational material.

BODY SYSTEMS (CHAPTERS 5 THROUGH 13) CAN BE STUDIED IN ANY SEQUENCE.

Instructors can easily change the sequence of the "body systems" chapters to their choice. **This flexibility is new to the fifth edition.**

FREQUENT REVIEWS REINFORCE LEARNING.

Section reviews help the student remember the meaning of word parts. A variety of question types are included in comprehensive end-of-chapter reviews. The software that is included introduces a gaming aspect and provides students with another way to determine how much they have learned and to prepare for the examination. Chapter 14 is a comprehensive review of basic terminology covered in the book.

SPANISH TRANSLATIONS ARE PRESENTED.

I lived in Venezuela years ago and learned the Spanish language. I am pleased to offer translation of many medical terms, and I am certain it will be helpful to some students.

THE BOOK ADAPTS WELL TO VARIOUS CLASSROOM LEARNING STRUCTURES.

The book is designed to teach medical terminology. Although pathology is given primary emphasis, this book can also be used as an introductory anatomy and physiology textbook.

PHARMACOLOGICAL TERMS AND ABBREVIATIONS ARE PRESENTED AT THE END OF MOST CHAPTERS.

Most chapters have a pharmacological section, new to the fifth edition. These sections, as well as those for abbreviations, are included for students who need them, but the author is aware that some classes will not choose to study these sections. As the instructor, you decide the importance of these two sections for your class.

LEARNING GOALS AND END-OF-CHAPTER EXERCISES ARE CLASSIFIED AS "BASIC" OR "GREATER COMPREHENSION."

Basic understanding requires labeling or simple recall of the meaning of word parts and medical terms. Greater comprehension includes spelling, pronunciation, classification (an application exercise), abbreviations, and drug classes. You determine and inform the students of your expectations. Instructors often have the students work all of the review questions, then exercise more specificity when choosing questions for the examination.

MORE ILLUSTRATIONS IN THE FIFTH EDITION HELP STUDENTS UNDERSTAND DIFFICULT CONCEPTS.

Two hundred illustrations enhance the written word and bring life to difficult terms.

INSTRUCTOR'S GUIDE IS AVAILABLE.

A comprehensive instructor's guide is available to instructors by contacting Harcourt Health Sciences. It includes a test-generating system with access to over 2000 questions that can be used to produce your own tests. Several types of questions are included, along with classroom exercises, transparency masters, flashcard templates, and several new summary tables designed especially for classroom use.

Contents

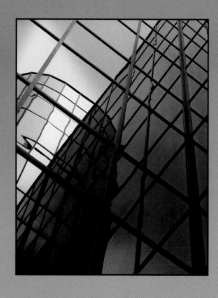

 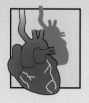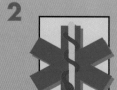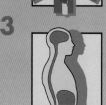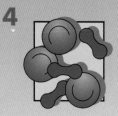

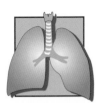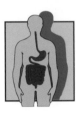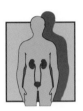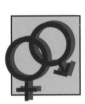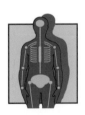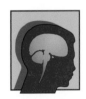

INTEGUMENTARY SYSTEM

 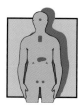
REVIEW

 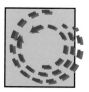

APPENDICES

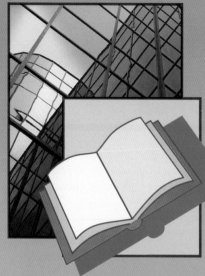

Programmed Learning and the Structure of Medical Terms

1

Outline

Learning Goals

In this chapter, you will learn to do the following:
1. Use the programmed learning format to learn medical terminology.
2. Identify the role and recognize examples of word roots, prefixes, suffixes, and combining forms.
3. Demonstrate correct usage of the combining vowel by correctly joining word parts to write medical terms.
4. Recognize the importance of spelling medical terms correctly.
5. Use the rules learned in this chapter to write the singular or plural forms of medical terms.
6. Pronounce medical terms correctly using the phonetic system that is presented in this book.

Learning by the Programmed Method

Programmed learning is a fast and effective means of becoming familiar with medical language, eliminating much of the tedium of memorization. It is important to study the first four chapters in the sequence presented, since these chapters are the foundation for learning terms presented in all other chapters. Material in this chapter is essential to your understanding of how to use the programmed format throughout the book.

1-1 Programmed learning consists of blocks of information, often containing blanks in which you will write answers. After writing an answer, you will check to see if it is correct by comparing your answer with that in the left column, called the answer column.

The answer column needs to be covered. To do this, use a bookmark or fold a piece of paper and position it so that it covers only the answer column.

1-2 A frame is a block of information preceded by a number. Each frame is given a separate number, and most frames contain one or more blanks in which you will write an answer.

After writing your answer in a blank, you will check to see if it is correct by sliding down the bookmark or folded paper enough to see the answer.

frame

1-3 You have just read two frames. Information contained in frames throughout this book will help you learn medical terms. A block of information with a number is called a _____ .

Write the answer in the preceding blank and check it immediately. Some students prefer to write their answers on a separate sheet of paper so that they can rework the material later.

It is important to *write* your answer, since writing it will help you to remember it better than if you just think of the answer.

Always check your answer immediately and say it aloud if possible. This is especially helpful when you are not familiar with the term. Saying an answer aloud helps you remember it.

1-4 Your answer needs only one word when you see only one blank.

The number of blanks indicates the number of words needed. For example:

_____ _____ requires how many words?

two

_____

1-5 When the answer consists of several words, the blank runs the full length of this column, as shown:

_____

Such a very long blank means that you need to write in _____ words.

several

If you make an error, look back at previous frames to see where you went wrong. Otherwise, you may repeat the error without realizing why it is incorrect.

1-6 You will also have frequent reviews to reinforce what you are learning. Answers to the reviews are in Appendix V, Solutions to Review Exercises. An end-of-the-chapter review helps integrate what you have learned in a chapter.

❑ SECTION A REVIEW *Learning* by the Programmed Method

This section review covers frames 1-1 through 1-6. Write answers in the blanks.

1. If you see two blanks (example: _____ _____), how many words do you write? _____

2. What does it mean if the blank in which to write the answer runs the full width of the column?

_____

(Use Appendix V to check your answers.)

SECTION B

*W*ord Building

Most medical terms are composed of word parts that have their origins in Greek or Latin. Although familiarity with either of the two languages would facilitate learning medical terms, it is not necessary. We will be learning the English translation of most Greek or Latin word parts used in medical terminology.

1-7 The material in this chapter is important because it is the foundation on which you will build a medical vocabulary. It explains word building and teaches you how to break down a word into its parts.

Each chapter introduces new terms and uses those you learned in previous chapters. You will gradually build a medical vocabulary that will enable you to recognize and write thousands of medical words. It is important to study material in the order that it is presented within a chapter. It is also important to study Chapters 1 through 4 in sequential order. These early chapters form the foundation for learning material about the body systems presented in Chapters 5 through 13.

word building

Word building is a system of learning the meaning of various word parts to understand and write new words. Because it is impractical to memorize the medical dictionary, you will use a system of _____ _____ to learn medical terms.

1-8 Correct spelling is essential. The exactness of medicine requires careful attention to writing a term correctly. An error of only one letter can result in a different term. For example, the ilium is a pelvic bone, and the ileum is part of the small intestine.

spelling

In addition to checking your answer each time, you will also check the _____.

❑ SECTION B REVIEW *W*ord Building

This section review covers frames 1-7 and 1-8. Write answers in the blanks.

1. Why is it important to study the first four chapters in the sequence presented?

_____

2. In your own words, what is meant by word building?

_____

(Use Appendix V to check your answers.)

Word Roots, Combining Forms, Prefixes, and Suffixes

Medical terms are composed of word roots, combining forms, prefixes, and suffixes. Learning the meaning of these *word parts* eliminates the necessity of memorizing each new term you encounter. In this chapter, it is important to learn to recognize word roots, prefixes, and suffixes in terms and how to combine them to write terms. In subsequent chapters, you will also be expected to remember the meaning of each word part.

root	**1-9** Most words have a word root, even ordinary words. The word root is the main body of the word. It is usually accompanied by a prefix or suffix or both. Word roots are the building blocks for many terms related to anatomy, diagnosis, and medical procedures. Most words have a word _____. Look at the Greek words and their associated word roots in Table 1-1. By adding prefixes and suffixes, you will soon begin writing medical terms.
eyelid **kneecap** **cephal(o)**	**1-10** Some compound words are composed of two word roots, or words, as in collarbone (collar and bone). Form a compound word using eye and lid: _____. Write another compound word, using knee and cap: _____. Many words would be difficult to pronounce if they were written without a vowel to join the word roots. A vowel [usually "o"] is often inserted between word roots to make the word easier to pronounce, as in speedometer. A combining form is recognized as a word part that ends in an enclosed vowel. In this example, the combining form, **speed(o),** is joined with another part of the word, meter. The parentheses are not included when the combining form joins other word parts. The term *cephalometer* is composed of two word roots, cephal and meter. Write the combining form for cephal: _____. The origin of several combining forms and their use in medical terms are shown in Table 1-2.
Latin	**1-11** You will sometimes learn two word roots that have the same meaning. Table 1-1 shows the Greek word root *nephr* for kidney, while Table 1-2 shows the Latin word root *ren* for kidney. Both nephric and renal mean pertaining to the kidney. Likewise, both dermal and cutaneous mean pertaining to the skin (see Figure 1-1). As a general rule, Latin roots are used to write words naming and describing structures of the body, whereas Greek roots are used to write words naming and describing diseases, conditions, diagnosis, and treatment. As with most rules, there are exceptions. When two medical terms have the same meaning but look very different, it is probably because the origin of the word roots comes from two different languages, Greek or_____.
prefix **without**	**1-12** A prefix is placed before a word to modify its meaning. When written alone, a prefix is usually followed by a hyphen (example: peri-). In anhydrous, **an-** is a prefix that means without. Hydrous means related to water. What type of word part is an-? _____. The prefix *an-* means _____.
without **water**	**1-13** In anhydrous, hydrous refers to water. Combining the two meanings, anhydrous means _____ _____.

TABLE 1-1 Examples of Word Roots

GREEK WORD	WORD ROOT
karkinos (crab, cancer)	carcin
lithos (stone)	lith
nephros (kidney)	nephr
stomatos (mouth)	stomat

TABLE 1-2 Examples of Word Roots and Combining Forms

LATIN WORD	WORD ROOT	COMBINING FORM	USE IN A WORD
articulus (joint)	articul	articul(o)	articulation
cauda (tail)	caud	caud(o)	caudal
fungi (fungus)	fung	fung(i)	fungicide
oris (mouth)	or	or(o)	oral
renes (kidney)	ren	ren(o)	renal

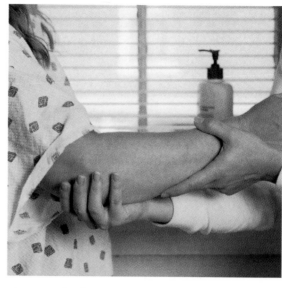

FIGURE 1-1

Examination of the skin. A patient's skin, the body's largest and most visible organ, can produce valuable information about his or her health. The scientific name of the skin is dermis, so named after the Greek term, *derma*. *Cutis* (Latin) also means skin. Both dermal and cutaneous mean pertaining to the skin. (From Polaski AL, Tatro SE: *Luckmann's core principles and practice of medical-surgical nursing*, Philadelphia, 1996, Saunders.)

sub- **below normal**	**1-14** In subnormal, **sub-** means below. In subnormal, which part of the word is the prefix? _____ Normal is a familiar word that we use to mean agreeing with the regular and established type. Its meaning is changed when a prefix is added. Subnormal means _____ _____.
root **suffix**	**1-15** A suffix is attached to the end of a word or word part to modify its meaning. Suffixes are joined to combining forms to write nouns, adjectives, and verbs. A suffix written alone is usually preceded by a hyphen, indicating that another word part precedes it. Carditis means inflammation of the heart. The word part *card* refers to the heart and is the word _____. The word part *-itis* means inflammation and is being used as what part of the word? _____
dyspnea **difficult breathing**	**1-16** Occasionally a word is composed of only a prefix and a suffix. Join dys- and -pnea to write a new word:_____. The prefix **dys-** means bad, painful, or difficult, and **-pnea** means breathing. Dyspnea means _____ _____.
combining forms **cyst(o)** **psych(o)**	**1-17** You will be learning the combining form for word roots because word roots are often combined with other word parts. In thermometer, *therm(o)* is the _____ _____. Which is a combining form, cyst or cyst(o) _____? In psychology, _____ is a combining form.

❏ SECTION C REVIEW   *W*ord Roots, Combining Forms, Prefixes, and Suffixes

This section review covers frames 1-9 through 1-17. Write CF (for combining form) or WR (for word root) after each of the following word parts:

1. aden(o) _____
2. bil(i) _____
3. cyan _____
4. derm(a) _____

5. duoden _____
6. electr _____
7. gloss(o) _____

8. hemat _____
9. ren _____
10. spir(o) _____

Circle the combining forms used to write the following words. Example: ⟨spin⟩al

11. adenopathy
12. biliary
13. cyanosis
14. dermal

15. duodenostomy
16. electrode
17. glossopathy
18. hematology

19. spirometry
20. tomography

Write CF (for combining form), P (for prefix), or S (for suffix) for each of the following:

21. brady- _____
22. -cele _____
23. eu- _____

24. -graphy _____
25. hydr(o) _____
26. -iasis _____

27. mal- _____
28. phon(o) _____
29. -pathy _____

A prefix or suffix is underlined in each of the following terms. Write P (for prefix) or S (for suffix) after each term:

30. <u>ad</u>hesion _____
31. adeno<u>pathy</u> _____
32. bili<u>ary</u> _____

33. derm<u>al</u> _____
34. <u>endo</u>cardial _____
35. hemato<u>logy</u> _____

36. <u>hypo</u>glossal _____
37. <u>micro</u>scope _____
38. <u>pre</u>natal _____

(Use Appendix V to check your answers.)

SECTION D

*C*ombining Word Parts to Write Medical Terms

You have learned that medical terms are composed of word roots, combining forms, prefixes, and suffixes. You will now learn to combine these word parts to write medical terms.

	1-18 One does not always use the vowel that is at the end of a combining form. A rule that will help you in writing medical terms is this: The combining vowel is used before suffixes that begin with a *consonant* and before another word root. (There are exceptions to the rule, and you will learn the exceptions as you progress through the material. For now, remember to drop the vowel before a suffix that begins with a vowel.)
consonant	The rule for using the combining vowel shows us that the combining vowel is used in two cases. In one case, the combining vowel is used before a suffix that begins with a _____.
	1-19 The combining vowel is also used to join two combining forms. Combine **gastr(o),** meaning stomach, and **enter(o),** meaning intestine:
gastroentero	_____. (Of course, this is not a complete word, since it needs a suffix.)
gastroenterology	Combine gastr(o) + enter(o) + -logy to write a term that means the study of the stomach, intestines, and related structures: _____.
carpal	**1-20** The wrist is also called the carpus. Write a word that means pertaining to the wrist by combining **carp(o),** meaning wrist, and -al: _____.
	A carpal support holds the wrist in a given position (see Figure 1-2).

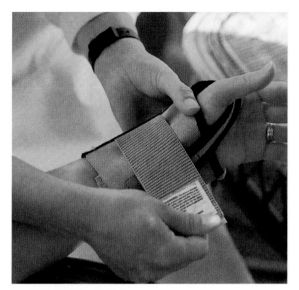

FIGURE 1-2

A carpal support. Maintaining the wrist in a resting position is important in preventing further irritation of the inflamed nerve in carpal tunnel syndrome, a painful disorder of the wrist and hand. It may develop spontaneously without a known cause or may result from disease or injury. A common cause is repetitive movements of the hands and wrists, such as factory work or typing. Surgery may be required to relieve severe symptoms of long duration. (From Polaski AL, Tatro SE: *Luckmann's core principles and practice of medical-surgical nursing*, Philadelphia, 1996, Saunders.)

aortitis	**1-21** The combining form *aort(o)* means aorta, and **-itis** means inflammation. Join the two word parts to write a term that means inflammation of the aorta: _____.
	(Check your spelling carefully.)
cardioaortitis	Join **cardi(o),** meaning heart, and aortitis: _____.
	Cardiaortitis is also an acceptable spelling of the term that you just wrote. Two spellings of the same term usually come about through popular use. As we progress through the material, such exceptions are noted.
tonsillitis	**1-22** Join the combining form *tonsill(o)* with -itis: _____. Imagine how cumbersome the pronunciation would be if you did not drop the vowel.
uremia	Combine **ur(o)** with **-emia** to form a new word: _____.
urogenital	Combine ur(o) with genital to form a new word: _____.
vowel	To summarize, one usually drops the combining vowel if the combining form is joined to a suffix that begins with a _____.
periappendicitis	**1-23** Notice that prefixes are not included in the rule concerning use of the combining vowel. That is because most prefixes require no change before they are joined with other word parts. (A few exceptions will be noted later.) Join **peri-** and appendicitis: _____.
enteritis	Let's be certain that you can apply this rule. Join enter(o) with -itis: _____.
enterocyst	Join enter(o) with cyst: _____.
unilateral	Join uni- and lateral: _____.
	1-24 If you were correct on the last few blanks, you have learned the rule for using word parts to write medical terms. In this program, you will be using combining forms, prefixes, and suffixes to build many new words. When a word part is first introduced, it will be in **bold type.**
combining form	A combining form will be recognized as a word part that has a vowel enclosed in parentheses as its ending. For example, you may not know the meaning of **thorac(o),** but you recognize that thorac(o) is which type of word part? _____ _____

anti-, tri-	**1-25** Prefixes will be designated by placing a hyphen after the word part, such as **pre-**. The hyphen indicates that something follows this word part. Which of the following word parts are prefixes: metr(o), anti-, tri-, -scope? _____ and _____
suffix	Remember that the hyphen follows the prefix when the prefix is shown alone. If the hyphen comes _before_ the word part, the word part is a suffix. This tells us that **-scope** is which type of word part? _____
-gram, -graph	Which of the following word parts are suffixes: -gram, -graph, chlor(o), post-? _____ and _____
	1-26 You will also learn to recognize word parts as components of other words. To help you distinguish the component parts of medical words, the words will often be divided by a diagonal between the component parts.
	For example, how many component parts are there in the word aden/oma? _____
two	
three	Chole/cysto/gram has _____ component parts.
	See Figure 1-3 to summarize what you have learned about writing and interpreting medical terms.

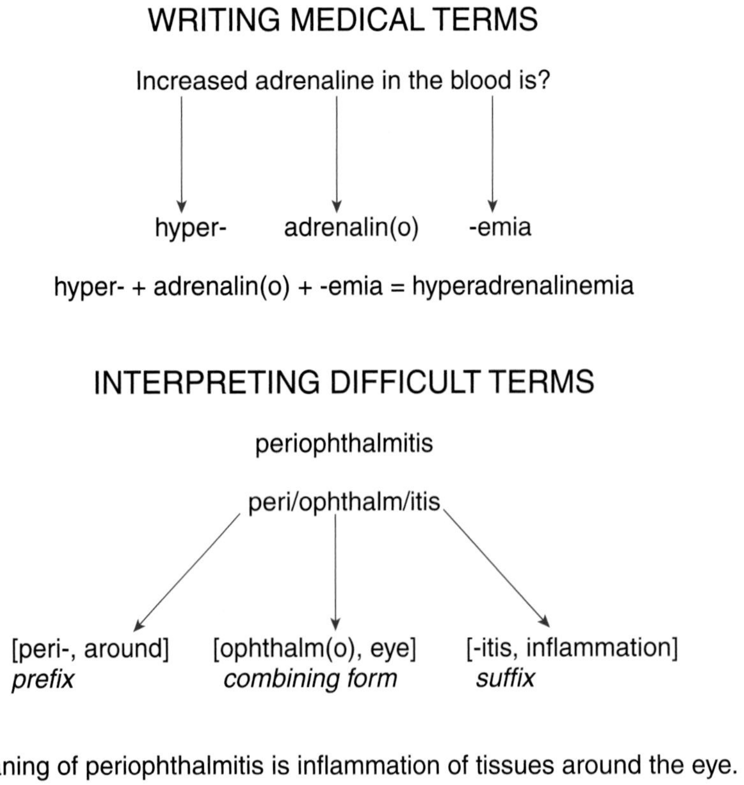

WRITING MEDICAL TERMS

Increased adrenaline in the blood is?

hyper-   adrenalin(o)   -emia

hyper- + adrenalin(o) + -emia = hyperadrenalinemia

INTERPRETING DIFFICULT TERMS

periophthalmitis

peri/ophthalm/itis

[peri-, around]   [ophthalm(o), eye]   [-itis, inflammation]
prefix   _combining form_   _suffix_

Meaning of periophthalmitis is inflammation of tissues around the eye.

FIGURE 1-3
Examples of using prefixes, suffixes, and combining forms to write and interpret medical terms.

❏ SECTION D REVIEW *C*ombining Word Parts to Write Medical Terms

This section review covers frames 1-18 through 1-26. Use CF (for combining form), P (for prefix), or S (for suffix) to designate each of the following word parts as a combining form, a prefix, or a suffix.

1. alkal(o) _____
2. bil(i) _____
3. -capnia _____
4. chol(e) _____
5. hypo- _____

6. neo- _____
7. -pepsia _____
8. post- _____
9. primi- _____
10. ven(o) _____

Combine the following word parts to write terms.

11. acid(o) + -osis _____
12. acr(o) + -megaly _____
13. anti- + -emesis _____
14. bronch(o) + -scopy _____
15. dys- + -phagia _____

16. hypo- + thyroid(o) + -ism _____
17. leuk(o) + cyt(o) + -osis _____
18. mal- + absorption _____
19. my(o) + metr(o) + -ium _____
20. thromb(o) + phleb(o) + -itis _____

(Use Appendix V to check your answers.)

SECTION E

*P*ronunciation of Medical Terms

A medical term is easier to remember when you know how to pronounce it. Pronunciations for newly introduced medical terms are shown in the following chapters. *If you have not already done so, study the rules for pronunciation that are found on the front inside cover of this book.* You will need to have done this before proceeding to the remaining frames of this chapter.

dren i an short	**1-27** In the term *adrenalin* (ə-**dren′**ə-lin), which syllable receives the primary accent? _____ In adrenalitis (ə-**dre″**nəl-i′**tis),** which syllable receives the primary accent? _____ Which syllable receives secondary emphasis in angiectomy (an″je-ek′tə-me)? _____ Is the "a" in angiectomy pronounced as a long or short "a"? _____
lo short	**1-28** In ang″kə-lo′sēz (ankylosis), which is the primary accented syllable? _____ Is the vowel in the "sis" syllable pronounced as a long or short "i"? _____
	1-29 Be aware that there are different ways to pronounce some medical terms. Pronunciation will be shown as new terms are introduced beginning with Chapter 2. In addition, a comprehensive alphabetical list of terms for all chapters that includes both pronunciations and definitions is presented in the Index/Glossary.

❏ **SECTION E REVIEW**   *Pronunciation of Medical Terms*

This section review covers frames 1-27 through 1-29. Write answers in the blanks to review your understanding of the rules of pronunciation used in this book.

1. List two sources in *Building a Medical Vocabulary* for learning the pronunciation of a medical term: _____ and _____

2. How many syllables does the term *hypercalcemia* (hi″pər-kal-se′me-ə) have? _____

3. Using the pronunciation of hypercalcemia shown in #2, which syllable receives the primary accent? _____

4. Using the pronunciation of hypercalcemia shown in #2, which syllable receives a secondary accent? _____

5. Using the pronunciation of hypercalcemia shown in #2, list all vowels that are pronounced as long vowels: _____
(Use Appendix V to check your answers.)

SECTION F

Plurals of Medical Terms

Although plurals of many medical terms are formed using the rules you may already know, it is important to learn rules that apply when terms have special endings. When you see a noun in its singular form, you will learn to write a plural for that term, but be aware that sometimes more than one plural is acceptable.

abrasions **lacerations**	**1-30** Plurals of many medical terms are formed using the rules you already know. Many plurals are formed by simply adding an "s" to the singular term. Write plurals by adding an "s" to these singular terms: abrasion _____ laceration _____
branches **brushes** **sinuses**	**1-31** Many nouns that end in "s", "ch", or "sh" form their plurals by adding "es." The plural of abscess is abscesses. Write plurals by adding "es" to these terms: branch _____ brush _____ sinus _____
capillaries **extremities** **ovaries**	**1-32** Singular nouns that end in "y" preceded by a consonant form their plurals by changing the "y" to "i" and adding "es." For example, the plural of allergy is allergies. Change the "y" to "i" and add "es" to write plurals of these nouns: capillary _____ extremity _____ ovary _____
	1-33 Use Table 1-3 to learn the rules for forming other plurals of medical terms, but be aware that there are a few exceptions and that only major rules are included. Many dictionaries show the plural form of nouns and can be used as a reference. Also notice that some terms have more than one acceptable plural.

TABLE 1-3 Forming Plurals of Nouns with Special Endings

IF THE SINGULAR ENDING IS	THE PLURAL ENDING IS	EXAMPLES (SINGULAR)	PLURAL
is	es	diagnosis, prognosis, psychosis (Some words ending in "is" form plurals by dropping the "is" and adding "ides," as in epididymis and epididymides.)	diagnoses, prognoses, psychoses
um	a	atrium, ileum, septum, bacterium	atria, ilea, septa, bacteria
us	i	alveolus, bacillus, bronchus (Some singular forms ending in "us" form plurals by dropping the "us" and adding either "era" or "ora," as in viscera and corpora. Others form plurals by simply adding "es", as in viruses.)	alveoli, bacilli, bronchi
a	ae	vertebra, patella, petechia	vertebrae, petallae, petechiae
ix	ices	appendix, varix, cervix (Through common use, appendixes and cervixes have become acceptable plural forms.)	appendices, varices, cervices
ex	ices	cortex	cortices
ax	aces	thorax	thoraces (Thoraxes is also acceptable.)
ma	s or mata	carcinoma, sarcoma	carcinomas or carcinomata, sarcomas or sarcomata
on	a	protozoon, spermatozoon (Some singular forms ending in "on" form plurals by adding "s," as in chorion and chorions.)	protozoa, spermatozoa
nx	nges	phalanx, larynx	phalanges, larynges

❑ SECTION F REVIEW 𝒫lurals of Medical Terms

This section review covers frames 1-30 through 1-33. Write the plural form for each of the following singular nouns.

1. capsule _____
2. cataract _____
3. calculus _____
4. cortex _____

5. diagnosis _____
6. neurosis _____
7. protozoon _____
8. virus _____

Write the singular form of each plural noun.

9. appendices _____
10. fungi _____
11. larynges _____

12. prognoses _____
13. sarcomata _____
14. spermatozoa _____

(Use Appendix V to check your answers.)

𝐸𝑠𝑝𝑎ñ𝑜𝑙 *Enhancing Spanish Communication*

Spanish translation of selected terms is presented at the end of each chapter beginning with Chapter 2. Appendix II of *Building a Medical Vocabulary* has a comprehensive list of both English-Spanish and Spanish-English translation for easy reference.

The sound of Spanish vowels does not vary and must be fully and distinctly pronounced. This does not apply to double vowels. Use these rules to pronounce vowels:

Spanish vowel	Pronounce as		Spanish vowel	Pronounce as
a	*a* in mama		*u*	*u* in rule or the sound of *oo* in spool (The u is generally silent in these syllables; que, gue, and gui.)
e	*a* in day			
i	*i* in police			
o	*o* in so		*y*	*e* in see

Some consonants have similar sounds in English and Spanish. Some significant differences are noted here.

Español *Enhancing Spanish Communication—cont'd*

Spanish	Pronunciation		Spanish	Pronunciation
c	sometimes as *k* or *s*		ñ	blending of *n* and *y*
d	sometimes as *th*		q	*k*
g	distinctly different g, sometimes *h*		r	trilled *r*
h	not pronounced		rr	strongly trilled *r*
j	*h*		z	*s*
ll	blending of *l* and *y*, or simply *y*			

Phonetic pronunciation is presented with the stressed syllable in upper case letters, as in the example, SAHN-gray. In this term, the first syllable is stressed.

English	Spanish (pronunciation)		English	Spanish (pronunciation)
adrenaline	*adrenalina (ah-dray-nah-LEE-nah)*		microscope	*microscopio (me-cros-CO-pe-o)*
breathing	*respiración (res-pe-ran-se-ON)*		mouth	*boca (BO-cah)*
calculus	*cálculo (CAHL-coo-lo)*		ovary	*ovario (o-VAH-re-o)*
cancer	*cáncer (CAHN-ser)*		psychology	*psicología (se-co-lo-HEE-ah)*
diagnosis	*diagnóstico (de-ag-NOS-te-co)*		skin	*piel (pe-EL)*
eyelid	*párpado (PAR-pah-do)*		stone	*cálculo (CAHL-coo-lo)*
heart	*corazón (co-rah-SON)*		water	*agua (AH-goo-ah)*
kidney	*riñon (ree-NYON)*		wrist	*muñeca (moo-NYAH-cah)*
kneecap	*rótula (RO-too-lah)*			

You have now learned the rules of the program. There is a review section at the end of each chapter. The review helps you to know if you learned the material. Work each section of the review and then check your answers with the solutions found in Appendix V. You will learn more if you work all of the review before checking your answers. (Don't be concerned about learning the meaning of the word parts for Chapter 1. All of these word parts will be included in subsequent chapters.)

CHAPTER REVIEW 1

REVIEWING WORD PARTS
I. Write a word for each clue or to complete a sentence.

CROSSWORD PUZZLE 1

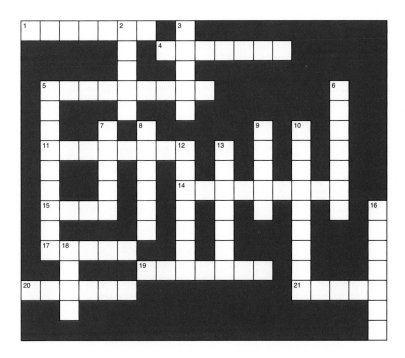

Across
1 plural of bacillus
4 plural of bronchus
5 singular form of carcinomata
11 plural of bacterium
14 plural of vertebra
15 plural of ileum
17 the origin of many medical terms
19 Which accent is represented by *sis'* in the pronunciation, sis'to pek"se?
20 the singular form of thoraces
21 the plural of septum

Down
2 language origin of many medical terms
3 block of information in programmed learning
5 A word part ending in an enclosed vowel is a _____ form.
6 plural of varix
7 plural of atrium
8 word part that is placed before a word to modify its meaning
9 A combining form ends with a _____ .
10 the plural of pharynx
12 plural of alveolus
13 singular form of sarcomata
16 syllable that receives the greatest emphasis
18 preliminary word part

IDENTIFYING WORD PARTS
II. Use CF (for combining form), P (for prefix), or S (for suffix) to designate each of the following terms as a combining form, a prefix, or a suffix.

1. bil(i)   _____
2. crani(o)   _____
3. -ectomy   _____
4. gigant(o)   _____
5. -iatrics   _____
6. intra-   _____
7. multi-   _____
8. -oid   _____
9. -plegia   _____
10. spher(o)   _____

COMBINING WORD PARTS

III. Using the rules you have learned in Chapter 1, combine the word parts to write terms.

1. alkal(o) + -osis _____
2. cardi(o) + -megaly _____
3. brady- + -pnea _____
4. bronch(o) + -scope _____
5. dys- + -phonia _____

6. hypo- + derm(o) + -ic _____
7. leuk(o) + -emia _____
8. melan(o) + -oid _____
9. my(o) + cardi(o) + -al _____
10. thromb(o) + -osis _____

SPELLING

IV. Use the index/glossary in the back of this book to check the spelling of the following terms. Circle all misspelled terms and write the correct spelling.

1. bulimia _____
2. catheterization _____
3. costektomy _____
4. ductus _____
5. gastroptosis _____

6. humeroskapular _____
7. intraneural _____
8. myxedema _____
9. phalangitis _____
10. splenomegaly _____

PRONUNCIATION

V. Pronunciation is shown for ten medical terms. Underline the primary-accented syllable in each term.

1. calcaneal (kal-ka′ne-əl)
2. diagnosis (di″əg-no′sis)
3. gastromegaly (gas″tro-meg′ə-le)
4. laparoscopy (lap″ə-ros′kə-pe)
5. myoplasty (mi′o-plas″te)

6. otalgia (o-tal′je-ə)
7. phrenic (fren′ik)
8. sclerotic (sklə-rot′ik)
9. trichosis (tri-ko′sis)
10. ureter (u-re′ter)

WRITING TERMS

VI. Complete the chart by writing either the singular or plural form as indicated.

Singular form	Plural form
1. adductor	_____
2. _____	alveoli
3. _____	appendices
4. bursa	_____
5. capillary	_____
6. cortex	_____
7. diagnosis	_____
8. ovary	_____
9. _____	phalanges
10. _____	thoraces

(Check your answers with the solutions in Appendix V. Pay particular attention to spelling.)

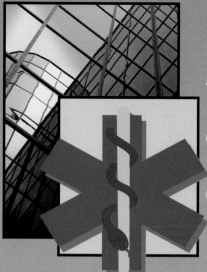

Medicine and Its Specialties

2

Outline

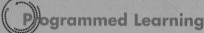
Principal Word Parts

COMBINING FORMS

algesi(o)	sensitivity to pain
bi(o)	life or living
cardi(o)	heart
crin(o)	to secrete
dent(o), odont(o)	tooth
derm(a), dermat(o)	skin
esthesi(o)	feeling
ger(a), ger(o), geront(o)	aged
gynec(o)	female
hist(o)	tissue
immun(o)	immune
laryng(o)	larynx
neur(o)	nerve or nervous system
obstetr(o)	midwife
onc(o)	tumor
ophthalm(o)	eye
opt(o), optic(o)	vision
or(o)	mouth
orth(o)	straight
ot(o)	ear
path(o)	disease
ped(o)	child or foot
pharmac(o)	drugs or medicine
pharmaceut(o)	drugs
physi(o)	nature
plast(o)	repair
pod(o)	foot
psych(o)	mind
radi(o)	radius or radiant energy
rheumat(o)	rheumatism
rhin(o)	nose
therapeut(o)	treatment
tom(o)	to cut
tox(o), toxic(o)	poison
ur(o)	urine or urinary tract

PREFIXES

an-	not or without
ana-	up or again
end-, endo-	inside
pes-	foot

SUFFIXES

-ac, -al, -ic	pertaining to
-crine	to secrete
-er, -ist	one who
-ia	condition
-iatrician	practitioner
-iatrics, -iatry	medicine
-ism	condition, theory, process
-logist	one who studies
-logy	study or science of
-opsy	to view
-pod	foot
-tomy	incision (cutting)

Learning Goals

These goals refer specifically to material covered in Chapter 2. With your instructor's guidance, determine which ones are appropriate for your needs.

▶ **BASIC UNDERSTANDING**

In this chapter, you will learn to do the following:
1. Recognize prefixes, suffixes, combining forms, and word roots in medical words.
2. Demonstrate understanding of the rules for using word parts to form medical terms.
3. Write the meaning of the word parts and use them to build and analyze terms.
4. Describe several medical specialties and name their associated specialists.
5. Recognize and define terms pertaining to sciences of the human body and fields of medicine.

▶ **GREATER COMPREHENSION**

6. Spell medical terms accurately.
7. Pronounce the terms correctly.
8. Write the meaning of the abbreviations.
9. Understand the meaning of drug administration, absorption, action, biotransformation, and addiction.
10. Identify the effects or uses of the drug classes presented in this chapter.

Art and Science of Medicine

Medicine is the art and science of the diagnosis and treatment of disease and the maintenance of health. Prospective physicians must study a number of "basic sciences" linked to the structure and function of the human body, but medicine is far more than the application of scientific principles. The focus of medicine is the patient, whose welfare is its continuing purpose. The physician is supported by a number of health professionals. This section introduces some of the sciences studied by individuals in health care.

An Overview of Principal Word Parts is presented at the beginning of Chapter 2 and the remaining chapters. You may wish to read through the list and their meanings before beginning the programmed portion of each chapter. It is also helpful to prepare flash cards to use as a review.

	2-1 The term *medicine* has several meanings, including a drug or a remedy for illness. A second meaning of medicine is the art and science of diagnosis, treatment, and prevention of disease. Prospective physicians study many sciences to understand the complexity of the human body.
	Sciences that involve the human body often have the ending **-logy,** which means the study or science of. It is a word part that is used in many common words, as well as in medical words. The introductory material in Chapter 1 described how to recognize prefixes, suffixes, and combining forms. Which type of word part is -logy? _____
suffix	
study	Embryo/logy (**em″bre-ol′ə-je**) is the_____ of the development of the embryo, a young organism in the early stages of growth and differentiation.

embryology	**2-2** Several branches of science are concerned with the study of the body. You have just learned that the study of the development of the embryo is _____.
	Be sure to check the pronunciation of a term when you first see it because pronunciation is not always obvious. The index/glossary in the back of the book also shows pronunciations and more formal definitions. When writing answers in the blank spaces, don't forget to slide down the bookmark or paper that covers the answer column and check your answer. Also carefully check each answer for correct spelling.
study **biology** (bi-ol′ə-je) **living** **bi(o)**	**2-3** The combining form **_bi(o)_** means life or living. Bio/logy is the _____ of life and living things. Stated simply, the study of life is _____. Bi/opsy (**bi′op-se**) is the examination of tissue from the _____ body. The suffix **_-opsy_** means to view. In a biopsy, tissue is removed, sectioned, and viewed through a microscope. A biopsy is performed to establish a precise diagnosis. The part of "biopsy" that means life or living is _____.
anatomy **cutting**	**2-4** Anatomy (**ə-nat′ə-me**) is the science of the structure of the body and the relationship of its parts. Its name is based on the combining form **_tom(o),_** which means to cut. Translated literally, anatomy means "cutting up" because the prefix **_ana-_** means up or again (cutting through tissue is implied in the term). The suffix **_-tomy_** means cutting (incision of). Dissection (**di-sek′shən**), to cut apart, plays an important role in the study of anatomy. The study of the structure of the body and the relationship of its parts ends in -tomy. The word that refers to the structure of the body and the relationship of its parts is _____. Many more words using tom(o) are formed in later chapters. The suffix -tomy means incision or _____.
study **-logy** **functions**	**2-5** Physio/logy (**fiz″e-ol′ə-je**) is the _____ of the function and activities of the living body; however, **_physi(o)_** refers to nature. The word _physician_ originated from physi(o). Physiology relates to the functions of the body. The part of physiology that means study is _____. Physiology is the study of the _____ of the body.
study **histology**	**2-6** Histo/logy (**his-tol′ə-je**) is the _____ of the structure, composition, and functions of tissues. Stated simply, histo/logy means the study of tissue; **_hist(o)_** means tissue. A microscope is used to study the minute cells that make up tissue. This detailed study of the structures, composition, and functions of tissue is known as _____.
pathology (pə-thol′ə-je) **pathology** **disease**	**2-7** You learned how to combine word parts to build medical words in Chapter 1. Those rules are summarized in Table 2-1. Combine path(o) and -logy to form a new word: _____. Pathology is the study of the causes and development of abnormal conditions and the structural and functional changes that occur as a result of these conditions. The combining form **_path(o)_** means disease. The medical specialty that deals with diseases and the changes they produce is _____. Patho/physiology (**path″o-fiz″e-ol′ə-je**) is the study of disordered function or, in other words, the physiology of _____. Human pathophysiology is the science that focuses on the illnesses of humans.

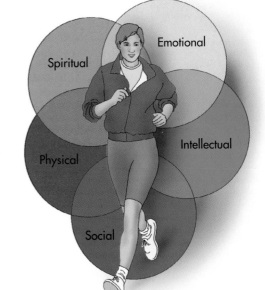

FIGURE 2-1
Holistic health, the concept that the physical, emotional, intellectual, social, and spiritual aspects of a person's life must be viewed as an integrated whole.

TABLE 2-1   Word Building Rules

Joining Combining Forms and Suffixes
- The combining vowel is usually retained when a combining form is joined with a suffix that begins with a consonant. Example: enter(o) + -logy = enterology
- The combining vowel is usually omitted when a combining form is joined with a suffix that begins with a vowel. Example: enter(o) + -ic = enteric

Joining Combining Forms
- The combining vowel is usually retained between combining forms. Example: gastr(o) + enterology = gastroenterology

Joining Other Word Parts to Prefixes
- Most prefixes require no change when they are joined with other word parts. Example: peri- + appendicitis = periappendicits

pathology	**2-8** A pathologist (**pə-thol′ə-jist**) is a specialist in _____. A medical pathologist usually specializes in either clinical or surgical pathology.
path(o)	A clinical pathologist is especially concerned with the use of laboratory methods in clinical diagnosis. The part of pathologist that means disease is _____.
pathologist	Tissues and organs that are removed in surgery are sent to the pathology laboratory. The physician who studies those tissues and organs to determine the cause of disease is a surgical _____.
holistic	**2-9** Medicine recognizes that a person is a composite of physical, social, spiritual, emotional, and intellectual needs (Figure 2-1). The holistic (**ho-lis′tik**)* viewpoint considers the human as a functioning whole. In illness, the components interact and influence one another. Recognizing that a person is a composite of physical, social, emotional, and intellectual needs is a _____ viewpoint. Both *-ic* and *-al* are suffixes that mean pertaining to.

*Holistic (Greek: *holos*, whole).

one who
-logist
one who studies or a specialist
bi(o)
biologist (bi-ol'ə-jist)
bio/logist (or bio/log/ist)
studies life
embryo/log/ist
one who studies embryos
bio/chem/ist
chemistry, living
a record of the electrical activity of the heart
one who physiologist (fiz"e-ol'ə-jist)
histology
histologist (his-tol'ə-jist)
neurology (noo-rol'ə-je)
neur(o)
neurologist (noo-rol'ə-jist)

2-10   The suffix *-ist* means one who. Many common words contain -ist. In words such as organ/ist, cycl/ist, and capital/ist, -ist means _____ _____. In medicine, -ist often refers to a specialist, one who has advanced education and training in a particular area of practice.

Combine log(o) and -ist to form a new suffix: _____. The suffix *-logist* means "one who studies" or "a specialist."

Some word parts have been combined and are so commonly used that they remain fixed and easily recognized. The suffix *-logist* is an example of this, and you need to recognize that -logist means _____.

2-11   You learned earlier in this chapter that the combining form for life is _____.

Combine bi(o) and -logist to form a word that means one who studies living organisms (life): _____.

2-12   You will also want to break down words into their components and analyze their meanings. Using a diagonal line, divide biologist into its components: _____.

To interpret a new word, begin by looking at the suffix. This identifies it as a noun, a verb, or an adjective. After deciding the meaning of the suffix, go to the beginning of the word and read across from left to right, interpreting the remaining elements to develop the full sense of the term.

The suffix in bio/log/ist indicates that the word is a noun because -ist means one who. A biologist is one who _____ _____.

2-13   Using diagonal lines, divide embryologist: _____.

An embryologist is _____.

Some terms require more than literal interpretation. Use diagonal lines to divide the term *biochemist*: _____.

Using the technique you have learned for breaking down words, you see that more interpretation is necessary. Direct analysis of biochemist yields "one who/living/chemical or chemistry." The meaning of biochemist is one who specializes in the _____ of _____ things.

Longer terms are not necessarily difficult if you recognize the word parts. For example, electrocardiogram can be divided as electro/cardio/gram. The suffix *-gram* means a record of information. Going back to the beginning of the term, **electr(o)** means electrical activity and **cardi(o)** means the heart. Write the meaning of electrocardiogram by interpreting the association of its parts (a record of information + electrical activity + the heart): _____.

2-14   An anatom/ist (ə nat'ə-mist) is _____ _____ is skilled in anatomy. What is the name given to one who is skilled in physiology (**fiz"e-ol'ə-je**)? _____

Use the combining form for tissue plus the suffix for study of to write a word that means the study of tissue: _____.

One who specializes in histology is a _____.

2-15   The combining form *neur(o)* means nerve. A nerve cell is called a neuron (**noor'on**) (Figure 2-2). In many words, neur(o) refers to the nervous system, which comprises the brain, spinal cord, and nerves. Build a word by combining neur(o) and -logy: _____

Neurology deals with the nervous system in both normal and diseased states. The word part that means the nervous system is _____.

One who studies and treats diseases of the nervous system is a _____.

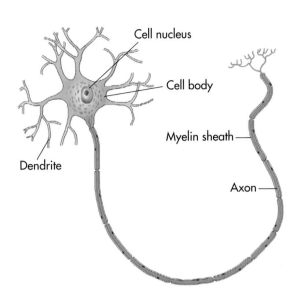

Cell nucleus

Cell body

Myelin sheath

Dendrite

Axon

FIGURE 2-2
The structure of a typical neuron, a type of nerve cell responsible for conducting nervous impulses. This neuron has a cell body and cytoplasmic projections, one axon, and several dendrites that are sometimes called nerve fibers. Unlike most cells in the body, the neuron cannot replicate.

Chapters throughout this book are divided into sections. Short reviews of new word parts are provided after each section. The line length in the review sections is the same regardless of the number of words needed for the answer. Try to complete all of the answers, but look back over the section to find the meaning of any word part that you cannot remember. After completion, check your answers with the solutions in Appendix V.

❑ **SECTION A REVIEW**   *A*rt and Science of Medicine

This section review covers frames 2-1 through 2-15. Complete the following table by writing the meaning of each word part listed:

Combining Form	Meaning		Suffix	Meaning
1. bi(o)	_____		8. -al	_____
2. hist(o)	_____		9. -ic	_____
3. neur(o)	_____		10. -ist	_____
4. path(o)	_____		11. -logist	_____
5. physi(o)	_____		12. -logy	_____
6. tom(o)	_____		13. -opsy	_____
			14. -tomy	_____
Prefix	**Meaning**			
7. ana-	_____			

(Use Appendix V to check your answers.)

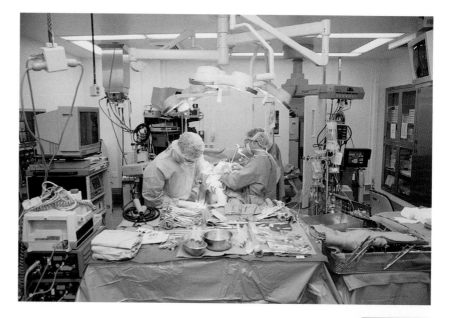

FIGURE 2-3
A typical operating room. The type of surgery determines the precise setup and specialized equipment that is needed. All persons in the operating room must wear surgical attire. (From Ignatavicius, DD, Workman, ML, Mishler, MA: *Medical-surgical nursing across the health care continuum*, ed 3, Philadelphia, 1999, WB Saunders.)

SECTION B

Surgery and Dentistry

Surgery includes several branches of medicine that treat disease, injuries, and deformities by manual or operative procedures. The term *surgery* also refers to the place where surgery is performed or the work performed by a surgeon. This section deals with several specialized areas of surgery. Oral surgery and other dental specialties are also included.

neurosurgeon (noo″ro-sur′jən) **neurosurgery** (noo′ro-sər″jər-e)	**2-16** General surgery deals with operations of all kinds. A surgeon treats diseases by manual or operative procedures. Surgery, or the operating room, is also where surgery is performed (Figure 2-3). Build a word combining neur(o) with surgeon that means a surgeon who specializes in surgery of the nervous system: _____. Use the combining form for nerve plus surgery to write a term that means the branch of surgery that specializes in the nervous system: _____. There are many other surgical specialties, such as those dealing only with the head and neck, hand, and urinary system.
repair (or recon-struction) **Reconstructive** **plastic surgeon**	**2-17** Plastic surgery is the repair or reconstruction of tissue or organs by means of surgery. The combining form **plast(o)** means repair. Plastic surgery is the surgical specialty that deals with _____ of tissue or organs. Reconstructive surgery is an aspect of plastic surgery. It includes everything from resetting broken facial bones to restoring parts of the body destroyed by cancer to correcting birth defects. _____ surgery restores body parts by plastic surgery. Aesthetic plastic surgery has greatly increased in the last few years, particularly that involving the face and breasts. Another notable trend is the increasing number of men who are having cosmetic surgery, with hair replacement leading the list. The medical specialist who performs plastic surgery is called a _____ _____.
oral **surgeon**	**2-18** Oral (or′əl) refers to the oral cavity, or the mouth. Oral is derived from **or(o)**, meaning mouth, plus -al, pertaining to. The science of operative procedures on the mouth is _____ surgery. If someone were having wisdom teeth pulled, it would probably be done by a specialist called an oral _____.

mouth	**2-19** A thermometer is an instrument for measuring temperature. An oral thermometer is placed in the _____.
	A rectal thermometer is inserted in the rectum. Most hospitals now use electronic thermometers that record temperatures rapidly and accurately. Newer instruments are capable of measuring body temperature on the skin surface.
mouth oral oral surgery	**2-20** If a medication is to be taken oral/ly, it is to be taken by _____. Another name for the mouth is the _____ cavity. The science of operative procedures on the mouth is _____ _____.
one who ortho/ped/ist orthopedics	**2-21** Ortho/pedics (or″tho-pe′diks) is a branch of surgery that deals with the preservation and restoration of the bones and associated structures. The specialist is called an orthopedic surgeon. An orthoped/ist (or″tho-pe′dist) is _____ _____ practices orthopedics. This is another name for an orthopedic surgeon. The combining form *orth(o)* means straight and *ped(o)* refers to child or foot [*pes-,* pod(o),* and *-pod* also refer to foot]. Divide orthopedist into three parts: _____. The orthopedist originally straightened children's bones and corrected deformities. Today an orthopedist specializes in disorders of the bones and associated structures in people of all ages. The specialty that is concerned with diseases and disorders of the bones and associated structures is _____.
orth(o) straight (or straightening) ortho orthodontist (or″tho-don′tist)	**2-22** You learned earlier that a combining form for straight is _____. Ortho/dontics (or″tho-don′tiks) is concerned with _____ teeth. Orthodontics is a branch of dentistry concerned with irregularities in tooth alignment and associated facial problems. The part of "orthodontics" that means straight is _____. One who specializes in orthodontics is an _____. (Hint: Change the ending of orthodontics to form the new word.)
teeth teeth endodontics (en″do-don′tiks)	**2-23** Both *odont(o)* and *dent(o)* mean tooth. An orth/odont/ist often uses braces to straighten _____. (Notice that when orth(o) is joined with odont(o) that one "o" is omitted to facilitate pronunciation.) An end/odont/ist (en″do-don′tist) is one who is concerned with the innermost parts of the _____. An endodontist is a dentist who specializes in the prevention and treatment of conditions that affect the tooth pulp and root and performs root canal therapy. (*Endo-* and *end-* are prefixes that mean inside. End- is generally used before a vowel.) An endodontist practices what specialty? _____
children pedodontics (pe-do-don′tiks)	**2-24** A ped/odont/ist (pe-do-don′tist) is interested in the teeth of whom? _____. (Careful: ped(o) has two meanings!) A pedodontist practices what specialty? _____ Pedodontics is a branch of dentistry that deals with the tooth and mouth conditions in children.
teeth dent	**2-25** Dent/istry is concerned with the teeth, the oral cavity, and associated structures, as well as the prevention, diagnosis, and treatment of disease and the restoration of defective or missing tissue. Dentistry is concerned with the treatment of _____. This includes the prevention of tooth and gum disease. A dentist has received a degree in dentistry and is authorized to practice. The part of "dentistry" that identifies the word's association with teeth is _____.

*Latin: (*pes:* foot).

2-26 An/esthesio/logy (**an″es-the″ze-ol′ə-je**) is an important part of surgery.

The prefix **an-** means not or without; **esthesi(o)** refers to feeling (nervous sensation). The term *anesthesia* is formed by combining an- + esthesi(o) + **-ia**, which means condition. (An "i" is dropped to avoid double "i" and to facilitate pronunciation.) Using your own words, an/esthes/ia is_____

_____.

Anesthesiology is the branch of medicine concerned with the administration of anesthetics (**an″es-thet′iks**) and with their effects. The physician who administers anesthetics during surgery is an _____.

An an/esthetist (**ə-nes′thə-tist**) is not a physician but is trained in administering anesthetics.

You have heard of the word esthetic, also spelled aesthetic, which pertains to the sense of beauty or the sense of sensation (feeling). An/esthetic means characterized by or producing anesthesia, and the same term is applied to a drug that brings about this numbing effect.

An/esthesia (**an″es-the′zhə**) is _____ feeling. Anesthesia is partial or complete loss of sensation, with or without loss of consciousness.

2-27 Anesthesia may be local, regional, or general. Local anesthesia is confined to one area of the body. Brief surgical or dental procedures can be performed when anesthesia is administered to a localized area; thus it is called _____ anesthesia.

When an anesthetic blocks a group of nerve fibers, regional anesthesia occurs. In this case, loss of feeling occurs in a certain region of the body. For this reason, it is called _____ anesthesia.

General anesthesia produces a state of unconsciousness with absence of sensation over the entire body. The drugs producing this state are called _____ anesthetics.

The anesthesiologist may need to administer additional drugs called neuromuscular blocking agents to stop muscle contraction during surgery. Neuro/muscular means pertaining to the nerves and muscles. Later you will study how the nerves and muscles interact to bring about movement. Curare was one of the first neuromuscular blocking agents that was studied (Figure 2-4).

---

loss of feeling or sensation

anesthesiologist (**an″es-the″ze-ol′ə-jist**)

without

local

regional

general

FIGURE 2-4

Curare is a deadly poison used by South American Indians to coat the tips of arrows used to kill animals. Wounded monkeys tend to grab hold of branches or tree trunks, but the curare relaxes their muscles and the monkeys fall to the ground. Curare was the forerunner of neuromuscular blocking agents that are used today to prevent contraction of muscle during general surgery.

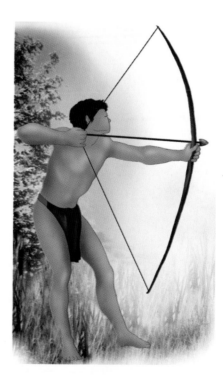

☐ SECTION B REVIEW   *Surgery and Dentisry*

This section review covers frames 2-16 through 2-27. Complete the following table by writing the meaning of each word part that is listed:

Combining Form	Meaning	Prefix	Meaning
1. dent(o)	_____	9. an-	_____
2. esthesi(o)	_____	10. end- or endo-	_____
3. odont(o)	_____	11. pes-	
4. or(o)	_____	**Suffix**	**Meaning**
5. orth(o)	_____	12. -ia	_____
6. ped(o)	_____	13. -pod	_____
7. plast(o)	_____		
8. pod(o)	_____		

(Use Appendix V to check your answers.)

SECTION C

Medical Specialties

A physician usually enters a hospital internship or residency program before beginning practice or further training in a specialty. Several medical specialties are presented in this section.

one who	**2-28** A family practice physician diagnoses and treats health problems in people of either sex and any age. A practitioner of family medicine is a general practitioner or GP. These physicians often act as the primary healthcare provider, referring complex disorders to a specialist. You have already learned that -ist means _____ _____. The suffix *-er,* used in practitioner and many terms, also means one who. Nurse practitioner, radiographer, health planner, and emergency medical technician dispatcher all end in -er, which means one who.
otology (o-tol′ə-je) **otologist** (o-tol′ə-jist)	**2-29** Physicians who specialize in ear, nose, and throat disorders are ENT specialists. The combining form for ear is *ot(o).* The study of the ear is _____. A physician who deals with diseases of the ear is an _____.
ear **otolaryngologist** (o″to-lar″ing-gol′ ə-jist) **ot(o)**	**2-30** *Laryng(o)* means the larynx (**lar′inks**), the organ of voice, but laryngo/logy (**lar″ing-gol′ə-je**) commonly refers to the study of not only the larynx, but also the trachea (windpipe) and the pharynx (throat). Oto/laryngo/logy (**o″to-lar″ing-gol′ə-je**) is the study of the larynx, the trachea (**tra′ke-əh**), the pharynx (**far′inks**), and the _____. A physician who practices otolaryngology is an _____. Otolaryngology deals with diseases of the ear, nose, and throat. Another name for otolaryngology is oto/rhino/laryngo/logy (**o″to-ri′no-lar″in-gol′ə-je).** The combining form *rhin(o)* means nose, but in otolaryngology it is understood that the nose is included, as well as the ear and throat. The word part in otolaryngology that means ear is _____.
larynx **larynx, trachea** **pharynx**	**2-31** The combining form laryng(o) means _____. Another name for the organ of voice is the _____. Another name for the windpipe is the _____. The throat is the _____.

ophthalmology (of″thəl-mol′ə-je) **ophthalm(o)**	**2-32** The combining form for eye is ***ophthalm(o).*** The study of the eye is _____. A physician who specializes in diseases of the eye is an ophthalmologist (of″thəl-mol′ə-jist). Look closely at the combining form for eye. Write the combining form, being careful of its spelling: _____.
urology (u-rol′ə-je) **urologist** (u-rol′ə-jist) **urinary tract** **urologist**	**2-33** The combining form ***ur(o)*** means urine or urinary tract. The medical specialty that is concerned with the urinary tract in both genders, and also the male genital tract, is _____. A specialist in urology is a _____. A uro/logic (u″ro-loj′ik) examination would have to do with what part of the body? _____ _____. A specialist who treats urinary tract infections is a _____.
cardiac **cardiologist** (kahr″-de-ol′ə-jist) **cardiology** (kahr″-de-ol′ə-je) **heart**	**2-34** In a cardiac (kahr′de-ak) arrest, the heart has stopped beating. In the term *cardiac,* ***cardi(o)*** means heart and ***-ac*** means pertaining to. If the heart stops beating, the patient has had a _____ arrest. A physician who specializes in diseases of the heart is a _____. The study of the heart and its function is _____. Cardi/ac means pertaining to the _____.
dermatology (dər″mə-tol′o-je) **skin**	**2-35** Both ***dermat(o)*** and ***derm(a)*** refer to skin. Use dermat(o) plus -logy to write a word that means the study of the skin: _____. A person with acne problems or skin allergies would be treated by a dermatologist (dər″mə-tol′o-jist). Derm/al (der′məl) means pertaining to the _____. Dermatologic (dər″mə-to-loj′ik) and dermatological both refer to the skin. Whether one chooses to say dermatologic or dermatological depends on one's preference. Remember that both -ic and -al mean pertaining to. The ending -ical makes use of both suffixes. Many adjectives accept either ending. You'll learn which ones they are through practice.
radiologist (ra″de-ol′ə-jist) **radiology**	**2-36** The combining form ***radi(o)*** means radiant energy. (Sometimes radi(o) is used to mean radius, a bone of the forearm, but usually it refers to radiant energy.) Radio/logy (ra″de-ol′ə-je) is the use of various forms of radiant energy (such as x-ray) in the diagnosis and treatment of disease. Radiology is an important part of cancer treatment. The physician who studies and interprets x-rays is a _____. Sometimes radiology is called roentgenology (rent″gən-ol′ə-je) after its discoverer, Wilhelm Conrad Röntgen. Roentgenology is really a branch of radiology dealing with the use of roentgen rays (x-rays). The branch of medical science that deals with the use of x-rays, as well as other forms or radiant energy, is _____. Unimpeded x-rays expose the silver coating of a photographic plate and cause it to blacken. X-ray radiation passes through different substances in the body with varying degrees. This results in four basic densities on a film: air appears black, fat appears dark gray, soft tissue appears light gray, and bone appears white (because of calcium). Other substances, such as metal, appear white, since they absorb the rays and prevent them from reaching the photographic plate (see thumbtack in Figure 2-5). Substances that do not permit the passage of x-rays or other radiant energy are described as radiopaque (ra″de-o-pāk′). When radi(o) is joined with the word opaque,* one "o" is omitted to facilitate pronunciation.

*Opaque (Latin: *opacus,* dark, obscure).

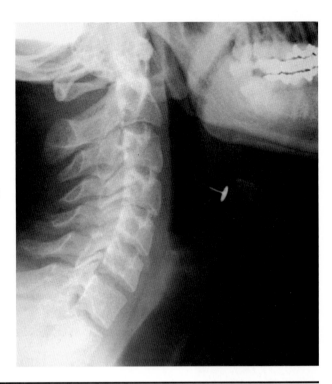

FIGURE 2-5
Radiograph of an aspirated thumbtack. The lodged tack appears white, since it absorbs the x-rays and prevents them from reaching the photographic plate. Also note the different appearances of air, soft tissue, bone, and teeth. (Ballinger PW, Frank ED: *Merrill's atlas of radiographic positions and radiologic procedures*, vol 1, ed 9, St Louis, 1999, Mosby.)

---

female **gynecologist** (gi″nə-kol′ə-jist) **female** **gynec(o)**	**2-37** The combining form **gynec(o)** means female. A medical specialty, gyneco/logy (**gi″nə-kol′ə-je**) is devoted to treating diseases of the _____ genital tract. A physician who specializes in the treatment of females is a _____. GYN is an abbreviation for gynecology. It refers to the _____ genital tract. The word part that means female is _____.
psychology (si-kol′ə-je) **psychiatry** (si-ki′ə-tre)	**2-38** Two suffixes, **-iatrics** and **-iatry,** mean medicine. A third suffix that is used in naming medical specialties is -logy. The ending of a medical specialty often depends on common usage. In some cases, both -logy and -iatry are used and differ mainly in the ways in which disease is treated. For example, **psych(o)** means mind. By adding two different suffixes to psych(o), write the names for the two areas that deal with mental or emotional disorders: _____ and _____.
mind **psychologist** (si-kol′ə-jist) **psychology** **psychiatry**	**2-39** You have heard many words that contain psych(o). In psycho/analysis, psycho/logical, and psycho/path, psych(o) means _____. The branch of psychology that deals with the diagnosis, treatment, and prevention of a wide range of personality and behavioral disorders is clinical psychology. One who is trained in this area is a clinical _____. Clinical psychology is not a branch of medicine but a branch of psychology. The two areas that deal with the mind and mental disorders are clinical _____ and _____. A medical specialist who deals with emotional disorders is called a psychiatrist (**si-ki′ə-trist**).
gerontology **gerontologist** (jer″on-tol′ə-jist)	**2-40** Three combining forms—**ger(a), ger(o),** and **geront(o)**—mean old age or the aged. The science that deals with the special problems of the elderly can be called by either of two names, geronto/logy or ger/iatrics (**jer″on-tol′ə-je, jer″e-at′riks**). The branch of medicine that deals with the problems of aging and the diseases of the elderly is geriatrics. The scientific study of the problems of aging in all of its aspects is _____. The science of treating diseases of the elderly is geriatrics. A physician who specializes in gerontology is a _____.

elderly	**2-41** Geront/al **(jer-on′tal)** means pertaining to the _____.
a dentist specializing in the dental problems of older people	Elderly persons have special dental problems. Ger/odont/ics **(jer″o-don′tiks)** is a branch of dentistry that deals with the dental problems of older people. Note that the vowel is dropped from ger(o) when it is combined with odont(o). A ger/odont/ist **(jer″o-don′tist)** is _____.
geriatrics	The medical specialty that deals with the diseases of elderly persons in general is _____. The selection of the correct combining form may be confusing. Common usage determines which term is proper. Practice will help you to remember.
children's	**2-42** The word root for child is ped(o). Ped/iatrics **(pe″de-at′riks)** is devoted to the study of _____ diseases.
pediatrics	Because diseases of children are often quite different from diseases encountered later in life, most parents prefer to take their children to a physician who specializes in _____.
children	The suffix -*iatrician,* which means practitioner, is used to write the name of the physician who specializes in pediatrics. A pediatrician **(pe″de-ə-tri′shən)** specializes in diseases of _____. The pediatrician is concerned not only with disease, but also with development of children.
children tooth pedodontist	**2-43** A dentist who specializes in pedodontics treats _____. Pedodontics is a branch of dentistry that deals with _____ and mouth conditions of children. A specialist in pedodontics is a _____.
obstetrician	**2-44** Obstetrics **(ob-stet′riks)** deals with pregnancy, labor, and delivery; however, **obstetr(o)** means midwife. Midwives assisted women during childbirth before obstetrics developed as a medical specialty. Physicians who specialize in obstetrics are obstetricians **(ob″stə-tri′shənz).** Two adjectives that mean pertaining to obstetrics are obstetric and obstetrical. A doctor may need to perform a cesarean section in some cases of difficult birth. According to legend, Julius Caesar, who later became emperor of Rome, was delivered by surgery from his mother's dead body. Today cesarean sections are performed by an _____.
internal structures internal internist	**2-45** Internal medicine is a nonsurgical specialty of medicine that deals specifically with the diagnosis and treatment of diseases of the internal structures of the body. The specialist is called an internist **(in-ter′nist).** It is important not to confuse internist with the term *intern.* An intern in many clinical programs is any immediate postgraduate trainee. A physician intern is in postgraduate training, learning medical practice under supervision before being licensed as a physician. An internist, however, is a licensed medical specialist. The internist treats diseases of _____ _____. The branch of medicine that deals solely with the diagnosis and treatment of internal structures is _____ medicine. A physician who practices internal medicine is an _____.
immunologist (im″u-nol′o-jist)	**2-46** Immunology **(im″u-nol′o-je)** represents one of the most rapidly expanding areas of science, and *immun(o)* is the combining form for immune. This branch of science involves assessment of the patient's immune defense mechanism against disease, hypersensitivity, and many diseases now thought to be associated with the immune mechanism. Use immun(o) plus the suffix for one who studies to form the name of the specialist in immunology: _____.
rheumatologist (roo″mə-tol′ə-jist)	Sometimes immunology is combined with the identification and treatment of allergies. At times a physician specializes in immunology and rheumato/logy **(roo″mə-tol′ə-je).** A specialist in rheumatology is a _____.

rheumatology	**2-47** Almost all words that contain the combining form ***rheumat(o)*** pertain to rheumatism (**roo′mə-tiz-əm**). Rheumato/logy is the branch of medicine that deals with rheumat/ic disorders. One may think of rheumatism as just one disease, but it is any of a variety of disorders marked by inflammation, degeneration, or other problems of the connective tissues of the body, especially the joints and related structures. This medical specialty is called _____.
rheumatism	Ancient Greeks believed that one's health was determined by the mixture of humors, certain fluids within the body. The word *rheum* meant a watery discharge; rheumatism was thought to be caused by a flowing of humors in the body and was thus named. Write the name of this variety of disorders of the connective tissues of the body: _____.
study of oncologist (ong-kol′ə-jist) oncology	**2-48** Onco/logy (**ong-kol′ə-je**), another rapidly changing specialty, is the _____ _____ tumors. The combining form ***onc(o)*** means tumor. Not all tumors are harmful. Oncology is particularly concerned with malignant tumors. Malignant* means tending to become worse, spread, and cause death. A specialist who practices oncology is an _____. An onco/logist is concerned with cancer and cancer therapy. The specialty that is concerned with tumors, particularly cancerous tumors, is _____.
gastroenterology gastroenterologist (gas″tro-en″tər-ol′ ə-jist)	**2-49** Gastro/entero/logy (**gas″tro-en″tər-ol′ə-je**) is the study of the stomach and intestines and their diseases. You will study the word components later. For now, learn that the specialty that deals with the stomach and intestines is _____. The specialist who practices gastroenterology is a _____.
epidemiologist (ep″ĭ-de″me-ol′ o-jist)	**2-50** An epidemic attacks several people in a region at the same time. The field of medicine that studies the factors that determine the frequency and distribution of diseases is epidemiology (**ep′ĭ-de″me-ol′o-je**). The specialist is an _____. A physician with this specialty may be assigned the responsibility of directing infection control programs within a hospital. An epidemiologist nurse also has special training and experience in the control of infections.
preventive emergency	**2-51** Preventive medicine is concerned with preventing the occurrence of both mental and physical illness and disease. The branch of medicine that aims at preventing disease is _____ medicine. Emergency room (ER) medicine deals with severely ill or injured patients who require immediate medical treatment. Emergency room specialists work in the _____ room of a hospital.
diagnosis	**2-52** Diagnosis is the use of scientific methods to establish the nature of a sick person's disease. The identification of the disease that the person has, or is believed to have, is also called the diagnosis. Physicians diagnose disease by evaluating the patient's history and the signs and symptoms present. Differentiating one disease from another is called the _____.
sign sign symptom	Symptoms are subjective evidence as perceived by the patient, such as pain. Signs are objective, or definitive, evidence of an illness or disordered function. Indisputable evidence, such as an abnormal radiology report, is which—a sign or a symptom? _____ Is a skin rash a sign or a symptom? _____ Is itching of the skin a sign or a symptom? _____

*Malignant (Latin: *malignus,* bad disposition).

endocrine

2-53 The endocrine (**en′do-krīn, en′do-krin**) glands secrete hormones (**hor′mōnz**) into the blood stream. These hormones play an important role in regulating the body's metabolism. The suffix *-ism* means condition, theory, or process. You learned earlier that endo- means inside. The suffix *-crine* from the combining form *crin(o),* means to secrete. Glands that secrete hormones into the blood stream are _____ glands.

The adrenal (**ə-dre′nəl**) gland secretes adrenaline (epinephrine) into the blood stream.

The adrenal gland is an example of an endocrine gland.

endocrinologist
(**en″do-krĭ-nol′ə-jist**)

The science of the endocrine glands and the hormones they produce is endocrinology. A specialist in endocrinology is called an _____.

2-54 Some physicians specialize in sports medicine, which is concerned with prevention, diagnosis, and treatment of sports injuries.

A specialist in forensic medicine is concerned with the application of medical knowledge to questions of law.

aerospace

Aerospace medicine studies the effects of space travel on animals. Its application is confined to government space programs. The effect of zero gravity on an astronaut's health would be an aspect of _____ medicine.

2-55

A physician assistant (PA) is a person certified by the American Academy of Physician Assistants. Depending on their skill, their experience, and legal regulations, physician assistants can deliver primary patient care much like a licensed physician. Sometimes they work under the supervision of a licensed physician. The PA can deliver primary patient care much like a licensed physician. PA stands for

physician assistant

_____ _____.

❏ SECTION C REVIEW   *M*edical Specialties

This section review covers frames 2–28 through 2–55. Complete the table by writing the meaning of each word part that is listed:

Combining Form	Meaning		Combining Form	Meaning
1. cardi(o)	_____		14. radi(o)	_____
2. crin(o)	_____		15. rheumat(o)	_____
3. derm(a), dermat(o)	_____		16. rhin(o)	_____
4. ger(a), ger(o)	_____		17. ur(o)	_____
5. geront(o)	_____		**Suffix**	**Meaning**
6. gynec(o)	_____		18. -ac	_____
7. immun(o)	_____		19. -crine	_____
8. laryng(o)	_____		20. -er	_____
9. obstetr(o)	_____		21. -iatrician	_____
10. onc(o)	_____		22. -iatrics	_____
11. ophthalm(o)	_____		23. -iatry	_____
12. ot(o)	_____		24. -ism	_____
13. psych(o)	_____			

(Use Appendix V to check your answers.)

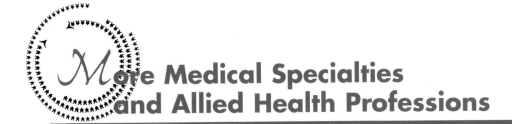

More Medical Specialties and Allied Health Professions

Sophisticated medical care would not be possible without the many specialties that provide total health care for the patient. Physicians now rely on the competence of co-workers, both those trained in medical specialties, as well as nurses and allied health workers, whose specialized knowledge is vitally important in the diagnosis and treatment of disease.

pharmacologist (fahr″mǝh kol′ǝ-jist) **pharmacist** (fahr′mǝh sist)	**2-56** Pharmaco/logy (**fahr″mǝ-kol′ǝ-je**) is the study of drugs, including their origin, nature, properties, and effects. The combining form ***pharmac(o)*** refers to drugs or medicine. One who studies drugs or medicine is a _____. One goes to a pharmacy to buy medicine. A pharmacy is a place for the preparation and dispensing of drugs and medicinal supplies by pharmacists and their assistants. The science of formulating, dispensing, and providing information on drugs is also called pharmacy. One who dispenses medicine is a _____.
medicine (drugs) **therapeutic** **drugs**	**2-57** Pharmaco/therapy (**fahr″mǝ-ko-ther′ǝ-pe**) is the treatment of diseases with _____. The combining form ***therapeut(o)*** means treatment. Therapy is another term for treatment. Write an adjective that means pertaining to treatment by combining therapeut(o) and -ic: _____. A second meaning of the term you just wrote is beneficial. Being familiar with the word parts of pharmaco/therapy tells us that it means treatment of disease with _____.
pharmaceutic **pain**	**2-58** Both pharmac(o) and ***pharmaceut(o)*** mean drugs or medicines. Pharmaceut/ic means pertaining to pharmacy or drugs, but prescribed drugs are commonly called pharmaceutics. Write this term that means a prescribed drug: _____. A prescribed drug with which you are familiar is an an/alges/ic. The combining form ***algesi(o)*** means sensitivity to pain. Knowing that an- means no, algesi(o) means pain, and -ic means pertaining to, you can interpret analgesic to mean relieving pain or a drug that relieves _____.
poison **toxic**	**2-59** You already have an idea of the meaning of toxic (**tok′sik**), which is another word for poisonous; the combining forms ***tox(o)*** and ***toxic(o)*** mean poison. The use of these word parts originates with a Greek word that means archery, or the archer's bow. Ancient Greeks used to smear poison on arrowheads that were used in hunting. In a regular dictionary, one finds the word *toxophilite*, one fond of archery. But in medical words, tox(o) almost always means _____. A tox/in (**tok′sin**) is a poison. If a substance is poisonous, it is said to be a _____ substance.
toxicology (tok″sĭ-kol′ǝ-je) **toxicologist** (tok″sĭ-kol′ǝ-jist) **poison**	**2-60** Combine toxic(o) and -logy to write a word that means the science or study of poisons: _____. A specialist in toxicology is a _____. A toxicology laboratory examines a substance to determine if it is a _____.

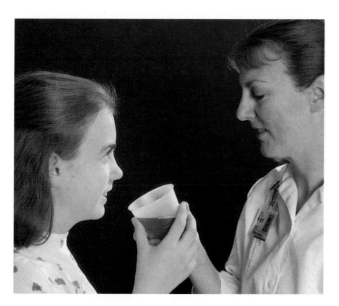

FIGURE 2-6
Nurse with young patient. The complexity of delivering excellent nursing care provides an even greater challenge as nursing is influenced by increased knowledge about disease, rapid changes in technology and health care, and greater promotion of wellness. (From Polaski AL, Tatro SE: *Luckmann's core principles and practice of medical-surgical nursing,* Philadelphia, 1996, WB Saunders.)

registered nurse

2-61 Nursing is one of the oldest and most familiar fields of medicine (Figure 2-6). The registered nurse (RN) is licensed to practice by a state board of nurse examiners or other state authority. The abbreviation RN means _____ _____.

licensed practical nurse

A licensed practical nurse (LPN) performs certain services for the sick under the supervision of a registered nurse. The LPN is a graduate of a school of practical nursing. LPN means

_____.

(LVN is licensed vocational nurse.)

Many nursing specialties have evolved as health care has become more complex, such as the nurse practitioner and the nurse midwife.

medical laboratory

2-62 Medical laboratory personnel are skilled in the performance of clinical laboratory procedures used in diagnosis and the evaluation of patient progress. In descending order of responsibility and education, laboratory personnel include medical technologists, medical technicians, and laboratory assistants. The place in which these people work is a _____ _____. (Laboratories make use of many instruments, including microscopes.)

x-rays

radiologist

2-63 A radio/logic (ra″de-o-loj′ik) technologist specializes in the use of _____ and other forms of radiant energy. A radio/logic technologist works under the supervision of a physician who specializes in radiology, a _____. The radiologist interprets x-rays as well as many other procedures, such as computed tomography.

Medical records, medical transcription, cytotechnology, and dietetics are only a few of the many other fields that are associated with health care.

physical therapist

2-64 Many hospitals employ a physical therapist, a professional who is not a physician but is specially trained to provide physical therapy to patients (Figure 2-7). A professional who is skilled in physical therapy is called a _____ _____.

physical therapy

2-65 Rehabilitation medicine is concerned with restoring the ability to live and work as normally as possible after an injury or illness. Physical therapy, which is often part of rehabilitation, is the treatment of body ailments by nonmedicinal means. It uses natural agents such as water, heat, massage, and exercise in the treatment of disease. This type of treatment is often written "PT," which is a way of abbreviating _____ _____.

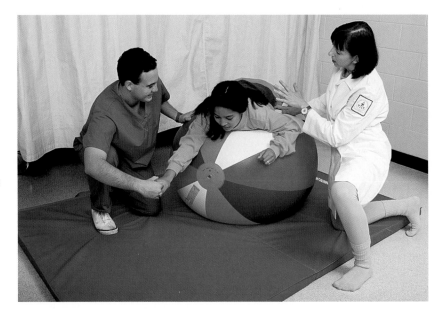

FIGURE 2-7
Physical therapists with young patient. The therapists are using exercise to help the patient strengthen and coordinate body movements. (From Gerdin J: *Health careers today,* ed 2 St Louis, 1996, Mosby.)

respiratory	**2-66** Respiratory therapy is the treatment of disorders in which breathing may be impaired. Any disease in which breathing is affected would be a concern of those who work in _____ therapy. A respiratory therapist is a specialist who holds a degree in respiratory therapy.
vision	**2-67** Both the combining forms *opt(o)* and *optic(o)* mean vision. A person who deals with optic/al (**op′ti-kəl**) glasses and other devices used to correct vision is an optician (**op-tish′ən**). An optic/ian specializes in _____.
vision	Opto/metry (**op-tom′ə-tre**) is the measurement of _____. Later you will study this suffix that means the "process of meaning."
vision	In optometry, the irregularities of vision are diagnosed. Corrective lenses are often prescribed. Optometry is concerned with _____.
specialist	**2-68** An opto/metr/ist (**op-tom′ə-trist**) is not a physician, but a _____ concerned with vision.
vision **optometrist**	You learned that ophthalm(o) means eye, and opt(o) and optic(o) refer to vision. An optic/al examination measures _____. The specialist who measures vision and prescribes corrective lenses is an _____.
	2-69 Medical care is fast-changing and influenced by increased knowledge about diseases, increased public awareness, and rapid advances in science and technology. Many new professions in the medical field have evolved in recent years, and no doubt they will continue to evolve as more emphasis is placed on health and the treatment of disease and the greater promotion of wellness.

❏ SECTION D REVIEW *More* Medical Specialties and Allied Health Professions

This section review covers frames 2-56 through 2-69. Complete the table by writing the meaning of each word part that is listed.

Combining Form	Meaning	Combining Form	Meaning
1. algesi(o)	_____	4. pharmaceut(o)	_____
2. opt(o) or optic(o)	_____	5. therapeut(o)	_____
3. pharmac(o)	_____	6. tox(o) or toxic(o)	_____

(Use Appendix V to check your answers.)

Terminology Challenge

This section introduces new medical specialties that contain word parts that are covered more extensively in later chapters. It also challenges you to use the word parts you have learned to write and to understand new terms.

neonatologist (ne″o-na-tol′ə-jist)	**2-70** Neonatology (**ne″o-na-tol′ə-je**) is the branch of medicine that specializes in the care, diagnosis, and treatment of the newborn child. You will study the meaning of the new word parts more extensively in later chapters. Write the name of the physician who specializes in neonatology: _____.
specialist perinatology (per″ĭ-na-tol′ə-je)	**2-71** Is a perinatologist (**per″ĭ-na-tol′ə-jist**) a medical specialty or a specialist? _____ A perinatologist is a physician who specializes in the diagnosis and treatment of disorders of pregnancy, childbirth, and the first few weeks after delivery. Write the name of the medical specialty of the perinatologist: _____.
microsurgery (mi′kro-sər′jər-e)	**2-72** Some surgeries are performed with the aid of a microscope to magnify tiny tissue structures. Later you will study that micro- is a prefix that means small. Form a new term for surgery that is performed under a microscope by combining micro- and surgery: _____.
biologic, biological pertaining to the skin adjective	**2-73** Adjectives are formed by changing the suffixes of many terms you have learned in this chapter. Biolog/ic and biologic/al (**bi-o-loj′ĭ-kəl**) are two adjectives that both mean pertaining to biology. The two suffixes -ic and -al mean pertaining to. They are used in many words that are already familiar to you, such as metric and metrical. Two words used interchangeably that mean pertaining to biology are _____ and _____. Derm/al means _____. When radiology is changed to radiologic by changing the ending, the noun has been changed to what part of speech? _____
radiologic radiological otic (o′tik) ear otic	**2-74** Using -ic and -al, write two terms that mean pertaining to radiology: _____ and _____. Combine ot(o) and -ic: _____. This new word means pertaining to the _____. Sometimes physicians prescribe medications to be used only in the ear. These medications for use in the ear are called _____ preparations.
eye eye medications	**2-75** An ophthalm/ic ointment is a medication for use in the _____. Ophthalmic (**of-thal′mik**) medications are often called ophthalmolog/ics (**of″thəl-mə-loj′iks**). The term *ophthalmologic* means pertaining to the _____. When the same word is plural, ophthalmologics, you need to recognize that it refers to _____ for the eye.
gynec(o) pertaining to females pertaining to the heart	**2-76** Write the combining form that means female: _____. Gynecolog/ic or gynecolog/ic/al means _____. The suffix -ac also means pertaining to. Cardiac means _____

disease pathogenic (path-o-jen′ik) disease	**2-77** Many words contain the word part *path(o)*. A patho/gen (**path′o-jən**) is any agent or microorganism that produces _____. Add -ic to pathogen to write a word that means capable of causing disease: _____. Patho/logic (**path-o-loj′ik**) means morbid, or pertaining to _____.
inside inside	**2-78** The prefix *endo-* means _____. Many words begin with endo-. Endo/genous (**en-doj′ə-nəs**) means produced _____ or caused by factors within the organism. (You will learn more about this suffix in Chapter 6.)
living	**2-79** Bio/hazards (**bi′o-haz″ərds**) are harmful or potentially harmful to humans, other organisms, or the environment. The combining form *bi(o)* in the word biohazard tells us that the agents under consideration are hazardous to _____ things. Laboratories that work with disease-causing organisms that require special conditions for containment post signs bearing a special biohazard symbol. This symbol is recognized internationally and warns of harmful or potentially harmful agents.
asymptomatic (a″simp-to-mat′ik)	**2-80** You know that subjective evidence of a disease or a change in condition as perceived by the patient is called a symptom. If patients have symptoms of a specific disease, they are said to be symptomatic (**simp″to-mat′ik**). The opposite of symptomatic is written by adding the prefix *a-* to the term. The prefix means "without" as used here. Write the term that means without symptoms: _____.
subnormal (səb-norm′əl)	**2-81** The prefix *sub-* means below and is used extensively in other chapters. Write a term that means below normal: _____. It is not unusual or harmful for some individuals to consistently have a subnormal temperature.
anesthesia	**2-82** Another prefix, *post-*, means behind in the term *post/anesthetic,* which refers to the period of time after _____.
post mortem examination of the organs and tissues of a dead body	**2-83** You may have already heard of a post/mortem examination. This is examination of the organs and tissues of a body to determine the cause of death or pathological conditions. Another name for postmortem examination is autopsy (**aw′top-se**). This may be written postmortem or as two words, _____ _____. What is an autopsy? _____ _____
endocrinotherapy (en″do-krĭ″no-ther′ə-pe)	**2-84** You learned in this chapter that therapy is another term for treatment. Combine endo- and crin(o) and therapy to write a term that means treatment of disease by administration of hormones: _____.

This is the end of programmed material for Chapter 2. There were no new word parts in this section, so a section review is not needed. Congratulations! You are well on your way to learning medical terminology.
- Study the following list of selected abbreviations.
- Then read through the **Chapter Pharmacology** section and be sure that you understand the introductory information, as well as the effects and uses of the six drug classes that are presented.
- Afterwards, work the **Chapter Review.** The written exercises are divided into Basic Understanding (I-VII) and Greater Comprehension (VIII-XII). Your instructor will advise you concerning parts of the review you are to work. After completing the exercises, check your answers with the solutions in Appendix V. It is preferable to work all of the exercises before checking your answers.

• You will find two additional items presented after the Chapter Review:

(1) **Listing of Medical Terms**

Review the terms in Chapter 2. Look at the spelling of each term and be sure that you know its meaning. If you cannot recall its meaning, look up the term in the glossary and reread the frames that pertain to the term. It is also helpful to click on Chapter 2 Pronunciations included on the CD (inside the back cover). Listen as the terms are pronounced.

(2) **Enhancing Spanish Communication**

Spanish translation is given for several terms found in this chapter.

Selected Abbreviations

a.c.	before meals *(ante cibum)*		LPN	licensed practical nurse
ad lib.	freely as needed, at pleasure *(ad libitum)*		LVN	licensed vocational nurse
AMA	American Medical Association		noct	night
aq.	water *(aqua)*		NPO, npo	nothing by mouth *(non per os)*
ARRT	American Registry of Radiologic Technologists		OB	obstetrics
b.i.d.	twice a day *(bis in die)*		OB-GYN	obstetrics and gynecology
b.i.n.	twice a night *(bis in noctis)*		OD	right eye *(oculus dexter)*, overdose
Bx	biopsy		OPS	outpatient service
C	Celsius, centigrade		OR	operating room
Ca	cancer		OT	occupational therapy
CDC	Centers for Disease Control		OTC	over the counter (drug that can be obtained without a prescription)
CICU	cardiology intensive care unit			
CS	central service or central supply, cesarean section		path	pathology
DOA	dead on arrival		po	by mouth *(per os)*
DOB	date of birth		p.r.n.	as the occasion arises, as needed *(pro re nata)*
Dx	diagnosis		PT	physical therapy
ENT	ear, nose, and throat		Pt	patient
ER	emergency room		Px	physical examination
F	Fahrenheit		q.d.	every day *(quaque die)*
GI	gastrointestinal		q.i.d.	four times a day *(quater in die)*
GP	general practice or practitioner		R	radiology, roentgen
Gyn	gynecology		rad	radiation absorbed dose
h/o	history of		RN	registered nurse
Hx	history		Rx	prescription
I & O	intake and output		stat	immediately *(statim)*
ICU	intensive care unit		t.i.d.	three times a day *(ter in die)*
IU	international unit			

Chapter Pharmacology

Pharmacology is the science that deals with the origin, nature, chemistry, effects, and uses of drugs. A drug may modify one or more of the body's functions. Drugs are used in medicine to prevent, diagnose, and treat disease and to relieve pain. Another term for medicines is *pharmaceuticals*. Radioactive pharmaceuticals that are used for medicinal diagnosis or treatment are called radiopharmaceuticals.

Drug abuse is use of any drug in a way that deviates from the manner in which it was prescribed. *Drug addiction* is caused by excessive or continued use of habit-forming drugs.

Giving a drug to a patient is called *drug administration.* The various ways a drug may be administered are called the *routes of administration.* Although most therapeutics are administered orally or by injection, they can sometimes be administered via the skin (transdermal patches) or mucous membranes (example, nasal spray). *Parenteral administration* includes all of the ways a drug may be administered except via the digestive tract.

Once administered, a drug may remain at the site of administration or it may enter the blood. The movement of the drug from the administration site into the blood is called *absorption* of the drug. The transportation of the drug to other body tissues is called the *distribution* of the drug. Where and how a drug combines with the tissue is called the *action* of the drug. If the effect is confined to the site of administration, the drug has a *local* effect. If it acts on many sites away from the administration site, the effect is said to be *systemic.* The drug eventually is chemically changed, a process called *biotransformation.*

A measured amount of a drug is called a *dose.* The greater the effect with a single dose, the more potent a drug is.

The *generic name* of a drug may be used by any company, while the trade name or *brand name* is the property of only one company and cannot be used by other companies. The first letter of the *trade name* is capitalized.

Drugs are generally grouped into several *classes* based on their major effects. The following list indicates the class of various drugs and gives some representative examples. Actions, reactions, and interactions with other drugs are often shared by drugs of the same class. Pharmacists provide information regarding a medication's possible side effects, reactions to or the consequences of taking the particular medication. Adverse drug reactions are harmful, unexpected reactions to a drug.

The drugs are listed by generic name with the trade name in parentheses. The trade name may be the only medication of its type available or the name more commonly used. The drugs listed for this chapter pertain to the whole body rather than to a particular body system. Rather than memorizing the names of the drugs, it is more important to remember the drug classes and their uses. Subsequent chapters also have a pharmacology section.

Drug Class	Effects and Uses	Drug Class	Effects and Uses
Analgesics	**Relief of Pain**	*General anesthetics*	*Loss of all body sensation, loss of consciousness*
Nonnarcotic analgesics	*No abuse potential*	Halothane (Fluothane)	Major surgery
Acetaminophen (Tylenol)	Mild to moderate pain	Ketamine	Major surgery
Aspirin (many trade names)	Mild to moderate pain	Nitrous oxide	Minor surgery
Ibuprofen (Motrin)	Mild to moderate pain	Propofol (Diprivan)	Major surgery
Ultram	Mild to moderate pain	Thiopental (Pentothal)	Minor surgery, induction anesthetic
Narcotic Analgesics	*Potential for abuse*		
Codeine	Mild to moderate pain		
Meperidine (Demerol)	Moderate pain	**Antineoplastic Drugs/**	
Methadone (Dolophine)	Drug detoxification	**Chemotherapeutics**	**Drugs Used to Treat Cancer**
Morphine	Moderate to severe pain	Cisplatin (Platinol)	Used for metastatic carcinoma
Propoxyphene (Darvon and Darvocet)	Mild to moderate pain	Cyclophosphamide (Cytoxan)	Used in myeloma and solid tumors
Oxycodone (Percodan)	Severe pain	Doxorubicin (Adriamycin)	Used in solid tumors
Sufentanil (Fentanyl)	Severe pain	Fluorouracil (5-FU)	Used in carcinoma of the colon
		Methotrexate	Used to treat trophoblastic neoplasms in women
Anesthetics	**Loss of Sensation**	Tamoxifen (Nolvadex)	Mainly used in mammary cancer
Local anesthetics	*Local loss of sensation*		
Benzocaine (Solarcaine)	Topical anesthetic		
Cocaine	Topical anesthetic (mucous membrane)		
Dibucaine (Nupercaine)	Nerve block, spinal anesthetic		
Lidocaine (Xylocaine)	Topical anesthetic, nerve block		
Procaine (Novocain)	Nerve block		
Tetracaine (Pontocaine)	Spinal anesthetic		

Chapter Pharmacology—cont'd

Drug Class	Effects and Uses
Neuromuscular Blocking Drugs	Used in Surgery to Cause Flaccid Paralysis So Surgeon Can Cut Through Muscles Without Reflex Contraction
Cisatracurium (Nimbex)	
Curare	
Dimethyltuboburarine (Metabine)	
Pancuronium (Pavulon)	Also used to produce respiratory paralysis in some patients who are on intermittent positive pressure respirators, as in the treatment of tetanus
Succinylcholine (Anectine)	Most widely used blocking drug in surgery
Tubocurarine	
Opioid antagonists	*Used to reverse narcotics*
Naloxone (Narcan)	Reverses opioid effects, including respiratory depression
Radiopharmaceuticals	*Used to assess many internal structures and to treat hyperfunction*
Iodine-131 (Iodotope)	Used in thyroid cancer
Strontium-89 (Metastron)	Used for metastatic bone pain

CHAPTER REVIEW 2

▶ ## BASIC UNDERSTANDING

REVIEWING WORD PARTS

I. Write a word (prefix, suffix, or combining form) for each clue. For the purpose of this exercise, omit hyphens and parentheses. For example, you will write *end, logist,* and *patho* instead of *end-, -logist,* and *path(o)*. Abbrev means abbreviation.

CROSSWORD PUZZLE 2

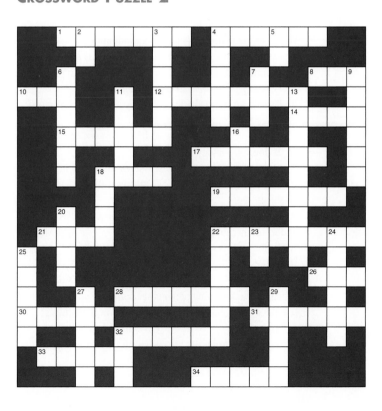

Across

1 larynx
4 vision
8 ear
10 life
12 feeling
14 child
15 immune
17 aged
18 incision (suffix)
19 skin
21 inside
22 drugs
26 urinary tract
28 medicine
30 radiant energy
31 nature
32 repair
33 disease
34 to secrete

Down

2 albumin (abbrev)
3 female
4 straight
5 pertaining to
6 poison
7 one who
9 tooth
11 nerve
13 eye
16 one who
18 poison
20 tumor
22 mind
23 without
24 heart
25 medicine
27 tissue
29 nose
32 foot

MATCHING

II. Match suffixes with their meanings (A-J).

_____ 1. -al   **A.** condition   _____ 6. -ist   **F.** one who
_____ 2. -crine   **B.** foot   _____ 7. -logist   **G.** one who studies
_____ 3. -ia   **C.** incision   _____ 8. -logy   **H.** study or science of
_____ 4. -iatrician   **D.** practitioner   _____ 9. -pod   **I.** pertaining to
_____ 5. -iatry   **E.** medicine   _____ 10. -tomy   **J.** secrete

III. Match combining forms (1-10) with their meanings (A-J).

_____ 1. dent(o)   **A.** aged   _____ 6. orth(o)   **F.** repair
_____ 2. esthesi(o)   **B.** drugs   _____ 7. ot(o)   **G.** straight
_____ 3. ger(a)   **C.** ear   _____ 8. pharmaceut(o) **H.** tooth
_____ 4. onc(o)   **D.** eye   _____ 9. plast(o)   **I.** treatment
_____ 5. ophthalm(o)   **E.** feeling   _____ 10. therapeut(o) **J.** tumor

IV. Match specialists (1-10) with the major area to which their practice is devoted (A-J):

_____ 1. cardiologist   **A.** children   _____ 6. neurologist   **F.** hormonal system
_____ 2. dermatologist   **B.** ear, nose, and throat _____ 7. ophthalmologist   **G.** nervous system
_____ 3. endocrinologist **C.** eye   _____ 8. otolaryngologist   **H.** older persons
_____ 4. gerontologist   **D.** females   _____ 9. pediatrician   **I.** radiant energy
_____ 5. gynecologist   **E.** heart   _____ 10. radiologist   **J.** skin

COMBINING WORD PARTS

V. Write medical terms by combining word parts that are indicated:

1. an- + esthesi(o) + -ia   _____   6. orth(o) + ped(o) + -ist   _____
2. ana- + -tomy   _____   7. ot(o) + -ic   _____
3. dermat(o) + -logy   _____   8. pharmac(o) + -logist   _____
4. endo- + -crine   _____   9. therapeut(o) + -ic   _____
5. ger(a) + -iatrics   _____   10. ur(o) + -logy   _____

MULTIPLE CHOICE

VI. Choose one answer (A-D) for each of the following multiple choice questions:

1. The term *oral* pertains to which of the following?
   A. tooth   C. throat
   B. mouth   D. windpipe

2. The word *neuron* means which of the following?
   A. A nerve cell
   B. A specialist in diseases of the nervous system
   C. Surgery that deals with the nervous system
   D. A branch of medicine that deals with the nervous system

3. Obstetrics deals with what type of problems?
   A. ear, nose, and throat
   B. emotional problems
   C. disorders of internal body structures
   D. pregnancy, labor, and delivery

4. Which of the following is true of endodontics?
   A. Deals with the tooth and mouth conditions of children
   B. Deals with irregularities of teeth alignment
   C. Deals with conditions that affect the tooth pulp and root
   D. Deals with all types of dental surgery

5. What does physiology mean?
   A. study of function   C. study of disease in general
   B. study of structure   D. study of tissue

6. Which of the following treatments for disease is used in endocrinotherapy?
   A. heat   C. massage
   B. water   D. hormones

7. Which of the following persons specializes in applying laboratory methods in the solution of clinical diagnosis?
   A. an internist   C. a clinical pathologist
   B. a gastroenterologist   D. a surgical pathologist

8. Which is true of the word *sign* as it relates to diagnosis?

    A. It is the same as symptom.

    B. It is subjective evidence of disease.

    C. It is objective evidence of disease.

    D. It is evidence as perceived by the patient.

9. What does histology mean?

    A. study of function

    B. study of structure

    C. study of disease in general

    D. study of tissue

10. Cardiology specializes in the treatment of which of the following structures?

    A. internal organs

    B. heart

    C. urinary system

    D. skin

WRITING TERMS

VII. Write a term for each of the following:

1. dentistry dealing specifically with children _____

2. below normal _____

3. pertaining to old age _____

4. pertaining to the eye _____

5. pertaining to treatment _____

6. physician specializing in the stomach and intestines _____

7. poisonous _____

8. relieving pain _____

9. removal and examination of tissue from the living body _____

10. the study of changes caused by disease _____

▶ GREATER COMPREHENSION

SPELLING

VIII. Circle all incorrectly spelled terms and write their correct spellings:

cardiak   gynecologic   orthodontics   sychiatry   therapeutic

INTERPRETING ABBREVIATIONS

IX: Write the meaning of each of these abbreviations:

1. ad lib. _____

2. Bx _____

3. Dx _____

4. Hx _____

5. I & O _____

6. noct _____

7. npo _____

8. OTC _____

9. q.d. _____

10. q.i.d. _____

MATCHING PHARMACEUTICS

X. Match these terms about pharmaceutics with their descriptions in the right column:

_____ 1. absorption

_____ 2. action

_____ 3. addiction

_____ 4. administration

_____ 5. biotransformation

A. chemical change that takes place in a drug after it is given

B. excessive or continued use of habit-forming drugs

C. giving a drug to a patient

D. movement of a drug from the administration site

E. where and how a drug combines with the tissue

FILL IN THE BLANK

XI. Write a word in each blank to complete these sentences:

1. The _____ name of a drug may be used by any company.

2. Drugs are generally grouped into several classes based on their major _____.

3. Unusual and unexpected adverse effects are drug _____.

4. Antineoplastics are a class of drugs used to treat _____.

5. Medicines that relieve pain are called _____.

6. The class of medicines that cause loss of feeling is _____.

7. Pharmaceuticals that are often used in diagnostic procedures and make use of radiant energy are placed in the drug class _____.

8. Drugs that prevent contraction of muscles during surgery are called neuromuscular _____ drugs.

9. All of the ways that a drug may be administered except via the digestive tract are called _____ administration.

PRONUNCIATION

XII. The pronunciation is shown for several medical words. Indicate which syllable has the primary accent by marking it with an ´:

1. an/esthesio/logy (**an es the ze ol ə je**)
2. gastro/entero/logy (**gas tro en tər ol ə je**)
3. histo/logy (**his tol ə je**)
4. ortho/dontics (**or tho don tiks**)
5. radio/logic (**ra de o loj ik**)

(Use Appendix V to check your answers.)

 Listing of Medical Terms

anatomist	embryology	larynx	orally
anatomy	endocrine	licensed practical nurse	orthodontics
anesthesia	endocrinologist	licensed vocational nurse	orthodontist
anesthesiologist	endocrinology	medical technologist	orthopedic surgeon
anesthesiology	endocrinotherapy	microsurgery	orthopedics
anesthetic	endodontics	neonatologist	orthopedist
anesthetist	endodontist	neonatology	otic
antineoplastic	endogenous	neurologist	otolaryngologist
asymptomatic	epidemiologist	neurology	otolaryngology
autopsy	epidemiology	neuromuscular blocking	otologist
biochemist	family practice	agent	otology
biohazard	gastroenterologist	neuron	otorhinolaryngology
biologic	gastroenterology	neurosurgeon	pathogen
biological	general practitioner	neurosurgery	pathogenic
biologist	general surgery	nurse midwife	pathologic
biology	geriatrics	nurse practitioner	pathological
biopsy	gerodontics	obstetric	pathologist
cardiac	gerodontist	obstetrical	pathology
cardiologist	gerontal	obstetrician	pathophysiology
cardiology	gerontologist	obstetrics	pediatrician
chemotherapeutics	gerontology	oncologist	pediatrics
clinical pathologist	gynecologic	oncology	pedodontics
clinical psychology	gynecological	ophthalmic	pedodontist
dentist	gynecologist	ophthalmologic	perinatologist
dentistry	gynecology	ophthalmologist	perinatology
dermal	histologist	ophthalmology	pharmaceutics
dermatologic	histology	opioid antagonists	pharmacist
dermatological	holistic	optical	pharmacologist
dermatologist	hormone	optician	pharmacology
dermatology	immunologist	optometrist	pharmacotherapy
diagnosis	immunology	optometry	pharmacy
dissection	internal medicine	oral	pharynx
electrocardiogram	internist	oral surgeon	physical therapist
embryologist	laryngology	oral thermometer	physical therapy

Listing of Medical Terms—cont'd

physician assistant	radiologic technologist	rheumatologist	therapy
physiologist	radiological	rheumatology	toxic
physiology	radiologist	roentgen	toxicologist
plastic surgery	radiology	roentgenology	toxicology
postanesthetic	radiopaque	subnormal	toxin
postmortem	radiopharmaceuticals	surgery	trachea
psychiatrist	registered nurse	surgical pathologist	urologic
psychiatry	rehabilitation medicine	symptom	urologist
psychologist	respiratory therapist	symptomatic	urology
psychology	respiratory therapy	therapeutic	
radiologic	rheumatism		

Español

Enhancing Spanish Communication

English	Spanish (pronunciation)	English	Spanish (pronunciation)
aged	envejecido (en-vay-hay-SEE-do)	nerve	nervio (NERR-ve-o)
anesthesia	anestesia (ah-nes-TAY-se-ah)	neurology	neurología (nay-oo-ro-lo-HEE-ah)
anesthetic	anestésico (ah-nes-TAY-se-co)	nose	nariz (nah-REES)
biopsy	biopsia (be-OP-see-ah)	orthodontist	ortodóntico (or-to-DON-te-co)
body	cuerpo (coo-ERR-po)	pathology	patología (pah-to-lo-HEE-ah)
bone	hueso (oo-AY-so)	physical examination	examen físico
brain	cerebro (say-RAY-bro)		(ek-SAH-men FEE-se-co)
breasts	senos (SAY-nos)	psychiatry	psiquiatría (se-ke-ah-TREE-ah)
child	niña (NEE-nya), niño (NEE-nyo)	psychology	psicología (se-co-lo-HEE-ah)
dentist	dentista (den-TEES-tah)	radiation	radiación (rah-de-ah-se-ON)
diagnosis	diagnóstico (de-ag-NOS-te-co)	skin	piel (pe-EL)
disease	enfermedad (en-fer-may-DAHD)	surgeon	cirujano(a) (se-roo-HAH-no) (na)
ear	oreja (o-RAY-hah)	surgery	cirugía (se-roo-HEE-ah)
eye	ojo (O-ho)	therapy	tratamiento (trah-tah-me-EN-to)
face	cara (CAH-rah)	throat	garganta (gar-GAHN-tah)
foot (pl., feet)	pie (PE-ay), pies (PE-ays)	tooth (pl., teeth)	diente (de-AYN-tay), dientes
gynecology	ginecología (he-nay-co-lo-HEE-ah)		(de-AYN-tays)
hand	mano (MAH-no)	trachea	tráquea (TRAH-kay-ah)
head	cabeza (cah-BAY-sah)	urinary system	sistema urinario
heart	corazón (co-rah-SON)		(sis-TAY-mah oo-re-NAH-re-o)
life	vida (VEE-dah)	urine	orina (o-REE-nah)
mind	mente (MEN-te)	urology	urología (oo-ro-lo-HEE-ah)
mouth	boca (BO-cah)	water	agua (AH-goo-ah)
narcotic	narcótico (nar-CO-te-co)	x-ray	radiografía (rah-de-o-grah-FEE-ah)
neck	cuello (coo-EL-lyo)		

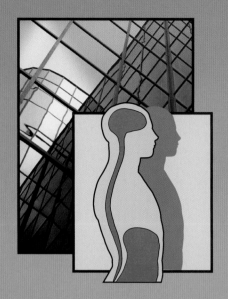

Body Structures

3

Outline

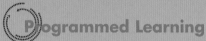
Principal Word Parts

COMBINING FORMS

abdomin(o)	abdomen
acr(o)	extremities
anter(o)	anterior
blephar(o)	eyelid
caud(o)	tail, lower portion of body
cephal(o)	head
chir(o)	hand
crani(o)	skull
cyan(o)	blue
dactyl(o)	digits (fingers and toes)
dist(o), tel(e)	distant
dors(o)	dorsal, back side
electr(o)	electricity
encephal(o)	brain
gigant(o)	large
gram(o)	to print or record

infer(o)	inferior, situated below
kinesi(o)	movement
later(o)	side
medi(o)	medial, middle
my(o)	muscle
omphal(o)	umbilicus
pelv(i)	pelvis
periton(o)	peritoneum
poster(o)	posterior
proxim(o)	near
som(a), somat(o)	body
spin(o)	spine
super(o)	superior, uppermost
thorac(o)	thorax (chest)
ventr(o)	ventral, belly

PREFIXES

anti-	against
bi-	two
brady-	slow
dys-	bad, painful, or difficult
en-	in or inside
mega-	large
tachy-	fast
uni-	one

SUFFIXES

-ad	toward
-dynia	pain
-eal	pertaining to
-gram	a record
-graph	recording instrument
-graphy	process of recording
-itis	inflammation
-megaly	enlargement
-osis	condition (sometimes, disease or abnormal increase)
-pathy	disease
-plasty	surgical repair
-pnea	breathing
-spasm	cramp or twitching

Learning Goals

▶ **BASIC UNDERSTANDING**

In this chapter you learn to do the following:

1. Identify the four abdominal quadrants.
2. Recognize directional terms and planes of the body.
3. Identify the body cavities.
4. Compare the two systems of identifying abdominopelvic regions.
5. Write the meanings of word parts pertaining to the body and use them to build and analyze medical terms.

▶ **GREATER COMPREHENSION**

6. Identify internal organs that are associated with the four abdominal quadrants.
7. Define the nine abdominopelvic divisions used by anatomists.
8. Spell medical terms accurately.
9. Pronounce medical terms correctly.
10. Write the meanings of the abbreviations.
11. Identify the effects or uses of the drug classes presented in this chapter.

SECTION A

Anatomic Position and Directional Terms

Anatomists use directional terms and planes to describe the position and direction of the body. Locations and positions are always described relative to the body in the anatomic position, that is, the position that a person has while standing erect with the arms at the sides and the palms forward. This position is used as a reference when describing the location or direction of various body structures or parts. Special anatomical terms are used to indicate the front, back, and sides of the body, as well as specific parts.

anatomic	**3-1** In the anatomic (**an″ə-tom′ik**) position, the body is erect and facing forward with the arms at the sides and the palms toward the front, as shown in Figure 3-1. The legs are parallel, with the toes pointing forward. This particular position is known as the _____ position.
anterior	Notice that in the anatomic position, the body is facing forward. Anterior (**an-tēr′e ər**) means nearer to or toward the front. The anatomic position is the _____ aspect, or front of the body. The combining form that means anterior is ***anter(o).***
front **anter(o)**	Antero/median (**an″tər-o-me′de-ən**) indicates the position of _____ and toward the middle. The combining form for anterior or front is _____.
anterior **ventral**	**3-2** In humans, the anterior or front side is also the ventral (**ven′trəl**) surface. Ventral refers to the belly side. The anatomic position in Figure 3-1 shows the _____ or _____ surface of the body. The combining form ***ventr(o)*** means ventral or belly. Ventro/median (**ven″tro-me′de-ən**) is another way of saying anteromedian, but the latter is more common.
belly (ventral) **ventral**	Ventr(o) means the _____ side of an organism. In humans, the anterior or front side is the same as the _____ surface.

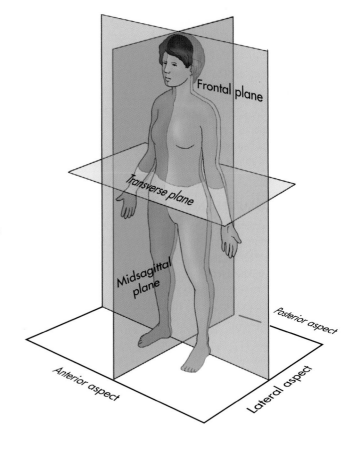

FIGURE 3-1
Anatomic position of the body (anterior view, palms forward) with reference systems (planes and aspects). The frontal, transverse, and midsagittal planes are shown. The anterior, posterior, and lateral aspects are used to describe locations of various structures or parts.

back	**3-3** The opposite of anterior is posterior (**pos-tēr′e-or**). Posterior means directed toward or situated at the back. The combining form *poster(o)* means behind or toward the _____.
behind, outside within (inside)	Postero/external (**pos″tər-o-ek-ster′nəl**) indicates that something is situated on the outside of a posterior part. Thus posteroexternal is situated _____ and _____. Postero/internal (**pos″tər-o-in-ter′nəl**) is situated behind and _____.
front back	Antero/posterior (**an″tər-o-pos-tēr′e-or**) pertains to both the _____ and the _____ sides. Anteroposterior means from the front to the back of the body.
front back	**3-4** In radiology, directional terms are used to specify the direction of the x-ray beam from its source to its exit surface before striking the film. In an anteroposterior projection, the x-ray beam strikes the anterior aspect of the body first. In other words, the beam passes from _____ to back. Postero/anterior (**pos″tər-o-an-tēr′e-or**) means from the posterior to the anterior surface, or, in other words, from _____ to front. Positions for some common radiographic projections of the chest are shown in Figure 3-2.
back belly (front)	**3-5** Dorsal (**dor′səl**), as well as posterior, means directed toward or situated on the back side. The combining form *dors(o)* means dorsal, or the _____ side of an organism. Dorso/ventral (**dor″so-ven′trəl**) pertains to the back and _____ surfaces. (Notice the order in which the two word parts are presented. The importance of the order becomes obvious when one is describing the path of a bullet, for example. Dorsoventral sometimes means passing from the back to the belly surface.)
behind posterolateral (pos″tər-o-lat′ər-əl)	Lateral means side, so dorso/lateral (**dor″so-lat′ər-əl**) means _____ and to one side of the body. Use the other word part that you learned that means behind to write another term that means behind and to one side: _____.

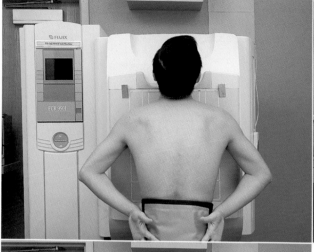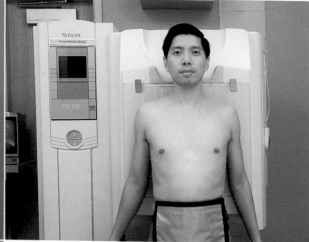
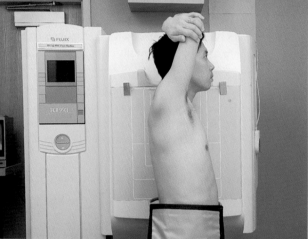

FIGURE 3-2

Patient positioning for a chest x-ray. **A,** In a posteroanterior (PA) projection, the anterior aspect of the chest is closest to the image receptor. **B,** In an anteroposterior (AP) projection, the posterior aspect of the chest is closest to the image receptor. **C,** In a left lateral chest projection, the left side of the patient is placed against the image receptor. (From Ballinger PW, Frank ED: *Merrill's atlas of radiographic positions and radiologic procedures,* vol 1, ed 9, St Louis, 1999, Mosby.)

side, behind **side**	**3-6** You saw in the last frame that lateral (**lat′ər-əl**) means side and denotes a position away from the midline of the body. The combining form for lateral is ***later(o).*** Later(o) means _____. You have already seen that dorso/lateral means _____ and to one _____.
anter(o) **anterolateral** (**an″tər-o-lat′ər-əl**) **situated in front** **and to one side**	Write the combining form for anterior: _____. Form a new word adding "lateral" to the combining form that you just wrote _____. The word you just wrote means _____.
side **uni-** **unilateral**	**3-7** The prefix ***uni-*** means one. Uni/lateral (**u′nĭ-lat′ər-əl**) means affecting only one _____. Uniform means always having the same form or one form. In many common words such as unite, union, and unit, the part that means one is _____. Write the word that means pertaining to only one side: _____.
sides	**3-8** The prefix ***bi-*** means two. It is used in many words that you already know, such as bicycle, bifocal, and bicentennial. In all of these words, bi-means two. Bi/lateral (**bi-lat′ər-əl**) pertains to two _____. In other words, bilateral refers to both sides of the body.

side	**3-9** The combining form *medi(o)* means medial (**me′de-əl**) or middle. Medio/lateral (**me″de-o-lat′ər-əl**) means in the middle and to one _____.
middle	
back	Postero/medial (**post″tər-o-me′de-əl**) means situated in the _____ of the _____ side of an organism.
situated in front and toward the middle or center	Antero/medial (**an″ter-o-me′de-əl**) means _____.
in front and above	**3-10** Anatomists use the term *superior* (**soo-pe′re-or**) to indicate uppermost or situated above. The combining form for superior is *super(o).* Antero/superior (**an″ter-o-soo-pēr′e-ər**) indicates what position? _____
posterosuperior (pos″tər-o-soo-pēr′e-or)	Using the combining form for posterior, build a word that means behind and above: _____.
above	Super/ficial (**soo″pər-fish′əl**) means situated on or near the surface. Superficial radiation therapy is sometimes used for surface lesions such as skin tumors. Superficial comes from a similar-appearing Latin word that contains super(o), the combining form that means uppermost or situated _____.
below	**3-11** The opposite of superior is inferior (**in-fēr′e-ər**). There may be certain products that you consider inferior to your favorite brand. When you consider something inferior, you believe that product is lower in value than something else. Inferior means lower or below. In anatomy, inferior means situated _____. It is often used in reference to the lower surface of a structure or the lower of two or more similar structures.
superior inferior	The right side of the heart receives blood from all parts of the body by way of two large veins called the venae cavae (plural of vena cava). One vena cava lies above the other and is called the _____ vena cava. The large vein that lies just below the superior vena cava is the _____ vena cava.
situated in the middle of the underside	**3-12** The combining form *infer(o)* means inferior. It is used in a few words such as infero/median (**in″fər-o-me′de-ən**), which means _____.
	Only a few medical words use the combining form *infer(o).* Later you will learn a prefix that means below and is more often used in medicine. But for now, recognize that infer(o) is a combining form that means _____.
inferior (or below)	The combining form *caud(o)* means toward the tail or the end of the body away from the head. Caudal (**kaw′dəl**) pertains to a _____ or tail-like structure. In human anatomy, it also means inferior.
tail	
caudal	Another word that means the same anatomically as inferior is _____, which also refers to the tail.
near	**3-13** The combining form *proxim(o)* means near. Proxim/al (**prok′si-məl**) refers to something that is _____.
proximal	Proximal describes the position of structures that are nearest their origin or point of attachment. The proximal end of the thigh bone joins with the hip bone. This means that the _____ end of this bone is near the hip bone.

3-14 Distal (**dis′təl**) is the opposite of proximal; *dist(o)* means distant or far. It also means away from the origin or point of attachment.

distal

If the upper end of the thigh bone is proximal, the lower end of the thigh bone is _____ to the hip bone.

proximal

Which is nearer its origin, a structure that is proximal or one that is distal? _____

distant

Another combining form, *tel(e),* also means distant. A tele/cardio/gram (**tel″ə-kahr′ de-o-gram**) registers the heart impulses of patients in _____ places. With a telecardiogram, the cardiologist and the patient may be in different cities, and the heart tracing is sent by phone. It will be easy to remember tel(e) if you think of the telephone, which allows someone distant to hear your voice.

3-15 The combining form *cephal(o)* means head, and the suffix -*ad* means toward. Cephalad (**sef′ə-ləd**) means toward the _____.

head

cephalic

Write another word using -ic that means pertaining to the head: _____.

head

Cephalic (**sə-fal′ik**) means pertaining to the _____, or to the head end of the body. Dorso/cephalad (**dor″so-sef′ə-lad**) means situated toward the

back of the head

_____.

❏ SECTION A REVIEW *A*natomic Position and Directional Terms

This section review covers frames 3–1 through 3–15. Complete the table by writing the meaning of each word part that is listed. Also write the corresponding anatomical term for 1 through 12. The first one is done as an example.

Combining Form	Meaning	Anatomical Term
1. anter(o)	front	anterior
2. caud(o)		
3. cephal(o)		
4. dist(o), tel(e)		
5. dors(o)		
6. infer(o)		
7. later(o)		
8. medi(o)		
9. poster(o)		
10. proxim(o)		
11. super(o)		
12. ventr(o)		

Prefix	Meaning
13. bi-	
14. uni-	

Suffix	Meaning
15. -ad	

(Use Appendix V to check your answers.)

Anatomical Reference Planes

Certain anatomical planes (frontal, sagittal, and transverse) are used to identify the position of various parts of the body. This section also introduces important combining forms for the head and the chest.

front, back	**3-16** The anatomical planes are labeled in Figure 3-1. Look again at this figure. A frontal (**frun′tǝl**) plane divides the body into anterior and posterior portions. In other words, a frontal plane divides the _____ of the body from the _____. The frontal plane is sometimes called the coronal (**kǝ-rōn′ǝl**) plane.
lower	A transverse (**trans vǝrs′**) plane divides the body into superior and inferior portions. In other words, a transverse plane divides the body into upper and _____ portions.
transverse	A plane that divides the body into upper and lower portions is a _____ plane.
right **left**	The midsagittal (**mid-saj′ĭ-tǝl**) plane divides the body into equal right and left halves. A sagittal plane lies parallel to the midsagittal line and divides the body into unequal _____ and _____ portions.
frontal	A plane that divides the body into anterior and posterior portions is known as a _____ plane.
	Study Figure 3-1 until you can identify the frontal, transverse, midsagittal, and sagittal planes. While studying the figure, also review the terms superior, inferior, lateral, anterior, and posterior.
palm	**3-17** In the anatomic position, the palms are forward. The palm* is the hollow of the hand. Palm/ar (**pahl′ mǝr**) pertains to the _____.
plantar	Plantar (**plan′tǝr**)† pertains to the sole. Write this word that means pertaining to the sole: _____.
chest (thorax)	**3-18** In the anatomic position, the chest faces forward. The combining form *thorac(o)* refers to the thorax (**thor′aks**), or chest. Thoraco/tomy (**thor″ǝ-kot′ ǝ-me**) is incision into the _____. Thoracotomy refers to any incision of the chest wall.
	The thorac/ic (**thǝ-ras′ik**) region is the area of the chest.
chest	**3-19** Hemo/thorax (**he″mo-thor′aks**) means blood in the _____. In other words, there is blood in the chest cavity owing to trauma (injury) or a ruptured blood vessel.
thorax **thorac(o)**	The scientific name of the chest is _____. The combining form for chest is _____.
pain, chest	**3-20** The suffix *-dynia* means pain. Thoraco/dynia (**thor″ǝ-ko-din′e-ǝ**) is a type of _____ in the _____. (It differs from angina pectoris (**an ji′nǝh pek′to res**), a heart disease in which the chest pain results from interference with the supply of oxygen to the heart muscle.)
thoracodynia	Another name for chest pain is _____.

*Palm (Latin: *palma*).
†Plantar (Latin: *planta,* sole).

❏ SECTION B REVIEW   𝒜natomical Reference Planes

This section review covers frames 3-16 through 3-20. Complete the table by writing the meaning of each word part that is listed:

Combining Form	Meaning		Suffix	Meaning
1. thorac(o)	_____		2. -dynia	_____

(Use Appendix V to check your answers.)

SECTION C

Body Regions and Body Cavities

The dorsal and ventral cavities are the spaces within the body that contain the internal organs. The major regions of the body are the head, neck, torso (also called the trunk), and the appendages. The torso includes the chest, abdomen, and pelvis. Because of the large area and numerous internal organs, these areas are frequently subdivided using imaginary lines to help describe the location of body organs or origin of pain.

---

abdomen

abdominothoracic
(ab-dom″ĭ-no-thə-ras′ik)

3-21 The combining form for abdomen (**ab′də-man, ab-do′mən**) is **abdomin(o).** The abdomen is that part of the body lying between the thorax and the pelvis. Abdomin(o) means _____.

Write a word that means pertaining to the abdomen and thorax by combining abdomin(o) and thorac(o) and -ic: _____.

---

upper
lower

quadrant

3-22 There are two methods of using imaginary lines to divide the abdomen into regions. Dividing the abdomen into four quadrants (**kwod′rənts**) is a convenient way to designate areas in the abdominal (**ab-dom′ĭ-nəl**) cavity (Figure 3-3, *A*). Refer to the diagram to answer the following:

RUQ and LUQ refer to the right and left _____ quadrants, respectively. RLQ and LLQ refer to the _____ quadrants. Quadrant is a term that means any one of four corresponding parts.

Abdominal quadrants are used to describe the location of pain or of body structures. The system of naming four abdominal areas that are determined by drawing two imaginary lines through the umbilicus is the four- _____ system. Principal organs contained in the four abdominal quadrants are shown in Table 3-1.

3-23 Anatomists describe the abdomen as having nine regions, shown in Figure 3-3, *B*. This nine-region system is also used particularly in the clinical and surgical settings. Some of the terms may be unfamiliar, but for now try to remember the divisions. When the terms are studied in later chapters in more detail, they will acquire more meaning. Look at Figure 3-3, *B* while working the next frame.

---

hypochondriac
(hi″po-kon′dre-ak)

epigastric
(ep″ĭ-gas′trik)

umbilical
(əm-bil′ĭ-kəl)

lumbar (lum′bahr)

hypogastric
(hi″po-gas′trik)

iliac (il′e-ak)

inguinal (ing′gwĭ-nəl)

3-24 The upper lateral regions beneath the ribs are the right and left _____ regions.

Between the hypochondriac regions lies the _____ region. The stomach is in this region.

The _____ region lies just below the epigastric region. The umbilical region is that of the navel, or umbilicus.

The right and left _____ regions lie on each side of the umbilical region.

The lower middle region is called the _____ region.

Finally, the two lower lateral regions are the right and left _____ or _____ regions.

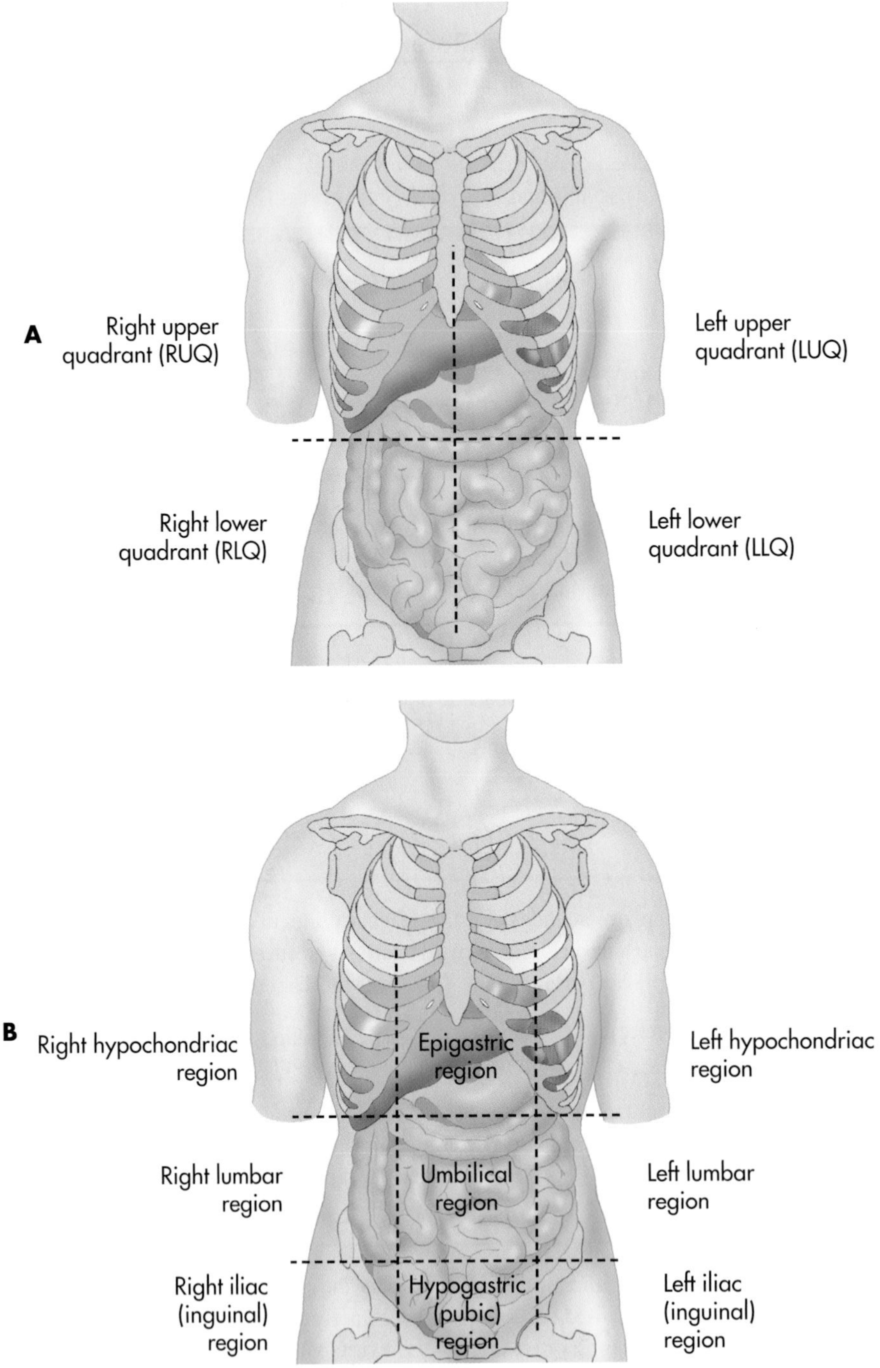

A, Right upper quadrant (RUQ)

Left upper quadrant (LUQ)

Right lower quadrant (RLQ)

Left lower quadrant (LLQ)

B, Right hypochondriac region

Epigastric region

Left hypochondriac region

Right lumbar region

Umbilical region

Left lumbar region

Right iliac (inguinal) region

Hypogastric (pubic) region

Left iliac (inguinal) region

FIGURE 3-3

Two systems of using imaginary lines to divide the abdomen into regions. **A,** Quadrants of the abdomen, four divisions of the abdomen determined by drawing a vertical and a horizontal line through the umbilicus. **B,** The nine anatomical regions of the abdomen, determined by four imaginary lines.

TABLE 3-1 **Abdominal Quadrants and Their Contents**

Right upper quadrant (RUQ)	Contains the right lobe of the liver, gallbladder, right kidney, and parts of the large and small intestines
Left upper quadrant (LUQ)	Contains the left lobe of the liver, stomach, pancreas, left kidney, spleen, and parts of the large and small intestines
Right lower quadrant (RLQ)	Contains the right ureter, right ovary and uterine tube, appendix, and parts of the large and small intestines
Left lower quadrant (LLQ)	Contains the left ureter, left ovary and uterine tube, and parts of the large and small intestines

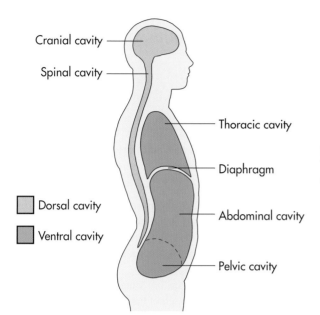

Cranial cavity
Spinal cavity
Thoracic cavity
Diaphragm
Dorsal cavity
Ventral cavity
Abdominal cavity
Pelvic cavity

FIGURE 3-4
The body has two principal body cavities, the dorsal and ventral cavities, each further subdivided.

abdomin(o) abdomen	**3-25** The first region that you named in the preceding frame was the hypochondriac region. (You have probably also heard the term *hypochondriac* applied to a person who has a false belief of suffering from some disease. Ancient Greeks believed that organs in the hypochondriac region of the abdomen were the cause of melancholy and imaginary diseases, hence the term *hypochondriac.*) Write the new combining form that you learned earlier for abdomen: _____. The hypochondriac region is just one of nine abdominal divisions. Abdomin/al means pertaining to the _____.
cavity back (posterior) front (belly)	**3-26** The body has two major cavities, spaces that contain internal organs. The space within the body that contains internal organs is called a body _____. The two principal body cavities are the dorsal cavity and the ventral cavity. We learned previously that dorsal means situated toward the _____ surface of the body. Ventral means situated toward the _____ surface.
cranial, spinal dorsal	**3-27** The dorsal and ventral cavities are subdivided as shown in Figure 3-4. The dorsal cavity is divided into the _____ cavity and the _____ cavity. The cranial (**kra′ne-əl**) cavity contains the brain, and the spinal (**spi′nəl**) cavity contains the spinal cord and the beginnings of the spinal nerves. A combining form *crani(o)* means skull and *spin(o)* means spine. The cranial and spinal cavities are divisions of the _____ body cavity.
chest	**3-28** The ventral cavity is the other principal body cavity. It is subdivided into the thoracic, the abdominal, and the pelvic (**pel′vik**) cavities. You have learned that thoracic means pertaining to the _____. The thoracic cavity contains several divisions, which you will learn in a later chapter. The abdominal and pelvic cavities are not separated by a muscular partition, and together they are frequently called the abdominopelvic (**ab-dom″ĭ-no-pel′vik**) cavity. The muscular diaphragm (**di′ə-fram**) divides the thoracic cavity and the abdominopelvic cavity.

pelvic	**3-29** The pelvis is the lower portion of the trunk of the body, and **pelv(i)** is the combining form for pelvis. The cavity formed by the pelvis is the _____ cavity.
abdominal	The pelvic cavity contains the urinary bladder, the lower portion of the large intestine, the rectum, and the male or female reproductive organs. However, organs such as the stomach, spleen, and liver are contained in the _____ cavity
peritoneum	**3-30** The abdominopelvic cavity is lined with a serous membrane called the peritoneum (**per″ĭ-to-ne′əm).** This membrane also invests the internal organs. Write the name of the serous membrane that lines the abdominopelvic cavity and is reflected over the internal organs: _____.
parietal **viscera (vis′ər-ə)** **visceral**	The peritoneum that lines the abdominal and pelvic walls is called parietal (**pə-ri′ə-tal**) peritoneum. The peritoneum that invests the organs is visceral (**vis′er-əl**) peritoneum. Organs within the ventral body cavity, especially the abdominal organs, are called viscera (singular, viscus). There are two types of peritoneum. That which lines the abdominopelvic cavity is _____ peritoneum. Organs within the ventral body cavity, especially the abdominal organs, are called _____. Peritoneum that invests the viscera is called _____ peritoneum. The peritoneum contains large folds that weave in between the organs, binding them to one another and to the walls of the cavity.
peritoneal **(per″ĭ-to-ne′əl)**	**3-31** The combining form for peritoneum is **periton(o).** You learned earlier that -al means pertaining to; however, **-eal** also means pertaining to. Build a word that means pertaining to the peritoneum using the suffix -eal: _____. Serous membranes such as the peritoneum secrete a lubricating fluid that allows the organs to slide against one another or against the cavity wall. The peritoneal cavity is the space between the parietal peritoneum and the visceral peritoneum.
abdomen	**3-32** Abdomino/centesis (**ab-dom″ĭ-no-sen-te′sis**) is surgical puncture of the _____. Abdominal paracentesis (**par″ə-sən-te′sis**) is another name for abdominocentesis. This procedure is performed to remove fluids or to inject a therapeutic agent. It is most often done to remove excess fluid (ascites [**ə-si′tēz**]) from the peritoneal cavity.
paracentesis	Ascites is abnormal accumulation of serous fluid in the peritoneal cavity, sometimes resulting in considerable distension (enlargement, stretching) of the abdomen. The removal of the excess fluid in the peritoneal cavity is called abdominal _____.

❑ SECTION C REVIEW   𝓑ody Regions and Body Cavities

This section review covers frames 3–21 through 3–32. Complete the table by writing the meaning of each word part that is listed:

Combining Form	Meaning	Suffix	Meaning
1. abdomin(o)	_____	6. -eal	_____
2. crani(o)	_____		
3. pelv(i)	_____		
4. periton(o)	_____		
5. spin(o)	_____		

(Use Appendix V to check your answers.)

Body Extremities

The body extremities are the four limbs. Each arm, wrist, hand, and associated fingers make up one of the body's upper extremities. Each thigh, kneecap, leg, ankle, and associated toes make up one of the lower extremities. Fingers and toes are digits. Many medical terms use combining forms for the body extremities—hands, feet, and phalanges (fingers and toes).

extremities acrocyanosis (ak″ro-si″ə-no′sis) extremities	**3-33** The combining form for extremities is **acr(o).** In acro/paralysis (**ak″ro-pə-ral′ĭ-sis),** movement of the _____ is impaired. Build a word by combining acr(o), cyan(o), and -osis: _____. This new word means a blue condition of the _____.
blue, blue skin	**3-34** The combining form *cyan(o)* means blue. In acrocyanosis, the extremities are _____. Cyano/derma (**si″ah-no-der′mah**) is a _____ discoloration of the _____.
blue condition blue or bluish skin condition (or disease)	**3-35** The suffix *-osis* means condition but sometimes implies a disease or abnormal increase. -osis usually indicates an abnormal noninflammatory condition. Inflammation is tissue reaction to injury and is recognized by pain, heat, redness, and swelling. -osis usually indicates an abnormal condition that is not associated with inflammation. -osis is usually affixed to a word part that indicates either the part affected or the nature of the abnormality. Cyanosis (**si″ə-no′sis**) is an abnormal _____ _____. If a person does not get enough oxygen, he or she may become cyano/tic (**si-ə-not′ik**) (Figure 3-5). The color of the person's skin would appear somewhat _____. Dermat/osis (**der″mə-to′sis**) means a _____ _____. Its true meaning is any disease of the skin in which inflammation is not present.
psych(o) psychosis condition, mind	**3-36** In Chapter 2, you learned that _____ means mind. Add -osis to the combining form for mind to form a word that means a major mental disorder: _____. The term *psychosis* is generally restricted to mental disorders of such magnitude that there is personality disintegration and gross impairment in reality testing, sometimes resulting in loss of contact with reality. Translated literally, psychosis is an abnormal _____ of the _____. A disorder is a disruption or interference with normal function.
extremities	**3-37** Acro/dermat/itis (**ak″ro-dər″mə-ti′tis**) is inflammation of the skin of the _____.

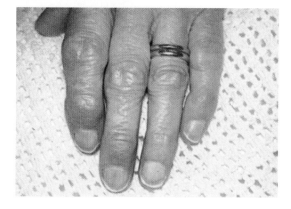

FIGURE 3-5

Cyanosis. The bluish discoloration is generally not as obvious as the extremely cyanotic skin of this patient. (From Kamal A, Brockelhurst JC: *Color atlas of geriatric medicine,* ed 2, St Louis, 1991, Mosby.)

extremities	**3-38** Acro/megaly (**ak″ro-meg′ə-le**) is a disorder in which there is enlargement of the _____. In acromegaly, there is excessive growth of the acral parts and the skull, a general coarsening of the facial features (nose and jaws), and enlargement of the fingers and toes.

It is caused by increased secretion of growth hormone by the pituitary gland. |
| finger
toe
digit
dactyl(o) | **3-39** The combining form *dactyl(o)* refers to a finger or toe. Fingers and toes are also called digits (**dij′its**). Whenever you see dactyl(o) or digit, immediately think of a _____ or_____.

The word that means finger or toe is _____. The combining form that means fingers or toes is _____. |
| dactyl(o)
dactylogram | **3-40** A dactylo/gram (**dak-til′o-gram**) is a mark or record of a fingerprint. The part of the word that refers to the finger is _____.

Write the word that means fingerprint: _____. |
| finger, toe
dactylospasm

finger, toe | **3-41** Dactylo/spasm (**dak′tə-lo-spaz-əm**) is a cramping or twitching of a digit. In other words, dactylospasm means cramping of a _____ or _____. Write this word that means cramping of a finger or toe: _____.

Spasm is a term for cramp or twitching, and it is frequently used as a suffix, **-spasm.**

Dactyl/itis (**dak″tĭ-li′tis**) is inflammation of a _____ or _____. |
| chirospasm
(**ki′ro-spaz-əm**) | **3-42** The combining form for hand is *chir(o).* Use chir(o) and -spasm to form a new word: _____.

Writer's cramp is a form of chirospasm. |
| hand

-plasty | **3-43** Chiro/plasty (**ki′ro-plas″te**) is surgical repair of the _____.

The suffix *-plasty* means surgical repair. It is derived from plast(o), which means repair. The suffix that means surgical repair is _____. |
| abdominoplasty
(**ab-dom″ĭ-no-plas′te**) | **3-44** Write a word using -plasty that means surgical repair of the abdomen: _____. (This type of plastic surgery, when done for aesthetic reasons, is commonly called a tummy tuck.) |
| ophthalmoplasty
(**of-thal′mo-plas″te**)
dermatoplasty
(**dər′mə-to-plas″te**) | **3-45** Write a word that means surgical repair of the eye: _____.

Write another word that, translated literally, means surgical repair of the skin: _____ In this surgery, skin grafts are used to cover destroyed or lost skin. |
| hands, feet
feet

podiatry
(**po-di′ə-tre**) | **3-46** You learned in Chapter 2 that pod(o) means foot. Chiro/pod/y (**ki-rop′ə-de**) literally refers to the _____ and _____, and was once a term for podiatry. A pod/iatrist (**po-di′ə-trist**) specializes in the care of _____.

The specialized field dealing with the foot, including its anatomy, pathology, and medical and surgical treatment, is _____. |
| print or record of
the foot

podogram | **3-47** The combining form *gram(o)* means to print or record. The associated suffix -gram means the print or record produced. A podo/gram (**pod′o-gram**) is a

_____.

The term *footprint* is more commonly used than _____. |

print (or record)	**3-48** Words using gram(o) refer to _____. Learn the following suffixes: *-gram* is the record itself. *-graph* refers to the instrument that is used to make the recording. *-graphy* is the process of recording.
dactylogram	Build a word for fingerprint: _____.
dactylography (dak″tə-log′rə-fe)	The process of taking fingerprints is _____.
electrogram (e-lek′tro-gram)	**3-49** The combining form for electricity is *electr(o)*. Build a word using *electr(o)* plus the suffix for record: _____.
heart	The most common electrograms are electrocardiograms (**e-lek″tro-kahr′de-o-grams″**), ECG or EKG, which trace the electrical impulses of the _____ (Figure 3-6). Either ECG or EKG is correct, but EKG has lost popularity along with the old spelling of electrocardiogram that had a "k."
electrocardiography (e-lek″tro-kahr″de-og′rəfe)	**3-50** The process of recording the electrical impulses of the heart is _____.
electrocardiograph (e-lek″tro-kahr′de-o-graf″)	The instrument used to record the electrical impulses of the heart is an _____.
myogram (mi′o-gram) **myograph** (mi′o-graf) **spasm (cramp)**	**3-51** The combining form *my(o)* means muscle. The process of recording muscle contractions is myo/graphy (**mi-og′rə-fe**). A record called a _____ is produced by an instrument called a _____. Most of us have experienced a myo/spasm (**mi′o-spaz-əm**), which is a muscle _____.

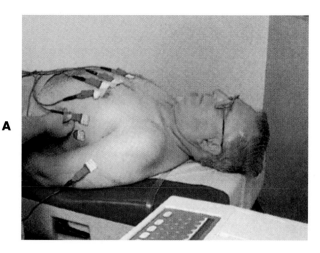 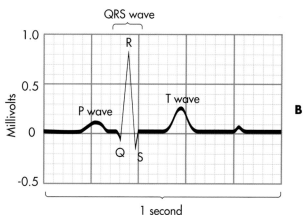

FIGURE 3-6

A, A patient undergoing electrocardiography, the making of graphic records produced by electrical activity of the heart muscle. The instrument, an electrocardiograph, is shown, as well as the ECG tracing, called an electrocardiogram. The electrical impulses that are given off by the heart are picked up by electrodes (sensors) and conducted into the electrocardiograph through wires. **B,** An enlarged section of an ECG, a tracing that represents the heart's electrical impulses, which are picked up and conducted to the electrocardiograph by electrodes or leads connected to the body. The pattern of the graphic recording indicates the heart's rhythm and other actions. The normal ECG is composed of the labeled parts shown in the drawing. Each labeled segment represents a different part of the heart beat. Electrocardiography is a valuable diagnostic tool. (**A,** From Bonewit-West K: *Clinical procedures for medical assistants,* ed 5, Philadelphia, 2000, Saunders).

❑ SECTION D REVIEW 𝓑ody Extremities

This section review covers frames 3–33 through 3–51. Complete the table by writing the meaning of each work part that is listed:

Combining Form	Meaning		Suffix	Meaning
1. acr(o)	_____		8. -graph	_____
2. chir(o)	_____		9. -graphy	_____
3. cyan(o)	_____		10. -osis	_____
4. dactyl(o)	_____		11. -plasty	_____
5. electr(o)	_____		12. -spasm	_____
6. gram(o)	_____			
7. my(o)	_____			

(Use Appendix V to check your answers.)

SECTION E

𝒜dditional Terms Related to the Body

Two word parts, som(a) and somat(o), refer to the body in general. The death of a person, somatic death, is usually defined as absence of electrical activity of the brain for a specified period of time under rigidly defined circumstances. Practice will help you learn which word part to use in writing terms about the body. Additional terms are presented for the eyelid and navel, as are several new prefixes and suffixes that are frequently used to write medical words.

body somat(o)	**3-52** Both *som(a)* and *somat(o)* refer to the body in general. Somato/genic (**so″mə-to-jen′ik**) means originating in the _____. The part of "somatogenic" that means body is _____. The suffix *-genic* comes from the same combining form as Genesis in the Bible, and both mean beginning or origin. You will study the combining form later.
body somatic	Somat/ic (**so-mat′ik**) cells are all the _____ cells of an organism except the reproductive cells. The death of a person is referred to as _____ death.
head	**3-53** You have already learned that cephal(o) refers to the head and that cephal/ad means toward the _____.
	The prefix *en-* means in or inside.
brain	The combining form *encephal(o)* means the brain and is so called because it is located inside the head. It is important to remember that encephal(o) means _____.
electroencephalog- raphy	Combine electr(o), encephal(o), and -graphy: _____. This new term is the process of recording electrical activity of the brain. Electroencephalography can be used to determine somatic death.
brain	**3-54** An electro/encephalo/gram (**e-lek″tro-en′sef′ə-lo-gram**) is a record produced by the electrical impulses of the _____. (You see why this is called an EEG!)
electroencephalo- graph (e-lek″tro-ən-sef′ ə-lo-graft)	The instrument used to record electrical impulses of the brain is an _____.
electroencephalog- raphy (e-tek″tro-ən-sef′ ə-log′rə-fe)	The process of recording electrical impulses of the brain is _____.

body	**3-55** Somato/megaly (**so″mǝ-to-meg′ǝ-le**) is increased size of the _____. The suffix *-megaly* has the same word root as a familiar prefix, ***mega-,*** which means large; *-megaly* means enlargement.
gigantism	Another name for somatomegaly is gigantism (**ji-gan′tiz-ǝm**), which is the more commonly used term. Gigantism (**gigant[o]** means large) is excessive growth of the body or a body part. It is caused by over-production of growth hormone occurring before the growing ends of bone have closed; thus excessive secretion of growth hormone can result in _____.
body feeling	**3-56** Som/esthetic (**so″mes-thet′ik**) pertains to _____ _____. Remember esthesi(o)? The "a" is dropped from som(a) to facilitate pronunciation.
	A particular part of the brain is the somesthetic area and is responsible for receiving and pinpointing where and what sensations occur in the body. A lesion in this part of the brain could affect one's ability to read, write, or speak, and also one's ability to recognize objects by touch.
body mind	**3-57** Somato/psych/ic (**so″mǝ-to-si′kik**) pertains to both _____ and _____. Somatopsychic disorders are physical disorders that influence mental activity. A brain lesion (physical disorder) often produces significant intellectual difficulties and memory loss (mental activities).
psychophysiologic (**si″ko-fiz-e-o-loj′ik**)	Psycho/physio/logic, also called psycho/somatic, disorders are just the opposite. Extreme or prolonged emotional states that influence the physical body's functioning are _____ disorders. Emotional factors may precipitate illnesses such as asthma and high blood pressure. You learned that physi(o) means nature. In psychophysiologic disorders, the natural functioning of the body is influenced by emotional factors.
	3-58 Psychosomatic (**si″ko-so-mat′ik**) is also the commonly used term that refers to the interaction of the mind or psyche and the body.
mind	You have learned that psych(o) means _____. Psych/ic has two meanings: A person said to be endowed with the ability to read the minds of others is called a psychic. Psychic also means pertaining to the mind.
cephal(o)	**3-59** Write the combining form for head: _____.
cephalometry	Cephalo/metry (**sef″ǝ-lom′ǝ-tre**) is measuring the dimensions of the head, perhaps for the purpose of a radiological procedure. Sometimes cephalometry is done to compare the size of the fetal head with that of the pelvis. In either case, _____ means measurement of the head.
encephal(o)	**3-60** Write the combining form for brain: _____.
	Encephal/itis (**en″sef ǝ-li′tis**) is inflammation of the brain. There are many types of encephalitis, but a large percentage of cases are caused by viruses. The symptoms include mild to severe convulsions, coma, and even death in some cases.
encephalitis	The suffix *-itis* means inflammation. Write the word that you just learned that means inflammation of the brain: _____.
brain disease **brain**	**3-61** Remember that path(o) means disease. The suffix *-pathy* means disease. Translated literally, encephalo/pathy (**en sef″ǝ-lop′ǝ-the**) is _____ _____. Encephalo/pathy is any disease of the _____.

pertaining to the umbilicus	**3-62** Omphalus (**om′fə-lus**) is another name for the umbilicus (**əm-bil′ĭ-kəs**) or navel. The combining form for umbilicus is **omphal(o).**
umbilicus	Omphalic means _____.
	An omphalo/cele (**om′fə-lo sēl″**) is a hernia of the _____. Babies are sometimes born with an omphalocele, protrusion of part of the intestine through a defect in the abdominal wall at the umbilicus.
omphalocele	The word part that means hernia will be used extensively in subsequent chapters. For now, learn the formal name for an umbilical hernia: _____.
umbilicus	**3-63** Omphal/oma (**om″fə-lo′mah**) is a tumor of the _____. You may have encountered other words that end in -oma. It probably means tumor in those words also. For now, remember that an
omphaloma	umbilical tumor is an _____.
plastic surgery (or surgical repair) of the umbilicus	**3-64** Omphalo/plasty (**om″fə-lo plas′te**) is _____.
	Omphaloplasty would be used to correct omphalocele.
umbilicus **omphalitis**	**3-65** Omphal/itis (**om″fə-li′tis**) is inflammation of the _____. Write the term that means inflammation of the umbilicus: _____.
otitis (o-ti′tis) **ophthalmitis (of″thəl-mi′tis)** **carditis (kahr-di′tis)** **neuritis (noo ri′tis)** **encephalitis** **dactylitis**	**3-66** Inflammation of the ear is _____.
	Inflammation of the eye is _____.
	Inflammation of the heart is _____.
	Inflammation of a nerve is _____.
	Inflammation of the brain is _____.
	Inflammation of a digit (finger or toe) is _____.
inflammation of the middle ear	**3-67** You wrote otitis to mean inflammation of the ear. Perhaps you have heard of otitis media (**me′de-ə**). Using the terminology you have learned, formulate a definition of otitis media: _____.
dermatitis (der″mə-ti′tis) **inflammation of the skin**	**3-68** Combine dermat(o) with -itis: _____
	The term you just wrote means _____.
inflammation of the eyelid	**3-69** The combining form **blephar(o)** means eyelid. Blephar/itis (**blef″ə-ri′tis**) is _____.
inflammation of both eyelids	Bilateral blepharitis is _____.
eyelid **blepharotomy (blef″ə-rot′ə-me)** **surgical repair of the eyelid**	**3-70** Blephar/al (**blef′ə-ral**) pertains to the _____. Write a word that means blepharal incision: _____.
	Blepharo/plasty (**blef′ə-ro-plas″te**) is _____.

blepharospasm (blef′ə-ro-spaz″əm) **twitching of the eyelid**	**3-71** Form a new word by joining blephar(o) and -spasm: _____. This new term means _____.
otopathy (o-top′ə-the) **disease of the ear**	**3-72** In Chapter 2, you learned that ot(o) means ear. Form a new word by combining ot(o) and -pathy: _____. The term you just wrote means _____.
ophthalmopathy (of″thəl-mop′ə-the) ur(o) **uropathy** (u-rop′ə-the)	**3-73** Ophthalm(o) means eye. Construct a word that means any disease of the eye: _____. Recall the combining form for urine or the urinary tract: _____. Form a new word that means any disease of the urinary tract: _____.
heart **cardiopathy** (kahr″de-op′ə-the)	**3-74** Cardi(o) is a combining form that means _____. (It may help you to remember the terms *cardiology, cardiologist,* and *cardiac.*) Any disease of the heart is a _____.
larynx **voice box** **laryngopathy**	**3-75** Laryngo/pathy (**lar″ing-gop′ə-the**) is any disease of the _____. The common name of the larynx is the _____ _____. Any disease or disorder of the larynx is called _____.
any disease of the brain **head** **headache**	**3-76** Encephalo/pathy is _____. Cephalo/dynia (**sef″ə-lo-din′e-ə**) is pain of the _____. A common name for cephalodynia is _____.
pain **ear pain** **pain, eye** **ophthalmodynia**	**3-77** You learned earlier that -*dynia* means pain. Dorso/dynia (**dor″so-din″e-ə**) is _____ in the back, or a backache. Oto/dynia (**o″to-din″e-ə**) is _____ _____, or earache. Ophthalmo/dynia (**of-thal″mo-din′e-ə**) is _____ of the _____. Write this new term that means painful eye: _____.
cardiodynia (kahr″de-o-din′e- ə)	**3-78** Write a word that means pain in the heart: _____. (This condition is commonly called angina or angina pectoris and usually results from an insufficient supply of oxygen to heart muscles.) Words indicating pain in different organs or structures can be formed by adding -dynia to various combining forms. You will learn many more words later.
fast **slow**	**3-79** Prefixes that mean fast and slow are **tachy-** and **brady-,** respectively.* Tachy/pnea (**tak″ip-ne′ə, tak″e-ne-ə**) is _____ breathing. Although tachypnea can be pathological, it is normal at other times, such as after running a long distance. Brady/pnea (**brad″e-ne′ə, brad-ip′ne-ə**) is _____ breathing.
bradypnea	**3-80** The suffix -*pnea* means breathing. The pronunciations of bradypnea and tachypnea are rather unusual. Note that two pronunciations are acceptable for these terms. Write the word that means slow breathing: _____.

*Brady- (Greek: *bradys,* slow). Tachy- (Greek: *tachys,* swift).

movement	**3-81** The combining form that means movement is *kinesi(o)*. When you see kinesi(o), it may remind you of kinetic energy, which is energy produced by movement.
slow movement bradykinesia	Kinesio/therapy (**ki-ne″se-o-ther′ə-pe**) is treatment of a disorder by _____ or exercise.
movement	Brady/kinesia (**brad″e-kĭ-ne′zhə**) is _____ _____. Abnormal slowness of movement or physical and mental responses is called _____.
	Dys/kinesia (**dis″kĭ-ne′zhə**) is difficult _____.

3-82 The prefix *dys-* means bad, painful, or difficult. Dysfunction (**dis-funk′shən**) means _____ or abnormal function. Any abnormality in the functioning of an organ is called a _____.

bad
dysfunction

Write a word that means difficult movement: _____.

dyskinesia

A dys/crasia (**dis-kra′zhə**) is a _____ or morbid condition. This is an old term that is roughly synonymous with disease; however, the term is usually used in describing certain conditions of the blood.

bad

3-83 You learned earlier that bi- means two. Bi/furcate (**bi-fər′kāt**) may be a new word for you. It means to divide into _____ branches.

two

Join bi- and concave to write a word that means having two concave surfaces. In other words, the object slants inward on two surfaces: _____.

biconcave
(bi-kon′kāv)

3-84 Pronation (**pro-na′shən**) and supination (**soo″pĭ-na′shən**) are terms used to describe the position of a person who is lying down. Pronation is the act of lying prone* or face downward. Pronation is also used to describe a position of the hand or foot. For example, the hand is in a prone position when the palm faces downward or backward. If a person is prone, is the face turned up or down? _____

down

Supination means lying flat on the back, but is also used to describe the turning of the palm to the front, or turning the foot inward and upward. If a person is supine,† is the face up or down? _____

up

3-85 Ambulation (**am″bu-la′shən**) means the act of walking. Ambulant describes a person who is able to _____.

walk

It is also accurate to say that the person is ambulatory.

3-86 A disease or a disorder in one structure can affect the functioning of the body as a whole. In the next chapter, you will learn how, even though the body has a remarkable defense against infectious microorganisms, an infectious disease such as influenza can spread from its host to someone else.

Infections are often preventable through proper hygiene and sanitation, and many infectious diseases can be avoided by the use of vaccination. Still, infection and infectious diseases remain a major cause of illness. An infection occurs when microorganisms invade the body.

Antiinfective means capable of killing infectious organisms or of preventing them from spreading. The same term is applied to an agent used to kill or prevent the spread of microorganisms. The prefix *anti-* means against. The literal translation of antiinfective is acting _____ infection.

against

3-87 Anti/microb/ial acts _____ microbes. It means the same as antiinfective.

against

There are many types of antiinfectives. Since the term anti/bio/tic contains the combining form *bi(o)*, we know that antibiotics act against _____ infectious organisms. Antibiotics are chemicals that are produced by microbes and can be used medicinally to treat infections, largely bacterial infections. Learn about other types of antiinfectives in the Chapter Pharmacology section.

living

*Prone (Latin: *pronare*, to bend forward).
† Supine (Latin: *supinus*, lying on the back).

against	**3-88** Antiinflammatory means acting _____ inflammation. In other words, it means counteracting or reducing inflammation.
against	Anti/pyretic (from G. *pyretos,* fever and related to pyr[o], meaning fire) pertains to a substance or procedure that acts _____ fever. Aspirin is a well-known antipyretic.

❑ SECTION E REVIEW ── 𝒜dditional Terms Related to the Body

This section review covers frames 3–52 through 3–88. Complete the table by writing the meaning(s) of each word part that is listed. Write all meanings of a term even though only one line is shown.

Word Part	Meaning	Prefix	Meaning	Suffix	Meaning
1. blephar(o)	_____	8. anti-	_____	14. -itis	_____
2. encephal(o)	_____	9. brady-	_____	15. -megaly	_____
3. gigant(o)	_____	10. dys-	_____	16. -pathy	_____
4. kinesi(o)	_____	11. en-	_____	17. -pnea	_____
5. omphal(o)	_____	12. mega-	_____		
6. som(a)	_____	13. tachy-	_____		
7. somat(o)	_____				

(Use Appendix V to check your answers.)

𝒯erminology Challenge

This section challenges you to read, write, and understand new terms about body structure that combine word parts that you know with unfamiliar word parts that are covered more extensively in later chapters.

fever **without fever** **fever** **effective against fever**	**3-89** Infections occur when the body is invaded by pathogenic microorganisms. Infection is just one of several causes of an abnormal elevation of the body temperature called fever or pyrexia (**pi-rek′se-ə**). The latter term is written using a combining form *pyr(o),* which means fire; however, pyrexia means a _____ or a febrile condition. Febrile pertains to fever. A/febrile means _____ _____. An anti/pyretic (**an″tĭ-pi-ret′ik**) is effective against _____. Anti/febrile (**an″tĭ-feb′ril**) and anti/pyretic both mean _____.
fever **hyperpyrexia**	**3-90** A pyro/gen (**pi′ro-jən**) is a substance that produces fever, such as some bacterial toxins. It is important to remember that a pyrogen causes _____. Hyper/pyrexia (**hi″pər-pi-rek′se-ə**) denotes a highly elevated body temperature, because *hyper-* means excessive or more than normal. A temperature of 106° F is considered to be hyperpyrexic. This can be produced by physical agents such as hot baths or hot air, or by reaction to infection. A body temperature that is much greater than normal is called _____.
trauma (injury) **atraumatic** **(a″traw-mat′ik)**	**3-91** You have learned that trauma means a wound or injury, whether physical or emotional. Traumatic means pertaining to or occurring as the result of _____. The prefix *a-*, like the prefix ***an-,*** means no or not. Write a word that means not inflicting or causing damage or injury: _____.

chest	**3-92** What part of the body is injured in a thoracic injury? _____
	Two directional terms that pertain to the chest are written by combining the prefixes *supra-* and *trans-*, which mean above and across, respectively. Write a term that means pertaining to a location above the
suprathoracic	chest: _____.
across	Trans/thorac/ic (**trans"thə-ras'ik**) means through the chest cavity or _____ the chest wall.
umbilicus	**3-93** Omphalorrhexis (**om"fə-lo-rek'sis**) means rupture of the _____ and is written using the suffix *-rrhexis*, which means rupture.
omphalorrhagia (**om"fə-lo-ra'je-ah**)	Write a term that means hemorrhage from the umbilicus by combining omphal(o) and *-rrhagia*, which means hemorrhage: _____.
eyelid	**3-94** Blephar/edema (**blef'ar-ə-de'mə**) is swelling of the _____. You will use the term *edema* both as a word and as a suffix to mean swelling that is caused by accumulation of fluid in an organ or place.
blepharoplegia (**blef"ə-ro-ple'je-ə**)	Using *-plegia*, which means paralysis, write a word that means paralysis of the eyelid: _____.
eyelid repair	Have you seen anyone whose eyelid appears to droop? This is called blephar/optosis (**blef'ə-rop-to'sis**), also simply called ptosis, and means drooping or sagging of the _____. This condition can be corrected by blephar/plasty, which means surgical _____ of the eyelid.
small ear microtia	**3-95** You will study many terms in the next chapter that use the combining form *micr(o)*, which means small. Combining micr(o), ot(o), and -ia results in microtia (**mi kro'shə**). The "o" in micr(o) is omitted to prevent "oo" in this term. Microtia is a condition of a _____ _____, if translated literally. Microtia is underdevelopment or absence of the external ear. Write this new term that uses micr(o): _____.
small head	Translated literally, micro/cephal/y (**mi"kro-sef'ə-le**) means a condition in which a person has a _____ _____. The size of the head is much smaller than normal and is usually associated with mental retardation.
large	**3-96** You will also learn that macr(o) means large. Macro/cephaly (**mak"ro-sef'ə-le**) means a _____ head or, in other words, abnormal largeness of the head as one might see in acromegaly and a few other conditions.
foot	Macro/pod/ia (**mak"ro-po'de-ə**) means a large _____, or abnormally large feet.

In the next few chapters, you will practice using the less familiar word parts in this last section. For now, be able to read and write the new terms in which the new word parts were used. There is no review for this section.

Study the following list of selected abbreviations. Then read through the Chapter Pharmacology section and be sure that you understand the effects and uses of the drug classes that are presented. When you are finished, work the Chapter Review. After completing the exercises, check your answers with the solutions in Appendix V.

You will find these items presented after the Chapter Review:

- Listing of Medical Terms
- Enhancing Spanish Communication

Selected Abbreviations

abd	abdomen, abdominal
AD	admitting diagnosis; right ear *(auris dextra)*
ADL	activities of daily living
AP	anteroposterior
AS	left ear *(auris sinistra)*
BMR	basal metabolic rate
BSA	body surface area
CXR	chest x-ray
D	dose, right *(dexter)*
ECG, EKG	electrocardiogram
EEG	electroencephalogram
EMG	electromyogram
lat	lateral
LLQ	left lower quadrant
LUQ	left upper quadrant
PA	posteroanterior
PE	physical examination
RLQ	right lower quadrant
RUQ	right upper quadrant
Sx	symptom
Vs, v.s.	vital signs
WNL	within normal limits

Chapter Pharmacology

Drug Class	Effects and Use	Drug Class	Effects and Use
Antiinfectives/Antimicrobials	**Used Against Microorganisms**	Clarithromycin (Biaxin)	
Amebicides	**Kill amebae**	Erythromycin (E-Mycin)	Streptococcal infections
Emetine	For amebic dysentery	Nitrofurantoin (Furadantin)	Urinary gram-negative microorganisms
Metronidazole (Flagyl)	Used in the treatment of trichomoniasis	Kanamycin (Kantrex)	Mainly gram-negative, some gram-positive
Paromomycin (Humatin)	Used to treat acute and chronic intestinal amebiasis		
		Penicillins	**Most gram-positive and gram-negative aerobes**
Aminoglycosides	**Generally active against gram-negative bacteria (neurotoxic, ototoxic, and nephrotoxic)**	Amoxicillin (Amoxil)	
		Ampicillin (Polycillin)	
Amikacin (Amikin)		Penicillin G (K-cillin)	Mainly gram-positive
Gentamicin (Garamycin)		Sulfas	Urinary tract infections
Kanamycin (Kantrex)		Sulfisoxazole (Gantrisin)	Urinary tract —mainly gram-positive
Tobramycin (Nebcin)		Tetracycline (Achromycin)	Gram-positive and gram-negative (broad spectrum)
Antibacterials	**Used in bacterial infections**	Vancomycin (Vancocin)	Life-threatening infections
Cephalosporins			
First generation	**Used mainly against gram-negative cocci**	**Antifungals**	**Used in fungal infections**
		Amphotericin B (Fungizone)	Parenteral drug used in severe fungal infections
Cefazolin (Kefzol)			
Cephalexin (Keflex)		Fluconazole (Diflucan)	
Cephalothin (Keflin)		Nystatin (Mycostatin)	Topical candidiasis infections
Second generation:	**Used mainly against gram-positive cocci and H. influenzae**	**Antihelmintics**	**Destroy worms**
		Mebendazole (Vermox)	Used for pinworms, whipworms
Cefaclor (Ceclor)		Pyrantel (Antiminth)	Used to treat *Ascaris*
Cefamandole (Mandol)			
Third generation:	**Expanded spectrum against gram-negative bacteria**	**Antimalarials**	**Used to treat malaria**
		Quinine	
Cefoperazone (Cefobid)		Quinacrine (Atabrine)	
Ceftazidime (Fortaz)			
Chloramphenicol (Chloromycetin)	Gram-positive and gram-negative (broad spectrum)		

Continued

Chapter Pharmacology—cont'd

Drug Class	Effects and Uses	Drug Class	Effects and Uses
Antituberculars Ethambutol (Myambutol) Isoniazid (INH) Rifampin (Rifadin)	**Used to treat organisms of genus Mycobacterium**	**Minerals—cont'd** Magnesium Manganese Phosphorus Potassium Sodium	 Essential for enzymes to function properly Essential for enzymes to function properly Essential for bone and tooth formation and for maintaining normal pH of body fluids Essential for normal cardiac and other muscle functions and for nervous system integrity Essential for normal cardiovascular function, maintenance of fluid balance, and nervous system function
Antivirals Acyclovir (Zovirax) Amantadine (Symmetrel) Zidovudine (Retrovir) Stavudine, D4T (Zerit) Dideoxyinosine, dDi (Videx) Zalcitabine, ddc (Hivid) Famciclovir (Famvir)	**Used in some viral infections** Herpes infection Influenza type A viruses HIV exposure		
Fluoroquinolones Ciprofloxacin (Cipro) Norfloxacin (Noroxin)	 Use with caution <18-year-old children	**Vitamins** A (beta carotene, retinol) **B-Complex**	 Prevents night blindness

Antiinflammatory Drugs
Aspirin
 	
Cyclooxygenase-2 (COX-2)
Celecoxib (Celebrex)
NSAIDs
  Diclofenac (Voltaren)
  Indomethacin (Indocin)
  Ibuprofen (Motrin)
Prednisone
	Reduce Inflammation
	
	New Group of NSAIDs with Fewer Side Effects
	
	Nonsteroidal antiinflammatory drugs
		Folic Acid
		
		Niacin, niacinamide
		
		Pantothenic acid
		
		Pyridoxine, B6
		
		Riboflavin, B2
		Thiamine, B1
		Cyanocobalamin, B12
			Used for megaloblastic and macrocytic anemias
			Used for the treatment of pellagra
			Used to stimulate intestinal peristalsis
			Prevents gastroenteritis, convulsions, neuritis
			Used to treat microcytic anemia
			Used to treat beriberi
			Used to treat pernicious anemia

Antipyretics Acetaminophen (Tylenol) Aspirin Ibuprofen (Motrin)	**Drugs Used to Reduce Fever**	C (ascorbic acid) D E K, menadione	Used to prevent scurvy Used to treat rickets Used as a vitamin supplement Used to treat hypoprothrombinemia
Minerals Calcium Iron, gluconate (Fergon), sulfate (Feosol)	 Essential for bone and tooth formation, for clotting of blood, and for normal nervous system activity, including heart Essential for hemoglobin formation and for function of certain enzymes		

CHAPTER REVIEW 3

▶ **BASIC UNDERSTANDING**

REVIEWING WORD PARTS
I. Write a word (prefix, suffix, or combining form) or abbreviation for each clue, omitting hyphens and parentheses.

CROSSWORD PUZZLE 3

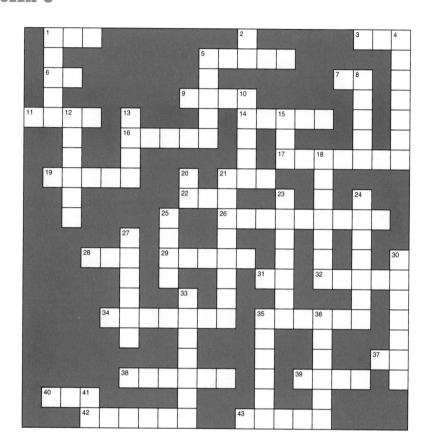

Across
1 chest x-ray (abbrev.)
2 type of vitamin
3 abdomen (abbrev.)
5 tooth
6 left ear (abbrev.)
7 toward
9 condition
11 incision (suffix)
14 pelvis
16 hand
17 chest
19 tail
21 basal metabolic rate (abbrev.)
22 pertaining to

26 brain
28 body surface area (abbrev.)
29 fast
30 near (abbrev.)
31 posteroanterior (abbrev.)
32 straight
34 near
35 body
37 surgery (abbrev.)
38 surgical repair (suffix)
39 child
40 brain tracing (abbrev.)
42 skull
43 back

Down
1 blue
2 without
4 digit
5 far
8 pain
10 cramp
12 enlargement (suffix)
13 extremities
15 lateral (abbrev.)
18 umbilicus
19 type of vitamin
20 physical examination (abbrev.)
21 eyelid
23 head

24 electric
25 against
27 side
30 posterior
33 movement
35 uppermost
36 anterior

LABELING

II. Label the body cavities that are indicated on the diagram.

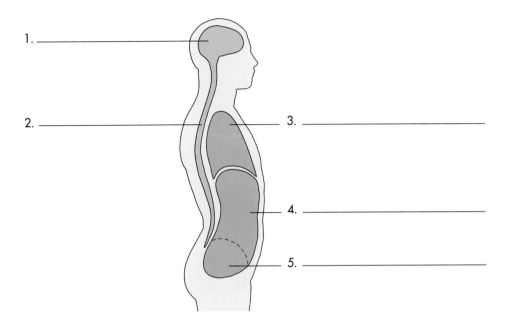

1. _____

2. _____   3. _____

4. _____

5. _____

III. Write the names or the abbreviations of the quadrants that are indicated on the diagram.

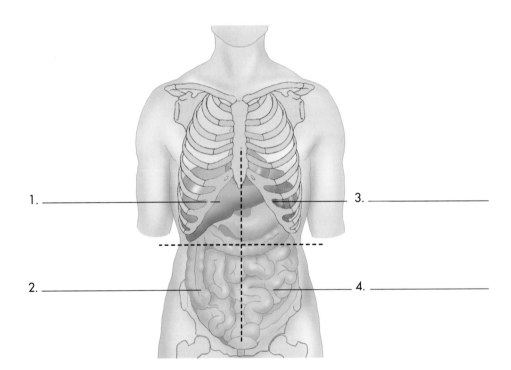

1. _____   3. _____

2. _____   4. _____

IV. Label the anatomical planes or aspects of the body as indicated on the illustration.

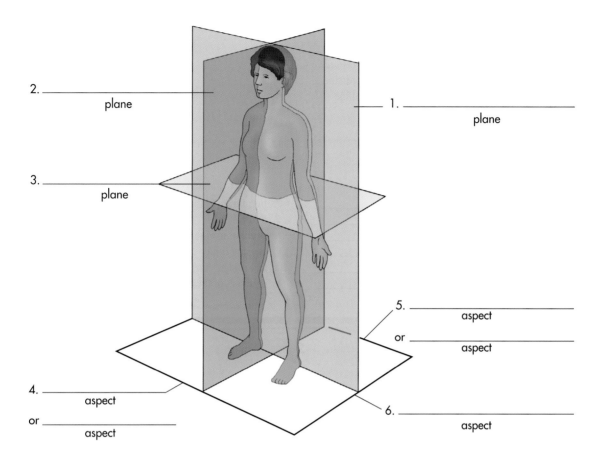

2. _____
plane

1. _____
plane

3. _____
plane

5. _____
aspect

or _____
aspect

4. _____
aspect

or _____
aspect

6. _____
aspect

MATCHING

V. Match each directional term with its meaning A through H:

_____ 1. anterior   **A.** above   _____ 5. lateral   **D.** far   _____ 8. posterior   **G.** near

_____ 2. distal   **B.** back   _____ 6. medial   **E.** front   _____ 9. superior   **H.** side

_____ 3. dorsal   **C.** below   _____ 7. proximal   **F.** middle   _____ 10. ventral

_____ 4. inferior

MULTIPLE CHOICE

VI. Choose one answer (A-D) for each of the following multiple-choice questions.

1. To what does mediolateral pertain?
   A. the middle of the back
   B. the middle and one side
   C. the back and one side
   D. the front and one side

2. Which of the following is a common name for chirospasm?
   A. eye twitch
   B. fingerprint
   C. spastic colitis
   D. writer's cramp

3. Which of the following words means "near the origin"?
   A. proximal
   B. distal
   C. medial
   D. lateral

4. How does a frontal plane divide the body?
   A. into upper and lower portions
   B. into anterior and posterior portions
   C. into equal right and left halves
   D. into unequal right and left portions

5. How does a sagittal plane divide the body?
   A. into upper and lower portions
   B. into anterior and posterior portions
   C. into equal right and left halves
   D. into unequal right and left portions

6. What is the location of dorsocephalad?
   A. toward one side of the head
   B. toward the front of the head
   C. toward the back of the head
   D. toward the middle of the back

7. Which of the following means inflammation of the brain?
   A. sephalitis
   B. cephaloitis
   C. encephalitis
   D. encephaloitis

8. What does dyskinesia mean?
   A. difficult breathing   C. difficult movement
   B. slow speech   D. slow breathing

9. What does cyanosis mean?
   A. a bluish condition of the   C. any condition caused
      hands   by drugs or medicine
   B. an abnormal bluish   D. enlargement of the
      discoloration   hands

10. What is the term that means lying face downward?
    A. paracentesis   C. proximation
    B. prone   D. supine

WRITING TERMS

VII. Write words for the following:

1. (abnormally) slow breathing   _____
2. any disease of the eye   _____
3. cramping of a muscle   _____
4. incision of the eyelid   _____
5. inflammation of the navel   _____
6. inflammation of the skin   _____

7. pertaining to the abdomen
   and pelvis   _____
8. pertaining to the chest   _____
9. causing injury   _____
10. recording electrical   _____
    impulses of the brain

▶ **GREATER COMPREHENSION**

SPELLING

VIII. Circle all incorrectly spelled terms and write their correct spelling:

abdominal   blepfaral   dorsocephalad   midsagital   omphalic   otodynia   peritoneum   somatogenic   superfishal   umbilical

MATCHING

IX. Identify the following abdominal regions with the letter (A-I) on the diagram that shows its location. The first region is done as an example.

1. epigastric   __B__
2. hypogastric   _____
3. left hypochondriac _____

4. left iliac   _____
5. left lumbar   _____
6. right hypochondriac _____

7. right iliac   _____
8. right lumbar   _____
9. umbilical   _____

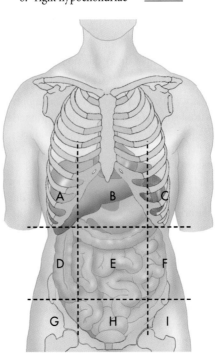

INTERPRETING ABBREVIATIONS

X. Write the meaning of each of these abbreviations:

1. abd _____
2. BMR _____
3. CXR _____
4. ECG _____

5. lat. _____
6. LUQ _____
7. PA _____
8. Sx _____

9. VS _____
10. WNL _____

IDENTIFYING SUBCLASSES

XI. Place a check mark by each of the following that represents a subclass of antiinfective.

_____ amebicides
_____ antibacterials
_____ antifungals

_____ antihelmintics
_____ antihistamines
_____ antiinflammatory drugs

_____ antimalarials
_____ antipyretics
_____ antituberculars

_____ antivirals

PRONUNCIATION

XII. The pronunciation is shown for several medical words. Indicate which syllable has the primary accent by marking it with an′.

1. **bilateral** (bi lat ər əl)
2. **cardiopathy** (kahr de op ə the)
3. **cephalic** (sə fal ik)
4. **dermatoplasty** (dər mə to plas te)
5. **lumbar** (lum bar)
6. **myography** (mi og rə fe)
7. **omphalic** (om fal ik)
8. **posterosuperior** (pos tər o soo pēr e or)
9. **supination** (soo pĭ na shən)
10. **visceral** (vis ər əl)

(Check your answers with the solutions in Appendix V.)

Listing of Medical Terms

abdomen	antihelmintic	caudal	dorsodynia
abdominal	antiinfective	cephalad	dorsolateral
abdominal paracentesis	antiinflammatory	cephalic	dorsoventral
abdominal quadrant	antimalarial	cephalodynia	dyscrasia
abdominocentesis	antimicrobial	cephalometry	dysfunction
abdominopelvic cavity	antipyretic	chiroplasty	dyskinesia
abdominoplasty	antitubercular	chiropody	edema
abdominothoracic	antiviral	chirospasm	electrocardiogram
acrocyanosis	ascites	coronal	electrocardiograph
acrodermatitis	atraumatic	cranial cavity	electrocardiography
acromegaly	biconcave	cyanoderma	electroencephalogram
acroparalysis	bifurcate	cyanosis	electroencephalograph
afebrile	bilateral	cyanotic	electroencephalography
ambulation	blepharal	dactylitis	encephalitis
anatomic position	blepharedema	dactylogram	encephalopathy
anatomical plane	blepharitis	dactylography	epigastric
angina pectoris	blepharoplasty	dactylospasm	febrile
anterior	blepharoplegia	dermatitis	fluoroquinolones
anterolateral	blepharoptosis	dermatoplasty	frontal
anteromedial	blepharospasm	dermatosis	gigantism
anteromedian	blepharotomy	diaphragm	hemothorax
anteroposterior	bradycardia	digit	hyperpyrexia
anterosuperior	bradykinesia	disorder	hypochondriac
antibacterial	bradypnea	distal	hypogastric
antibiotic	cardiodynia	dorsal	iliac
antifebrile	cardiopathy	dorsal cavity	inferior
antifungal	carditis	dorsocephalad	inferomedian

Continued

Listing of Medical Terms—cont'd

inguinal	omphalorrhexis	posterointernal	supine
kinesiotherapy	omphalus	posterolateral	suprathoracic
laryngopathy	ophthalmitis	posteromedial	tachypnea
lateral	ophthalmodynia	posterosuperior	telecardiogram
lumbar	ophthalmopathy	pronation	thoracic
macrocephaly	ophthalmoplasty	prone	thoracic cavity
macropodia	otitis	proximal	thoracodynia
medial	otitis media	psychic	thoracotomy
median	otodynia	psychophysiologic	thorax
mediolateral	otopathy	psychosis	transthoracic
microcephaly	palmar	psychosomatic	transverse
microtia	paracentesis	ptosis	trauma
midsagittal	parietal peritoneum	pyrexia	traumatic
myogram	pelvic cavity	pyrogen	umbilical
myograph	pelvis	sagittal	umbilicus
myography	peritoneal cavity	somatic	unilateral
myospasm	peritoneum	somatogenic	uropathy
neuritis	plantar	somatomegaly	ventral
omphalic	podiatrist	somatopsychic	ventral cavity
omphalitis	podiatry	somesthetic	ventrolateral
omphalocele	podogram	spinal cavity	ventromedian
omphaloma	posterior	superficial	viscera
omphaloplasty	posteroanterior	superior	visceral peritoneum
omphalorrhagia	posteroexternal	supination	

Español Enhancing Spanish Communication

English	Spanish (pronunciation)	English	Spanish (pronunciation)
abdomen	abdomen (ab-DOH-men), vientre (ve-EN-tray)	leg	pierna (pe-ERR-nah)
antibiotic	antibiótico (an-te-be-O-te-co)	liver	hígado (EE-ga-do)
arm	brazo (BRAH-so)	muscle	músculo (MOOS-coo-lo)
belly	barriga (bar-REE-gah)	navel	ombligo (om-BLEE-go)
bladder	vejiga (vah-HEE-gah)	palm	palma (PAHL-mah)
blood	sangre (SAHN-gray)	rectum	recto (REK-to)
blue	azul (ah-SOOL)	rib	costilla (cos-TEEL-lyah)
breathing	respiración (res-pe-rah-se-ON)	skull	cráneo (CRAH-nay-o)
chest	pecho (PAY-cho)	sole	planta (PLAHN-tah)
electricity	electricidad (ay-lec-tre-se-DAHD)	spasm	espasmo (es-PAHS-mo)
eyelid	párpado (PAR-pah-do)	thigh	muslo (MOOS-lo)
fever	fiebre (fe-AY-bray)	toe	dedo del pie (DAY-do del PE-ay)
finger	dedo (DAY-do)	trauma	daño (DAH-nyo), herida (ay-REE-dah)
fingerprint	impresión digital (im-pray-se-ON de-he-TAHL)	uterus	útero (OO-tay-ro)
		vein	vena (VAY-nah)
hip	cadera (cah-DAY-rah)	wrist	muñeca (moo-NYAY-cah)

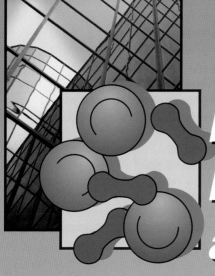

Blood, Other Body Fluids, and Immunity 4

Outline

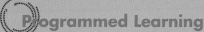
Principal Word Parts

COMBINING FORMS

aer(o)	air or gas
cellul(o)	little cell or compartment
chlor(o)	green
chrom(o)	color
coagul(o)	coagulation
cyt(o)	cell
erythr(o)	red
fibrin(o)	fibrin
hem(a), hem(o), hemat(o)	blood
hemoglobin(o)	hemoglobin
hydr(o)	water
immun(o)	immunity
is(o)	equal
kary(o), nucle(o)	nucleus
leuk(o)	white
log(o)	words or study
lys(o)	destruction or dissolving
macr(o), megal(o)	large or enlarged
melan(o)	black
micr(o)	small
morph(o)	shape; form
muc(o)	mucus
norm(o)	normal
phag(o)	to eat
phil(o)	attraction
poikil(o)	irregular
scop(o)	to view or examine
spher(o)	round
thromb(o)	thrombus; clot
vascul(o)	vessel
xanth(o)	yellow

PREFIXES

a-	no, not, or without
extra-	outside
hyper-	excessive; more than normal
hypo-	beneath; below normal
inter-	between
intra-	within
poly-	many
trans-	across

SUFFIXES

-ant	that which causes
-ar	pertaining to
-ate	to cause an action or the result of an action
-cyte	cell
-ectomy	removal of; excision
-emia	blood

SUFFIXES—CONT'D

-lysin	substance that dissolves or destroys
-lysis	destruction
-lytic	capable of destroying
-oid	like or resembling
-opia	vision
-ous	pertaining to or characterized by
-penia	decreased; deficient

-phylaxis	protection
-poiesis	production
-poietin	that which causes production
-scope	instrument used to view or examine
-scopy	viewing
-tic	pertaining to
-y	state or condition

Learning Goals

▶ **BASIC UNDERSTANDING**

In this chapter you learn to do the following:
1. Understand the important role of body fluids.
2. Recognize the meaning of word parts pertaining to body fluids and immunity and use them to write terms.
3. Identify the functions and principal conditions that affect erythrocytes, leukocytes, and blood platelets.
4. Describe several important processes and characteristics of blood.
5. Define active versus passive immunity, natural versus artificial immunity, and nonspecific versus specific body defense mechanisms.

▶ **GREATER COMPREHENSION**

6. Understand several characteristics of anemia, body defense mechanisms, and factors involved in healing.
7. Name several nonspecific body defense mechanisms and describe the two aspects of specific immune response.
8. Differentiate terms as being related to diagnosis, anatomy, surgery, therapy, or radiology.
9. Spell medical terms accurately.
10. Pronounce medical terms correctly.
11. Write the meanings of the abbreviations.
12. Identify the effects or uses of the drug classes presented in this chapter.

Body Fluids and the Composition of Blood

Fluids constitute over half of an adult's weight under normal conditions. These fluids are vital in the transport of nutrients to all cells and removal of wastes from the body. Fluid balance is maintained through intake and output of water. Water is obtained by drinking fluids and eating foods. Water leaves the body via urine, feces, sweat, tears, and other fluid discharges (i.e., pus, sputum, and mucus). Blood and lymph, two of the body's main fluids, are circulated through two separate but interconnected vascular networks. Blood is given emphasis in this chapter. Other fluids are studied more in depth with their related body systems.

intracellular	**4-1** Water is the most important component of body fluids. These fluids are not distributed evenly throughout the body, and they move back and forth between compartments that are separated by cell membranes. Body fluids are found either within the cells, intra/cellul/ar, or outside the cells, extra/cellul/ar (Figure 4-1). The prefix **intra-** means within, the combining form **cellul(o)** means little cell or compartment, and the suffix **-ar** means pertaining to. Combine intra- + cellul(o) + -ar to write the adjective that means within a cell: _____.
extracellular	Extra/cellul/ar fluid is not contained inside the cells. The prefix **extra-** means outside. Write this adjective that means outside the cell: _____.
intravascular	Only about one fourth of the extracellular fluid is plasma, the liquid portion of the blood. Blood remains inside blood vessels (intravascular) in humans, so it is an intravascular fluid. Write the term that means within a vessel by combining intra-, **vascul(o),** meaning vessel, and -ar: _____. Besides blood plasma, the remaining extracellular fluid is located between cells and tissue spaces. This type of fluid is called interstitial* fluid. Knowing that **inter-** means between should be helpful.
intracellular extracellular interstitial intravascular	Look again at Figure 4-1. Review these new terms that are used to describe body fluids by choosing either extracellular, intracellular, intravascular, or interstitial to complete these sentences: More than one half of all body fluid is contained within cells and is called _____ fluid. Body fluid is classified as either intracellular or _____ fluid. There are two types of extracellular fluid. The majority of extracellular fluid is found between cells and tissue spaces and is called _____ fluid. The remaining extracellular fluid is blood plasma. Plasma is an _____ fluid.
fluid	**4-2** The regulation of the amount of water in the body is called fluid balance. This balance depends on the proper intake of water and the elimination (output) of body wastes, including excess water (Figure 4-2). The fluid balance depends on proper functioning of several body systems, particularly the urinary system. Dehydration or generalized edema (swelling caused by excessive accumulation of fluid in the body tissues) can occur if the body cannot maintain fluid balance. This regulation of the amount of water in the body is called _____ balance.
study	**4-3** Blood, the most studied of all body fluids, is composed of a liquid portion, plasma, and several formed elements (cells or cell fragments). The study of blood and blood-forming tissues is called hematology (hem″ə-tol′ə-je). You have learned that -logy means _____ of.
hemat(o) blood	The blood-forming tissues are bone marrow and lymphoid tissue (spleen, thymus, tonsils, and lymph nodes). The combining form **hemat(o)** means blood, but in the word *hematology,* the definition includes the blood-forming tissues. Write this new word part that means blood: _____. Hemato/logic (hem″ə-to-loj′ik) means pertaining to hematology or the study of the _____. You already know the meaning of -logy and -logist. These suffixes are formed using **log(o),** which means words or study.
hematologist (hem″ə-tol′ə-jist)	Change the ending of hematology to create a word that means one who studies blood: _____.

*Interstitial (Latin: *interstitium,* space or gap in a tissue or structure).

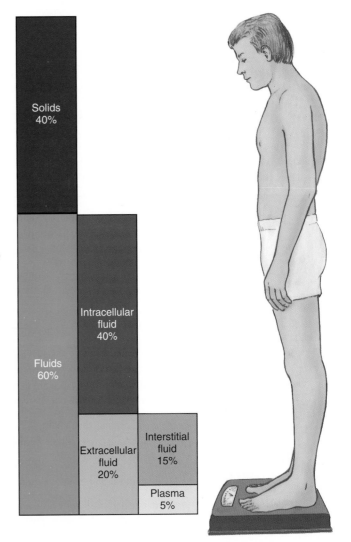

FIGURE 4-1

The body's fluid compartments. Fluid makes up 60% of the adult's body weight and most of that is intracellular fluid. Two types of extracellular fluid are interstitial fluid and plasma. Accumulation of fluid in the interstitial compartment results in a condition called edema. (From Applegate EJ, Thomas P: *The anatomy and physiology learning system: textbook,* Philadelphia, 1995, WB Saunders.)

TOTAL INTAKE—2500 mL

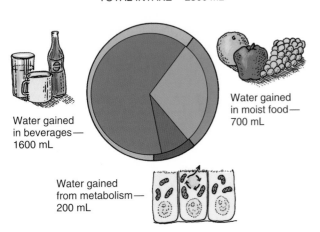

Water gained in beverages— 1600 mL

Water gained in moist food— 700 mL

Water gained from metabolism— 200 mL

TOTAL OUTPUT—2500 mL

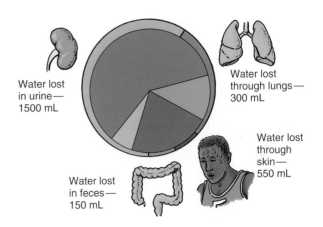

Water lost in urine— 1500 mL

Water lost through lungs— 300 mL

Water lost through skin— 550 mL

Water lost in feces— 150 mL

FIGURE 4-2

Avenues of fluid intake and output. The kidneys are the main regulators of fluid loss. Generally, fluid intake equals fluid output so that the total amount of fluid in the body remains constant. Water is the most important constituent of the body and is essential to every body process. Depriving the body of needed water eventually leads to dehydration. (From Applegate EJ, Thomas P: *The anatomy and physiology learning system: textbook,* Philadelphia, 1995, WB Saunders.)

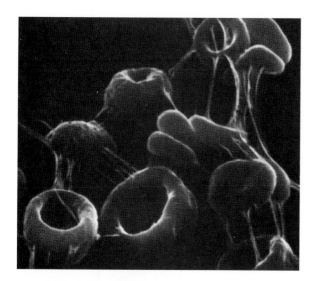

FIGURE 4-3

Blood coagulation. Scanning electron micrograph of fibrin threads and red blood cells at a magnification of 5000×. Fibrin, a whitish protein, entangles the formed elements of the blood, and the whole forms a coagulum, or blood clot. Note the thin center and the thick edges that give the cells a concave appearance. (Courtesy of Fisher Scientific Company.)

production **hematopoiesis**	**4-4** The suffix *-poiesis* means production. Hemato/poiesis (**hem″ə-to-poi-e′sis**) is the _____ of blood, specifically the formation and development of its cells. Write this new word that means the formation and development of blood cells: _____.
against **coagulation** **anticoagulant**	**4-5** Blood clots when removed from the body. Coagulation (**ko-ag″u-la′shən**) is the formation of a clot (Figure 4-3). Blood transfusions and many hematologic studies require blood that has not coagulated. An anti/coagulant (**an″tĭ-ko-ag′u-lənt**) is used to prevent blood from clotting. You have learned that *anti-* is a prefix that means against. An anti/coagulant acts _____ coagulation. In other words, it prevents blood from clotting. Another word for blood clotting is _____. A coagul/ant promotes or accelerates coagulation, for *-ant* means that which causes. A substance that prevents coagulation is called an _____. Another suffix, *-ate,* means to cause an action or the result of an action. Thus coagulate has two meanings, either to cause to clot or to become clotted. When you read that blood coagulates when removed from the body, it means that the blood clots.
coagulopathy (**ko-ag″u-lop′ə-the**) **coagulation**	**4-6** The combining form *coagul(o)* refers to coagulation. Write a word that means any disease (disorder) of coagulation: _____. Blood coagulation is a series of chemical reactions in which special fibers (fibrin) entrap blood cells, resulting in a blood clot. Exposure to air is not the reason that blood coagulates when removed from the body. A circulating anticoagulant normally prevents blood from clotting within the body. An anticoagulant can also be placed in blood as soon as it is removed from the body to prevent _____.
in vitro (**in ve′tro**) **clotting** **(coagulation)**	**4-7** In vitro* means occurring in a laboratory test tube (or glass) or occurring in an artificial environment. Because the anticoagulant is placed in the blood in an artificial environment (outside the body), this is in vitro use of an anticoagulant. A Latin term meaning in an artificial environment or outside the body is _____. Some patients tend to form clots within blood vessels, a serious condition that can result in death. For these patients, a physician prescribes in vivo (**in ve′vo**) anticoagulants to prevent _____. In vivo is a Latin term that means occurring in a living organism.

*Latin: *in vitro* (Latin: *in,* within; *vitreus,* glassware).

FIGURE 4-4

The blood in this test tube has been treated with anticoagulant to prevent clotting and centrifuged to separate its components. Red blood cells, the heaviest of the three components, make up the bottom layer. The middle layer of white blood cells and platelets is often called the buffy coat. The liquid part of treated blood, plasma, constitutes the upper layer. Any of these blood components can be given in a transfusion. (From Applegate EJ, Thomas P: *The anatomy and physiology learning system: textbook*, Philadelphia, 1995, WB Saunders.)

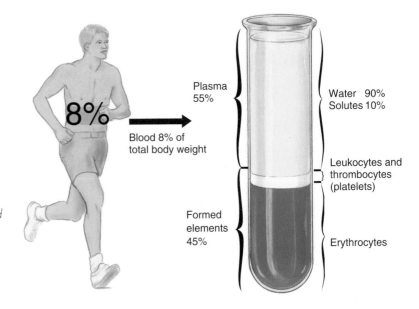

Blood 8% of total body weight

Plasma 55%

Water 90%
Solutes 10%

Leukocytes and thrombocytes (platelets)

Formed elements 45%

Erythrocytes

hemato	**4-8** Laboratory tests often require treating blood with an anticoagulant to prevent clotting (Figure 4-4). The hemato/crit (**he-mat′ə-krit**) is such a test. It measures the percentage of red blood cells in a volume of blood. The part of "hematocrit" that means blood is _____. (Hematocrit is often abbreviated HCT.) The hematocrit is not a difficult concept. It simply tells us what percentage of the blood is made up of red blood cells. Normal values are based on packed red cell volume, which is determined by centrifuging the blood. Exact normal values vary among children, men, and women, but they usually range between 37% and 54%. (The concept of the hematocrit can also be calculated based on the size and number of red cells in a minute sample of blood.)
blood	**4-9** The combining form hemat(o) means blood. Two other combining forms that mean blood are *hem(a)* and *hem(o)*. A hemo/cyte (**he′mo-sīt**) is a _____ cell. (Hemocyte is not commonly used. Instead, different combining forms are joined to -cyte to indicate types of cells. The suffix *-cyte* means cell.) There are many types of blood cells, and each type is given a particular name.
pertaining to erythrocytes (or red blood cells) **erythrocytes** **red**	**4-10** A frequently used combining form for cell is **cyt(o)**. There are two major types of cells in the blood. Erythro/cytes (**ə-rith′ro-sītz**) are red blood cells, often simply called red cells and abbreviated RBC. Erythrocytes are also called red corpuscles (**kor′pəs-əls**). A corpuscle is defined as any small mass or cell. Many structures, including red blood cells, are corpuscles. Normally, erythrocytes are biconcave disks that have no nucleus when seen in circulating blood (Figure 4-5). Their major function is transportation of oxygen and carbon dioxide. The combining form *erythr(o)* means red. Erythro/cyt/ic (**ə-rith″ro-sit′ik**) means _____. Erythro/poiesis (**ə-rith″ro-poi-e′sis**) is the production of _____. Erythro/poietin (**ə-rith″ro-poi′ə-tin**) is a hormone that stimulates erythropoiesis. (Notice the slight change in the suffix *-poiesis* The suffix *-poietin* means a substance that causes production.) Erythropoietin acts on stem cells of the bone marrow to produce what type of cells? _____ cells

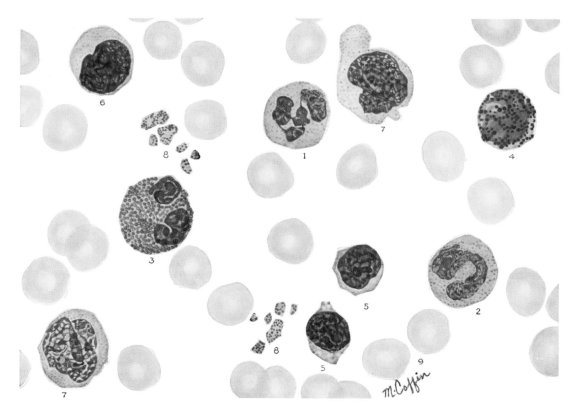

FIGURE 4-5

Types of human blood cells, stained: 1 to 7 are white cells (or leukocytes). These cells play an active role in immune response, or defense against disease. There are several different types of leukocytes, identified by the shape of the nucleus and the size and color of granules in the cytoplasm: *1* is a segmented neutrophil; *2* is a nonsegmented neutrophil called a neutrophilic stab; *3* is an eosinophil; *4* is a basophil; *5* are small lymphocytes; *6* is a large lymphocyte; *7* are monocytes; *8* are platelets (thrombocytes), which are involved in clotting; and *9* are red blood cells (erythrocytes), which carry oxygen. (From Custer RP [editor]: *An atlas of the blood and bone marrow,* ed 2, Philadelphia, 1974, WB Saunders.)

leukocyte	**4-11** The leukocyte (**loo′ko-sīt**) is another type of blood cell, also called a white corpuscle. The combining form ***leuk(o)*** means white. A white blood cell (WBC), often simply called a white cell, is a _____.
disease	The primary function of leukocytes is to protect the body against pathogenic organisms. You remember from Chapter 2 that patho/genic means capable of causing _____.
leukocyte erythrocyte	**4-12** There are normal numbers of erythrocytes and leukocytes in the blood of healthy people. This number is determined by blood counts. A determination of the number of white blood cells is a _____ count. What is an evaluation of the number of red blood cells? _____ count

❑ SECTION A REVIEW   𝐵ody Fluids and the Composition of Blood

This section review covers frames 4–1 through 4–12. Complete the table by writing the meaning of each word part that is listed:

Combining Form	Meaning		Prefix	Meaning
1. coagul(o)	_____		9. extra-	_____
2. cellul(o)	_____		10. inter-	_____
3. cyt(o)	_____		11. intra-	_____
4. erythr(o)	_____		**Suffix**	**Meaning**
5. hem(a), hem(o), or hemat(o)	_____		12. -ant	_____
6. leuk(o)	_____		13. -ar	_____
7. log(o)	_____		14. -ate	_____
8. vascul(o)	_____		15. -cyte	_____
			16. -poiesis	_____
			17. -poietin	_____

(Use Appendix V to check your answers.)

SECTION B

𝒜bnormalities of the Formed Elements of Blood

Erythrocytes, leukocytes, and thrombocytes (more commonly called blood platelets) are the formed elements of the blood. There is a normal range in number of these three elements. Anemia and polycythemia represent abnormalities in the number of erythrocytes. Leukemia, leukocytosis, and leukopenia are abnormalities in the number of leukocytes. An increase or a decrease in blood platelets is also abnormal.

---

thrombocyte

4-13 Thrombo/cyte (**throm′bo-sīt**) is another name for a blood platelet. The suffix in the term *thrombocyte* implies that it is a cell; however, thrombocytes are not typical cells but simply cell fragments without a nucleus (see Figure 4-5).

The combining form ***thromb(o)*** means thrombus (**throm′bəs**), a blood clot that obstructs a blood vessel or a cavity of the heart. You should be aware that some specialists differentiate between a blood clot (occurring outside the body) and a thrombus (occurring internally).

A thrombo/cyte is not a cell that has clotted. It is a cell fragment that initiates the formation of the clot and is commonly called a blood platelet. Another name for a blood platelet is a _____ .

---

clot

4-14 Thrombo/genesis (**throm″bo-jen′ə-sis**) is the formation of a blood _____ . You will learn more about the suffix -*genesis* in Chapter 6. For now, remember -genesis as the beginning, and in this particular term, it represents the beginning or formation of the thrombus.

When a clot forms inside a blood vessel or the heart, the clot itself is called a thromb/us (plural, thrombi).

---

thrombus

4-15 Thrombo/lysis (**throm-bol′ī-sis**) is dissolution or destruction of a clot that has formed in a blood vessel. In other words, thrombolysis is destruction of a _____ .

Distinguish the difference in these word parts: ***lys(o)*** means destruction or dissolving; -*lysis* is used to form words that describe the act of dissolving or destruction.

thrombolytic
(throm″bo-lit′ik)

-*lytic* is a suffix used to form adjectives describing dissolution or destruction. Write a word that means capable of dissolving a thrombus: _____ .

Thrombolysin
(throm-bol′ī-sin)

-*lysin* means a substance that dissolves or destroys. A word that is a trade name for a substance capable of dissolving a thrombus is _____ .

thrombus	**4-16** Thromb/osis (**throm-bo′sis**) is the presence of a _____. The thrombus forms inside a blood vessel or a chamber of the heart.
thrombolysis	The dissolving of a thrombus is known as _____. If a clot does not dissolve spontaneously, or if a thrombolytic agent cannot be used, the clot may need to be surgically removed, a procedure known as a thromb/ectomy (**throm-bek′tə-me**).
surgical removal of a thrombus	The suffix, **-ectomy** means surgical removal or excision. Perhaps remembering that an appendectomy is surgical removal of the appendix will be helpful. For now, remember that a thromb/ectomy means _____.
destruction of blood	**4-17** If thrombo/lysis is destruction of a clot, what is hemo/lysis (**he-mol′ə-sis**)? _____
hemolysis	Because you have learned three combining forms that mean blood, you may be wondering how one knows which form to use. Common usage determines the proper form. Even though hemato/lysis is a word, hemolysis is much better known. The most common word for the destruction of blood (actually red blood cells) is _____.
destruction of red blood cells	A hemo/lysin (**he-mol′ə-sin**) is a substance that causes _____.
	When blood is placed in water or another substance that hemolyzes it, the destruction refers to the dissolving of the erythrocytes, which burst and release their red pigment.
blood	**4-18** Use **-emia** as a suffix to mean blood. Literal translation of leuk/emia (**loo-ke′me-ə**) is white _____, so called because of the large number of white cells in the blood of patients with this disease. Leukemia is a progressive, malignant disease of the hemato/poietic (blood-forming) organs, characterized by a sharp increase in the number of leukocytes, as well as the presence of immature forms of leukocytes in the blood and bone marrow. A disease in which there is a sharp increase in the number of
leukemia	leukocytes is _____.
blood	An/emia (**ə-ne′me-ə**) literally means without _____. Because no one can live without blood, the name anemia is an exaggeration of the condition.
leukocytopenia **decrease**	**4-19** The suffix **-penia** means decreased or deficient. Write a word using leuk(o) + cyt(o) + -penia: _____. This is often shortened to leukopenia (**loo″ko-pe′ne-ə**). Either word means a _____ or deficiency in the number of leukocytes.
deficiency of erythrocytes	Erythro/cyto/penia (**ə-rith″ro-si″to-pe′ne-ə**) is a _____.
	Erythrocytopenia can be shortened to erythropenia (**ə-rith″ro pe′ne-ə**). Either word means a deficiency in the number of red blood cells. Anemia, however, is a deficiency in the number of red blood cells, or a deficiency in hemoglobin (**he′mo-glo″bin**), or sometimes, a reduction in both red cells and hemoglobin. Hemoglobin is the red pigment of blood.
	4-20 Anemia is not a disease, but a sign of various diseases. The severity of signs and symptoms depends on the severity of the anemia. Table 4-1 lists classic signs and symptoms of anemia.
	Several new terms are included in Table 4-1. Note that pallor, named after the Latin term, refers to an unnatural paleness or absence of color.
fast	Tachycardia (**tak″ĭ-kahr′de-ə**), which means an increased pulse rate, will be studied in the next chapter. Analyzing its word parts, tachy- means _____, cardi(o) means heart, and -ia means condition. One "i" is omitted to facilitate pronunciation. You learned in the last chapter that dys/pnea is
difficult	_____ breathing.
fainting **ringing**	The table defines syncope* (**sing′kə-pe**) as _____ and tinnitus† (**tin′ĭ-təs**) as _____ in the ears.

*Syncope (Greek: *synkoptein,* to cut short).
†Tinnitus (Latin: *tinnire,* to tinkle).

TABLE 4-1   Classic Signs and Symptoms of Anemia

Pallor (color of nail beds, palms, and mucous membranes of the mouth and conjunctivae are more reliable than skin color for assessing paleness)
Tachycardia
Heart murmur
Angina (chest pain)

SEVERE ANEMIA
Congestive heart failure
Dyspnea
Shortness of breath
Fatigue on exertion
Headache
Dizziness
Syncope (fainting)
Tinnitus (ringing in the ears)
Gastrointestinal symptoms (anorexia, nausea, sore tongue and mouth)
Constipation or diarrhea

TABLE 4-2   Factors Affecting Inflammation and Healing

Normal blood circulation to the affected area is essential for rapid healing
Liberal supply of leukocytes in the circulating blood is important in defense
Inadequately functioning leukocytes retard healing
Deficiency of antibodies retards healing
Patients who are malnourished heal slowly
Infection, presence of foreign material, or necrotic tissue in the wound retards healing
Incomplete immobilization of wound slows the healing process

---

iron deficiency

4-21 Iron deficiency anemia results when there is a greater demand for iron than the body can supply. It can be caused by blood loss or insufficient intake or absorption of iron from the intestinal tract. Iron deficiency anemia is often treated successfully with iron tablets and a well-balanced diet.

Ancient Greeks drank water in which iron swords had been allowed to rust, thinking that they derived strength from the sword. The French steeped iron filings in wine and then drank it! Like the French wine with added iron, some modern products contain iron and vitamins with substantial alcohol.

It is said that long ago, Ozark mountain people stuck nails in apples and let the nails rust. They removed the nails and fed the apples to their children. If the children's anemia improved after eating the apples, it is possible that they had _____ _____ anemia.

thrombocytes

increased

4-22 Thrombo/cyto/penia (**throm″bo-si″to-pen′ne-ə**) is a decrease in the number of _____. This is also called thrombopenia (**throm″bo-pe′ne-ə**). Because thrombo/cytes are important in the process of blood coagulation, thrombocytopenia, if severe, results in a bleeding disorder.

Thrombo/cyt/osis (**throm″bo-si-to′sis**) means an increase in the number of thrombocytes in the circulating blood. In Chapter 3, you learned that -osis means condition, but sometimes it implies an _____ condition.

anemia

4-23 Because coagulation involves several factors, a bleeding disorder can result from any number of deficiencies. Using the combining form **phil(o),** which means attraction, hemo/philia (**he″mo-fil′e-ə**) is a hereditary bleeding disorder in which there is deficiency of one coagulation factor called antihemophilic factor VIII. In hemophilia, there is spontaneous bleeding or prolonged bleeding after a minor injury. (Perhaps the naming of hemophilia came about because of excessive and prolonged bleeding that occurs in the disorder, thus leading to an inaccurate conclusion that affected individuals had an affinity or attraction to blood.)

Prolonged bleeding leads to a deficiency of both red blood cells and hemoglobin. We call this condition _____.

erythrocytes
leukocytosis
(**loo″ko-si-to′sis**)

4-24 Often words ending in -osis describe more than just a condition. Erythro/cyt/osis (**ə-rith″ro-si-to′sis**) means an increase in the number of _____.

An increase in the number of leukocytes is _____.

leukocytes

4-25 You learned earlier that leukemia is characterized by leukocytosis. But there is a major difference between leukemia and leukocytosis owing to infection. In leukemia, the production of leukocytes is uncontrolled, and many of the leukocytes produced are immature and nonfunctional.

Leukocytosis may be transitory, but it is often associated with an infection. Because the main function of leukocytes is protection against harmful invading microorganisms such as bacteria, this should help you remember which type of cell is likely to increase during an infection: _____.

inflammation

4-26 Infection is sometimes confused with inflammation. Inflammation is a beneficial and defensive phenomenon, often resulting in elimination of offending agents and establishment of conditions necessary for repair. Inflammation is a striking response of the body to injury. Infection (the presence of living microorganisms within the tissue) is but one cause of inflammation. Which of these two words is part of the body's natural defense? _____

The cardinal signs of inflammation are redness, heat, swelling, and pain, sometimes accompanied by loss of function. The severity, timing, and character of inflammation depend on other factors besides the cause. Table 4-2 lists several factors that affect inflammation and healing.

erythrocytes

4-27 One disorder in which there is an increase in erythrocytes is polycythemia. There are two forms of this condition, primary polycythemia (also called polycythemia vera [pol″e-si-the′me-ǝ ver′ǝ]) and secondary polycythemia. In both there is an increase in the number of _____.

Primary polycythemia is a serious disorder in which the bone marrow overproduces many types of cells and is associated with a chromosomal defect. Secondary polycythemia occurs as a physiologic response to prolonged exposure to high altitude, or lung or heart disease. In the described situations, insufficient oxygen in the tissue brings about the response. Sometimes the cause of secondary polycythemia is not known.

There is also an increase in the number of leukocytes in this disease, as well as the more marked erythrocytosis. The increased red cell mass leads to several secondary alterations, such as elevated blood pressure, increased viscosity, and thrombotic tendencies. Viscosity is the ability or inability of a fluid solution to flow well. A solution with high viscosity is thick and flows more slowly than one of lower viscosity. The suffix *-tic* means pertaining to. Thrombo/tic means _____ _____ a thrombus.

pertaining to

thrombi

Thrombotic tendencies favor formation of _____.

polycythemia

The name of the disorder characterized by marked erythrocytosis, which leads to increased viscosity (stickiness) of the blood, is _____.

**many, cell
blood, condition**

4-28 The prefix *poly-* means many. The term poly/cyt/hem/ia comes from poly-, which means _____; cyt(o), which means_____; hem(o), which means _____; and -ia, which means _____. In polycythemia, there are more cells than are normally produced by the bone marrow. This increased cell mass results in a sluggish flow of blood through the blood vessels.

**nucleus
large nucleus**

4-29 A normal red cell in circulating blood has matured and lost its nucleus; however, a white blood cell still has a nucleus. The word part for nucleus is *nucle(o)* or *kary(o).* A nucleo/protein (noo″kle-o-pro′tēn) is a protein found in the _____. Karyo/megal/y (kar″e-o-meg′ǝ-le) indicates a _____ _____. Karyomegaly is abnormal enlargement of a cell nucleus.

nucleus

Nucle/oid (noo′kle-oid) means resembling a _____; *-oid* means like or resembling.

TABLE 4-3   **Principal Conditions Affecting Blood Cells and Platelets**

CONDITIONS INVOLVING ERYTHROCYTES	CONDITIONS INVOLVING LEUKOCYTES	CONDITIONS INVOLVING BLOOD PLATELETS
Anemia	Leukocytosis	Disseminated intravascular coagulation
Bone marrow failure	Leukopenia	Thrombocytopenia
Hemolysis	Agranulocytosis	Thrombocytosis
Polycythemia	Leukemia (acute or chronic)	

many

form (or shape)

nucleus

polymorphonuclear

4-30 Poly/morpho/nuclear (**pol″e-mor″fo-noo′kle-ər**) is a word often encountered when one is reading about leukocytes. There are several types of leukocytes, and the most abundant type is polymorphonuclear, meaning it has a nucleus that is divided in such a way that the cell may appear to have several nuclei. The combining form *morph(o)* means form or shape. In the term *polymorphonuclear,* poly- means _____, morph(o) means _____, and nuclear pertains to a _____.

A leukocyte with a nucleus that is divided in such a way that it appears multiple is _____.

It is also called a polymorph (**pol′e morf**) and is abbreviated PMN. The cytoplasm of polymorphs typically contains small granular structures that stain lavender, black, or reddish orange. As a result, these cells may be referred to as granulocytes (**gran′u-lo-sīts″**).

granulocyte

any defect in coagulation

4-31 Principal conditions that are associated with abnormalities in the blood cells and platelets are listed in Table 4-3. The table lists a few terms that you have not yet studied. A/granulo/cyt/osis means absence of what type of blood cell? _____

Disseminated (meaning scattered or distributed over a considerable area; that is, an organ or the body) intra/vascul/ar coagulation is a grave coagulopathy in which there is generalized intravascular clotting. A coagulopathy is _____.

❑ SECTION B REVIEW   *A*bnormalities of the Formed Elements of Blood

This section review covers frames 4-13 through 4-31. Complete the table by writing the meaning of each word part that is listed:

Combining Form	Meaning		Suffix	Meaning
1. kary(o)	_____		8. -ectomy	_____
2. lys(o)	_____		9. -emia	_____
3. morph(o)	_____		10. -lysin	_____
4. nucle(o)	_____		11. -lysis	_____
5. phil(o)	_____		12. -lytic	_____
6. thromb(o)	_____		13. -oid	_____
Prefix	**Meaning**		14. -penia	_____
7. poly-	_____		15. -tic	_____

(Use Appendix V to check your answers.)

Anemias and Abnormal Hemoglobins

Hemoglobin, the iron-containing pigment of erythrocytes, carries oxygen from the lungs to tissues throughout the body. Microscopic variations in the erythrocytes are frequently observed in anemias, including those caused by a deficiency of hemoglobin. Electrophoresis helps identify many kinds of hemoglobin, including some abnormal types that cause anemias of varying severity.

small cell microcyte microcytosis (mi″kro-si-to′-sis)	**4-32** A microscope is used to view cells and other objects too small to be seen with the naked eye. The combining form **micr(o)** means small. A micro/cyte (**mi′kro-sīt**) is a _____ _____. Microcytes are undersized red blood cells sometimes seen in anemia. A small erythrocyte is a _____. A condition in which there is an increase in the number of undersized red blood cells can be named by combining micr(o), cyto/(o), and -osis: _____.
macrocyte (mak′ro-sīt) macrocytosis (mak″ro-si-to′sis)	**4-33** The opposite of micr(o) is **macr(o),** and it means large. A large cell is a _____. Macro/cyte usually refers to a large erythrocyte. Macrocytes are seen in certain types of anemia. An increase in the number of larger-than-normal erythrocytes is called _____.
scope instrument	**4-34** The combining form **scop(o)** means to view or examine. You are familiar with the word *micro/scope,* which means an instrument used to examine something small. The part of "microscope" that is closely related to examine is _____. When words end in **-scope,** they refer to an instrument used to view or examine something. A tele/scope is an _____ used to view something that is distant.
small large	**4-35** The suffix that means the act of viewing is **-scopy.** Micro/scopy (**mi-kros′kə-pe**) is examining something _____. Macro/scopy (**mə- kros′kə-pe**), as opposed to micro/scopy, is examining something _____. We can see a macro/scopic object with the naked eye. The term *macroscopic examination* is used more commonly than macroscopy.
large cells large cell (usually large erythrocyte)	**4-36** You have already learned that macr(o) means large. Now remember that **megal(o)** is another combining form that means large or enlarged. Megalocytes (**meg′ə-lo-sīts″**) are _____ _____. Macrocyte and megalocyte both mean _____ _____.
normal cells (actually normal red cells)	**4-37** In the laboratory, cells are observed using a microscope. Erythro/cytes are studied to determine if they appear normal. The combining form **norm(o)** means normal. Normo/cytes (**nor′mo-sīts**) are _____ _____. If erythrocytes appear normal, we refer to them as normocytes, or we describe them as normocytic (**nor″mo-sit′ik**).
cells of equal size anisocytosis (an-i″so-si-to′sis) iso	**4-38** Iso/cyt/osis (**i″so-si-to′sis**) means that all cells are of equal size. The combining form **is(o)** means equal. Iso/cytes are _____. Using an- as a prefix, write a word that means that cells are not of equal size: _____. Anisocytosis is common in the blood of people who are anemic. The part of the word that means equal is _____.

TABLE 4-4   **Two Classifications of Anemia**

MORPHOLOGICAL CLASSIFICATION	ETIOLOGICAL CLASSIFICATION
(Based on the appearance of red cells in stained smear) 1. Normocytic normochromic (from sudden blood loss, hemolytic anemias, kidney disorders, and certain chronic diseases) 2. Macrocytic normochromic (deficiency of vitamin B_{12} or folic acid is a leading cause of certain chronic diseases) 3. Microcytic hypochromic (insufficient iron or hemoglobin production, chronic blood loss)	(Pathophysiology) 1. Increased loss or destruction of red cells (bleeding or hemolysis owing to heredity or change in the red cell environment) 2. Decreased or defective production of red cells, called dyserythropoiesis (deficiencies in diet, defective absorption, bone marrow interference such as malignancies, toxic drugs, or irradiation)

equal isotonic	**4-39** Perhaps you are familiar with an isosceles triangle. In this case, "iso" means that two sides of the triangle are equal. Iso/tonic (**i″so-ton′ik**) means _____ tension. Isotonic also denotes a solution in which body cells can be bathed without damage to the cells through diffusion of water into or out of the cells. A solution in which cells can be placed without damage to the cells or change in their general appearance is an _____ solution.
round cell round spherocytosis (sfer′-o-si-to′sis)	**4-40** The combining form **spher(o)** means round. A sphere is round. A sphero/cyte (**sfer′o-sīt**) is a _____ _____. A normal red blood cell is biconcave, resembling a disk indented on opposite sides. A sphero/cyte is a red blood cell that is less concave than normal and appears _____. Using spherocyte and -osis, write a term that means the presence of spherocytes in the blood: _____.
poikilocyte poikilocytosis (poi″kĭ-lo-si-to′sis)	**4-41** Poikilo/cytes (**poi′kĭ-lo-sīts**) are red blood cells that have an abnormal shape. The combining form **poikil(o)** means irregular. If a red blood cell has an irregular shape, we call it a _____. The presence of poikilocytes in the blood is _____. Poikilocytes are seen in several disorders, including sickle (**sik′əl**) cell anemia. People with sickle cell anemia, a hereditary anemia that mainly afflicts blacks, inherit an abnormal type of hemoglobin. Their red blood cells appear elongated and sickled and are highly fragile. In vivo hemolysis occurs, resulting in hemolytic anemia. Sickle cells are irregularly shaped erythrocytes, so they are called poikilocytes.
below normal hyperchromic (hi″pər-kro′mik) blood	**4-42** Two important prefixes that are frequently used are **hyper-,** meaning excessive or more than normal, and **hypo-,** meaning beneath or below normal. **chrom(o)** means color. Hypo/chrom/ia (**hi″po-kro′me-ə**) is a condition in which the blood cells have a _____ _____ amount of color. This is the same as saying hypochromic (**hi″po-kro′mik**) cells. Cells that have more than the normal amount of color, in other words, excessive pigmentation, are called _____ cells. Hemo/globin is the red pigment found inside erythrocytes that gives blood its red color. Globins or globulins are types of proteins; therefore, hemo/globin is a type of protein found in _____. Hemoglobin is often abbreviated Hb or Hgb.
smaller, larger size shape	**4-43** Figure 4-6 shows several abnormal types of erythrocytes. You can see that microcytes are _____ than normal, macrocytes are _____ than normal, anisocytes are erythrocytes that vary in _____, and poikilocytes are erythrocytes that have an unusual _____. In anemia, erythrocytes usually do not have a normal appearance. Table 4-4 shows two ways in which anemias are classified, one on the basis of appearance of red cells and the other on the basis of cause.

A   B   C

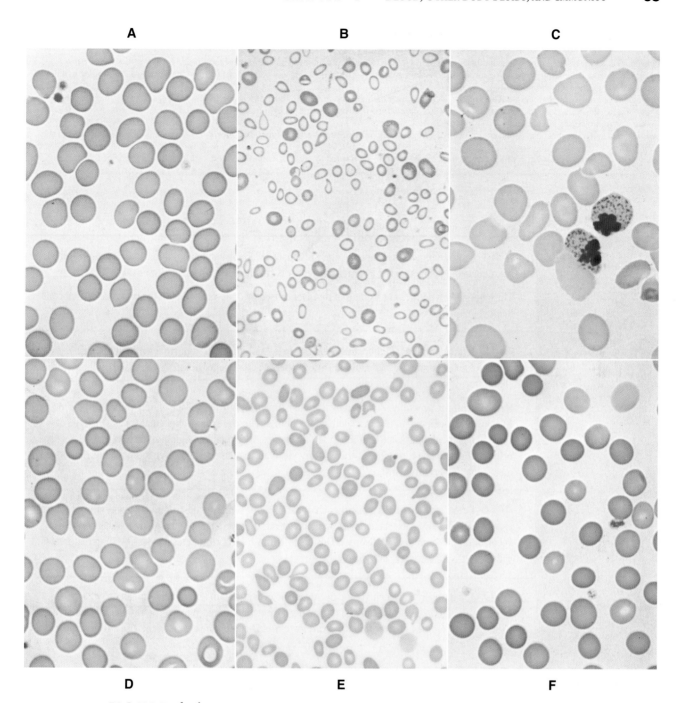

D   E   F

FIGURE 4-6

Morphologic variations of red blood cells in a stained blood smear. **A,** Normal erythrocytes.
B, Hypochromic microcytes. A few cells are normal, but most have central paleness and small
diameter. **C,** Macrocytes in pernicious anemia. In addition to erythrocytes of a larger size than
normal, two immature ones still have a nucleus. These cells also show anisocytosis and
poikilocytosis. **D,** Anisocytosis. Note the varying sizes of erythrocytes. **E,** Poikilocytes. Several
erythrocytes have abnormal shapes. **F,** Spherocytes. About half of the cells show dense staining
and a small diameter. (From Hayhoe FGJ, Flemans RJ: *Color atlas of hematological cytology,* ed
3, London, 1992, Mosby-Wolfe.)

TABLE 4-5   Additional Diseases or Disorders of the Blood

Blood parasites: any of several parasites that invade the blood stream. Malaria is one of the more familiar blood parasites.

Christmas disease: a hereditary bleeding disorder that is due to a deficiency of factor IX; it was named for Stephen Christmas, an English boy in whom the disease was first studied in detail

Hemophilia: a group of hereditary disorders of coagulation, which includes classic hemophilia A, the most common type, and Christmas disease

Malaria: a febrile disease caused by protozoa of the genus *Plasmodium* that are transmitted by infected mosquitoes. In its acute form, the disease is characterized by fever, anemia, enlarged spleen, chills, and sweating

Septicemia: a systemic infectious condition caused by pathogenic microorganisms (bacteria, fungi, parasites, viruses) or their enzymes or toxins in the blood

Vitamin K deficiency: a disorder in which there is insufficient vitamin K, essential to the coagulation of blood, resulting in hemorrhagic tendencies

hemoglobinopathy (he″mo-glob″bin-op′ə-the)	**4-44** Some anemias are hereditary and are caused by abnormal hemoglobins. Use ***hemoglobin(o),*** meaning hemoglobin, to write a word that literally is any disease of the hemoglobins: _____. The hemoglobinopathies are a group of diseases caused by or associated with the presence of abnormal hemoglobin in the blood.
dissolve	**4-45** Hemoglobin electrophoresis (e-lek″tro-fə-re′sis) identifies abnormal hemoglobin. Because hemoglobins are proteins, they move at various speeds across paper or starch gel, based on their electrical charge, their size, and their mobility. Hemoglobins are generally identified by letters or sometimes by their place of occurrence and discovery. Normal adult hemoglobin is designated hemoglobin A. There are many abnormal types. One type of abnormal hemoglobin, S, is found in sickle cell anemia. Abnormal hemoglobins such as Hb S generally result in distortion and fragility of the erythrocytes, causing them to hemolyze more readily. Hemo/lyze means that the erythrocytes _____.
hemolytic	**4-46** Hemo/lytic anemia is a disorder characterized by premature destruction of the erythrocytes. This type of anemia may be associated with some infectious diseases, may be a response to drugs or a toxic agent, or may be an inherited disorder. This disorder in which erythrocytes are destroyed prematurely is called _____ anemia.
without **aplastic** **without repair**	**4-47** You have already learned that an- means no or without. In an/emia, an- means _____. A similar prefix, ***a-,*** means no, not, or without. When a- or an- is used as a prefix, there is a special rule to determine which prefix to use: Use a- before a consonant. Use an- before a vowel or the letter "h." Write a word that means the opposite of plastic by using either a- or an-: _____. You previously learned that plast(o) means repair. A/plastic is _____ _____. Aplastic means heaving no tendency to develop new tissue. In aplastic anemia, the bone marrow is diseased and produces few cells. Irregularities in the blood often indicate abnormal conditions of various body systems; however, certain diseases or disorders are associated mainly with the blood or bone marrow and are called dyscrasias (dis-kra′ zhəz).* Some examples of the latter, such as leukemia and aplastic anemia, have already been discussed. Additional disorders of the blood are discussed in Table 4-5.

*Dyscrasia (Greek: *dys,* bad; *krasis,* mingling).

❏ SECTION C REVIEW *A*nemias and Abnormal Hemoglobins

This section review covers frames 4-32 through 4-47. Complete the table by writing the meaning of each word part that is listed:

Combining Form	Meaning
1. chrom(o)	_____
2. hemoglobin(o)	_____
3. is(o)	_____
4. macr(o)	_____
5. megal(o)	_____
6. micr(o)	_____
7. norm(o)	_____
8. poikil(o)	_____
9. scop(o)	_____
10. spher(o)	_____

Prefix	Meaning
11. a-	_____
12. hyper-	_____
13. hypo-	_____

Suffix	Meaning
14. -scope	_____
15. -scopy	_____

(Use Appendix V to check your answers.)

SECTION D

*B*lood Coagulation

Coagulation of the blood is a series of chemical reactions that results in a blood clot. Clotting is also a natural body defense mechanism when a person is cut. Bleeding generally stops within 5 minutes. An internal clot, a thrombus, can form within a vessel if the inner wall has been roughened by injury or disease, as seen in varicose veins.

resembling fibrin destruction of fibrin fibrinolysin (fi″brə-nol′ə-sin) blood clot	**4-48** Fibrin is formed when blood clots. The word part for fibrin is **fibrin(o)**. Fibrin/oid (**fi′brĭ-noid**) means _____ fibrin. Fibrino/gen (**fi-brin′o-jən**) is a precursor of _____. Fibrinogen is a protein that is changed into fibrin in the process of coagulation. Fibrino/lysis (**fi″brĭ-nol′ə-sis**) is the _____. Write a word that describes a substance that can dissolve fibrin: _____. A fibrinolysin can dissolve a thrombus, which is another name for a _____ _____.
stoppage of blood flow	**4-49** Blood coagulation saves lives when it occurs in response to injury but can result in death if it occurs in the circulating blood. A thrombus is particularly life-threatening if the clot occurs in the heart. Blood coagulation brings about hemo/stasis (**he″mo-sta′sis**). Stasis means stoppage of flow. You will learn later that the suffix *-stasis* means stopping or controlling. Hemo/stasis is _____ _____. Hemo/stasis also means interruption of blood flow through a vessel or to any part of the body. (Some abnormalities of hemostasis and coagulation are presented in Table 4-6). Malfunction or absence of any of the coagulation factors causes at least some degree of bleeding tendency. Hemostasis may be delayed in these cases, resulting in the loss of large amounts of blood. A transfusion may be necessary to replace the lost blood.

TABLE 4-6   Selected Abnormalities of Hemostasis and Coagulation

Defects in blood vessels (owing to injury or disease)
Thrombocytosis: primary thrombocytosis is observed in certain bone marrow disorders; platelet function is abnormal
Thrombocytopenia:
(1) Decreased production (any condition that interferes with bone marrow function, such as leukemia or aplastic anemia)
(2) Increased destruction of platelets (could be the result of many conditions that cause an enlarged spleen, such as lymphoma; also certain antibodies acting against one's own tissues)
Hemophilia: inherited plasma factor disorder
Acquired plasma factor deficiencies (severe liver impairment, disseminated intravascular coagulation, or fibrinolysis)

---

across

visible to the naked eye

agglutination

transfusion

4-50 The prefix *trans-* means through or across. In the earliest trans/fusions, blood was passed _____ from one person to another.

When blood is used for transfusion, grouping or typing of the blood is necessary. Blood typing determines the blood group of a person. There are four main blood groups (A, B, O, and AB) and an Rh system that are always considered. Tests determine a person's blood type by mixing blood with specially prepared sera and observing for agglutination (ə-gloo″tĭ-na′shən). In this type of agglutination, clumps or masses of erythrocytes form, which are visible macro/scopically. Macro/scopically means _____.

Write this term that is another name for blood clumping: _____.

The introduction of whole blood or blood components into the blood stream of a person is called a blood _____.

---

destruction

4-51 A transfusion reaction is an adverse reaction to the blood a person receives in a transfusion. Among the most common reactions are those that result from blood group incompatibilities. In other words, something in the donor's blood is not compatible with the blood of the recipient. Blood group incompatibilities often result in agglutination or hemolysis of the erythrocytes. Hemo/lysis is _____ of the erythrocytes.

Symptoms of transfusion reactions vary in degree from mild to severe. Some are manifested immediately, whereas others may not occur for several days. Infectious hepatitis and acquired immunodeficiency syndrome (AIDS) can be transmitted through blood from an infected person. Screening tests help to detect blood from infected people, and thus the use of such blood can be avoided. These diseases are discussed in later chapters.

❏ **SECTION D REVIEW**   𝐵lood **Coagulation**

This section review covers frames 4–48 through 4–51. Complete the table by writing the meaning of each word part that is listed.

Combining Form	Meaning	Prefix	Meaning
fibrin(o)	_____	trans-	_____

(Use Appendix V to check your answers.)

Immune System

Our bodies have many defenses, including an immune system that usually protects us from pathogenic organisms and other foreign substances. The immune response includes an initial nonspecific defense against the invader and, if needed, specific defense against the particular invader.

disease	**4-52** The immune reaction that can occur in a blood transfusion is part of the same system that provides protection against disease-causing organisms. We are continually exposed to pathogens and other harmful substances. Patho/gens are microorganisms that are capable of causing _____.
resistance **susceptibility**	Many substances that the body does not recognize are perceived to be foreign and may elicit the body's defensive mechanisms. The body's ability to counteract the effects of the foreign invader is called resistance. Susceptibility (sə-sep″tĭ-bil′ĭ-te) is a lack of resistance. For example, when we are exposed to the influenza virus, we do not become ill if our body has sufficient _____. The term for lacking resistance (or being susceptible) is _____.
ingest (or eat)	**4-53** Two types of body defenses are nonspecific resistance and specific resistance. Nonspecific defensive mechanisms are directed against all pathogens and include unbroken skin, phagocytes, inflammation, and proteins such as complement (kom′plə-mənt) and interferon (in″tər-fēr′on) (Figure 4-7). Interferon is of particular importance because it is formed when cells are exposed to a virus. Phagocytosis (fag″o-si-to′sis) is the ingestion and destruction of microorganisms and cellular debris by certain cells. The combining form *phag(o)* means to eat. Certain tissue cells called macrophages (mak′ro-fāj-ez) and leukocytes are the primary phago/cyt/ic cells. Phago/cyt/ic means pertaining to phagocytes or phagocytosis. Phagocytes (fag′o-sīts) are cells that _____ microorganisms and cellular debris.
immunity	**4-54** The second type of defense, specific defense mechanisms, is selective (specific) for particular pathogens. This specific resistance is called immunity, and it protects us from a particular disease or condition. Both specific and nonspecific defenses occur simultaneously and work together to overcome pathogens. Resistance to a particular disease is called _____. Specific defense incorporates cell-mediated immunity and antibody-mediated immunity. A type of white blood cell, T-lymphocytes (also called T cells), are responsible for cell-mediated immunity. B-lymphocytes (also called B cells) are responsible for antibody-mediated immunity.
against **against**	**4-55** Anti/bodies (an′tĭ-bod″ez) are formed _____ foreign substances. People do not generally form antibodies against their own body cells, although this may happen in a few cases. Antibodies are formed to act _____ other cells or substances that our bodies recognize as being foreign.
against **antibodies**	**4-56** Antibodies are immuno/globulins (im″u-no-glob′u-linz). The combining form *immun(o)* means immune. Globulins are an important type of plasma protein; special globulins called immuno/globulins are proteins formed in response to foreign substances. Immuno/globulins, or antibodies, are found in the liquid part of the blood, the blood plasma. Antibodies act _____ harmful invading microorganisms. Specific antibodies provide us with immunity against disease-causing organisms. We generally acquire antibodies either by having a disease or by receiving a vaccination. A vaccination causes our bodies to produce _____.

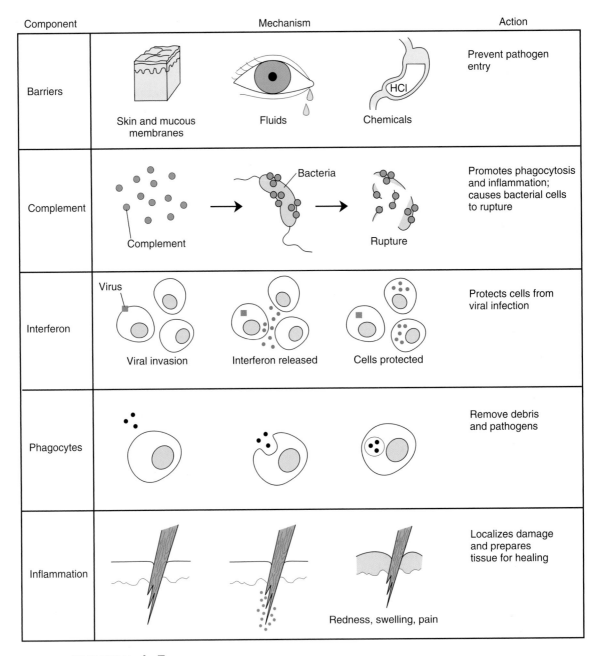

FIGURE 4-7

Nonspecific defense mechanisms. This is the body's initial defense against pathogens and foreign substances. Unlike cell-mediated immunity or antibody-mediated immunity, these defense mechanisms are nonspecific and directed against all types of invaders. (From Applegate EJ, Thomas P: *The anatomy and physiology learning system: textbook*, Philadelphia, 1995, WB Saunders.)

antibodies **immunized**	**4-57** A foreign substance that induces production of antibodies is called an antigen (**an′tĭ-jən**). Polio vaccine contains polio antigen, which causes the formation of polio _____. After receiving polio vaccine, one is _____ against polio.
	Occasionally the interaction of our defense mechanisms with an antigen results in injury. This excessive reaction to an antigen is called hyper/sensitivity (**hi″pər-sen″sĭ-tiv′ĭ-te**).
hypersensitivity	Write the word that means a heightened reaction to an antigen: _____.
	Anaphylaxis or anaphylactic reactions are exaggerated, life-threatening hypersensitivity reactions to a previously encountered antigen. The suffix -**phylaxis** means protection. With a wide range in the severity of symptoms, the reactions may include generalized itching, difficult breathing, airway obstruction, and shock. Insect stings and penicillin are two common causes of anaphylactic shock, a severe and sometimes fatal systemic hypersensitivity reaction. Systemic means pertaining to the whole body rather than to a localized area.
	4-58 Allergies (**al′ər-jēz**) are conditions in which the body reacts with an exaggerated immune response to common, harmless substances, most of which are found in the environment. A substance that can produce an allergic reaction but is not necessarily harmful is called an allergen (**al′ər-jēn**).
allergens	Some common environmental substances that may cause allergic reactions are certain foods, pollen, animal dander, feathers, and house dust. These essentially harmless substances that cause allergies are called _____.
against	In an allergic reaction, injured cells release a substance called histamine (**his′tə-mēn**), which causes dilation of the capillaries (the smallest blood vessels), an increase of gastric secretion, and contraction of smooth muscle of several internal organs. Histamine is responsible for the symptoms of hayfever: teary eyes, sneezing, and swollen membranes of the upper respiratory tract. An anti/histamine (**an″tĭ-his′tə-mēn**), a preparation that acts _____ histamine, usually relieves the symptoms.
active **passive**	**4-59** Immunization is the process by which resistance to an infectious disease is induced or augmented. Active immunity occurs when the individual's own body produces an immune response to a harmful antigen. Passive immunity results when the immune agents develop in another person or animal and then are transferred to an individual who was not previously immune. This second type of immunity is borrowed immunity that provides immediate protection but is effective for only a short time. Immunity that an individual develops in response to a harmful antigen is _____ immunity. Borrowed immunity that is effective for only a short time is _____ immunity.
	4-60 In both active and passive immunity, the recognition of specific antigens is called specific immunity. The terms *natural* and *artificial* refer to how the immunity is obtained (Figure 4-8).
	A vaccination is any injection or ingestion of inactivated or killed microbes or their products that is administered to induce immunity. Vaccinations are available to immunize against many diseases such as typhoid, diphtheria, polio, measles, and mumps. Depending on its type, vaccine is administered orally or by injection. Vaccination is a form of prophylaxis* (**pro″ fə-lak′sis**), prevention of or protection against disease.
antibodies	**4-61** Toxoids (**tok′soidz**) contain toxins, which are antigens. Toxoids cause our bodies to produce _____, thus providing us with immunity.
toxin (or poison)	You have already learned that tox(o) means toxin or poison. Tox/oid, when broken down into its components, means resembling a _____. Actually, a toxoid is simply a toxin that has been treated to eliminate its harmful properties without destroying its ability to stimulate antibody production.

*Prophylaxis (Greek: *prophylax*, advance guard).

Natural   Artificial

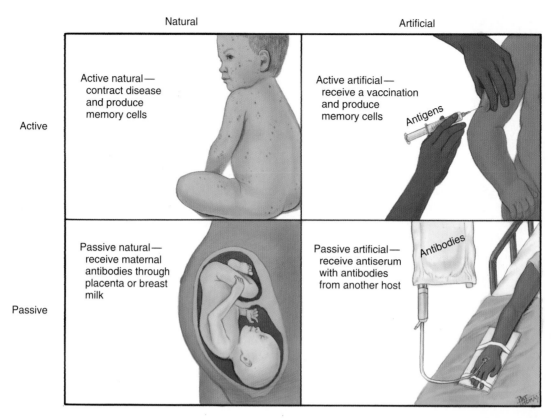

Active

Active natural—
contract disease
and produce
memory cells

Active artificial—
receive a vaccination
and produce
memory cells

Antigens

Passive

Passive natural—
receive maternal
antibodies through
placenta or breast
milk

Passive artificial—
receive antiserum
with antibodies
from another host

Antibodies

FIGURE 4-8
Four types of specific immunity. Active natural and passive natural immunities, as the names
imply, occur through the normal activities of either an individual contracting a disease or a fetus
being exposed to maternal antibodies. Both active artificial and passive artificial immunities
require deliberate actions of receiving vaccinations or antibodies. (From Applegate EJ, Thomas
P: *The anatomy and physiology learning system: textbook*, Philadelphia, 1995, WB Saunders.)

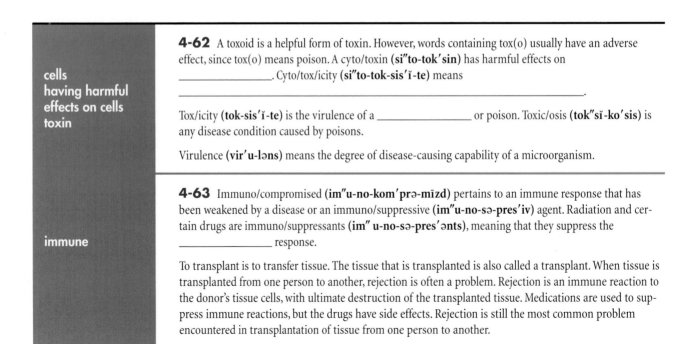

**cells
having harmful
effects on cells
toxin**

4-62 A toxoid is a helpful form of toxin. However, words containing tox(o) usually have an adverse
effect, since tox(o) means poison. A cyto/toxin (**si″to-tok′sin**) has harmful effects on
_____. Cyto/tox/icity (**si″to-tok-sis′ĭ-te**) means
_____.

Tox/icity (**tok-sis′ĭ-te**) is the virulence of a _____ or poison. Toxic/osis (**tok″sĭ-ko′sis**) is
any disease condition caused by poisons.

Virulence (**vir′u-ləns**) means the degree of disease-causing capability of a microorganism.

immune

4-63 Immuno/compromised (**im″u-no-kom′prə-mīzd**) pertains to an immune response that has
been weakened by a disease or an immuno/suppressive (**im″u-no-sə-pres′iv**) agent. Radiation and certain drugs are immuno/suppressants (**im″ u-no-sə-pres′ənts**), meaning that they suppress the
_____ response.

To transplant is to transfer tissue. The tissue that is transplanted is also called a transplant. When tissue is
transplanted from one person to another, rejection is often a problem. Rejection is an immune reaction to
the donor's tissue cells, with ultimate destruction of the transplanted tissue. Medications are used to suppress immune reactions, but the drugs have side effects. Rejection is still the most common problem
encountered in transplantation of tissue from one person to another.

❑ **SECTION E REVIEW**   𝒥mmune System

This section review covers frames 4–52 through 4–63. Complete the table by writing the meaning of each word part that is listed:

Combining Form	Meaning	Suffix	Meaning
1. phag(o)	_____	2. -phylaxis	_____

(Use Appendix V to check your answers.)

SECTION F

Cellular Needs and Analysis of Body Fluids

Cells throughout the body need metabolic waste disposal and a continuous supply of oxygen and nutrients. Blood is the primary transport medium. Since blood is contained within a vascular network, needed substances move across the vessel walls into the fluid that surrounds the body cells. Such is the purpose of some body fluids, whereas others primarily rid the body of waste. Many body fluids are available for chemical and microscopic study to determine the body's internal status. This information can be useful in diagnosing abnormal conditions in various body systems.

water

4-64 Cells depend on certain physical factors from the body fluids that surround them. Water, oxygen, and nutrients are essential to life.

The combining form **hydr(o)** means water. In chemistry, hydr(o) refers to hydrogen, but more commonly hydr(o) means water. Hydr/ant is a familiar word to you, so when you see hydr(o), think of hydrant and you will remember that hydr(o) means water.

The suffix **-ous** means pertaining to or characterized by. Hydr/ous means pertaining to _____.

water, head

shunt

4-65 The suffix **-y** means state or condition. Hydro/cephaly (hi″dro-sef′ə-le) appears to mean _____ in the _____. In medical terms, some interpretation is needed in dividing words into their components. Hydrocephaly is more commonly called hydrocephalus (hi″dro-sef′ə-ləs). Hydrocephalus means a condition characterized by abnormal accumulation of cerebrospinal fluid within the skull, enlargement of the head, mental retardation, and convulsions (Figure 4-9).

Treatment of hydrocephalus generally consists of surgical intervention to correct the cause or to shunt the excess fluid away from the skull. Shunt (shunt) means to redirect the flow of a body fluid from one cavity or vessel to another. The device that is implanted in the body to redirect the fluid is also called a shunt. Write this new term for what is often used in treating hydrocephalus: _____.

air

4-66 Two meanings of aerobic (ār-o′bik) are requiring oxygen (air) to maintain life and growing or occurring in the presence of oxygen. **aer(o)** means air or gas. Perhaps knowing that an aeroplane is the same as airplane will help you remember that aer(o) means air or gas. The combining form **aer(o)** in a term will mean _____ or gas, but sometimes the definition is extended to mean oxygen.

resembling

mucoid

4-67 Mucus is the slimy material produced by mucous membranes.

Muc/oid (mu′koid) means _____ mucus, because **muc(o)** means mucus.

Write the word that means resembling mucus: _____.

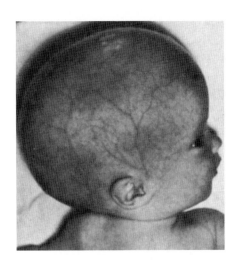

FIGURE 4-9
Four-month-old child with hydrocephalus. Hydrocephalus is usually caused by obstruction of the flow of cerebrospinal fluid. If hydrocephalus occurs in an infant, the soft bones of the skull push apart as the head increases progressively in size. (From Jacob SW, Francone CA, Lossow WJ: *Structure and function in man*, ed 5, Philadelphia, 1982, WB Saunders.)

pus	**4-68** Many body fluids such as urine, feces, sweat, sputum, and tears will be studied in their respective chapters. One particular body fluid, pus, is the result of tissue breakdown owing to infection.
	Pus is the liquid product of infection and comprises protein substances, fluid, bacteria, and leukocytes (or their remains). It is generally yellow; if it is red, this suggests blood from the rupture of small vessels. The liquid product of infection is called _____.
	A localized collection of pus in a cavity formed by disintegration of the tissue is called an abscess (**ab′ses**).
	Abscesses are slow to heal. One reason is the difficulty of delivering medication to the site of infection, since it is walled off from the other tissue. Some abscesses have to be surgically drained. Factors affecting healing in general are shown in Table 4-2.
hemat or hemat(o)	**4-69** A hemat/oma (**hem″ə-to′mə**) is a localized collection of blood, usually clotted, in an organ, space, or tissue, resulting from a break in the wall of a blood vessel. The part of the word that means blood is _____.
	Hematomas can occur almost anywhere in the body. They are especially dangerous when they occur inside the skull, but most hematomas are not serious. Bruises are familiar forms of hematomas.
hematoma	Later you will use the suffix *-oma* to write words for tumors of many kinds. The word *hematoma* is derived from the old meaning of tumor, a swelling, as there is a raised area wherever a hematoma exists. For now, combine hemat(o) and -oma to write the new word you have learned: _____.
blood, chest **blood in the chest**	**4-70** You learned that hem(o) means _____ and thorac(o) means _____.
	Translated literally, hemo/thorax is _____.
	(Hemothorax is blood or bloody fluid in the pleural cavity that surrounds the lung.)
	4-71 Laboratory analysis yields vital information about the cellular and chemical composition of body fluids. Laboratory tests detect, identify, and quantify substances, evaluate organ functions, and establish the nature of a condition or disease. They are commonly used to help establish or confirm a diagnosis and aid in the management of disease. Sometimes, a simple observation or deviation from the expected color of a body fluid or of the individual can provide helpful information. The next several frames will introduce several combining forms for specific colors. You have already learned that the combining form for color is
chrom(o)	_____.
red, white	You have also learned that erythr(o) means _____ and leuk(o) means _____.

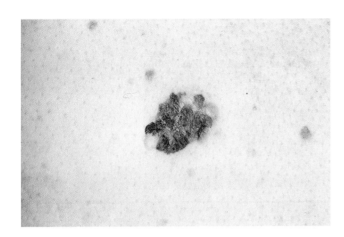

FIGURE 4-10

Melanoma, a pigmented lesion originating in the melanin-producing cells of the epidermis. Unlike most skin cancers, melanomas are malignant, and a person's survival depends on early diagnosis and treatment. (From Ignatavicius DD, Workman ML, Mishler MA: *Medical-surgical nursing across the health care continuum*, ed 3, Philadelphia, 1999, WB Saunders.)

blue	**4-72** Cyan/osis is caused by a deficiency of oxygen and an excess of carbon dioxide in the blood, as in severe conditions that interfere with normal breathing or circulation. The color of the person's skin appears bluish in cyanosis, so named because cyan(o) means _____.
black **melan(o)**	**4-73** You have heard of melancholy (**mel′ən-kol″ə**). A melancholy person is sad or depressed. In ancient times, it was thought that melancholy people produced a black bile that caused sadness, thus the origin of the word melan/choly. The combining form ***melan(o)*** means the color black. Melan/oid (**mel′ə-noid**) is like or resembling _____. Melan/in (**mel′ə-nin**) is the dark pigment of the skin and hair. It is a dark brown to black pigment, and the word is derived from the combining form that means black, which is _____.
melanoma **black cell**	**4-74** A melan/oma (**mel″ə-no′mə**) is a tumor composed of masses of cells that appear black (Figure 4-10). Melanomas are malignant, meaning they have a tendency to spread. Thus melanomas are often surgically removed to prevent them from spreading. Write this name for a malignant, pigmented (black) tumor: _____. A melano/cyte (**mel′ə-no-sīt**) is a _____ _____.
green **green**	**4-75** To what color do you think *chloro* in chloro/phyll refers? _____ Thus, ***chlor(o)*** means green. Chlor/opia (**klor-ōp′e-ə**) is _____ vision. (This is defective vision in which all things appear green, as sometimes occurs in certain drug toxicities.) A chloro/plast is a special structure found in plant cells and is so named because it is green.
yellow skin **yellow** **yellow** **yellowish**	**4-76** The combining form ***xanth(o)*** means yellow. Xantho/derma (**zan″tho-der′mə**) is _____ _____. Xanth/osis (**zan-tho′sis**) is a _____ condition. Xanth/ous (**zan′thəs**) pertains to _____ or yellowish. The skin often appears xanthous in patients with jaundice. In jaundice, the sclerae (whites of the eye) may also appear yellow. Xantho/chromia (**zan″tho-kro′me-ə**) means any _____ discoloration. Xanthochromia may be discoloration of the skin or of the spinal fluid.

4-77 The suffix *-opia* means vision.

Combine word parts for various colors with -opia to form words that mean different types of defective vision in which objects appear these colors.

blue vision: _____

cyanopia
(si"ə-no′pe-ə)

red vision: _____

erythropia
(er"ə-thro′pe-ə)

chloropia

green vision: _____

4-78 Form words for the following by using the combining form for the particular color plus -derma:

blue discoloration of skin (blue skin): _____

cyanoderma
(si"ə-no-der′mə)

patchy skin discoloration caused by increased production of melanin or melanocytes (black skin): _____

melanoderma
(mel"ə-no-der′mə)

leukoderma
(loo"ko-dər′mə)

deficient skin pigmentation, especially in patches (white skin): _____

erythroderma
(ə-rith"ro-dər′mə)

abnormal redness of the skin (red skin): _____

❏ **SECTION F REVIEW**   𝒞**ellular Needs and Analysis of Body Fluids**

This section review covers frames 4-64 through 4-78. Complete the table by writing the meaning of each word part that is listed:

Combining Form	Meaning		Suffix	Meaning
1. aer(o)	_____		7. -opia	_____
2. chlor(o)	_____		8. -ous	_____
3. hydr(o)	_____		9. -y	_____
4. melan(o)	_____			
5. muc(o)	_____			
6. xanth(o)	_____			

(Use Appendix V to check your answers.)

𝒯erminology Challenge

This section challenges you to read, write, and understand new terms about body fluids and immunity. You will combine word parts that you know with unfamiliar word parts that are covered more extensively in later chapters.

4-79 Immunodeficiency diseases are a group of health conditions caused by a defect in the immune system and are generally characterized by susceptibility to infections and chronic diseases. One of the most publicized immunodeficiency diseases is AIDS (acquired immunodeficiency syndrome). Additional information about this disease is presented in Chapter 9. AIDS, a viral disease that is transmitted by sexual intercourse or exposure to contaminated body fluid of an infected person, weakens the body's _____ to infection.

immunity

Trans/mission means passing from one point to another (transfer). When contagious diseases are passed from one person to another, there is transmission of the disease.

increase, white	**4-80** Infectious mononucleosis (**mon″o-noo″kle-o′sis**) is an acute viral disease that is characterized by fever, sore throat, swollen lymph glands, and leukocytosis with atypical lymphocytes, a particular type of leukocyte. Leukocytosis means an _____ in the number of _____ blood cells. Young people are most often affected. Treatment is primarily symptomatic, with enforced bed rest to prevent complications.
cytometry (si-tom′ə-tre) **cytometer (si-tom′ə-tər)** **study of cells** **cytologist (si-tol′ə-jist)** **cytoscopy**	**4-81** Two suffixes that you will study later are *-metry*, which means the measuring of, and *-meter*, meaning the instrument used to measure. Using cyt(o), write a term that literally means the measuring of cells: _____. Cytometry means the counting and measuring of cells, specifically blood cells. Write the term that means the instrument for counting and measuring the number of blood cells: _____. Cyto/logy (**si-tol-ə-je**) is the _____. Write a word that means a specialist in cytology: _____. Cyto/scopy (**si-tos′kə-pe**) is the microscopic study of the characteristics of cells. Studying the characteristics of cells differs from counting the number of cells. Write the term that means the study of cells: _____.
inter- **intercellular (in″tər-sel′u-lər)**	**4-82** Cellular means pertaining to cells. You learned earlier that the prefix that means between is _____. Write a term that means between cells, specifically pertaining to the area between or among cells: _____.
autologous	**4-83** Autologous and homologous* are terms that are frequently associated with blood transfusions or skin grafts. In an autologous (**aw-tol′ə-gəs**) transfusion, blood is removed from a donor and stored for a variable period before it is returned to the donor's circulation. In an _____ graft, tissue is transferred from one site to another on the same body. In contrast, a homologous (**ho-mol′o-gəs**) graft is a tissue removed from a donor for transplantation to a recipient of the same species.
polyuria (pol″e-u′re-ə) **absence**	**4-84** You have learned many word parts in the last two chapters. Combine the prefix that means many plus ur(o) plus -ia to write a term that means excessive urination: _____. An/uria (**an-u′re-ə**) means _____ of urination. The amount of urine excreted by the kidneys helps regulate the fluid levels within the body.
water **anhydrous (an-hi-drəs)**	**4-85** If a compound is described as hydrous, this means that it contains _____. Use either the prefix a- or an- to write a term that means without, or lacking, water: _____. Hydro/therapy (**hi″dro-ther′ə-pe**) is treatment using water.
poison	**4-86** Literal translation of tox/emia (**tok-se′me-ə**) is _____ in the blood; however, you need to remember that the term means a general intoxication of the body caused by absorption of bacterial toxins. The blood stream distributes the toxins throughout the body in toxemia, hence the name *toxemia*.

*Autologous (Greek: *autos,* self). Homologous (Greek: *homos,* same).

transdermal **(trans-dərm′əl)**	**4-87** Write a term that means entering through (across) the skin by combining trans, derm(a), and -al: _____. Perhaps you are familiar with transdermal patches that are worn to prevent motion sickness. There is no review for this section.

Study the following list of selected abbreviations. Then read through the Chapter Pharmacology section and be sure you understand the effects and uses of the drug classes that are presented. When you are finished, work the Chapter Review. After completing the exercises, check your answers with the solutions in Appendix V.

You will find these items presented after the Chapter Review:

- Listing of Medical Terms
- Enhancing Spanish Communication

 # ℞ *Selected Abbreviations*

ABO	blood groups
AHF	antihemophilic factor
ALL	acute lymphoblastic leukemia
AML	acute myelogenous leukemia
CBC	complete blood count
CLL	chronic lymphocytic leukemia
CML	chronic myelocytic leukemia
diff	differential count (WBCs)
DIC	disseminated intravascular coagulation
ELISA	enzyme-linked immunosorbent assay (commonly used in AIDS diagnosis)
ESR	erythrocyte sedimentation rate
Hb, Hgb	hemoglobin
HCT	hematocrit
HgA	hemoglobin A
HgC	hemoglobin C
HgE	hemoglobin E
HgF	hemoglobin F
HgS	hemoglobin S

IgA, IgD, IgG, IgM, IgE	immunoglobulins
MCH	mean corpuscular hemoglobin (amount of hemoglobin in each RBC)
MCHC	mean corpuscular hemoglobin concentration (amount of hemoglobin per unit of blood)
MCV	mean corpuscular volume (size of individual red cell)
PCV	packed cell volume
PMN	polymorphonuclear
PT	prothrombin time
PTT	partial thromboplastin time
RBC	red blood cell, red blood count
RES	reticuloendothelial system
Rh	rhesus factor in blood
segs	segmented neutrophils
WBC	white blood cell, white blood count
WNL	within normal limits

Chapter Pharmacology

Drug Class	Effects and Use
Anticoagulants	**Prevent Clotting of Blood**
Indirect acting *of clotting factors*	*Act in liver to prevent synthesis*
Dicumarol	
Warfarin (Coumadin)	Can be administered orally or by IV
Direct acting	*Act in blood to prevent activation of clotting factors*
Heparin (Panheprin)	
Aspirin (many trade names)	
Antihistamines	**Oppose the Action of Histamine**
H1 types	*Inhibit most actions of histamine, particularly block allergic reactions*
Diphenhydramine (Benadryl)	Drowsiness is the main side effect
Fexofenadine (Allegra)	Much less drowsiness
Triprolidine (Actidil)	Much less drowsiness
H2 types	*Inhibit histamine action on parietal cells, thus reducing gastric acid secretion*
Cimetidine (Tagamet)	Used in the treatment of gastric ulcers
Omeprazole (Prilosec)	Used in the treatment of gastric ulcers
Ranitidine (Zantac)	A proton pump inactivator used in gastric reflux
Antiplatelet Drugs (Platelet Aggregation Inhibitors)	**Reduce Risk of Arterial Thrombin Formation**
Aspirin	The most commonly used drug
Dipyridamole (Persantine)	
Ticlopidine (Ticlid)	
Hemostatics	**Control Bleeding**
Aminocaproic acid	Used in acute life-threatening situations
Phytonadione (Vitamin K)	Used to control bleeding, an oral preparation

Drug Class	Effects and Use
Immunosuppressants	**Adjuncts for Prevention of Graft Rejection**
Azathioprine	Used to prevent kidney transplant rejection
Cyclosporine	Used to prevent rejection of kidney, liver, and heart allografts
Vaccines	**Used to Prevent or Modulate Diseases**
BCG vaccine (bacille Calmette-Guérin vaccine)	Used to promote active immunity to tuberculosis
Cholera vaccine	Used for prevention of cholera
Hepatitis B virus vaccine	Used to promote immunity in persons at high risk of potential exposure to hepatitis B
Influenza virus vaccine	Used to promote active immunity to influenza
Measles virus vaccine	Used to promote active immunity to measles
Mumps vaccine	Used to promote active immunity to mumps
Plague vaccine	Used to promote active immunity in persons at high risk of infection following exposure
Pneumococcal vaccine	Used to promote active immunity to pneumonia
Polio virus	Used to promote active immunity to polio
Rabies vaccine	Used to promote active immunity to persons who have been exposed to rabies
Rubella vaccine	Used to promote active immunity to rubella
Typhoid vaccine	Used to promote active immunity to persons at risk
Yellow fever vaccine	Used to promote active immunity to yellow fever

CHAPTER REVIEW 4

▶ **BASIC UNDERSTANDING**

REVIEWING WORD PARTS

I. Write a word (prefix, suffix, or combining form) for each clue.

CROSSWORD PUZZLE 4

Across

1 outside
5 black
6 cell
9 production
11 excessive
12 fibrin
13 small
14 heart
17 repair (suffix)
19 coagulation
21 between
24 thrombus
25 tooth
26 to eat
27 color
29 red
34 cramp
37 body
38 shape
39 characterized by
40 round
43 substance that destroys
44 inflammation
45 yellow
49 slow
51 many
52 to cut
53 viewing

Down

2 pertaining to
3 air or gas
4 sensitivity to pain
5 large
6 hand
7 nucleus
8 head
9 irregular
10 within
11 blood
15 nerve, but not nervo
16 mucus
17 posterior

18 deficiency
19 green
20 that which causes
21 equal
22 one
23 large
25 back
28 large
30 water
31 umbilicus
32 condition
33 instrument used to
    examine

35 capable of destroying
36 destruction
39 vision
41 blood
42 fast
46 across
47 beneath or below normal
48 ear
49 two
50 living

MATCHING

II. Select A, B, or C for each item 1 through 5:

_____ 1. body defense   **A.** leukocyte
_____ 2. blood platelet   **B.** erythrocyte
_____ 3. contains hemoglobin   **C.** thrombocyte
_____ 4. initiates coagulation
_____ 5. transports oxygen

III. Match each of the types of immunity with its description in the right column.

_____ 1. active natural   **A.** contracting a disease
_____ 2. active artificial   **B.** exposure of the fetus to maternal antibodies
_____ 3. passive artificial   **C.** receiving a vaccination
_____ 4. passive natural   **D.** receiving an injection of antibodies

MULTIPLE CHOICE

IV. Select one answer (A-D) for the following multiple-choice questions:

1. What does nucleoid mean?
   A. a round nucleus
   B. absence of a nucleus
   C. an enlarged nucleus
   D. resembling a nucleus

2. How do the erythrocytes appear in spherocytosis?
   A. larger than normal
   B. lighter than normal
   C. round
   D. sickled

3. What is the name of the substance from which fibrin originates?
   A. fibrinogen
   B. fibrinolysis
   C. thrombogen
   D. thrombolysis

4. What does virulence mean?
   A. a virus that evokes an immune response
   B. increased susceptibility by the host
   C. pertaining to a virus
   D. the degree of disease-causing capability of an organism

5. What color is the pigment melanin?
   A. bluish white to gray
   B. dark brown to black
   C. red
   D. yellowish green

6. What is the major function of an erythrocyte?
   A. defends the body against disease
   B. initiates coagulation
   C. manufactures antibodies
   D. transports oxygen

7. To what does the term *xanthosis* refer?
   A. an exaggerated immune response
   B. general intoxication of the body
   C. requiring oxygen for life
   D. yellowish discoloration

8. Which of the following means "having no tendency to repair itself or develop into new tissue"?
   A. analytic
   B. anisocytosis
   C. aplastic
   D. hemolytic

9. Which of the following is true of leukocytosis?
   A. an increase in the number of leukocytes
   B. characterized by a deficiency of hemoglobin
   C. the same as leukemia
   D. usually associated with anemia

10. What is the name of the surgical procedure whereby living organs are transferred from one part of the body to another or from one individual to another?
    A. rejection
    B. transmission
    C. transplant
    D. transreaction

11. Where is intracellular fluid found in the body?
    A. between cells
    B. inside cells
    C. outside cells
    D. within plasma

12. What is the most important function of body fluids?
    A. to bring anticoagulant to keep blood from clotting
    B. to protect against harmful microorganisms
    C. to provide natural immunity
    D. to transport nutrients and remove wastes

13. Which of the following is a specific body defense mechanism?
    A. cell-mediated immunity
    B. intact skin
    C. interferon
    D. phagocytosis

14. Which of the following is a normal response by the body to a pathogen?
    A. erythropia
    B. infection
    C. inflammation
    D. xanthoderma

15. Which body fluid is most abundant?
    A. extracellular
    B. interstitial
    C. intracellular
    D. plasma

WRITING TERMS

V. Write a term for each of the following meanings:

1. excessive urination _____
2. an erythrocyte of irregular shape _____
3. an increase in number of white blood cells _____
4. a blood platelet _____
5. any disease (disorder) of coagulation _____

6. any disease condition caused by poisons _____
7. blood clotting _____
8. dissolving of a thrombus _____
9. between cells _____
10. the study of cells _____

▶ **GREATER COMPREHENSION**

SPELLING

VI. Circle all incorrectly spelled terms and write their correct spelling:

aglutination   anarobic   antigen   chloropia   fibrinolisis   polymorfonuclear   toxisity   vacination   zanthochromia

TRUE OR FALSE

VII. Mark each statement T for true or F for false:

_____ 1. Body fluids move back and forth between compartments that are separated by cell membranes.
_____ 2. Blood is an intravascular fluid.
_____ 3. Water loss through respiration is the main source of water loss in the body.

_____ 4. Most extracellular fluid is plasma.
_____ 5. Interstitial fluid is located between cells and tissue spaces.

VIII. Several factors that affect healing are listed. Write T for true by each factor that assists healing. Write F for false by each factor that retards or delays healing.

_____ 1. immobilization of the wound
_____ 2. inadequately functioning leukocytes
_____ 3. infection

_____ 4. leukopenia
_____ 5. malnutrition

MATCHING

IX. Match the signs and symptoms of severe anemia in the left column with the correct meaning in the right column:

_____ 1. dyspnea
_____ 2. pallor
_____ 3. syncope
_____ 4. tinnitus

A. difficult breathing
B. fainting
C. loss of appetite
D. nausea
E. paleness
F. ringing in the ears
G. sore mouth

LISTING

X. Name five nonspecific body defenses:

1. _____
2. _____
3. _____
4. _____
5. _____

XI. Name two types of specific body defenses:

1. _____
2. _____

INTERPRETING ABBREVIATIONS

XII. Write the meaning of these abbreviations:

1. AHF _____
2. ELISA _____
3. HCT _____
4. Hgb _____
5. HgS _____

6. IgG _____
7. PMN _____
8. PT _____
9. Rh _____
10. WBC _____

PRONUNCIATION

XIII. The pronunciation is shown for several medical words. Indicate which syllable has the primary accent by marking it with ′.

1. erythropoiesis (**ə rith ro poi e sis**)
2. fibrinolysis (**fi brĭ nol ə sis**)
3. hematoma (**hem ə to mə**)

4. hypochromic (**hi po kro mik**)
5. toxicity (**tok sis ĭ te**)

CATEGORIZING TERMS

XIV. Terms are sometimes placed in the following categories:

- Anatomical (names of structures and related terms)
- Diagnostic (names of diseases, signs and symptoms, and related terms)
- Radiological (terms related to the use of radiant energy in medicine)

- Surgical (operative procedures and related terms)
- Therapeutic (terms pertaining to treatment of the patient)

In each of the following words, categorize the term by writing A, D, or S to indicate anatomical, diagnostic, or surgical. The first term is done as an example.

Category (A, D, S)

1. leukocyte _____A_____
2. cytometry _____
3. thrombectomy _____
4. blood platelet _____
5. polycythemia _____
6. anemia _____
7. dyscrasia _____

DRUG CLASSES

XV. Match the drug classes in the left column with their effects or use in the right column.

_____ 1. anticoagulants
_____ 2. antihistamines
_____ 3. hemostatics
_____ 4. immunosuppressants
_____ 5. platelet aggregation inhibitors
_____ 6. vaccines

A. control bleeding
B. inhibit histamine action
C. prevent blood from clotting
D. prevent or modulate disease
E. prevent rejection of grafts
F. reduce risk of thrombin formation

(Check your answers with the solutions in Appendix V.)

Listing of Medical Terms

abscess	erythropoietin	infectious mononucleosis	polymorph
aerobic	extracellular	intercellular	polymorphonuclear
agglutination	fibrin	interferon	polyuria
agranulocytosis	fibrinogen	interstitial fluid	prophylaxis
allergen	fibrinoid	intracellular	pus
allergy	fibrinolysin	intravascular	rejection
anaphylactic	fibrinolysis	isotonic	resistance
anaphylaxis	graft	karyomegaly	septicemia
anemia	granulocyte	leukemia	shunt
anhydrous	hematocrit	leukocyte	sickle cell anemia
anisocytosis	hematologic	leukocytopenia	spherocyte
antibody	hematologist	leukocytosis	spherocytosis
anticoagulant	hematology	leukoderma	susceptibility
antigen	hematoma	leukopenia	syncope
antihistamine	hematopoiesis	macrocyte	tachycardia
anuria	hematopoietic	macrocytosis	thrombectomy
aplastic	hemocyte	macrophage	thrombocyte
autologous	hemoglobin	macroscopy	thrombocytopenia
chloropia	hemoglobinopathy	malaria	thrombocytosis
coagulant	hemolysin	megalocyte	thrombogenesis
coagulate	hemolysis	melancholy	Thrombolysin
coagulation	hemolytic	melanin	thrombolysis
coagulopathy	hemolyze	melanocyte	thrombolytic
complement	hemophilia	melanoderma	thrombopenia
corpuscle	hemostasis	melanoid	thrombosis
cyanoderma	hemostatic	melanoma	thrombotic
cyanopia	hemothorax	microcyte	thrombus
cyanosis	histamine	microcytosis	tinnitus
cytologist	homologous	microscope	toxemia
cytology	hydrocephalus	microscopy	toxicity
cytometer	hydrocephaly	mucoid	toxicosis
cytometry	hydrotherapy	mucus	toxoid
cytoscopy	hydrous	normochromic	transdermal
cytotoxicity	hyperchromic	normocyte	transfusion
cytotoxin	hypersensitivity	normocytic	transmission
dyscrasia	hypochromia	nucleoid	transplant
dyspnea	hypochromic	nucleoprotein	vaccination
electrophoresis	immunity	pallor	vaccine
erythrocyte	immunization	pathogen	virulence
erythrocytic	immunocompromised	phagocyte	viscosity
erythrocytopenia	immunoglobulin	phagocytosis	xanthochromia
erythrocytosis	immunosuppressant	plasma	xanthoderma
erythroderma	immunosuppressive	poikilocyte	xanthosis
erythropenia	in vitro	poikilocytosis	xanthous
erythropia	in vivo	polycythemia	
erythropoiesis	incompatibility		

Español *Enhancing Spanish Communication*

English	Spanish (pronunciation)
allergy	alergia (ah-LEHR-he-ah)
anemia	anemia (ah-NAY-me-ah)
antibiotic	antibiótico (an-te-be-O-te-co)
blood	sangre (SAHN-gray)
clot	coágulo (co-AH-goo-lo)
constipation	estreñimiento (es-tray-nye-me-EN-to)
destruction	destrucción (des-trooc-se-ON)
diagnosis	diagnosis (de-ag-NO-ses)
diagnostic	diagnóstico (de-ag-NOS-te-co)
diarrhea	diarrea (de-ar-RAY-ah)
disease	enfermedad (en-fer-may-DAHD)
dizziness	vértigo (VERR-te-go)
fainting	languidez (lan-gee-DES), desmayo (des-MAH-yo)
fatigue	fatiga (fah-TEE-gah)
fiber	fibra (FEE-brah)
fluid	fluido (floo-EE-do)
hair	pelo (PAY-lo)
headache	dolor de cabeza (do-LOR day cah-BAY-sa)
heart	corazón (co-rah-SON)
inflammation	inflamación (in-flah-mah-se-ON)
influenza	gripe (GREE-pay)
injection	inyección (in-yec-se-ON)
injury	daño (DAH-nyo)
instrument	instrumento (ins-troo-MEN-to)
leukemia	leucemia (lay-oo-SAY-me-ah)
microscope	microscopio (me-cros-CO-pe-o)

English	Spanish (pronunciation)
mouth	boca (BO-cah)
mucus	moco (MO-co)
murmur	murmullo (moor-MOOL-lyo)
oxygen	oxígeno (ok-SEE-hay-no)
parasite	parásito (pah-RAH-se-to)
ringing	zumbido (zoom-BEE-do)
saliva	saliva (sah-LEE-vah)
sweat	sudor (soo-DOR)
tears	lágrimas (LAH-gre-mahs)
tests	pruebas (proo-AY-bahs)
tongue	lengua (LEN-goo-ah)
transfusion	transfusión (trans-foo-se-ON)
urine	orina (o-REE-nah)
vessel	vaso (VAH-so)
water	agua (AH-goo-ah)
wound	lesión (lay-se-ON)

Colors	Colores
black	negro (NAY-gro)
blue	azul (ah-SOOL)
gray	gris (grees)
green	verde (VERR-day)
orange (color)	anaranjado (ah-nah-ran-HAH-do), naranjado (nah-ran-HAH-do)
red	rojo (ROH-ho)
white	blanco (BLAHN-co)
yellow	amarillo (ah-mah-REEL-lyo)

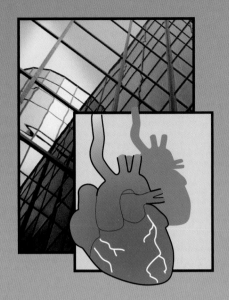

Cardiovascular and Lymphatic Systems

5

Outline

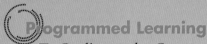
Principal Word Parts

COMBINING FORMS

aden(o)	gland
adenoid(o)	adenoids
aneurysm(o)	aneurysm
angi(o), vas(o), vascul(o)	vessel
aort(o)	aorta
arter(o), arteri(o)	artery
arteriol(o)	arteriole
ather(o)	yellowish, fatty plaque
atri(o)	atrium
cancer(o), carcin(o)	cancer
cardi(o)	heart
coron(o)	crown
ech(o), son(o)	sound
endocardi(o)	endocardium
immun(o)	immune
lymph(o)	lymph, lymphatics
lymphaden(o)	lymph node
lymphangi(o)	lymph vessel
lymphat(o)	lymphatics
mediastin(o)	mediastinum
myocardi(o)	myocardium
ox(i)	oxygen
pericardi(o)	pericardium
phleb(o), ven(i), ven(o)	vein
phot(o)	light
pulmon(o)	lung
rhythm(o), rrhythm(o)	rhythm
scler(o)	hard, hardening
sept(o)	septum; partition
sin(o)	sinus
splen(o)	spleen
steth(o), thorac(o)	chest
thym(o)	thymus
tonsill(o)	tonsil
valv(o), valvul(o)	valve
ventricul(o)	ventricle
venul(o)	venule

PREFIXES

de-	down; from; reversing
epi-	above or upon
peri-	around
tri-	three

SUFFIXES

-ary	pertaining to
-edema	swelling
-ium	membrane
-meter	instrument used to measure
-metry	process of measuring

SUFFIXES—CONT'D

-ole	small	-stenosis	narrowing; stricture
-oma	tumor; swelling	-stomy	artificial opening
-phobia	abnormal fear	-tome	cutting instrument
-sclerosis	abnormal hardening		

Learning Goals

▶ BASIC UNDERSTANDING

In this chapter you will learn to do the following:

1. Recognize names of the structures of the cardiovascular system and define terms associated with these structures.
2. Differentiate between the functions of systemic circulation and pulmonary circulation.
3. Understand how coronary heart disease and myocardial infarction are related.
4. Demonstrate understanding of the significance of the lymphatic system and analyze associated terminology.
5. Write the meaning of word parts associated with the cardiovascular and lymphatic systems and use the word parts to build and analyze terms.

▶ GREATER COMPREHENSION

6. Describe the flow of blood through the major structures of the cardiovascular system.
7. Name several factors that cause blood pressure to increase.
8. Recognize the major structures and functions of the lymphatic system.
9. Differentiate terms as being related to diagnosis, anatomy, surgery, therapy, or radiology.
10. Spell the terms accurately.
11. Pronounce the terms correctly.
12. Know the meaning of the abbreviations.
13. Identify the effects or uses of the drug classes presented in this chapter.

Cardiovascular Components and Blood Circulation

SECTION A

The heart, arteries, veins, and capillaries make up the cardiovascular system. This network of blood vessels delivers oxygen, nutrients, and vital substances to the interstitial fluids surrounding all of the body's cells. This same network transports cellular waste products to organs where they can be excreted. As blood circulates, interstitial fluid accumulates in the tissue spaces. This excess fluid is normally transported away from the tissues by another vascular network that helps maintain the internal fluid environment—the lymphatic system.

5-1 Circulation means movement in a regular or circular fashion. The pumping action of the heart propels blood through a network of vessels that complete the circuit by taking blood to all parts of the body and returning it to the heart. This is called systemic circulation. The amount of time required for this to be accomplished is called blood circulation time and can be determined by injecting a substance into a vessel and timing its reappearance.

System/ic* means pertaining to or affecting the body as a whole. The route that blood takes when it leaves the heart, travels throughout the body, and returns to the heart is called _____ circulation.

systemic

*Systemic (Greek: *systema,* a complex or organized whole).

vessel heart	**5-2** You learned previously that cardi(o) means heart and vascul(o) means vessel. Vascul/ar means pertaining to a _____, specifically a blood vessel. The cardio/vascular system is made up of the _____ and the network of blood vessels that pump blood throughout the body (Figure 5–1). This system delivers oxygen, nutrients, and other materials to the fluids surrounding the cells (interstitial fluids) and transports waste products to special organs, such as the kidneys, for excretion. Excretion* is the normal process that the body uses to get rid of wastes. Figure 5-1 oversimplifies blood circulation, but it will help you remember that in general, arteries carry oxygen-rich blood to body tissues and veins carry oxygen-poor blood back to the heart.
lungs arterioles, capillaries venules veins	**5-3** If you study blood circulation more closely, you learn that it consists of many events that occur simultaneously. Two important types of circulation that occur each time the heart beats are systemic circulation and pulmonary circulation (Figure 5-2). The combining form **pulmon(o)** means lung, and the suffix **-ary** means pertaining to. Pulmon/ary means pertaining to the _____. The upper left part of the schematic drawing in Figure 5-2 shows pulmonary circulation, and the remainder represents systemic circulation. Look at the drawing as you complete these sentences: In systemic circulation, oxygen-rich blood leaves the left side of the heart via the largest artery in the body, the aorta. The aorta subdivides several times to form arteries, which in turn branch many times to become _____. The smallest vessels, the _____, form the connection between the arteries and the _____. Venules join, and the blood flows into larger and larger _____ until it reaches the heart.
artery arterioles capillaries venules, veins	**5-4** Pulmonary circulation provides the means for the blood to take on oxygen from air that we take into our lungs. Oxygen-deficient blood leaves the heart via the pulmonary _____. Arteries branch many times to become _____. These vessels also branch many times to become lung _____. While in the lung capillaries, the blood releases carbon dioxide and picks up a new supply of oxygen. After blood passes through the capillaries, it enters structures called _____. Blood then flows into progressively larger vessels called _____, which transport it back to the heart.
arteries	**5-5** You already know the combining form that means heart. You also need to remember that **arter(o)** and **arteri(o)** mean artery. Arteri/al (ahr-tēr′e-əl) means pertaining to one or more _____. Arteri/ole means little artery when translated literally, because **-ole** means little. The combining form for arteriole is **arteriol(o)**. Capillaries are so named because the Latin word *capillaris* means hairlike. Capillaries are so small that erythrocytes must pass through them in single file.
vein incision veins venules	**5-6** You will be using three combining forms that mean vein: **phleb(o), ven(i),** and **ven(o).** Phleb(o) is used more often to write medical terms, but you will need to remember that veni/puncture means puncture of a _____. Both venipuncture (ven′ĭ-punk″chər) and phlebo/tomy (flə-bot′ə-me) mean opening of a vein to draw blood for laboratory analysis. Translated literally, phlebotomy means _____ of a vein. Phlebotomists (flə-bot′ə-mists) are persons with special training in the practice of drawing blood. Ven/ous means pertaining to the_____. Venules join the capillaries and veins. The combining form **venul(o)** means venule.† Venul/ar means pertaining to, composed of, or affecting _____.

*Excretion (Latin: *excretio,* separate out).
†Venule (Latin: *venula,* small vein).

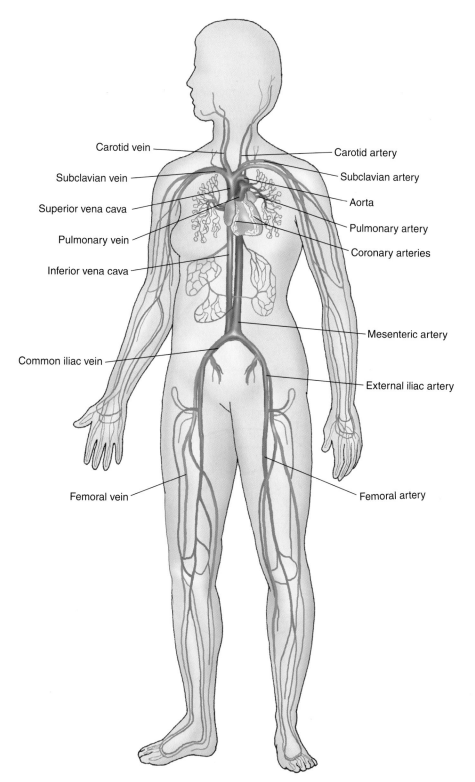

FIGURE 5-1

The cardiovascular system, the heart, and blood vessels. Two major components of the vascular network are shown, the arteries (red) and the veins (blue). Only the larger or more common blood vessels are labeled.

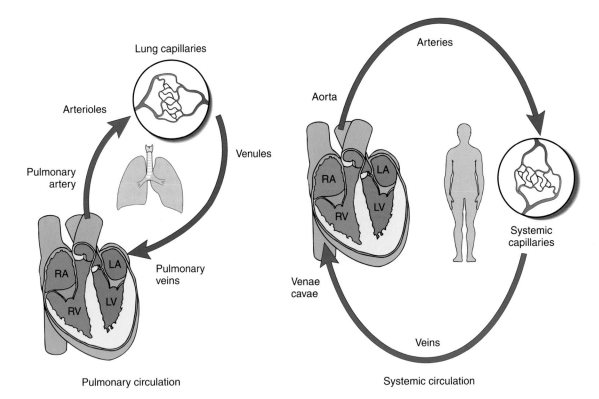

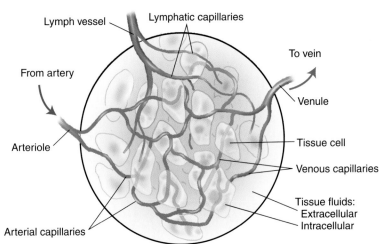

FIGURE 5-2

Schematic drawing of blood circulation and the relationship of blood vessels. Pulmonary circulation is the means by which blood picks up oxygen from air that is taken in by the lungs. Systemic circulation is the way in which oxygen-rich blood is carried from the heart to all parts of the body, where it gives up much of its oxygen before returning to the heart. RA, RV, LA, and LV are abbreviations for the four chambers of the heart: Right atrium, right ventricle, left atrium, and left ventricle. A capillary bed is shown in detail.

❏ SECTION A REVIEW 　*C*ardiovascular Components and Blood Circulation

This section review covers frames 5–1 through 5–6. Complete the table by writing the meaning of each word part that is listed:

Combining Form	Meaning		Suffixes	Meaning
1. arter(o), arteri(o)	_____		8. -ary	_____
2. arteriol(o)	_____		9. -ole	_____
3. phleb(o)	_____			
4. pulmon(o)	_____			
5. ven(i)	_____			
6. ven(o)	_____			
7. venul(o)	_____			

(Use Appendix V to check your answers.)

SECTION B

*T*he Heart

The muscular heart is the center of the cardiovascular system. It beats normally about 70 times per minute, or over 100,000 times per day. In the adult, it weights 230 grams to 340 grams (about one-half pound) and is the size of a clenched fist.

chest	**5-7** The pumping structure of the cardiovascular system, the heart, lies in the thorac/ic cavity. You learned earlier that the thoracic cavity is the _____ cavity.
media	The heart lies just left of the midline of the body, between the lungs, in a space called the mediastinum (me″de-əs-ti′ nəm). The media/stinum is an area in the middle of the chest cavity. The part of media/stinum that indicates that it is in the middle is _____. The mediastinum contains the heart and its large vessels, the trachea, the esophagus, and nearby structures such as the lymph nodes.
mediastinum	Write this new word, which refers to the area between the lungs: _____.
mediastinoscopy (me″de-as″tĭ-nos′ kə-pe)	The combining form ***mediastin(o)*** is used to form words concerning the mediastinum. Combine medi-astin(o) with the suffix for viewing or visually inspecting: _____.
mediastinoscope (me″de-ə-sti′no-skōp)	Mediastinoscopy allows visual inspection of structures in the mediastinum, using an instrument that is inserted through a small incision. Write the name of the instrument that is used in mediastinoscopy: _____.
coronary	**5-8** Special arteries supply blood to the heart itself. The combining form ***coron(o)*** means crown. Coronary (kor′ə-nar″ e) means encircling in the manner of a crown. Blood vessels that supply oxygen to the heart encircle it in a crownlike fashion (Figure 5-3). Arteries that supply blood to the heart are _____ arteries.
	The wall of the heart consists primarily of cardiac muscle tissue, myocardium (mi″o-kahr′ de-əm). You probably remember that my(o) means muscle. The term *myocardium* is the product of combining my(o) with cardi(o) and a new suffix, **-ium,** that means membrane. (One "i" is dropped to facilitate pronunciation.) My(o) and cardi(o) are often used together, so it is easier to remember that ***myocardi(o)*** means myocardium.
muscle	The important thing to remember about myocardium is that it composes most of the heart and is what type of tissue? _____

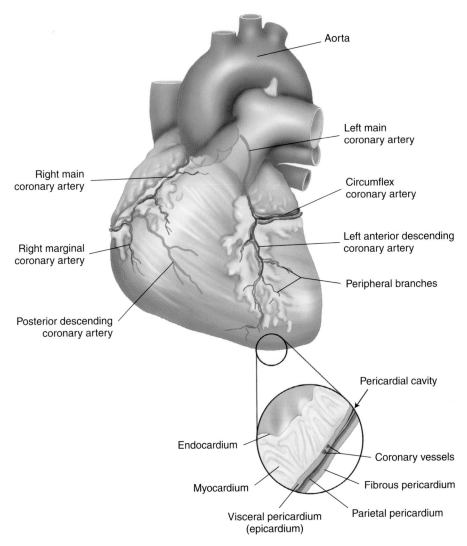

Aorta

Left main
coronary artery

Right main
coronary artery

Circumflex
coronary artery

Left anterior descending
coronary artery

Right marginal
coronary artery

Peripheral branches

Posterior descending
coronary artery

Pericardial cavity

Endocardium

Coronary vessels

Myocardium

Fibrous pericardium

Parietal pericardium

Visceral pericardium
(epicardium)

FIGURE 5-3
Coronary arteries and heart tissues. The two main coronary arteries are the left coronary artery
(LCA) and right coronary artery (RCA). The three layers of the heart, beginning with the
innermost layer, are endocardium, myocardium, and epicardium (also called the visceral
pericardium).

5-9 A membranous sac, the pericardium (**per″ĭ-kahr′de-um**), encloses the heart, as shown in Figure 5-3. The pericardium, which is attached to the heart, is composed of an inner layer (visceral pericardium or epicardium) and an outer, tougher layer (parietal pericardium). The prefix *epi-* means above or upon. Epi/cardium is so named because it lies upon the surface of the heart. The fibrous pericardium, a tough fibrous tissue that constitutes the outermost sac, fits loosely around the heart and protects it.

around the heart

The prefix **peri-** means around. Peri/card/ium is a membrane _____.

(Again, when cardi[o] is combined with -ium, one "i" is dropped.)

Peri- is used in some words you already know. For example, peri/meter is the measurement around the outside of an object.

around

Peri/cardial (**per″ĭ-kahr′de-əl**) means _____ the heart and pertains to the pericardium. The space between the two pericardial layers is the pericardial cavity.

pericardial

Because peri- and cardi(o) are frequently combined, it is easier to learn that **pericardi(o)** means the pericardium. Write a term that means pertaining to the pericardium using the suffix *-al:* _____.

pericarditis
(per″ĭ-kahr-di′tis)

Using -itis, build a word that means inflammation of the pericardium: _____.

In pericarditis, the pericardium becomes inflamed, owing to an infectious microorganism, a cancerous growth, or a variety of other causes.

Hemo/pericardium (**he″mo-per″ĭ-kahr′de-əm**) is an effusion (**ə-fu′zhən**)* of blood into the pericardial space. Effusion means the escape of fluid into a part, such as a cavity.

hemopericardium

Blood in the pericardial space is called _____.

inside the heart

5-10 Translated literally, endo/card/ium (**en″do-kahr′de-um**) is the membrane _____.

It is the membrane that forms the lining inside the heart. The combining form **endocardi(o)** means endocardium. Inflammation of the inner lining of the heart is _____.

endocarditis
(en″do-kahr-di′tis)

Endocarditis is frequently caused by infectious microorganisms that invade the lining of the heart, quite frequently the valves. Endo/cardial (**en″do-kahr′de-əl**) means situated or occurring inside the heart and also means pertaining to the endocardium.

5-11 The middle and thickest tissue of the heart, which is composed of cardiac muscle, is the _____. The myocardium is made up of muscle fibers that contract, resulting in a wringing type of movement that squeezes blood from the heart with each beat. Write a word that means pertaining to the myocardium: _____.

myocardium
myocardial
(mi″o-kahr′de-əl)

myocarditis
(mi″o-kahr-di′tis)

Inflammation of the myocardium is _____. This may be caused by a large variety of microorganisms.

5-12 The four-chambered heart is separated into right and left chambers by a partition called the septum (**sep′təm**). The combining form **sept(o)** means septum. The term *septum* is used in other terms as well and always means a dividing wall or _____.

partition

septal (sep′təl)

Using the suffix *-al,* write a term that means pertaining to the septum: _____.

*Effusion (Latin: *effusio,* pour out).

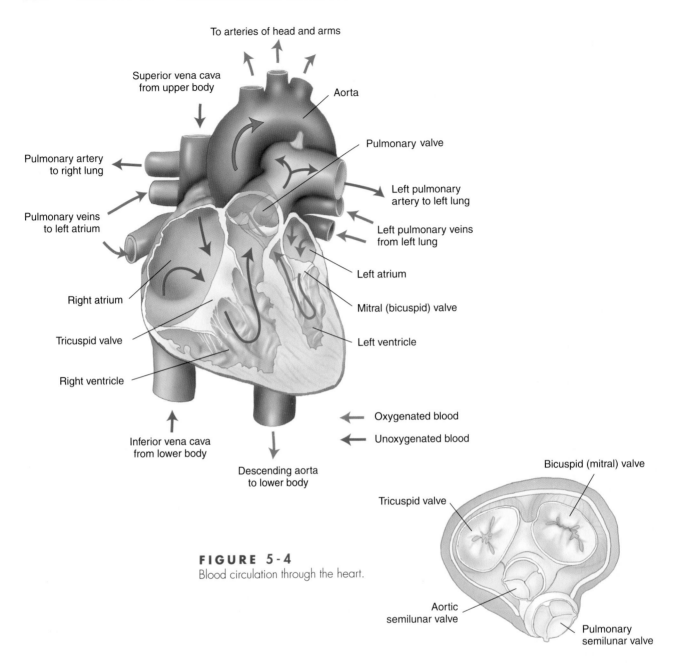

FIGURE 5-4
Blood circulation through the heart.

5-13 In addition to being divided longitudinally into right and left chambers by a septum, each side of the heart is further divided into an atrium (**a′tre-əm**) (plural: atria) and a ventricle (**ven′trĭ-kəl**). This can be seen in the simple drawing of blood circulation in Figure 5-2, but also locate these four chambers in Figure 5-4.

The two upper chambers of the heart are the right and left _____.

The two lower chambers of the heart are the right and left _____.

The combining form ***atri(o)*** means atrium or atria. Using septal as a model, write a term that means pertaining to the atrium: _____.

atria

ventricles

atrial

heart
brain
ventricular
atrioventricular
(a″tre-o-ven′trik′
u-lər)
right
atrium
atrium
ventricle
lungs
mitral (or bicuspid)
two
tricuspid

5-14 The combining form for ventricle is **ventricul(o),** but ventricle is a term that is also applied to a chamber of the brain. Therefore ventricul(o) refers to a ventricle of either the _____ or the _____. The heart has both a left ventricle and a right ventricle. Using the suffix -*ar,* write a term that means pertaining to a ventricle: _____.

By analyzing other parts of the term or the sentence, one can often determine which organ is affected, the brain or the heart. Combine atri(o), ventricul(o), and -ar to write a term that means pertaining to an atrium and a ventricle of the heart: _____.

5-15 Study the pattern of blood flow through the heart in Figure 5-4. Blood that has had much of its oxygen removed enters the heart on the right side of the body through its two largest veins. The large vein by which blood from the trunk and legs enters the heart is the inferior vena cava (**ve′nə ka′və**).*

Blood from the head and arms enters the heart by way of the large vein, the superior vena cava. The venae cavae (plural of vena cava) bring the blood to which chamber of the heart? _____ _____.

5-16 The right atrium contracts to force blood through a valve to the right ventricle. The name of this valve is the tricuspid valve, and it is located between the right _____ and the right _____.

Contraction of the right ventricle forces blood through the pulmonary artery, which branches and carries blood to the _____. As blood flows through the lungs, it picks up a fresh supply of oxygen and returns to the left side of the heart by way of the pulmonary veins. The pulmonary veins bring the blood to the left atrium.

The left atrium contracts and forces blood into the left ventricle. The flow of blood from the left atrium to the left ventricle is controlled by the _____ valve. This richly oxygenated blood is then pumped into the aorta (**a-or′tə**) from the left ventricle. The aorta is the largest artery of the body. It branches into smaller arteries to carry blood all over the body.

5-17 In normal heart function, valves close and prevent backflow of blood when the heart contracts. Valves between the atria and ventricles are atrioventricular valves—the tricuspid valve on the right side and the bicuspid or mitral valve on the left side (Figure 5-4). Cuspid refers to the little flaps of tissue that make up the valve. Remembering that bi- means two, the bi/cuspid valve has _____ flaps. The left atrioventricular valve is generally called the mitral (**mi′trəl**) valve in medicine, so named because the two valve flaps are shaped somewhat like the mitered corner joints of a picture frame. Weakening of one or both cusps when the heart contracts is called mitral valve prolapse (MVP). Symptoms vary from absent to severe, and the condition may be associated with sounds heard through a stethoscope, including a clicking sound or heart murmur.

The prefix *tri-* means three. These last two prefixes will not be difficult if you remember that bi/cycles and tri/cycles have two and three wheels, respectively. The valve that regulates the flow of blood between the right atrium and the right ventricle is the _____ valve.

*(Latin: *vena,* veins, *cava,* cavity.)

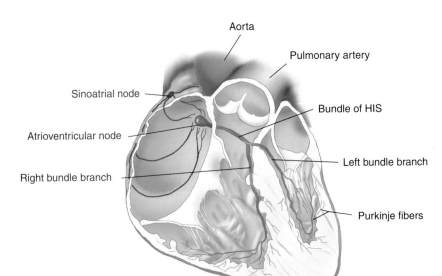

Aorta

Pulmonary artery

Sinoatrial node

Bundle of HIS

Atrioventricular node

Left bundle branch

Right bundle branch

Purkinje fibers

FIGURE 5-5
Conduction system of the heart. The electrical impulse originates in the heart, and contraction of the heart's chambers is coordinated by specialized heart tissues.

pulmonary **pulmonary artery** **pulmonary vein**	**5-18** Once again, look at Figure 5-4 and locate the pulmonary valve. It regulates the flow of blood from the right ventricle to the pulmonary trunk, which divides into _____ arteries that lead to the lungs. Pulmonary (**pool′mo-nar″e**) means pertaining to the lungs, and the vessel that carries blood to the lungs is the _____ _____. Note that the vessel that carries blood from the lungs back to the heart is the _____ _____.
aortic (a-or′tik) **pulmonary, aortic**	After flowing from the left atrium to the left ventricle, blood leaves the heart by way of the _____ valve, which regulates the flow of blood into the aorta. The pulmonary and aortic valves are also called semilunar (**sem″e-loo′nər**) valves (because of the half-moon appearance of the valve cusps). A semilunar valve may be either the _____ or the _____ valve.
valve **valvate**	**5-19** The combining form *valv(o)* means valve. Only a few words use this combining form, but all pertain to a valve. Valv/al (**val′vəl**) and valv/ar (**val′vər**) both pertain to a _____. Valv/ate means pertaining to or having valves. Valvula is a term meaning a valve, especially a small valve. *valvul(o)* is also used in words to mean valve. Valvul/ar (**val′vu-lər**), having valves, is a synonym for _____.
	5-20 It is important to remember that both atria contract simultaneously, followed by simultaneous contraction of both ventricles. The cardiac conduction system, composed of highly specialized tissue that is capable of producing and conveying electrical impulses, is responsible for the coordinated contraction (Figure 5-5). Find the sino/atrial (SA) node, located at the junction of the right atrium and the superior vena cava. Electrical impulses arise spontaneously in the SA node and stimulate contraction. The SA node is the natural pacemaker of the heart. The SA node is also called the sinus node. The combining form *sin(o)* means sinus. A sinus* is a cavity or channel. Perhaps you are more familiar with the sinuses near the nose (air cavities that sometimes drain or become inflamed in sinus/itis). The term *sinusitis* does not use the combining form.
sinoatrial	Use this new combining form plus atrial to write the name of the natural pacemaker of the heart, the _____ node.

*(Latin: *sinus,* a hollow.)

5-21 The electrical impulse generated by the SA node travels through both atria to the atrio/ventricul/ar node (AV node), which in turn conducts the impulse to the atrioventricular bundle (AV bundle, called also the bundle of His) and then to the Purkinje fibers and walls of the ventricles. This highly specialized system results in simultaneous contraction of the atria, followed by contraction of the ventricles.

atrioventricular

AV node means the _____ node. This special type of cardiac tissue is located near the septal wall between the left and right atria. The atria contract while the electrical impulse is briefly delayed in the AV node.

Another name for the atrioventricular bundle or AV bundle is the bundle of His, named after the Swiss physician Wilhelm His, Jr. The Purkinje fibers are the termination of the bundle branches. These fibers, spread throughout the right and left ventricles, are specialized to carry the impulse at a high velocity, and

ventricles

cause the _____ to contract.

heart

5-22 The impulses arising in the SA node and carried by the cardiac conduction system produce electrical currents that can be measured in electro/cardio/graphy, the process of recording the electrical currents of the _____. Write the name of the record produced in electrocardiography: _____.

electrocardiogram

electrocardiograph

The name of the instrument used in electrocardiography is an _____.

❏ SECTION B REVIEW   *The* Heart

This section review covers frames 5–7 through 5–22. Complete the table by writing the meaning of each word part that is listed:

Combining Form	Meaning	Prefix	Meaning
1. atri(o)	_____	12. epi-	_____
2. coron(o)	_____	13. peri-	_____
3. endocardi(o)	_____	14. tri-	_____
4. mediastin(o)	_____		
5. myocardi(o)	_____	**Suffix**	**Meaning**
6. pericardi(o)	_____	15. -ium	_____
7. sept(o)	_____		
8. sin(o)	_____		
9. valv(o)	_____		
10. valvul(o)	_____		
11. ventricul(o)	_____		

(Use Appendix V to check your answers.)

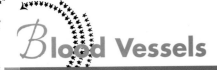

Blood Vessels

The heart and blood vessels work together to provide a continuous supply of oxygen and nutrients to cells throughout the body. The blood vessels form a network of tubes that carry blood away from the heart, transport it to the tissues, and then return it to the heart. Although all blood vessels (arteries, veins, arterioles, venules, and capillaries) are responsible for transport, they differ from each other both structurally and functionally.

artery **vein** phleb(o) **arteriopathy** (ahr-tēr″e-op′ə-the) **arteries** **arteritis** (ahr″tə-ri′tis)	**5-23** You learned earlier that arteries carry blood away from the heart and veins transport blood back to the heart. The combining forms *arter(o)* and *arteri(o)* mean _____. The combining forms *ven(i)* and *ven(o)* mean _____. Write a third combining form that means vein: _____. Using arteri(o) + the suffix that is related to path(o), build a word that means any disease of the arteries: _____. Arterial (**ahr-tēr′e-əl**) pertains to _____. Use arter(o) to write a word that means inflammation of an artery: _____.
arteriography (ahr″tēr-e-og′rə-fe) **arteriogram** (ahr-tēr′e-o-gram)	**5-24** Use arteri(o) to build a word that means radiography of arteries after injection of radiopaque material into the blood stream. Literally, this word means recording of the arteries: _____. Build a word that means the film produced in arteriography: _____. Through common usage, arteriograph (**ahr-tēr′e-o-graf**) is used interchangeably with arteriogram, just as photo/graph is used to mean the record produced (picture) in photography. The combining form ***phot(o)*** means light. Coronary arteriography is a radiographic procedure used to study coronary arteries.
arteriol(o) **venul(o)** **vessel** **inflammation, heart** **vessel** **any disease of** **vessels (specifically,** **blood or lymph** **vessels)** **angioplasty** (an′je-o-plas″te)	**5-25** You have learned combining forms for other vessels that make up the cardiovascular system. The combining form for arterioles is _____. The combining form for venule is _____. There are two additional combining forms that mean vessels, in general: ***vas(o)*** and ***angi(o).*** The combining form *vas(o)* also refers to a duct, such as the vas deferens, which is discussed in Chapter 9. Practice will help you determine which meaning is intended. You learned earlier that vascul(o) also means _____. Angio/card/itis (**an″je-o-kahr-di′tis**) is _____ of the _____ and great blood vessels. Angio/spasm (**an′je-o-spaz″əm**) is a cramping or twitching of a blood _____. Angio/pathy (**an-je-op′ə-the**) is _____. Use angi(o) to write a word that means surgical repair of blood vessels: _____.

vessel	**5-26** Vaso/dilation (**vas″o-di-la′shən**) is stretching or dilation of a _____. In the word *vasodilation,* dilation means expansion or stretching. Dilation is also used to mean expansion of an orifice with an instrument called a dilator. Dilatation (**dil″ə-ta′shən**) is a synonym for dilation. An increase in the diameter of a blood vessel is _____. Dilators are used to enlarge an orifice or canal by stretching. Some medications are vasodilators (**vas″o-di-la′tərz**). Write a word using vas(o) that means an agent that causes dilation of the blood vessels: _____.
vasodilation	
vasodilator	
vasoconstriction	The opposite of vasodilation is vaso/constriction (**vas″o-kən-strik′shən**). When blood vessels constrict, they become narrow. A decrease in the diameter of blood vessels is _____.
vessels	The dilation and constriction of blood vessels influence blood pressure and the distribution of blood to various parts of the body. The measurement and significance of changes in blood pressure are discussed in the next section. Vasoconstriction and vasodilation are regulated by the vaso/motor center located in the brain. The vaso/motor center regulates the size of the blood _____.
	5-27 The aorta is the main trunk of the systemic arterial system (Figure 5-6). Arteries branch out either directly or indirectly from the aorta, which arises from the left ventricle of the heart. Each artery is responsible for conveying oxygen and nutrients to specific organs and tissues as indicated in Figure 5-7.
	To identify and discuss location, anatomists divide the aorta into three major portions: the ascending aorta, the arch of the aorta, and the descending aorta. The descending aorta is further divided into the abdominal and the thoracic aorta.
ascending **heart** **arch of the aorta**	**5-28** As the aorta emerges from the left ventricle, it stretches upward. At this point it is called the _____ aorta. It gives off two branches, the right and left coronary arteries, that transport blood to the _____. The ascending aorta then turns to the left, forming an arch that is called the _____, also called the aortic arch.
thoracic **chest** **abdominal** **abdomen**	The descending aorta is a continuation of the aortic arch. The portion of the descending aorta in the thorax is called the _____ aorta. You learned in the previous chapter that thorac/ic means pertaining to the _____. The portion of the descending aorta in the abdomen is called the _____ aorta. Abdomin/al means pertaining to the _____.
aorta **within**	**5-29** Use **aort(o)** to build words about the aorta. Aort/ic pertains to the _____. Intraaortic means _____ the aorta.
hardening **aortosclerosis** (a-or″to-sklə-ro′sis) **aortitis** (a″or-ti′tis) **aortopathy** (a″or-top′ə-the) **narrowing**	**5-30** The combining form *scler(o)* means hard or hardening. Scler/osis is a condition characterized by _____ of tissue. The suffix *-sclerosis* means hardening. Build a word that means hardening of the aorta: _____.
	Build a word that means inflammation of the aorta by using the combining form for aorta plus the suffix for inflammation: _____.
	Any disease of the aorta is an _____.
	Stenosis means narrowing or stricture.
	Aortic stenosis is _____ of the aorta.
	In aortic stenosis (AS), blood cannot flow as efficiently from the left ventricle into the aorta.

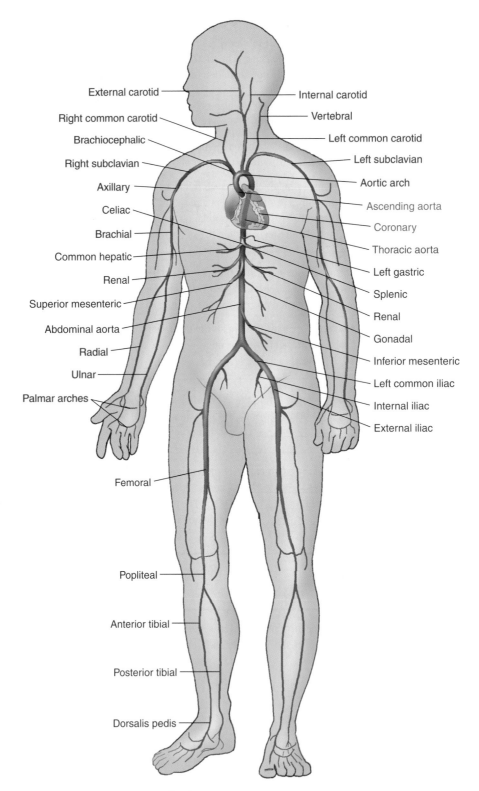

FIGURE 5-6
Anterior view of the aorta and its principal arterial branches.

THE AORTA AND ITS BRANCHES

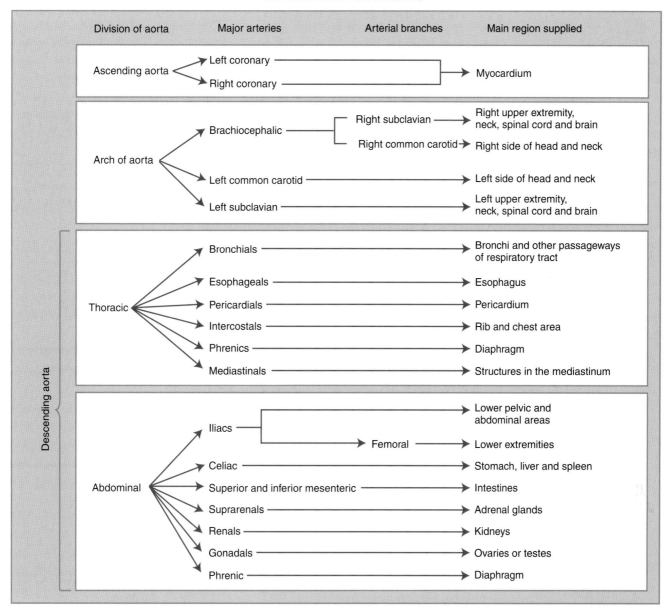

FIGURE 5-7
Schematic presentation of the divisions of the aorta and the corresponding regions of the body to which blood is supplied.

aortogram
(a-or′to-gram″)

aortography

aneurysm

5-31 Aortography (a″or-tog′rə-fe) is radiography of the aorta after introducing a contrast medium. The film produced by aortography is an _____. All of the divisions of the aorta could be visualized in aortography, but general areas are frequently studied. Thoracic, abdominal, and renal aortography are examples. Radiology of the aorta in the abdominal area is called abdominal _____.

Aortography is one method used to diagnose an aortic aneurysm **(an′u-rizm).** An aneurysm is a sac formed by localized dilation of an artery or vein, or of the heart itself. The potential danger is that the aneurysm will rupture. A ballooning out of the wall of some part of the aorta is called an aortic _____.

arteries

aneurysm

5-32 Aneurysms can occur in many blood vessels, but most aneurysms are arterial. In other words, aneurysms occur most often in _____. This is because pressure is higher in the arteries, particularly the aorta. Use the combining form **aneurysm(o)** to write words about aneurysms. Aneurysm/al means pertaining to an _____.

arteriolitis
(ahr-tēr″e-o′li′tis)

arteries, veins
phlebitis (flə-bi′tis)
venography
(ve-nog′rə-fe)
venogram
(ve′no-gram)

5-33 The aorta branches out to form arteries, which in turn branch out into the arterioles. Arterioles are minute arterial branches. Inflammation of the arterioles is _____.

Arterioles carry blood to the smallest of all blood vessels, the capillaries. Capillaries connect with venules, the minute veins that carry blood to the veins.

Note that venous **(ve′nəs)** means pertaining to the veins. Arterio/ven/ous **(ahr-tēr″e-o-ve′nəs)** means pertaining to both _____ and _____. Using phleb(o), build a word that means inflammation of a vein: _____.

Use ven(o) to write a word that means roentgenography (radiology) of the veins: _____.

The record produced in venography is called a _____.

clot
formation of a
thrombus within a
vein
thrombus
inflammation
vein
clot

5-34 Remembering that thromb(o) means thrombus, or blood clot, thrombo/phleb/itis **(throm″bo-flə-bi′tis)** is inflammation of a vein associated with a blood _____, or a thrombus.

Venous thrombosis is _____.

Venous thrombosis may be a complication of phleb/itis. This means that a _____ in the vein may be a result of _____. Venous thrombosis may also result from an injury to the leg or prolonged bed confinement. Venous pertains to a _____, and thrombosis means the presence of a blood _____.

phlebosclerosis
(fleb″o-sklə-ro′sis)

5-35 Write a word using phleb(o) plus sclerosis: _____.

The word you just wrote means a fibrous thickening and hardening of the walls of the veins.

plastic surgery of
a vein

varicose

5-36 Phlebo/plasty **(fleb′o-plas″te)** is _____.

Varicose **(var′ĭ kōs)** veins are swollen and knotted and occur most often in the legs. They result from sluggish blood flow in combination with weakened walls and incompetent valves in the veins. Unlike arteries that have substantially more muscle and elastic tissue, veins have flaplike valves that prevent blood from flowing backward. Defective valves allow the blood to collect in the veins, which become swollen and knotted (Figure 5-8).

This condition is called _____ veins.

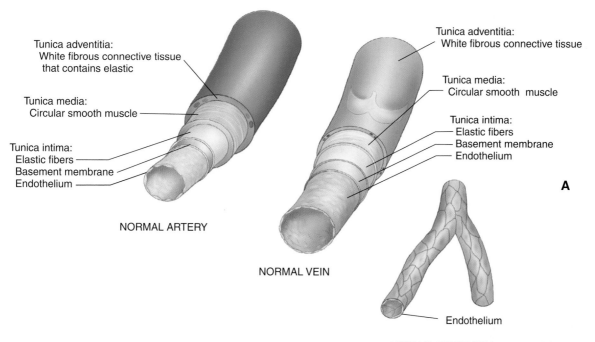

Tunica adventitia:
  White fibrous connective tissue
  that contains elastic

Tunica media:
  Circular smooth muscle

Tunica intima:
  Elastic fibers
  Basement membrane
  Endothelium

NORMAL ARTERY

Tunica adventitia:
  White fibrous connective tissue

Tunica media:
  Circular smooth muscle

Tunica intima:
  Elastic fibers
  Basement membrane
  Endothelium

A

NORMAL VEIN

Endothelium

NORMAL CAPILLARY
(microscopic)

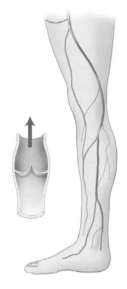

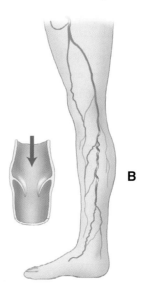

B

NORMAL VEINS
Functional valves aid in flow
of venous blood back to heart

VARICOSE VEINS
Failure of valves and pooling
of blood in superficial veins

FIGURE 5-8

A, The comparison of the structure of blood vessels. Note the external elastic membrane that is present in arteries. **B,** Normal veins versus varicose veins. Sluggish blood flow, weakened walls, and incompetent valves contribute to varicose veins in the legs, a common location for these enlarged and twisted veins near the surface of the skin.

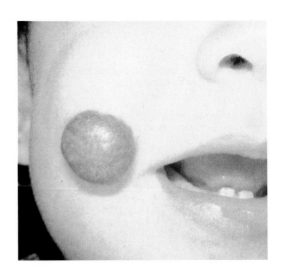

FIGURE 5-9
Hemangiona. This capillary hemangioma, often called a birthmark because it is commonly found during infancy, consists of closely packed small blood vessels. It grows at first but may spontaneously disappear in early childhood. It can be surgically removed if bleeding or injury is a problem, or later for cosmetic reasons. (From Zacarian SA: *Cryosurgery*, St Louis, 1985, Mosby.)

removal of a vein	**5-37** Phleb/ectomy (**flə-bek′to-me**) is _____.
	This procedure may involve removing only a segment of the vein.
-tomy	Remembering that -ectomy means removal or excision, write the suffix that means incision: _____.
	Both of these suffixes mean cutting into; however, -ectomy also implies removal of an organ or part.
-tome	**5-38** The suffix *-tome* is used to write words that mean an instrument used for cutting. The suffix is formed by simply changing the ending of -tomy, which means incision. Write this new suffix that means an instrument used for cutting: _____.
forming a new opening into a blood vessel	**5-39** Another suffix, *-stomy,* means formation of an opening and usually implies forming a new or artificial opening.
	Angio/stomy (**an″je-os′tə-me**) is _____.
angiectomy (an″je-ek′tə-me)	**5-40** Use angi(o) to form words that mean the following: removal (excision) of a vessel: _____.
angiotomy (an″je-ot′ə-me)	incision of a vessel: _____.
angiostomy (an″je-os′tə-me)	making a new opening in a vessel: _____.
blood	**5-41** An angi/oma (**an″je-o′mə**) is a tumor of either blood or lymph vessels. Angiomas are not malignant and sometimes disappear spontaneously. The suffix *-oma* means tumor.
	An angioma is either a hem/angi/oma (**he-man″je-o′mə**) or a lymph/angi/oma (**lim-fan″je-o′mə**). A hemangioma is a tumor of _____ vessels (Figure 5-9). (Note that the vowel is dropped from hem(a) and lymph(o) when they are joined with combining forms that begin with a vowel.)
hemangioma	A lymph/angi/oma is a tumor composed of lymph vessels. Knowing that angioma is a tumor composed of vessels, write the word that means a tumor consisting of blood vessels: _____.

hardening

5-42 Cardiovascular disease is the leading cause of death in the United States. A heart attack is often preceded by coronary artery disease (CAD), an abnormal condition of the coronary arteries that causes a reduced flow of oxygen and nutrients to the myocardium.

Arterio/scler/osis means _____ of the arteries.

Arterio/sclerosis (**ahr-tēr″e-o-sklə-ro′sis**) is a thickening and loss of elasticity of the walls of the arteries.

arteriosclerotic

5-43 Arterio/sclero/tic (**ahr-tēr″e-o-sklə-rot′ik**) heart disease (ASHD) is hardening and thickening of the walls of the coronary arteries. This reduces the oxygen supply to the myocardium and may lead to a heart attack. Write the adjective that means pertaining to hardening of an artery: _____.

atherosclerosis

Athero/sclerosis (**ath″er-o-sklə-ro′sis**) is a form of arteriosclerosis characterized by the formation of fatty deposits on the walls of arteries. The combining form ***ather(o)*** means yellow, fatty plaque. Only a few words use the combining form *ather(o)*. A form of arteriosclerosis characterized by the formation of fatty deposits on the walls of arteries is _____.

There is often a relationship between advanced atherosclerosis and a heart attack, which is called a myocardial infarction and is explained in the next section.

inside

5-44 End/arter/ectomy (**end-ahr″tər-ek′tə-me**) is removal of arteriosclerotic plaque from any obstructed artery. You learned that endo- means _____.

artery

Arteriosclerotic plaque tends to accumulate with age. Endarterectomy is removal of plaque from the inner wall of an obstructed _____. Endarterectomy does not designate a particular artery. There are several sites in the body where plaque commonly forms. One of these is the carotid artery, and this occlusion causes restricted blood flow to the brain. Removal of arteriosclerotic plaque from an obstructed carotid artery is called _____.

endarterectomy

5-45 The systemic blood vessels are the connection between the heart and the rest of the body. Thousands of miles of blood vessels transport oxygen and nutrients to all of the body cells every hour of every day.

❑ SECTION C REVIEW $\mathcal{B}$lood Vessels

This section review covers frames 5–23 through 5–45. Complete the table by writing the meaning of each word part that is used.

Combining Form	Meaning	Suffix	Meaning
1. aneurysm(o)	_____	8. -oma	_____
2. angi(o)	_____	9. -sclerosis	_____
3. aort(o)	_____	10. -stomy	_____
4. ather(o)	_____	11. -tome	_____
5. phot(o)	_____		
6. scler(o)	_____		
7. vas(o)	_____		

(Use Appendix V to check your answers.)

Cardiovascular Diagnosis, Pathology, and Treatment

Diagnosis and treatment of cardiovascular disorders have improved rapidly in the past decade, but cardiovascular disease remains the major cause of death in the United States. Several vascular disorders, including coronary artery disease that can lead to a heart attack, were discussed in the previous section. Heart disease can be classified in many ways. One method is based on whether the cause of the heart dysfunction developed away from the heart (as in CAD) or if the heart itself was the primary site of the dysfunction.

bad	**5-46** Abnormal, inadequate, or impaired function of an organ or part is termed a dysfunction (**dis-funk′shən**). You learned earlier that dys- means bad, painful, or difficult. In dys/function, dys- means _____ .
arteries	**5-47** The heart rate and blood pressure (BP) give a preliminary indication of how the heart is functioning. Arteries are popularly used to measure blood pressure, and the reading is a reflection of cardiac output and arterial resistance. In other words, the blood pressure reading is a reflection of the quantity of blood flow from the heart and resistance in the walls of the _____ .
	Arteries have more muscle and elastic fibers than do veins. This is a necessary structural characteristic, since the pressure of blood is much higher in arteries.
	Blood pressure measures the amount of pressure on the walls of the arteries.
	5-48 Hyper/tension (**hi″pər-ten′shən**) is increased blood pressure.
	The prefix *hyper-* means excessive or more than normal. Hyper is used as slang to mean more than normal activity or excitable.
excessive **against**	Hyper/tension means _____ tension and is commonly called high blood pressure. Anti/hyper/tensive (**an″tĭ-hi″pər-ten′siv**) means _____ hypertension.
antihypertensive	Antihypertensive means counteracting high blood pressure. The term is also applied to agents that reduce high blood pressure. An agent that reduces hypertension is called an _____ .
hypotension (hi″po-ten′shən)	Elevated blood pressure is hypertension; therefore decreased blood pressure is _____ .
	5-49 Blood pressure is measured using an apparatus called a sphygmomanometer (**sfig″mo-mə-nom′ə-ter**) (Figure 5-10). This very long word, sphygmomanometer,* refers to the instrument used to measure blood pressure indirectly. The suffix *-meter* refers to an instrument used for measuring, and *-metry* means the process for measuring. A direct measurement can be obtained only by measuring pressure within a vessel or the heart itself, as in heart catheterization, which is described later in this section.
systolic (sis-tol′ik)	Blood pressure is at its highest point when the ventricles contract. This is known as the systolic (Gk. *systolē*, contraction) pressure. The blood pressure measured during ventricular contraction is _____ pressure.
diastolic (di″ə-stol′ik)	Relaxation of the ventricles is diastole (**di-as′to-le**) (Gk. *diastolē*, expansion). The blood pressure measured during diastole is the diastolic pressure. The blood pressure measured when the ventricles are relaxed is called the _____ pressure.

*(Greek: *sphygmos*, pulse + *manos*, thin + *metron*, measure.)

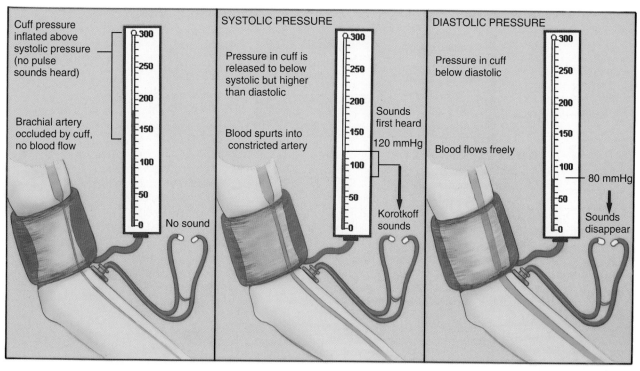

FIGURE 5-10

Measurement of blood pressure. Systolic pressure is due to ventricular contraction. Diastolic pressure occurs when the ventricles relax. The sounds resulting from blood flow that are heard through the stethoscope are called Korotkoff sounds. The first sound heard represents the systolic pressure. As the pressure declines, the last sound heard represents the diastolic pressure. This example represents a normal blood pressure reading of 120/80. In arteriosclerosis the arteries lose their elasticity and cannot expand when blood is pumped into them. (From Applegate EJ: *The anatomy and physiology learning system: textbook,* Philadelphia, 1995, WB Saunders.)

systolic diastolic	**5-50** Blood pressure is usually expressed as a fraction. The standard unit of measurement is millimeters of mercury (mm Hg). For example, a healthy young person has a blood pressure of approximately 120/80. The higher reading is the systolic pressure, and the lower reading is the diastolic pressure. In the example of a BP reading of 120/80, the _____ pressure is 120 mm Hg and the _____ pressure is 80 mm Hg.
hypertension	Increased BP is _____. Factors that cause the BP to increase are shown in Figure 5-11.
cardiac, increased increased, arterial	Four factors that increase blood pressure are increased _____ output, _____ blood volume, _____ blood viscosity, or loss of elasticity of the _____ walls.
hypotension	Decreased BP is _____.
stethoscope (steth'o-skōp)	**5-51** Used less often than thorac(o), another combining form, **steth(o),** also means chest. (You have already learned that scop(o) means to examine or view.) The stetho/scope is placed on the chest to listen to heart sounds. What is heard through the stethoscope is the closing of the heart valves. Heart murmurs are abnormal sounds produced by improper functioning of the valves. Write the name of this instrument placed on the chest to hear heart sounds: _____.
chest	It is also used to hear sounds of breathing and intestinal action and to take blood pressure. Steth(o) in stethoscope means _____.

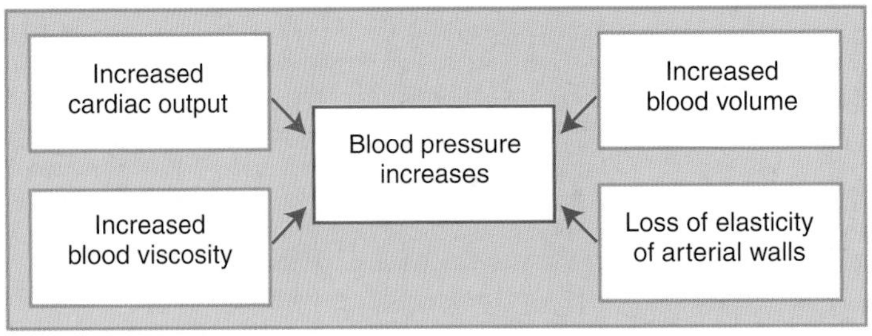

FIGURE 5-11
Factors that increase blood pressure. An increase in any of these four factors causes the arterial blood pressure to increase. **A,** Cardiac output is the principal determinant of blood pressure. It is the amount of blood ejected into the aorta each minute. (Normal, resting cardiac output is approximately 5 liters per minute.) **B,** Normal blood volume for an adult is approximately 5 liters. High salt intake can cause water retention, thereby increasing blood pressure. **C,** Blood viscosity is the stickiness or resistance to flow. Dehydration or an unusually high number of erythrocytes increases blood pressure. **D,** The smaller the diameter of an artery, the more resistance it offers to blood flow. When the heart contracts, arterial walls stretch outward to receive the extra blood. When the heart contraction is completed, vessels recoil inward, because of their elasticity, resuming their normal shape.

bradycardia
(brad″e-kahr′de-ə)

without

arrhythmia

bad

dysrhythmia

sinoatrial

heart block

5-52 The rhythmic expansion of an artery lying near the surface of the skin can be felt with the finger. This is known as the pulse. All arteries have a pulse, but the one most often used is the radial artery on the inside of the wrist.

A normal pulse rate in a resting state is 60 to 100 beats per minute. An increased pulse rate is tachy/cardia (**tak″ĭ-kahr′de-ə**). Using brady-, write a word that means a decreased pulse rate: _____.

Normally the intervals between pulses are of equal length. Remembering that a- means no or without, a/rhythmia is _____ rhythm. The combining forms **rrhythm(o)** and **rhythm(o)** mean rhythm. Arrhythmia (ə-rith′me-ə) is the same as arhythmia and is the more common spelling.

A variation in the normal rhythm of the heartbeat is an _____. Although this term is more commonly used, dysrhythmia (**dis-rith′me-ə**) would be more technically correct. Dysrhythmia is a disturbance of rhythm. Translated literally, it means _____ rhythm. Common usage generally determines whether one uses one or two *r*s in medical terms that pertain to rhythm. Write this new term that means an abnormal, disordered, or disturbed rhythm: _____.

5-53 You learned earlier that the heart has a special structure, the _____ node, where electrical impulses arise and stimulate contraction.

The SA node is called the pacemaker of the heart. If the SA node is not functioning properly, arrhythmia results. In certain arrhythmias, an artificial pacemaker can be used. An artificial pacemaker is a device designed to stimulate contraction of the heart. Depending on the patient's need, a cardiac pacemaker may be permanent or temporary and may fire only on demand or at a constant rate.

The brain can speed the heart up or slow it down to meet the demands of changing conditions, but the brain does not cause the heartbeat.

An impairment in the conduction of the impulse from the SA node to other parts of the heart is known as heart block. When the electrical impulse is not conducted throughout the heart, normal heart contraction does not occur. This condition is known as a _____ _____.

fibrillation	**5-54** Ventricular fibrillation (**fĭ brĭ-la′shən**) is a severe cardiac arrhythmia in which ventricular contractions are too rapid and uncoordinated for effective blood circulation. A cardiac arrhythmia marked by rapid, uncoordinated contractions is called _____.
fibrillation	Sometimes a defibrillator is used to alleviate fibrillation. (The prefix ***de-*** is used to mean down, from, or reversing. It is in the latter sense that it is used here.) A defibrillator (**de-fib″rĭ-la′tər**) is an electronic apparatus used to shock the heart, often through the placement of electrodes on the chest. The process, defibrillation (**de-fib″rĭ-la′shən**), stops _____.
absence of heart-beat or contraction	Ventricular fibrillation is frequently a cause of cardiac arrest. Systole refers to contraction of the heart. Another name for cardiac arrest is a/systole (**a-sis′to-le**), which means _____.
cardiopulmonary resuscitation	**5-55** When the heart stops, cardiopulmonary resuscitation (**re-sus-ĭ-ta′shən**) (CPR) is recommended as an emergency first aid procedure to reestablish heart and lung action. Pulmonary refers to the lungs, so cardio/pulmonary pertains to the heart and lungs. Resuscitation means restoring life or consciousness to one whose heartbeat or breathing has ceased. CPR is an abbreviation for _____ _____.
	CPR consists of closed heart massage and artificial respiration. It provides basic life support until it is no longer needed or until more advanced life support is available.
arrest	One indication for the use of CPR is a cardiac _____.
heart	**5-56** Primary cardiac diseases include those caused by structural cardiac defects, as well as inflammation and infection that originate within the heart. Defects are sometimes present in one of the four chambers of the heart, in one of the heart valves, or in the septum that divides the two sides of the heart. If heart disease is present at birth, it is a congenital (**kən-jen′ ĭ-təl**) _____ disease. Congenital* means existing at, and usually before, birth.
atri(o)	Write the combining forms for the heart chambers and the septum. The combining form for atrium is _____.
ventricul(o)	Write the combining form for ventricle: _____.
sept(o)	Write the combining form for septum: _____.
atrium	Atrio/megaly (**a″tre-o-meg′ə-le**) is abnormal enlargement of an _____ of the heart.
atria	Atrio/septo/plasty (**a″tre-o-sep″to-plas′te**) is surgical repair of the septum in the area between the right and left _____.
ventricles	**5-57** A ventricular septal defect (VSD) is an abnormal opening in the septum dividing the right and the left _____. Look at Figure 5-3 and be sure that you can locate where a ventricular septal defect would occur. This defect is a type of congenital heart disease, meaning an abnormality of the heart that is present at birth.
atria	An atrial septal defect (ASD) is also a congenital heart disease. An atrial septal defect is an abnormal opening in the part of the septum that separates the right and the left _____.
blue (or bluish)	There are other congenital heart diseases, but atrial septal defects and ventricular septal defects account for 30% to 40% of heart diseases that are present at birth. Almost all congenital heart defects interrupt the normal flow of blood through the heart and vessels. Heart murmurs—abnormal heart sounds—are often heard. Cyan/osis may also be present. Cyan/osis is a _____ discoloration of the skin and mucous membranes that results from insufficient oxygen to the tissues.

*Congenital (Latin: *congenitus*, born together).

narrowing
inflammation of a valve
cardiovalvulitis (kahr″de-o-val″vu-li′tis)
inflammation of the valves of the heart
myocardium
cardiomyopathy
inflammation of the myocardium
coronary
closed (or obstructed)
oxygen
myocardial infarction
ischemia
bypass

5-58 Heart valves can also be defective and result in the valves not opening fully as in valvul/ar stenosis. Valvular stenosis is _____ of the opening created by the valve.

Valves may also become inflamed and infected.

Valvul/itis (**val″vu-li′tis**) is _____, especially a heart valve. Build a new word by using a combining form that means heart + valvulitis: _____.

The new word that you just wrote means
_____.

Cardio/myo/pathy (**kahr″de-o-mi-op′ə-the**) is a general diagnostic term that designates primary myocardial disease. In other words, the disease originated in the _____.

This disease of the myocardium that is not attributable to outside causes that results in insufficient oxygen, damaged valves, or high blood pressure is called a _____. Myocarditis is an example of a cardiomyopathy.
Myocard/itis means _____.

5-59 Formation of a blood clot in a coronary artery is coronary thrombosis (**throm-bo′sis**).

Coronary occlusion (**o-kloo′zhən**) is a closing off of a _____ artery. The occlusion may result from a thrombus, but it is more likely due to a narrowing of the lumen (cavity) of the blood vessel.

An occlusion* is an obstruction or closure. Occlusion is also used in other terms, but it always means _____. In a coronary occlusion, the heart does not receive sufficient oxygen.

If occlusion is complete and no blood is being supplied to an area of the myocardium, myocardial infarction (**in-fahrk′shən**) results. Cells die when deprived of oxygen. The death of cells in an area of the myocardium because of oxygen deprivation is myocardial infarction. A myocardial infarction (MI) is a heart attack. The combining form *ox(i)* means oxygen, so when translated literally, an/ox/ia means an abnormal condition characterized by absence of _____. A localized area of damaged tissue resulting from anoxia is called an infarct† (**in′fahrkt**).

MI is the most frequent cause of death in the United States. Whether death occurs after MI largely depends on the resulting damage to the myocardium. Those who survive often suffer complications of heart function. When areas of the myocardium die because of lack of oxygen, this is called _____
_____.

5-60 Insufficient blood flow to an area is termed *ischemia* (**is-ke′me-ah**). If the myocardial demand for oxygen exceeds the capability of diseased coronary arteries, myocardial _____ results and, if prolonged, leads to myocardial infarction.

Rest is an important part of recovery after a heart attack. The patient is usually left with some heart damage, often resulting in failure of the heart to function normally. This deficiency of the heart is called cardiac insufficiency. If the damage is too severe, surgical intervention may be necessary. A coronary artery bypass graft (CABG) uses a vessel from elsewhere in the patient's body to provide an alternate route for the blood to circumvent obstruction of a coronary artery. The vessels that are generally used are a segment of the saphenous vein from the patient's leg or the mammary artery. A bypass is also called a shunt. One that circumvents a vessel that supplies blood to the heart is called a coronary _____.

*(Latin: *occludere,* to close up.)
†(Latin: *infarcire,* to stuff.)

extracorporeal	**5-61** The term *bypass* is also used in other ways. During heart surgery, the heart itself may be bypassed by providing an extracorporeal* (**eks"trə-kor-por'e-əl**) (outside the body) device to pump blood. The term that means "outside the body" is _____.
heart	Cardio/pulmonary (**kahr"de-o-pul'mə-nar-e**) bypass diverts blood away from the heart while surgery of the heart and major vessels is performed. A cardio/pulmonary machine is a special _____-lung machine that collects the blood, adds oxygen, and then pumps the blood to all parts of the body.
bypass	Surgeries involving the heart and major vessels generally require cardiopulmonary _____. New developments in cardiac surgery are heart transplantation and use of an artificial heart. Research continues, and many improvements in these two types of surgeries will no doubt occur.
enlarged heart	**5-62** In many types of heart disease, the heart attempts to compensate for its deficit by working harder. Cardio/megaly (**kahr"de-o-meg"ə-le**) may result. Cardio/megaly is an _____ _____.
smallness	Micro/cardia (**mi-kro-kahr'de-ə**), the opposite of cardiomegaly, is abnormal _____ of the heart.
inflammation of the heart	Carditis (**kahr-di'tis**) is another term related to the heart. In this term, cardi(o) plus -itis, one "i" and the "o" are omitted to facilitate pronunciation. Card/itis is _____.
stenosis, stricture	**5-63** Stenosis (**stə-no'sis**) means constriction or narrowing of a passage or orifice. Stricture (**strik'chər**) is also used in this sense. Two terms often have the same meaning because we have taken the words from both the Latin and the Greek languages. Two words that mean constriction of a passage or opening are _____ and _____.
narrowing, vessel	The suffix *-stenosis* means stricture or narrowing. Angio/stenosis (**an"je-o-stə-no'sis**) is _____ of the diameter of a _____.
	Stenosis of the coronary arteries reduces blood flow to the heart. In some cases blood flow can be increased by using methods that do not require extensive surgery. These methods are intravascular thrombolysis, intraarterial infusion of vasodilators, and percutaneous transluminal angioplasty. We will look at them individually in the next few frames. If conservative methods are not helpful, coronary artery bypass is generally performed.
catheter	**5-64** In the cardiac procedures that are being described in the next few frames, catheters are generally used. A catheter (**kath'ə-tər**) is inserted into a major artery and advanced toward the heart. They are used for a variety of purposes in a hospital. A catheter is a tube passed through the body for evacuating or injecting fluids. In the cardiac procedures described here, a _____ is placed in a major artery and advanced toward the heart (Figure 5-12).
angiography (**an"je-og'rə-fe**) coronary	The catheter enables the use of contrast dyes that enhance x-ray images of the heart and its vessels. A radiographic procedure that produces an angiogram is called _____. Radiography of the coronary arteries is _____ angiography. Cardiac angiography is radiology of the heart and its vessels.
thrombus	**5-65** Intra/vascular (**in"trə-vas'ku lər**) thrombolysis is the application of a thrombolytic agent directly to a _____ within a vessel. This technique is primarily used to treat myocardial infarction and acute thrombotic occlusion of vessels. Success mainly depends on age, size, and location of the thrombus.
within dissolve	The thrombolytic agent is administered through the catheter. Intra/vascular means _____ a vessel. The purpose of intravascular thrombolysis is to _____ the thrombus within a coronary artery.

*(Latin: *corpus,* body.)

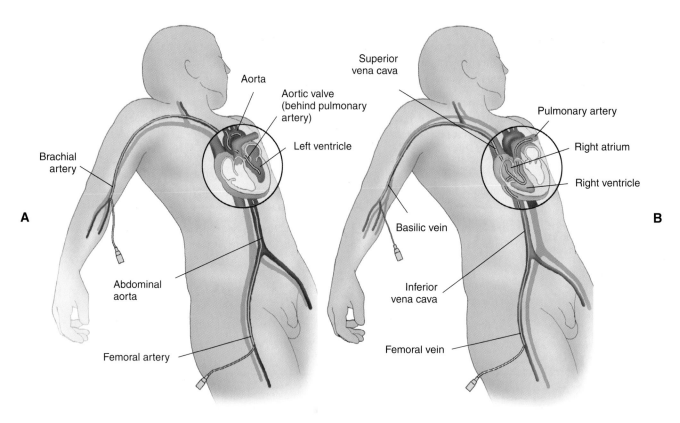

FIGURE 5-12
Heart catheterization. **A,** Left-sided. **B,** Right-sided. Progress of the catheter is monitored by fluoroscopy as it is threaded through blood vessels to reach the heart. Fluoroscopy gives the physician immediate images of the location of the catheter throughout the procedure. The right side of the heart may be the only side examined, since left-sided heart catheterization is riskier.

within	**5-66** Intra/arterial (**in"trə-ahr-ter-e-əl**) means _____ an artery. Intraarterial infusion of a vasodilator into an artery is limited to specific cases.
dilate the vessels	You need to remember that the purpose of vasodilators is to _____.
repair a vessel	**5-67** Because angioplasty is included in percutaneous (**per"ku-ta′ne-əs**) transluminal angioplasty (PTA), we know that the purpose of the procedure is to _____.
percutaneous	In analyzing other parts of PTA, percutaneous means through the skin, or removal or injection by needle. (Cutaneous means pertaining to the skin.) In PTA the word that means through the skin is _____.
	Percutaneous transluminal coronary angioplasty (PTCA) is performed on coronary arteries and is done to improve blood circulation to the heart. After angiography enhances the x-ray images of the heart and vessels, a small balloon on the end of the catheter is inflated at a point where the lumen of the artery is narrowed. The inflated balloon compresses fatty deposits or plaque, thus allowing blood to flow more freely through the vessel. Percutaneous transluminal angioplasty is also called balloon catheter dilation.
angiocardiography (**an"je-o-kahr"de-og′rə-fe**)	Angiography is an integral part of the cardiac procedures just described. Form a new word that means the same as cardiac angiography by combining angi(o), cardi(o), and -graphy: _____.

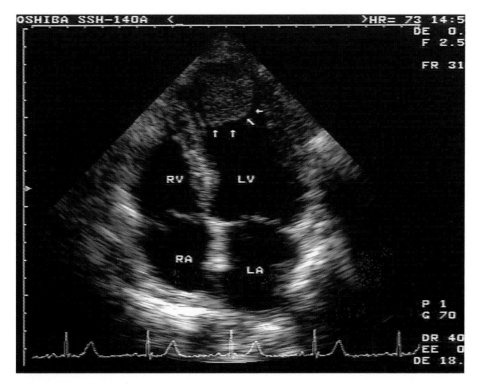

FIGURE 5-13
Echocardiogram. The heart is viewed from the top, and the four chambers (RV, RA, LV, LA) are visible, as well as a large thrombus, indicated by the arrows. (From Ballinger PW, Frank ED: *Merrill's atlas of radiographic positions and radiologic procedures*, vol 3, ed 9, St Louis, 1999, Mosby.)

---

stress

5-68 Many diagnostic techniques are used to help assess heart disease. Electrocardiography (**e-lek″tro-kahr″de-og′rə-fe**) and angiocardiography have already been mentioned. Pressures and patterns of blood flow can be determined by cardiac catheterization (**kath″ə-tər-ĭ-za′shən**). The stress test, sometimes called the treadmill stress test, measures the heart's response during exercise (stress). An electrocardiogram (ECG) and other measurements are taken while the patient is exercising (walking or jogging) on a treadmill. Measuring the heart's response while exercising in this manner is called the _____ test.

---

record

sonogram
(so′no-gram)
echogram
(ek′o-gram)

echocardiography
(ek″o-kahr″de-og′
rə-fe)

5-69 Diagnostic procedures are often able to detect abnormalities before the heart is damaged. Each procedure has special benefits, and several may be performed to determine diagnosis.

Two combining forms, *son(o)* and *ech(o),* refer to sound. They are frequently combined with gram(o) and various related suffixes that mean to _____. Sono/graphy (**sə-nog′rə-fe**), also called ultrasound or echography, bounces ultrasonic waves off tissues to produce a record.
The record produced by sonography or echography is a _____

or an _____.

Echo/cardio/gram is the term generally associated with the use of ultrasonography in diagnosing heart disease (Figure 5-13). An echocardiogram is a record of the heart obtained by directing ultrasonic waves through the chest wall. The procedure that produces an echocardiogram is called _____.

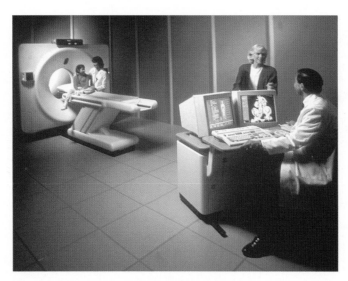

FIGURE 5-14

Computed tomography. The major components of the CT scanner are shown. The young patient awaits her turn while the CT technologist examines an image on the monitor. (Courtesy of GE Medical Systems, Waukesha, Wisc.)

---

computed tomography cut	**5-70** Another noninvasive diagnostic procedure is computed tomography **(to-mog′rə-fe),** abbreviated CT. This procedure produces images of organ cross sections similar to what one would see if the organ were actually cut into sections. This procedure is called _____ _____. The tom(o) in tomo/graphy means to _____. In this case, it refers to images that appear as though the organ were cut into cross sections. In CT, x-ray transmission patterns are recorded by electronic detectors and stored in a computer's memory. After recording a large number of directions and positions, the computer reconstructs a three-dimensional view of the internal structures of the body (Figure 5-14).
tomogram (to′mo-gram) **tomograph** (to′mo-graf)	The record produced by tomography is a _____. In addition to a computer, a special apparatus is needed to position the x-ray tube for tomography. The apparatus (instrument) associated with tomography is a _____. CT was once called computerized axial tomography (CAT) or computerized transverse axial tomography. CT is now the more commonly used term.
a record of the heart **electrocardiography electrocardiograph** (e-lek″tro-kahr′de-o-graf″)	**5-71** A cardio/gram is _____. An electrocardiogram **(e-lek″tro-kahr′de-o-gram″)** is a record of the electric currents generated by the heart. Electrodes placed on the body are able to detect electric currents generated by the heart. This procedure is called _____ and is abbreviated ECG or EKG. The instrument that records electrical impulses of the heart is an _____.

TABLE 5-1 Additional Cardiovascular Diseases or Disorders

Angina pectoris: Severe pain and constriction about the heart caused by an insufficient supply of blood to the heart; actually not a disease of the heart, but a symptom

Cardiac block: Interferences with the heart's contractions owing to failure of the impulses to pass through the conductile tissue

Congestive heart failure: A condition characterized by weakness, breathlessness, and edema in lower portions of the body resulting from venous stasis and reduced outflow of blood

Peripheral vascular disease: An unspecific term indicating diseases of the arteries and veins of the extremities, especially those conditions that interfere with adequate flow of blood to or from the extremities (e.g., varicose veins)

Shock: A serious condition in which blood flow is inadequate to return sufficient blood to the heart for normal function, particularly transport of oxygen to all organs and tissues; may be caused by a variety of conditions such as hemorrhage, drug reaction, injury, infection, myocardial infarction, and dehydration

Valvular heart disease: Any of a number of disorders of the heart valves, including mitral stenosis, mitral insufficiency, mitral valve prolapse, aortic stenosis, and aortic insufficiency

---

5-72 Before leaving this section, look at the additional cardiovascular diseases or disorders presented in Table 5-1.

In general, a disorder is defined as a disruption or interruption in normal functions of established systems. Disease has two definitions: a condition of abnormal function, or a specific illness or disorder characterized by a recognizable set of signs and symptoms. The choice of which to use is often determined by common use. Most psychological dysfunctions are classified as disorders because they represent a disruption of normal function. Phobias and terms using the suffix *-phobia,* meaning abnormal fear, are generally classified as disorders. Conditions involving infectious microorganisms are generally called infectious diseases.

pain

Angina pectoris (L. *angor,* quinsy; *pectus,* breast or chest) (**an-ji′nə pek′tə-ris**) is often simply called angina, a term now used primarily to denote cardiac _____ caused by anoxia to the myocardium.

failure

Weakness, breathlessness, and edema (**ə-de′mə**) in the lower portion of the body are signs of congestive heart failure (CHF). Edema is an abnormal accumulation of fluid in the interstitial spaces of tissue. This condition is called congestive heart _____.

Sclerosis or stenosis of any of the heart's valves can decrease blood circulation.

narrower

You have learned that stenosis means narrowing. When a valve is stenos/ed, it becomes _____.

hardened

You know that sclerosis means hardening. When a valve becomes scleros/ed, it is _____.

Prolapse means sagging. When a valve prolapses, such as in mitral valve prolapse (MVP), the valve sags rather than opening fully. Symptoms vary from absent to severe.

In aortic insufficiency (AI), blood flows back into the left ventricle during systole. The heart will work harder in an attempt to deliver needed oxygen and nutrients to all of the body's cells.

Shock is a life-threatening condition in which blood flow is inadequate. Although there are many other cardiovascular disorders, you now have a working knowledge of the ones you are most likely to encounter.

❏ SECTION D REVIEW   *C*ardiovascular Diagnosis, Pathology, and Treatment

This section review covers frames 5–46 through 5–72. Complete the table by writing the meaning of each word part that is used. Write all of the meanings of a word part (for example, for de-.)

Combining Form	Meaning		Prefix	Meaning
1. ech(o)	_____		6. de-	_____
2. ox(i)	_____		**Suffix**	**Meaning**
3. rrhythm(o)	_____		7. -meter	_____
4. son(o)	_____		8. -metry	_____
5. steth(o)	_____		9. -phobia	_____
			10. -stenosis	_____

(Use Appendix V to check your answers.)

Lymphatic System

The lymphatic system is an important part of circulation because it normally returns excess interstitial fluid to the bloodstream. It can be considered a separate system, however, because it consists of a set of vessels and organs that work together to perform a vital function. The absorption of fats and fat-soluble vitamins from the small intestine is another function of the lymphatics. The lymphatics also are part of the immune system that helps defend the body against microorganisms and disease.

	5-73 The lymphatic (**lim-fat′ik**) system is composed of lymphatic vessels, a fluid called lymph (**limf**), lymph nodes, and three organs: the spleen, thymus, and tonsils.
study of the lymphatics	The combining form ***lymphat(o)*** refers to the lymphatics, also called the lymphatic system. Lymphato/logy (**lim″fə-tol′ə-je**) is the _____.
destruction	Lymphato/lysis (**lim″fə-tol′ĭ-sis**) is _____ of the lymphatics (tissue or vessels are implied).
	5-74 Study the major parts of the lymphatic system (Figure 5-15). Only the major lymph vessels and nodes are shown.
interstitial	The smallest vessels of this system are lymph capillaries that are found in almost all regions of the body. Look at the detailed drawing of the proximity of the lymphatic capillaries to the cardiovascular capillaries, venules, and arterioles. The lymphatic capillaries pick up _____ fluid that has collected from the normal course of blood circulation.
	Lymphatic capillaries are constructed in such a way that fluid enters but does not leave the capillaries. Fluid moves in only one direction in lymph vessels because of valves that carry the fluid away from the tissue. The whole system depends on muscular contraction because there is no pump; transport of fluid is slow. Lymph ducts eventually empty the lymph into the subclavian veins, thus returning the fluid to the systemic circulation.
	5-75 Note the bean-shaped lymph nodes along the course of the lymph vessels shown in Figure 5-15. The cisterna chyli and the ducts are structures that are formed by the merging of many lymph vessels and their trunks.
chest	As its name indicates, the thorac/ic duct is located in the _____.
neck	There are three types of lymph nodes shown in the drawing. The cervic/al lymph nodes are located in the area of the _____. In later chapters, you will study the combining forms *axill(o)* and *inguin(o)*, which mean armpit and groin, respectively. For now, remember the locations of the cervical, axillary (**ak′sĭ-lar″e**), and inguinal (**ing′gwĭ-nəl**) lymph nodes.
	5-76 Lymph is the fluid transported by the lymphatic vessels. Sometimes ***lymph(o)*** is used to mean lymphatics, but it is also a combining form for lymph. The fluid transported by the lymphatic vessels is
lymph	called _____.

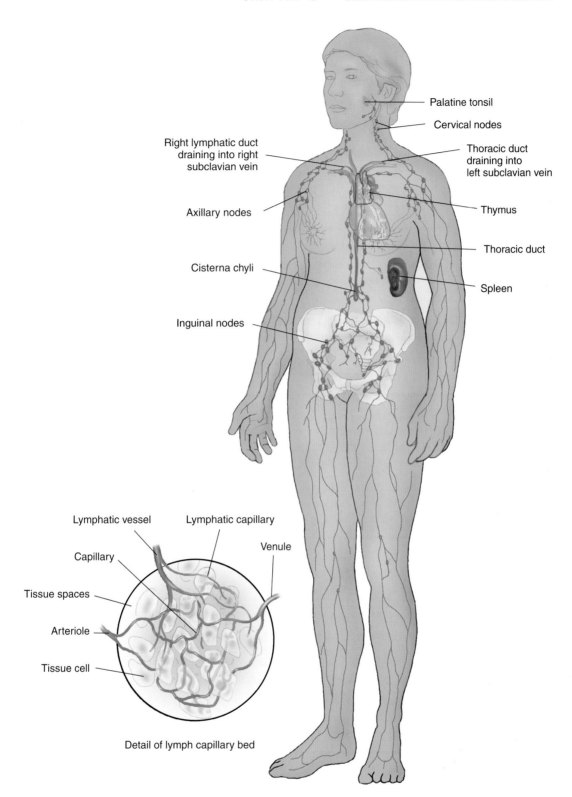

Palatine tonsil

Cervical nodes

Right lymphatic duct
draining into right
subclavian vein

Thoracic duct
draining into
left subclavian vein

Axillary nodes

Thymus

Thoracic duct

Cisterna chyli

Spleen

Inguinal nodes

Lymphatic vessel   Lymphatic capillary

Capillary   Venule

Tissue spaces

Arteriole

Tissue cell

Detail of lymph capillary bed

FIGURE 5-15

Lymphatic system. The close relationship to the cardiovascular system is shown in the detailed drawing. Lymph capillaries merge to form lymphatic vessels that join other vessels to become trunks that drain large regions of the body. The right lymphatic duct receives fluid from the upper right quadrant of the body and empties into the right subclavian vein. The thoracic duct, which begins with the cisterna chyli, collects fluid form the rest of the body and empties it into the left subclavian vein. The lymph nodes are small, bean-shaped structures distributed along the vessels. Also shown are the lymphatic organs: tonsils, thymus, and spleen.

lymphatic	**5-77** A lympho/cyte (**lim′fo-sīt**) is a blood cell that matures in the _____ system. Lymphocytes originate in the bone marrow and are carried by the blood to the lymphatic organs, where they become part of the immune response.
lymphocytes phagocytes (**fag′o-sīts**) **it is large and in-gests material**	Lymphocytes are part of the body's defense against disease, as are phagocytes, another type of cell. Phagocytes and some lymphocytes are capable of destroying harmful microorganisms. These cells are found in the tonsils, the spleen, the thymus, and the lymph nodes. Two types of cells found in the lymph nodes that trap harmful organisms are _____ and _____.
	One of the most important phagocytic cells found in the lymph nodes is the macro/phage. What can we learn about a macro/phage by analyzing its word parts? _____
lymph nodes	**5-78** Lymph nodes also filter the lymph and prevent many harmful products from entering the general circulation. Sometimes these nodes become inflamed or swollen and may be felt or seen. Small knots of tissue found at intervals along the course of the lymphatic vessels are called _____ _____.
	The lymphatic system is also important in the absorption of fats from the digestive tract. Although not as well known as other body systems, the lymphatic system is essential to normal body function.
lymph	Lympho/stasis (**lim-fos′tə-sis**) is stoppage of _____ flow. (Stasis means stoppage or diminution of flow.)
	5-79 The lymphatic system frequently becomes involved in the spread of cancer. If cancer cells wander into a lymphatic vessel, the cells may be trapped by the lymph nodes and begin growing there, or the cells may be carried to sites far from their origin. To determine if cancer has spread to the lymphatic system, lymph nodes are often examined.
lymphogram (**lim′fo-gram**)	The lymphatic channels and lymph nodes can be x-rayed after injection of radiopaque material into a lymphatic vessel. This procedure is called lymphography. Write a word that means the picture produced in lymphography (**lim-fog′rə-fe**): _____.
lymphatics	**5-80** Lymph/edema means swelling of the subcutaneous tissue of an extremity as a result of obstruction of the lymphatics. The meaning of lymphedema (**lim″fə-de′mə**) is implied. You will need to remember that lymphedema means swelling of an extremity owing to obstruction of the _____.
	In lymphedema, the swelling results from obstruction of a lymphatic vessel (Figure 5-16).
	Edema (**ə-de′mə**) means swelling (caused by an accumulation of fluid). The suffix *-edema* means swelling.
	You will be using this suffix to write many terms. Its intended meaning is not related to obstructed lymph vessels unless -edema is joined to lymph(o), as in lymph/edema.
	Elephantiasis (**el″ə-fən-ti′ə-sis**) is a disease in which swelling of the lymphatics causes monstrous enlargements of parts of the body, such as the legs. The lymphatics are clogged by the parasites that cause the disease, and lymph/edema results.

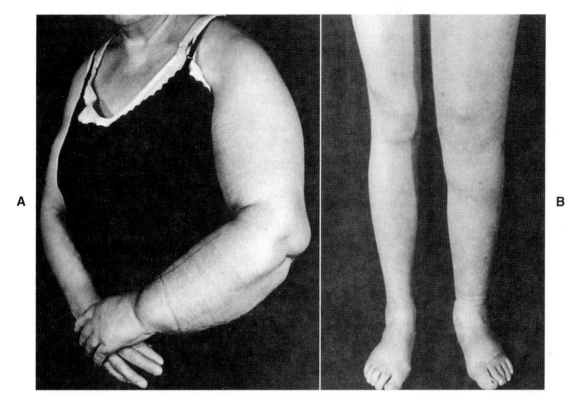

FIGURE 5-16
Two examples of lymphedema. **A,** Lymphedema of the arm may develop after surgical excision of the axillary lymph nodes, done sometimes when a cancerous breast is removed. **B,** Lymphedema of the lower limb. The cause of obstructed lymphatic vessels is sometimes an inherited trait but is not always known. (From Polaski AL, Tatro SE: *Luckmann's core principles and practice of medical-surgical nursing,* Philadelphia, 1996, WB Saunders.)

lymphatic	**5-81** Lymph/ang/itis (**lim″fan-ji′tis**) is inflammation of a _____ vessel. (Note the spelling of lymphangitis, which uses the combining forms for lymph, vessel, and inflammation. Some of the vowels are omitted in the spelling of lymphangitis to facilitate pronunciation.) The combining form ***lymphangi(o)*** means lymph vessel.
thrombolym- phangitis (thromb″bo- lim″fan-ji′tis)	Combine thromb(o) and lymphangitis to form a new word that means inflammation of a lymph vessel resulting from a blood clot: _____.
lymphatic	A lymph/oma (**lim-fo′mə**) is a _____ tumor. This word is a general term for growth of new tissue in the lymphatics, but lymphomas are almost always malignant.
	A lymph/angi/oma is a tumor composed of newly formed lymph vessels.
radiography	Lymph/angio/graphy (**lim-fan″je-og′rə-fe**) is _____ of the lymphatic vessels after the injection of contrast medium.

5-82 A few words use *cancer(o),* meaning cancer. You will also learn another combining form that is used more often in medical terms that refer to cancer.

cancer

Cancer/ous means pertaining to _____.

tumor

Carcin/oma (**kahr″sĭ-no′mə**) means a cancerous _____. A carcinoma is a malignant growth, meaning it has a tendency to spread.

The combining form, *carcin(o),* also means cancer. Write this word that means cancerous tumor by joining carcin(o) and the suffix for tumor: _____.

carcinoma

carcinoma

The presence of a cancerous tumor in the lymphatic system is lymphatic _____.

tumor

An aden/oma (**ad″ə-no′mə**) is a _____ of a gland, but this term does not indicate whether the tumor is cancerous.

5-83 The combining form *aden(o)* means gland. This combining form does not designate a particular gland but refers to an aggregation of cells specialized to secrete or excrete materials not related to their ordinary needs. You have heard of many glands already, such as the adrenal gland and the thyroid gland. Lymph nodes were originally thought to be lymph glands and were named accordingly. The combining form *lymphaden(o)* means lymph node.

inflammation of a
lymph node

Lymph/aden/itis (**lim-fad″ə-ni′tis**) is _____.

any disease of the
lymph nodes

Lymph/adeno/pathy (**lim-fad″ə-nop′ə-the**) is _____.

tumor

A lymph/aden/oma (**lim-fad″ə-no′mə**) is a _____ of a lymph node. This term is used interchangeably with lymphoma.

5-84 Three organs that are part of the lymphatic system are the spleen, the tonsils, and the thymus, shown in Figure 5-15. The spleen is a large organ situated in the upper left part of the abdominal cavity. The combining form *splen(o)* means spleen. Splen/ic (**splen′ik**) refers to the _____.

spleen

The spleen destroys red blood cells when their usefulness is ended. The average life of an erythrocyte is approximately 4 months, at which time it is destroyed by the spleen and its materials are reused to make new red blood cells. In addition, the spleen is important in defending the body against disease. Diseases of the spleen can profoundly affect one's health. Any disease of the spleen is called a _____.

splenopathy
(sple-nop′ə-the)

enlargement of the
spleen
splenectomy
(sple-nek′tə-me)
spleen
lymph

5-85 Spleno/megaly (**sple″no-meg′ə-le**) is _____.

Surgical removal of the spleen is _____.

Spleno/lymphatic (**sple″no-lim-fat′ik**) pertains to the _____ and the _____ nodes.

splenalgia
(sple-nal′jə)

Write a term using splen(o) and -algia that means pain in the spleen: _____.

5-86 When writing words about the thymus, use *thym(o).* The thymus is also called the thymus gland because it is a glandlike body. It is located in the anterior mediastinal cavity. It is important in the production of antibodies, a crucial part of our immune system. Thymic (**thi′mik**) means

pertaining to the
thymus

_____.

thymectomy
(thi-mek′tə-me)

Write a word that means removal of the thymus: _____.

tumor
thymopathy
(thi-mop′ə-the)

A thym/oma (**thi-mo′mə**) is a _____ of the thymus. Any disease of the thymus is a _____.

tonsil
tonsillitis
(ton″sĭ-li′tis)
tonsillectomy
(ton″sĭ-lek′tə-me)

5-87 When we see the word tonsil, we think of the small masses located at the back of the throat. These are the palatine (**pal′ə-tĭn**) tonsils (the palate is the roof of the mouth) and are usually what one is referring to when the term tonsil is used. But one should be aware that there are other types of tonsils.

The combining form **tonsill(o)** means tonsil. Tonsillo/tomy (**ton″sĭ-lot′ə-me**) is incision of a

_____.

Inflammation of the tonsils is _____.

Excision of the tonsils is a _____.

removal of the adenoids

5-88 A tonsillectomy is performed to treat a chronic infection of the tonsils. An adenoidectomy (**ad″ə-noid-ek′tə-me**) is often performed at the same time as a tonsillectomy, since both the adenoids and the tonsils become enlarged after repeated bouts of tonsillitis. Adenoid/ectomy is

_____.

A tonsillectomy and adenoidectomy performed at the same time is called a tonsilloadenoidectomy. (**ton″sĭ-lo-ad″ə-noid-ek′tə-me**) and is usually written T & A.

The combining form **adenoid(o)** means adenoids, a type of tonsils, located high in the pharynx behind the nose.

adenoiditis
(ad″ə-noid-i′tis)

Inflammation of the adenoids is _____.

❏ SECTION E REVIEW   𝓛ymphatic System

This section review covers frames 5–73 through 5–88. Complete the table by writing the meaning of each word part that is listed.

Combining Form	Meaning		Combining Form	Meaning
1. aden(o)	_____		8. lymphat(o)	_____
2. adenoid(o)	_____		9. splen(o)	_____
3. cancer(o)	_____		10. thym(o)	_____
4. carcin(o)	_____		11. tonsill(o)	_____
5. lymph(o)	_____		**Suffix**	**Meaning**
6. lymphaden(o)	_____		12. -edema	_____
7. lymphangi(o)	_____			

(Use Appendix V to check your answers.)

Terminology Challenge

This section challenges you to read, write, and understand new terms or concepts about the cardiovascular and lymphatic systems. You will combine word parts that you know with less familiar word parts. It is important to remember the new terms introduced in this section.

tumors	**5-89** The suffix *-oma* usually denotes an abnormal growth of tissue, called a neoplasm or a tumor. But sometimes it means only an abnormal or diseased condition, such as in glaucoma, a destructive eye disease caused by increased intraocular pressure. Occasionally -oma means a swelling, as in the word *hematoma;* however, most terms that pertain to swelling caused by an accumulation of fluid use the suffix *-edema*. Sometimes -oma is affixed to a word part that denotes location, as in the word *neuroma* (noo-ro′mə). At other times the word part to which it is affixed tells something about the nature of the growth. A melan/oma (mel″ə-no′mə) is composed of melanin-forming cells. Benign tumors are usually not serious and can be removed without further problems. They are not malignant and therefore are not cancerous. In contrast, cancerous tumors are capable of spreading to other parts of the body. Carcinomas are cancerous _____ that occur in epithelial tissue, the cells that form the outer surface of the body and line the cavities and the passageways leading to the exterior. Cancerous tumors that arise in bones, muscles, or other connective tissues are called sarcomas* (sahr-ko′məz).
blood	**5-90** Translated literally, hyper/emia (hi″pər-e′me-ə) means excessive _____. You need to know that hyperemia is an excess of blood in part of the body caused by increased blood flow, as one often sees in inflammation. In hyperemia, the overlying skin usually becomes reddened and warm.
cardiodynia **cardiotomy (kahr″de-ot′ə-me)** **heart** **cardiodiaphragmatic (kahr″de-o-di″ə-frag-mat′ik)**	**5-91** Using -dynia, write a term that, translated literally, means heart pain: _____. This is more commonly called angina or angina pectoris. Cardi/algia (kahr″de-al′jə) is a synonym for cardiodynia. The suffix *-algia* also means pain. Write a word that means incision of the heart: _____. (Be aware that there is a second meaning of this term that pertains to a specific surgical operation on the stomach.) Cardio/centesis (kahr″de-o-sən-te′sis) is surgical puncture of the _____. The suffix *-centesis* means surgical puncture. Diaphragmatic means pertaining to the diaphragm, the dome-shaped muscular partition that separates the thoracic and abdominal cavities. Use diaphragmatic to write a term that means pertaining to the heart and the diaphragm: _____.
extravascular (eks″trə-vas′ku-lar) **vessel** **artery**	**5-92** Vascular pertains to blood vessels. Situated or outside a vessel or the vessels is _____. Angi/ectasis (an″je-ek′tə-sis) is dilation or stretching of a _____. The suffix *-ectasia* means dilation or stretching. Arteri/ectasis (ahr″tə-re-ek′tə-sis) is dilation of an _____.

*Sarcoma (Greek: *sarx*, flesh + -oma).

5-93 Five suffixes that begin with -rrh that you need to recognize are the following:

Suffix	Meaning
-rrhage	excessive bleeding
-rrhagia	hemorrhage
-rrhaphy	suture
-rrhea	flow or discharge
-rrhexis	rupture

Use information about these suffixes to complete the following blanks:

hemorrhage

Arterio/rrhagia (**ahr-tēr″e-o-ra′jə**) is arterial _____.

**hepatorrhagia
(hep″ə-to-ra′jə)**

Using *hepat(o),* build a term that means hemorrhage from the liver: _____.

**arteriorrhexis
(ahr-tēr″e-o-rek′sis)**

Using arteri(o), build a term that means rupture of an artery: _____.

**cardiorrhexis
(kahr″de-o-rek′sis)**

Write a term that means rupture of the heart: _____.

**angiorrhaphy
(an″je-or′ə-fe)**

Suture means uniting a wound by stitches or other means to hold cut or torn edges of tissue in place. Use angi(o) to write a term that means suture of a vessel: _____.

**splenorrhaphy
(sple-nor′ə-fe)**

Write a word using splen(o) and -rrhaphy that means suture of the spleen: _____.

spleen

Spleno/rrhagia (**sple″no-ra′jə**) is hemorrhage from the _____.

5-94 When used as a suffix, -stasis* means stopping or controlling.

**stopping
(or controlling)**

Phlebo/stasis (**flə-bos′tə-sis**) is _____ the flow of blood in a vein.

Phlebostasis may be a spontaneous slowing down of blood flow in a vein or the result of a deliberate act in which one compresses the vein to control the flow of blood temporarily. In many words, -stasis will be used for either of these two meanings.

blood

Hemo/stasis (**he″mo-sta′sis**) is stopping or arresting the flow of _____.

5-95 Cardio/plegia (**kahr″de-o-ple′jə**) means the arrest of myocardial contraction, as may be induced by the use of chemicals in the performance of surgery on the heart. The suffix -plegia† means paralysis, and some interpretation of the term cardioplegia is needed.

**cardioplegic
(kahr″de-o-plej′ik)**

Solutions used to stop the heart's action so that surgery may be performed on the heart are called _____ solutions.

5-96 Lympho/genous means both forming lymph or derived from lymph or the lymphatics. Write this word that means originating in the lymphatics: _____.

**lymphogenous
(lim-foj′ə-nus)**

The lymphatic system is composed of lymphatic vessels, nodes, fluid, and three organs: the spleen, the tonsils, and the _____.

thymus

Using supra- and the suffix -ar, write a word that means above the tonsil: _____.

**supratonsillar
(soo″prə-ton′sĭ-lər)**

Combine splen(o) and -ptosis‡ to write a term that means a downward displacement (sagging) of the spleen: _____

**splenoptosis
(sple″nop-to′sis)
spleen**

A displaced spleen can be surgically corrected by spleno/pexy (**sple′no-pek″se**), which is surgical fixation of the _____.

---

*(Greek: *stasis,* a standing.)
†-plegia (Greek: *plege,* stroke).
‡(Greek: *ptosis,* a dropping.)

In the next chapters, you will practice using the less familiar word parts in this section. For now, be able to read and write the new terms. There is no review for this section.

Study the following list of selected abbreviations. Then read through the Chapter Pharmacology section and be sure you understand the effects and uses of the drug classes that are presented. When you are finished, work the Chapter Review. After completing the exercises, check your answers with the solutions in Appendix V.

You will find these items presented after the Chapter Review:
- Listing of Medical Terms
- Enhancing Spanish Communication

Selected Abbreviations

AI	aortic insufficiency	ECG, EKG	electrocardiogram
ASD	atrial septal defect	LA	left atrium
ASHD	arteriosclerotic heart disease	LCA	left coronary artery
AST (SGOT)	aspartate aminotransferase (enzyme elevated after MI)	LDH	lactate dehydrogenase (enzyme elevated after MI)
		LV	left ventricle
AV, A-V	atrioventricular	MI	myocardial infarction
BP	blood pressure	MVP	mitral valve prolapse
CA	carcinoma	PAT	paroxysmal atrial tachycardia
CABG	coronary artery bypass graft	PTA	percutaneous transluminal angioplasty
CAD	coronary artery disease	PTCA	percutaneous transluminal coronary angioplasty
CCU	critical care unit	PVC	premature ventricular contraction
CHF	congestive heart failure	RA	right atrium; rheumatoid arthritis
CK (CPK)	creatine kinase (formerly called creatine phosphokinase), enzyme released by damaged heart or other skeletal muscle)	RCA	right coronary artery
		RV	right ventricle
		SA	sinoatrial
CPR	cardiopulmonary resuscitation	T & A	tonsillectomy and adenoidectomy
CT, CAT	computed tomography	VSD	ventricular septal defect

Chapter Pharmacology

Class	Effect and Uses	Class	Effect and Uses
Antihypertensives	**Reduce Blood Pressure to Treat Hypertension**	*Calcium Channel Blockers*	*Inhibit Movement of Calcium Ions Across Cell Membranes*
ACE inhibitors (angiotensin-converting enzyme inhibitors)	*Block formation of angiotensin II*	nifedipine (Procardia)	
captopril (Capoten)		bepridil (Vascor)	
ramipril (Altace)		isradipine (DynaCirc)	
fosinopril (Monopril)		amlodipine (Norvasc)	
lisinopril (Zestril)		diltiazem (Cardizem)	
quinapril (Accupril)		verapamil (Calan)	
enalapril (Vasotec)			

Chapter Pharmacology—cont'd

Drug Class	Effects and Uses	Drug Class	Effects and Uses
Beta Adrenergic Blocking Agents	*These Exert a Quinidine-like Effect*	**Antiarrhythmic Drugs—cont'd**	**Regulate Cardiac Arrhythmias—cont'd**
atenolol (Tenormin)		propafenone (Rythmol)	
pindolol (Visken)		adenosine (Adenocard)	
metoprolol (Lopressor)			
nadolol (Corgard)		**Blood Flow Agents**	**Peripheral Vasodilators**
propranolol (Inderal)		cyclandelate (Cyclospasmol)	Used for intermittent cramping of legs
		isoxsuprine (Vasodilan)	Used for relief of symptoms of cerebral vascular insufficiency
Diuretics	*Used for Edema and Hypertension*		
hydrochlorothiazide, HCTZ (HydroDiuril)		**Cardiac Drugs**	**Used in CHF, Atrial Fibrillation, Atrial Flutter**
indapamide (Lozol)		digoxin (Lanoxin)	
metolazone (Zaroxolyn)		amrinone (Inocor)	
furosemide (Lasix)	Inhibit reabsorption of water in renal tubules		
bumetanide (Bumex)	Inhibit reabsorption of water in renal tubules	**Cholesterol Reducing Agents (Antihyperlipidemics)**	**Reduce Lipids (Cholesterol) in the Blood**
spironolactone (Aldactone)	A potassium-sparing diuretic	cholestyramine (Questran)	
triamterene (Dyrenium)	A potassium-sparing diuretic	colestipol (colestid)	
		lovastatin (Mevacor)	
Carbonic Anhydrase Inhibitors	*Used in Glaucoma*	simvastatin (Zocor)	
acetazolamide (Diamox)	Decreases intraocular pressure	pravastatin (Pravachol)	
methazolamide (Neptazane)	Decreases intraocular pressure	atorvastatin (Lipitor)	
		gemfibrozil (Lopid)	
Antianginal Drugs	**Used to Relieve Pain of Acute Angina Pectoris and for Prophylaxis**		
isosorbide mononitrate (ISMO)	Used for angina pectoris	**Ophthalmic Vasoconstrictors**	**Reduce the Amount of Aqueous Humor in the Eye and Dilate the Pupil**
nitroglycerin (Nitrostat)	Used for the management of angina pectoris	tetrahydrozoline (Visine)	Used in the eye (over the counter)
isosorbide dinitrate (Isordil)	Used for the management of angina pectoris	phenylephrine (Neo-Synephrine)	Used in the eye and nose
		naphazoline (Naphcon)	Used in the eye
Antiarrhythmic Drugs	**Regulate Cardiac Arrhythmias**		
moricizine (Ethmozine)		**Vasoconstrictors**	**Used in Shock to Support Blood Circulation**
ibutilide fumarate (Corvert)			
quinidine (Quinora)		isoproterenol (Isuprel)	
procainamide (Pronestyl)		dobutamine (Dobutrex)	
disopyramide (Norpace)		epinephrine (Adrenalin)	
lidocaine (Xylocaine)		methoxamine (Vasoxyl)	
tocainide (Tonocard)			

CHAPTER REVIEW 5

▶ BASIC UNDERSTANDING

REVIEWING WORD PARTS

I. Write a word (prefix, suffix, or combining form) for each clue.

CROSSWORD PUZZLE 5

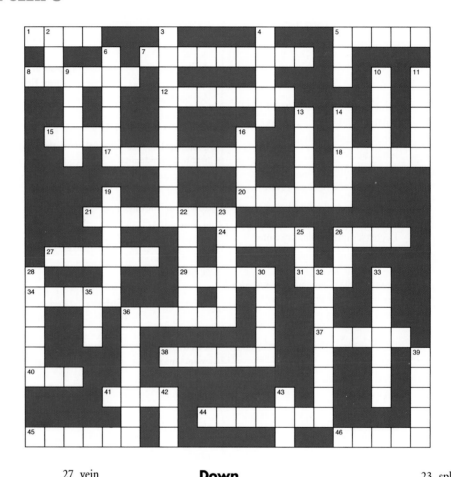

Across

1 vessel
5 fast
7 myocardium
8 lymphatics
12 lung
15 around
17 adenoids
18 thymus
20 excision
21 narrowing
24 light
26 incision
27 vein
29 swelling
31 above
34 vessel
36 crown
37 between
38 venule
40 tumor
41 sinus
44 electricity
45 chest
46 pain

Down

2 pertaining to
3 lymphatic vessel
4 gland
5 pertaining to
6 abnormal fear
9 instrument used to measure
10 artificial opening
11 septum
13 aorta
14 process of measuring
16 cutting instrument
19 yellowish, fatty plaque
22 hard
23 spleen
25 small
26 three
28 heart
30 atrium
32 peritoneum
33 production
35 membrane
36 cancer
39 skin
42 oxygen
43 to cause an action
46 L. *dexter*, right (abbrev.)

LABELING

II. Using this illustration of a capillary bed, write combining forms for the structures that are indicated. Line 1 is done as an example.

Write two combining forms for line 2 (artery) and three combining forms for line 4 (vein) as indicated on the drawing.

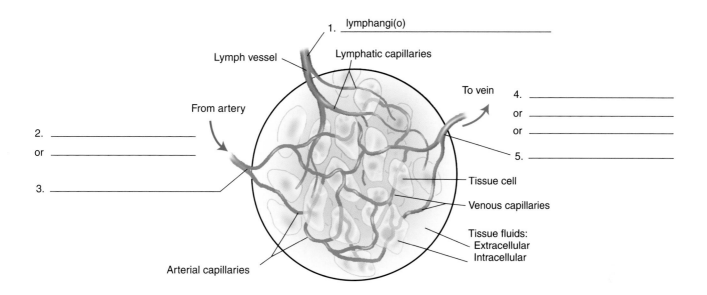

1. lymphangi(o) _____

Lymph vessel   Lymphatic capillaries

To vein   4. _____

or _____

or _____

From artery

5. _____

2. _____

or _____

Tissue cell

3. _____

Venous capillaries

Tissue fluids:
  Extracellular
  Intracellular

Arterial capillaries

LISTING

III. Name three functions of the lymphatic system:

1. _____
2. _____
3. _____

MULTIPLE CHOICE

IV. Select one answer (A-D) for each of the following:

1. Which of the following is an abnormal opening in part of the septum dividing the two ventricles?

   A. coronary heart disease   C. ventriculitis
   B. ventricular septal defect   D. ventriculoplasty

2. Which of the following is more likely to occur in a coronary occlusion?

   A. arteriosclerotic heart   C. myocardial infarction
      disease
   B. congenital heart disease   D. rheumatic fever

3. What is the term for inflammation of the sac that encloses the heart?

   A. coronary heart disease   C. myocarditis
   B. endocarditis   D. pericarditis

4. How many flaps of tissue does a tricuspid valve have?

   A. one   C. three
   B. two   D. four

5. Which of the following combining forms refers to a SPE-CIFIC type of blood vessel?

   A. angi(o)   C. phleb(o)
   B. lymph(o)   D. vas(o)

6. What is a coronary thrombosis?

   A. a myocardial infarction in   C. formation of a blood clot in a coronary artery
   B. closing off of a coronary artery   D. narrowing of the lumen of a blood vessel

7. What does hypertension mean?

   A. decreased blood pressure   C. increased blood pressure
   B. decreased pulse   D. increased pulse

8. What does excision mean?

   A. a mouthlike opening   C. formation of an artificial opening
   B. cut out or remove   D. to cut into but not remove

9. What is a lymphangioma?
   - A. a tumor composed of blood vessels
   - B. a tumor composed of lymph vessels
   - C. an echocardiogram
   - D. computed tomography of the lymphatic system

10. What is the meaning of asystole?
    - A. absence of a heart beat
    - B. contraction of the heart at maximum strength
    - C. relaxation of the heart between contractions
    - D. variation in the normal rhythm of the heart

11. What is the origin of the electrical impulse that causes the heart to contract?
    - A. brain
    - B. cisterna chyli
    - C. Purkinje fibers
    - D. sinoatrial node

12. Which of the following is a harmless tumor that consists of closely packed small blood vessels?
    - A. hemangioma
    - B. lymphadenopathy
    - C. lymphoma
    - D. vasoconstriction

13. Which term means hardening of the aorta?
    - A. aortography
    - B. aortosclerosis
    - C. aortostenosis
    - D. aortic insufficiency

14. What is the term for a ballooning out of the wall of a vessel or the heart?
    - A. aneurysm
    - B. angiocarditis
    - C. stenosis
    - D. stricture

15. What is the term for the blood pressure reading when the ventricles are relaxed?
    - A. arrhythmia
    - B. diastole
    - C. dysrrhythmia
    - D. systole

FILL IN THE BLANK

V. Write one word in each blank to complete the sentences.

1. The route that blood takes when it leaves the heart, travels throughout the body, and returns to the heart is called _____ circulation.

2. The route that oxygen-poor blood takes when it leaves the heart and picks up oxygen in the lungs is called _____ circulation.

3. The heart and the blood vessels that transport blood throughout the body are called the _____ system.

4. In general, the blood vessels that carry oxygen-rich blood to all of the body cells are called _____.

5. The smallest blood vessels are called _____.

6. The largest artery is the _____.

7. The wall of the heart consists primarily of a tissue called _____.

8. The upper chambers of the heart are called _____, and the lower chambers are called _____.

9. Blood vessels that supply blood to the heart are called _____ arteries.

10. The thymus, the spleen, the tonsils, lymphatic vessels, lymph nodes, and a special fluid make up the _____ system.

WRITING TERMS

VI. Write one word for each of the following clues:

1. any disease of the aorta _____
2. inflammation of a lymph node _____
3. obstruction _____
4. absence of a heart beat _____
5. membrane that lines the heart _____
6. outside a vessel _____
7. cancerous tumor _____
8. removal of the tonsils _____
9. decreased pulse _____
10. swelling of the lymphatics _____

▶ **GREATER COMPREHENSION**

LABELING
VII. Write the names of the parts of the lymphatic system that are indicated on the diagram.

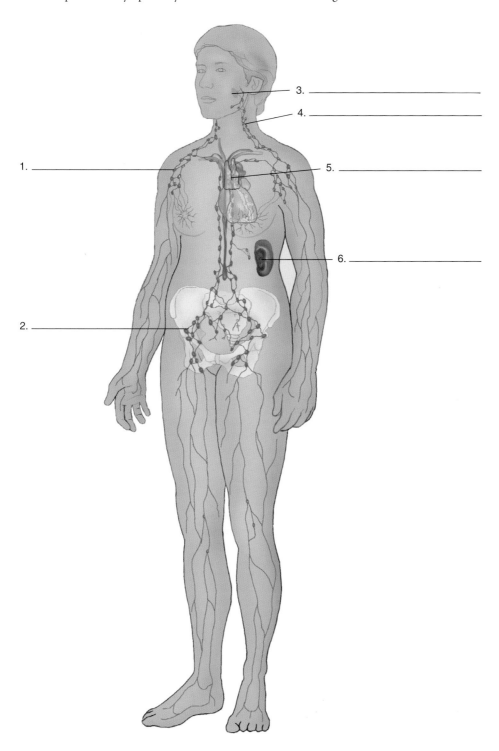

3. _____

4. _____

1. _____

5. _____

6. _____

2. _____

SPELLING
VIII. Circle all incorrectly spelled terms and write their correct spelling:

adenoidectomy   athrosclerosis   diastole   iskemia   mediastinum

FILL IN THE BLANK

IX. Write a word in each blank to complete these sentences that describe circulation.

Oxygen-poor blood is delivered to the right side of the heart via the two largest veins, the superior and inferior (1) _____

_____. The blood from these two largest veins is emptied into the chamber of the heart called the right

(2) _____. When the heart contracts, blood is forced through the tricuspid valve to the lower chamber called the

(3) _____ _____. Another contraction of the heart forces the blood into the pulmonary artery, which

branches and carries blood to the (4) _____, where it picks up oxygen. The pulmonary veins take blood back to the heart

chamber called the (5) _____ _____. The flow of blood from the left atrium to the left ventricle is controlled

by the (6) _____ valve. Blood is then pumped into the largest artery in the body, the (7) _____. This vessel

branches many times to become arteries, which again branch many times to become the smallest arteries, called (8) _____,

which in turn branch to become the smallest vessels, where oxygen is delivered to body tissues. These vessels, called

(9) _____, are composed of only a single layer of cells and are continuous with venules, which in turn are continuous

with larger vessels called (10) _____. These vessels are directly or indirectly connected with the vena cavae.

As blood circulates, interstitial fluid accumulates in the tissue spaces. This excess fluid is normally transported away from the tissues by

a vascular network called the (11) _____ system. The system is composed of vessels, nodes, the spleen, thymus, tonsils, and

a fluid called (12) _____. The fluid flows in one direction only, away from the tissue, and is eventually emptied into the

subclavian (13) _____, thus returning the fluid to the (14) _____ circulation.

LISTING

X. Name four factors that cause the blood pressure to increase:

1. _____   3. _____
2. _____   4. _____

INTERPRETING ABBREVIATIONS

XI. Write the meaning of these abbreviations:

1. ASHD _____   6. CPR _____
2. A-V _____   7. LV _____
3. CA _____   8. MI _____
4. CABG _____   9. RA _____
5. CAD _____   10. VSD _____

CASE STUDY

XII. Answer questions 1 through 5 after reading the case study.

> B.W., a 70-year-old man with a history of CHF, is seen in the ER. He complains of getting progressively weaker. He is dyspneic and has edema in the lower extremities. The records at the time of admission show the following:
>
> P: 130
> BP: 92/60
> CXR: No change from previous admission 3 months ago
> Lab work: Normal
> ECG: No change
> Rx: O_2 4 L/min per nasal prongs
> Lasix 40 mg q.d. po
> Vasotec 5 mg q.d. po
> See cardiologist in coming week.

1. What does CHF mean? _____
2. What does CXR mean? _____
3. Write the meaning of *dyspneic:* _____
4. Write the meaning of *edema:* _____
5. Interpret how each prescription is to be used: _____

PRONUNCIATION

XIII. The pronunciation is shown for several medical words. Indicate which syllable has the primary accent by marking it with an ´.

1. cardiomyopathy (**kahr de o mi op ə the**)
2. lymphadenopathy (**lim fad ə nop ə the**)
3. lymphography (**lim fog rə fe**)
4. pericardial (**per ĭ kahr de əl**)
5. vasodilation (**vas o di la shən**)

CATEGORIZING TERMS

XIV. Using definitions for anatomical, diagnostic, surgical, and radiological classification presented in exercises at the end of Chapter 4, categorize the following terms by writing A, D, S, or R after the term. (The first term is done as an example.)

Category (A, D, S, or R)

1. angiography _____R_____
2. angiostenosis _____
3. atrioseptoplasty _____
4. aortosclerosis _____
5. sarcoma _____

Category (A, D, S, or R)

6. lymphangitis _____
7. lymphography _____
8. phlebectomy _____
9. splenomegaly _____
10. venule _____

DRUG CLASSES

XV. Match the descriptions in the left column with the therapeutics A, B, C, or D.

_____ 1. decrease the diameter of blood vessels
_____ 2. may be used to control dysrhythmia
_____ 3. reduce blood pressure
_____ 4. reduce lipids in the blood

A. antiarrhythmic drugs
B. antihypertensives
C. cholesterol reducing agents
D. vasoconstrictors

(Check your answers with the solutions in Appendix V.)

Listing of Medical Terms

adenoidectomy	atrioventricular	electrocardiography	mitral valve
adenoiditis	atrium	elephantiasis	myocardial
adenoma	axillary node	endarterectomy	myocardial infarction
aneurysm	bicuspid valve	endocardial	myocarditis
aneurysmal	bradycardia	endocarditis	myocardium
angiectasis	cancerous	endocardium	pacemaker
angiectomy	capillary	epicardium	palatine tonsil
angina pectoris	carcinoma	extracorporeal	parietal pericardium
angiocardiography	cardiac catheterization	extravascular	percutaneous transluminal
angiocarditis	cardialgia	fibrillation	angioplasty
angiography	cardiocentesis	heart block	pericardial
angioma	cardiodiaphragmatic	hemangioma	pericarditis
angiopathy	cardiodynia	hematoma	pericardium
angioplasty	cardiomegaly	hemopericardium	phagocyte
angiorrhaphy	cardiomyopathy	hemostasis	phlebectomy
angiospasm	cardioplegia	hepatorrhagia	phlebitis
angiostenosis	cardioplegic	hyperemia	phleboplasty
angiostomy	cardiopulmonary bypass	hypertension	phlebosclerosis
angiotomy	cardiopulmonary	hypotension	phlebostasis
anoxia	resuscitation	infarct	phlebotomist
antiangina drug	cardiorrhexis	infarction	plaque
antiarrhythmic drug	cardiotomy	inguinal node	pulmonary circulation
antihypertensive	cardiovalvulitis	interstitial fluid	Purkinje fibers
aorta	cardiovascular	intraarterial	sclerosis
aortic	carditis	ischemia	semilunar valve
aortitis	catheter	lymph	septal
aortogram	catheterization	lymph node	septum
aortography	cervical lymph node	lymphadenitis	sinoatrial node
aortopathy	computed tomography	lymphadenoma	sonogram
arrhythmia	congenital heart disease	lymphadenopathy	sonography
arterial	congestive heart failure	lymphangiography	sphygmomanometer
arteriectasis	coronary artery disease	lymphangioma	splenalgia
arteriogram	coronary occlusion	lymphangitis	splenectomy
arteriograph	coronary thrombosis	lymphatic carcinoma	splenic
arteriography	defibrillation	lymphatics	splenolymphatic
arteriole	defibrillator	lymphatology	splenomegaly
arteriolitis	diastole	lymphatolysis	splenopathy
arteriopathy	diastolic	lymphedema	splenopexy
arteriorrhagia	dilatation	lymphocyte	splenoptosis
arteriorrhexis	diuretic	lymphogenous	splenorrhagia
arteriosclerosis	dysfunction	lymphogram	splenorrhaphy
arteriosclerotic	dysrhythmia	lymphography	stenosis
arteriovenous	echocardiogram	lymphoma	stethoscope
arteritis	echocardiography	lymphostasis	stricture
artery	echogram	macrophage	supratonsillar
asystole	echography	mediastinoscope	systemic circulation
atherosclerosis	edema	mediastinoscopy	systole
atrial septal defect	effusion	mediastinum	systolic
atriomegaly	electrocardiogram	mesenteric artery	tachycardia
atrioseptoplasty	electrocardiograph	microcardia	thoracic duct

Listing of Medical Terms—cont'd

thrombolymphangitis	tonsilloadenoidectomy	valvular	venipuncture
thrombophlebitis	tonsillotomy	valvulitis	venogram
thymectomy	tricuspid valve	varicose veins	venography
thymic	tunica adventitia	vascular	venous thrombosis
thymoma	tunica intima	vasoconstriction	ventricle
thymopathy	tunica media	vasoconstrictor	ventricular septal defect
thymus	ultrasonography	vasodilation	venular
tomogram	ultrasound	vasodilator	venule
tomograph	valval	vein	visceral pericardium
tonsillectomy	valvar	vena cava	
tonsillitis	valvate	venesection	

Español Enhancing Spanish Communication

English	Spanish (pronunciation)	English	Spanish (pronunciation)
artery	arteria (ar-TAY-re-ah)	narrow	estrecho (es-TRAY-cho)
benign	benigno (bay-NEEG-no)	obstruction	obstrucción (obs-trooc-se-ON)
blood pressure	presión sanguínea (pray-se-ON san-GEE-nay-ah)	oxygen	oxígeno (ok-SEE-hay-no)
		prolapse	prolapso (pro-LAHP-so)
cancer	cáncer (CAHN-ser)	pulse	pulso (POOL-so)
capillary	capilar (cah-pe-LAR)	rhythm	ritmo (REET-mo)
catheter	catéter (cah-TAY-ter)	sound	sonido (so-NEE-do)
cholesterol	colesterol (co-les-tay-ROL)	spleen	bazo (BAH-so)
edema	hidropesía (e-dro-pay-SEE-ah)	swelling (to swell)	hinchar (in-CHAR)
gland	glándula (GLAN-doo-lah)	tonsil	tonsila (ton-SEE-lah), amígdala (ah-MEEG-dah-lah)
heart	corazón (co-rah-SON)		
high blood pressure	hipertensión, presión alta (e-per-ten-se-ON, pray-se-ON AHL-tah)	varicose veins	venas varicosas (VAH-nahs vah-re-CO-sas)
lymph	linfa (LEEN-fah)	vein	vena (VAY-nah)
lymphatic	linfático (lin-FAH-te-co)	vessel	vaso (VAH-so)
malignant	maligno (mah-LEEG-no)	weakness	debilidad (day-be-le-DAHD)

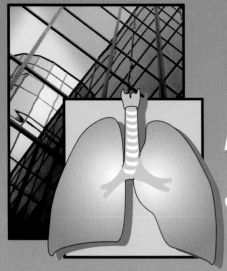

Respiratory System

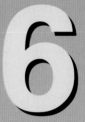

6

Outline

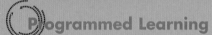

Principal Word Parts

COMBINING FORMS

acid(o)	acid
alkal(o)	alkaline, basic
alveol(o)	alveoli
anthrac(o)	coal
atel(o)	imperfect or incomplete
bronch(o), bronchi(o)	bronchi
bronchiol(o)	bronchioles
coni(o)	dust
embol(o)	embolus
epiglott(o)	epiglottis
gen(o)	origin or beginning
fibr(o)	fiber or fibrous

lith(o)	stone or calculus
lob(o)	lobe
malac(o)	softness, softening
nas(o), rhin(o)	nose
or(o)	mouth
ox(i)	oxygen
palat(o)	palate
pharyng(o)	pharynx
phas(o)	speech
phon(o)	voice
phren(o)	diaphragm or mind
plas(o)	formation or development
pleg(o)	paralysis
pleur(o)	pleura
pneum(o)	lungs or air
pulm(o), pulmon(o), pneumon(o)	lungs
spir(o)	to breathe
thorac(o)	chest
trache(o)	trachea

PREFIXES

epi-	above or upon
ex-	out, without, away from
in-	in, inside, or negative
meta-	change; next, as in a series
neo-	new
sym-, syn-	joined or together

SUFFIXES

-algia	pain
-ation	process
-capnia	carbon dioxide
-centesis	surgical puncture
-ectasia, -ectasis	stretching or dilation
-gen, -genesis, -genous	origin or beginning
-iasis	condition
-lith	stone or calculus
-malacia	softness
-ole	little or small

SUFFIXES—CONT'D

-plasia	formation or development	-ptosis	prolapse
-plasm	formation	-ptysis	spitting
-plegia	paralysis	-rrhea	flow or discharge
-pnea	breathing	-stasis	stopping or controlling

Learning Goals

▶ **BASIC UNDERSTANDING**

In this chapter, you will learn to do the following:

1. Recognize names of the structures of the respiratory system and define terms associated with these structures.
2. Sequence the flow of air from the atmosphere through the respiratory structures.
3. Distinguish between the upper respiratory tract and the lower respiratory tract.
4. Identify the functions of external respiration and its association with the acid-base balance.
5. Analyze data concerning death rates in the United States and see the significance of lung cancer incidence and deaths.
6. Write the meaning of word parts associated with the respiratory system and use them to build and analyze terms.

▶ **GREATER COMPREHENSION**

7. Differentiate terms as being related to diagnosis, anatomy, surgery, therapy, or radiology.
8. Spell the terms accurately.
9. Pronounce the terms correctly.
10. Know the meaning of the abbreviations.
11. Identify the effects or uses of the drug classes presented in this chapter.

SECTION A

*R*espiration and Its Functions

The respiratory system cooperates with the circulatory system to provide oxygen and expel waste carbon dioxide by breathing. The exchange of these gases is involved in both internal and external respiration. This chapter focuses on external respiration, the processes involved in ventilating the lungs and the exchange of oxygen and carbon dioxide between the air in the lungs and the blood. In addition to supplying oxygen for the metabolic needs of body cells, respiration helps maintain proper blood pH, body water concentration, and body temperature.

	6-1 The process of exchanging oxygen (O_2) and carbon dioxide (CO_2) is called respiration. This chapter focuses on external respiration,* the means by which the body takes in atmospheric oxygen and releases carbon dioxide.
	External respiration is the exchange of oxygen and carbon dioxide between air in the lungs and the blood. The delivery of oxygen by the blood to body cells with the removal of carbon dioxide is internal respiration.
	6-2 Breathing is one of the activities involved in respiration. Breathing is alternate inspiration (in″spĭ-ra′shən) and expiration (ek-spĭ-ra′shən) of air into and out of the lungs. The prefix **-in** means in or into. Sometimes in- means no or negative, but in in/spir/ation, in- means _____ or
in **into**	_____. The suffix **-ation** means process.
inspiration	Inspiration is the process of breathing in. The drawing of air into the lungs is _____. It is also called in/halation.
	Expelling air from the lungs is expiration. The act of breathing out or letting out one's breath is
expiration	_____. This is the same as exhalation. The prefix **ex-** means out, without, or away from.
out	Ex/piration is breathing _____.

*(Latin: *respirare*, to breathe.)

6-3 In studying the respiratory system, you will frequently see breathing referred to as pulmonary ventilation (L. *ventilare,* to fan), or simply, ventilation. You learned earlier that pulmon/ary pertains to the

lungs

_____.

Write this term that means the process by which gases are moved into or out of the lungs:

ventilation

_____.

6-4 You learned earlier that -pnea is a suffix that means breathing. Choose either a- or an- to write a word that means absence of breathing: _____. (Remember to use a- before a consonant; use an- before a vowel or the letter "h.")

apnea
(ap′ne-ə)

Sleep apnea is a sleep disorder characterized by an absence of breathing occurring five or more times an hour. The most common type in adults is obstructive sleep apnea and involves an obstruction in the upper air passageways.

breathing
dyspnea

Dys/pnea (**disp′ne-ə**) is labored or difficult _____. Dys/pne/ic (**disp-ne′ik**) is an adjective that means pertaining to or caused by _____.

6-5 Asphyxia* (**as-fik′se-ə**) or asphyxiation (**as-fik″se-a′shən**) is a condition caused by insufficient intake of oxygen. Extrinsic† causes, those originating outside the body, include drowning, crushing injuries of the chest, and inhalation of carbon monoxide. Intrinsic‡ causes include hemorrhage into the lungs or pleural cavity, foreign bodies in the throat, and diseases of the air passages. Asphyxia is caused by lack of _____.

oxygen

Cyanosis, dyspnea, and tachycardia accompanied by mental disturbances are seen in asphyxia. In extreme cases, convulsions, unconsciousness, and death may occur.

blue discoloration
of the skin

Cyanosis is _____.

difficult breathing

Dyspnea is _____ _____.

rapid pulse

Tachycardia is _____ _____.

asphyxia or
asphyxiation

Write the term that means a condition caused by insufficient intake of oxygen: (Be careful with the spelling!) _____.

6-6 Under normal conditions, the average adult takes in about one pint of air in about 12 to 15 breaths a minute.

Hyperpnea (**hi″pərp-ne′ə**) is an exaggerated deep or rapid respiration. It occurs normally with exercise and abnormally in several conditions, including pain, fever, hysteria, or inadequate oxygen. The latter can occur in cardiac or respiratory disease. A literal translation of hyper/pnea is _____

increased
breathing

_____.

Hyper/pnea may lead to hyper/ventilation (**hi″per-ven″tĭ-la′shən**)—increased aeration of the lungs—which commonly reduces carbon dioxide levels in the body. Carbon dioxide contributes to the acidity of body fluids. Alkalosis (**al″kə-lo′sis**) is a pathologic condition resulting from the accumulation of basic substances or from the loss of acid by the body. Transient§ means not lasting or of brief duration.

hyperventilation
carbon dioxide

Transient alkalosis can be caused by _____. In this case, alkalosis is caused by loss of

_____ _____.

hyperpnea

A word that means an abnormal increase in the depth and rate of respiration is _____.

---

*(a, no + Greek, *phyxis,* pulse.)
†(Latin: *extrinsecus,* situated on the outside.)
‡(Latin: *intrinsecus,* situated on the inside.)
§(Latin: *trans,* to go by.)

alkaline	**6-7** The abbreviation pH means potential hydrogen, a calculated scale that represents the relative acidity or alkalinity of a solution, in which a value of 7.0 is neutral, below 7.0 is acidic, and above 7.0 is alkaline. The normal pH of body fluids (plasma, intracellular, and interstitial fluids) is 7.35 to 7.45. Is normal plasma slightly acid or alkaline? _____
balance	Cellular metabolism produces substances such as excess carbon dioxide that would upset the pH were it not for buffer systems of the blood and functions of the respiratory and urinary systems that help keep the pH constant. The state of equilibrium of the blood pH is called the acid-base balance. The expelling of carbon dioxide when one exhales is part of the regulatory mechanism that maintains the constancy of the pH, that is, the acid-base _____ .
alkaline blood	**6-8** The combining form *alkal(o)* means alkaline or basic. Alkal/osis is an alkaline condition. Alkal/emia (al″kə-le′me-ə) is _____ _____ , or increased alkalinity of the blood.
acid	Alkal/emia is an aspect of alkalosis, the general term for accumulation of basic substances in the body fluids. The opposite of alkalosis is acidosis. The combining form *acid(o)* means acid. Acid/osis is an _____ condition of the body.
acidosis (as″ĭ-do′sis)	A pathologic condition that results from accumulation of acid or depletion of alkaline substances is called _____ .
hypercapnia (hi″pər-kap′ne-ə)	**6-9** The suffix *-capnia* refers to carbon dioxide. Build a word using hyper- that means excessive carbon dioxide: _____ . (It is understood that this term means excessive carbon dioxide in the blood.)
lowering	Carbon dioxide contributes to the acidity of blood. Does hypercapnia result in lowering or increasing the blood pH? _____ .
	Within minutes, the lungs begin to compensate for any acid-base imbalance by increasing the excretion of carbon dioxide through faster or deeper breathing.
hypocapnia (hi″po-kap′ne-ə)	**6-10** The opposite of hypercapnia is _____ .
absence of carbon dioxide	Acapnia (ə-kap′ne-ə) is a synonym for hypocapnia, although in its strictest sense a/capnia means _____ .
hypocapnia	Hyperventilation would lead to which, hypercapnia or hypocapnia? _____
acidemia	**6-11** Acid/emia (as″ĭ-de′me-ə) is an arterial blood pH below 7.35, while alkal/emia is recognized as a blood pH above 7.45. Either of these conditions can be considered an acid-base imbalance. Look at some conditions listed in Table 6-1 that can lead to an acid-base imbalance.
	Asphyxia leads to which condition, alkalemia or acidemia? _____
alkalemia	Vomiting of gastric acid leads to which, alkalemia or acidemia? _____

TABLE 6-1 Acid-Base Imbalances

	ACIDEMIA	ALKALEMIA
	Ingestion of highly acidic drugs	Ingestion of alkaline drugs
	Severe diarrhea	Intense hyperventilation
	Severe diabetes	Vomiting of gastric acid
	Asphyxia	Metabolic problems
	Vomiting of lower intestinal contents	Disease
	Disease, particularly respiratory or kidney failure	

below

blood

6-12 Acute (ə-kūt′) diseases begin abruptly with intensity and subside after a short period of time. Symptoms are also described as acute. Chronic (kron′ik) symptoms or disease, persist over a long period of time.

Acute respiratory failure is a sudden inability of the lungs to maintain normal respiratory function. It may be caused by an obstruction in the airways or failure of the lungs. Respiratory failure leads to hyp/ox/ia. Hypoxia (hi-pok′se-ə) is a reduction of oxygen in body tissues to levels below those required for normal metabolic functioning. Hypoxia is _____ normal levels of oxygen in the body tissue. Remember *ox/i* means oxygen. Note the spelling of hyp/ox/ia (the "o" of hypo- has been dropped).

Hyp/ox/emia (hi″pok-se′me-ə) is decreased oxygen in the _____. Once again, notice the spelling.

excessive

6-13 You learned earlier that asphyxia is caused by insufficient intake of oxygen. This leads to hypoxemia, hypercapnia, loss of consciousness, and death, if not corrected. Hyper/capnia is _____ carbon dioxide in the blood. A laboratory blood gas determination would show a low pH, increased carbon dioxide, and a low oxygen level.

Corrective measures are removal of any obstruction of the airway and provision of artificial ventilation and oxygen. Artificial respiration may be manual, as in the lifesaving procedure cardiopulmonary resuscitation (CPR) or provided by a mechanical ventilator, a device used to provide assisted respiration and usually a temporary life-support.

oxygen

across the trachea

6-14 In chronic obstructive pulmonary disease (COPD) or other problems in hypoxic patients, oxygen therapy may be prescribed by the physician. Hyp/ox/ic means pertaining to hypoxia, or deficient _____ in the blood. Oxygen is sometimes administered after general surgery.

In patients who can breathe but are hypoxic, oxygen is delivered through tubing via a mask, nasal prongs, or a flexible catheter placed directly into the trachea (windpipe). The latter is called transtracheal (trans-tra′ke-əl) oxygen delivery. Remembering that trans- means across, the literal translation of trans/trache/al is _____.
Transtracheal means passage through the wall of the trachea.

The use of transtracheal oxygen (TTO) is an alternative for patients who require long-term use of oxygen. It is more efficient and avoids irritation of the nose, and some patients think it is more cosmetically acceptable. Three means of administering oxygen are illustrated in Figure 6-1. The term *cannula* (kan′u-lə) means a flexible tube that may be inserted into a duct or cavity to deliver medication or drain fluid. The nasal cannula shown in Figure 6-1, *B*, delivers oxygen.

straight, breathing

straight

6-15 In ortho/pnea (or″thop-ne′ə, or″thop′ne-ə), breathing is difficult except in an upright position. Analyze ortho/pnea:

orth(o) means _____; -pnea means _____.

In orthopnea, breathing may be impossible except when the person is sitting up or in a _____ position.

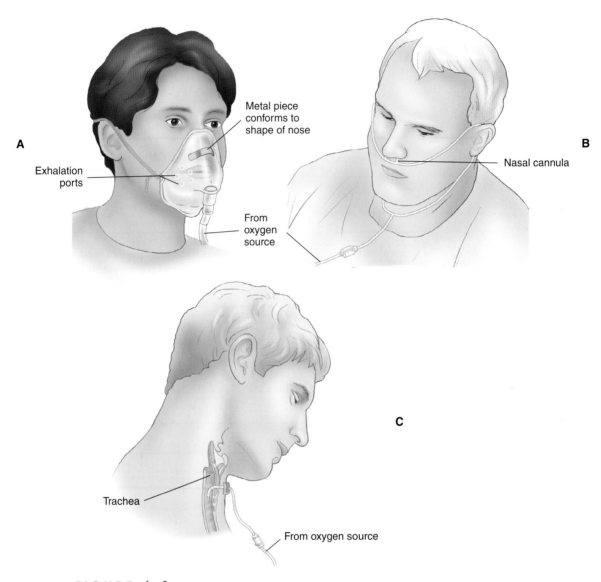

A

Metal piece
conforms to
shape of nose

Exhalation
ports

From
oxygen
source

B

Nasal cannula

C

Trachea

From oxygen source

FIGURE 6-1

Three means of administering oxygen. **A,** A simple oxygen mask delivers high concentrations of oxygen and is used for short-term oxygen therapy or in an emergency. **B,** The nasal cannula, a device that delivers oxygen by way of two small tubes that are inserted into the nostrils, is frequently used for long-term oxygen maintenance. Nasal means pertaining to the nose. **C,** Transtracheal oxygen is a long-term method of delivering oxygen directly into the lungs. It is more efficient and is an alternative to the nasal cannula.

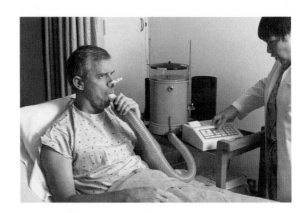

FIGURE 6-2
Spirometry. Evaluation of the air capacity of the lungs uses a spirometer, such as the one shown. The spirometer is used to assess pulmonary function by measuring and recording the volume of inhaled and exhaled air. (From Wilson SF, Thompson JM: *Respiratory disorders*, St Louis, 1990, Mosby.)

fast **bradypnea** **(brad″e-ne′ə)**	**6-16** One normally takes about 12 to 15 breaths per minute. If one were breathing at a rate of 25 breaths per minute at rest, this would be tachypnea. The word tachy/pnea (**tak″ip-ne′ə, tak″e-ne′ə**) means _____ breathing. The opposite of this is slow breathing, or _____.
spirometer **(spi-rom′ə-tər)** **spirometer**	**6-17** The lung volume in normal quiet breathing is approximately 500 ml; however, forced maximum inspiration raises this level considerably. Spiro/metry (**spi-rom′ə-tre**) is a measurement of the amount of air taken into and expelled from the lungs (Figure 6-2). The combining form *spir(o)* means breath or breathing. The instrument used is a _____. The largest volume of air that can be exhaled after maximal inspiration is the vital capacity (VC). A reduction in vital capacity often indicates a loss of functioning lung tissue. Vital capacity is measured by an instrument called a _____. Spirometry is one type of pulmonary function test (PFT) that helps determine the capacity of the lungs to exchange oxygen and carbon dioxide effectively.

❑ SECTION A REVIEW   *R*espiration and Its Functions

This section review covers frames 6–1 through 6–17. Complete the table by writing either the word part or its meaning in the blank spaces.

Combining Form	Meaning	Prefix	Meaning
1. acid(o)	_____	4. _____	in, into, or not
2. alkal(o)	_____	5. _____	out, without, away from
3. spir(o)	_____	**Suffix**	**Meaning**
		6. _____	process
		7. _____	carbon dioxide

(Use Appendix V to check your answers.)

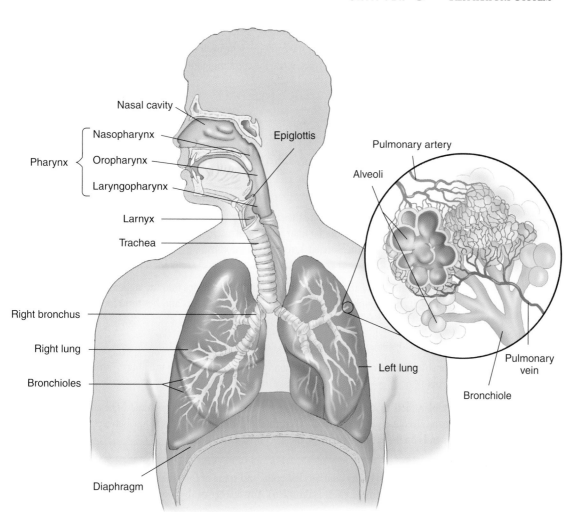

FIGURE 6-3
Structures of the respiratory system.

*S*tructures of the Respiratory Tract

The respiratory tract is the complex of organs and structures that perform pulmonary ventilation and the exchange of oxygen and carbon dioxide between the air and the blood as it circulates through the lungs. It is divided into the upper respiratory tract and the lower respiratory tract.

6-18 The primary function of the respiratory system is to provide oxygen for the body and to remove carbon dioxide. Secondary functions are maintaining acid-base balance, producing speech, facilitating smell, and maintaining the body's heat and water balance. The conducting passages of this system are known as the upper respiratory tract and the lower respiratory tract. See the names of the structures in Figure 6-3.

upper
lower

The nose, pharynx **(far′inks),** and larynx **(lar′inks,)** comprise the _____ respiratory tract. The trachea, bronchi, bronchioles, and lungs belong to the _____ respiratory tract.

rhin(o)	**6-19** You have already learned the combining forms for some of these structures. Beginning with structures of the upper respiratory tract, write the combining forms for the following structures: nose _____ pharynx ___**pharyng(o)**___ larynx _____

6-19 ... (see side column)

rhin(o)

laryng(o)

lung

The combining form **trache(o)** means trachea (tra´ke-ə) or windpipe. You learned in a previous chapter that pulmon(o) means _____. Three additional combining forms that mean lungs are presented in the next section.

Three names that may be new are the right and left bronchi (plural of bronchus), the bronchioles, and the alveoli. Most people are more familiar with the structures of the upper respiratory tract, because those of the lower respiratory tract are enclosed within the chest.

6-20 In the mediastinum, the trachea (windpipe) divides into the right and left primary bronchi; **bronch(o)** and **bronchi(o)** mean bronchi. Bronchial tubes is another term for bronchi (singular is bronchus).

pertaining to the bronchi

little

pertaining to alveoli

Bronchi/al means _____.

Bronchioles are small airways that extend from the bronchi into the lungs. Translated literally, bronchi/ole means _____ bronchus.

Alveolar ducts that end in clusters of alveoli extend from the bronchioles. The combining form **alveol(o)** means alveolus (plural is alveoli). Oxygen and carbon dioxide exchange between the air and the blood depends on these tiny structures, the alveoli. Alveol/ar means _____.

thoracopathy (tho″rə-kop´ə-the)

thoracoplasty

6-21 The chest cavity contains the lungs and some of the other organs of respiration. Remember that the combining form for chest is thorac(o). Any disease of the thoracic organs or tissues is a _____.

Thoraco/plasty (tho″rə-ko-plas´te) is a surgical procedure that involves removing ribs and allowing the chest wall to collapse a diseased lung. The procedure that collapses a diseased lung is called a _____.

diaphragm

6-22 The formal anatomic name for the diaphragm is diaphragma (di″ə-frag´mə). Diaphragma/tic means pertaining to the _____.

Long ago, people believed that the midriff was the seat of emotions; the Greek word *phren* was applied to this area as a structure, as well as the center of emotions. For this reason diaphragm and mind have the same combining form.

The combining form **phren(o)** means the diaphragm, the muscular partition that separates the thoracic and abdominal cavities. It is pierced by several openings which pass the aorta, the venae cavae, and the esophagus. It aids respiration by moving up and down (Figure 6-4). The combining form *phren(o)* also means mind, which is studied in Chapter 11.

diaphragm

When one is studying respiration, phren(o) probably refers to the muscular partition that separates the chest and abdominal cavities, the _____.

phrenitis (frə-ni´tis)
pertaining to the diaphragm
pain in the diaphragm

6-23 Write a word that means inflammation of the diaphragm: _____.

Phren/ic (fren´ik) means _____.
(Phrenic also means pertaining to the mind.)

Phreno/dynia (fren″o-din´e-ə) is _____.

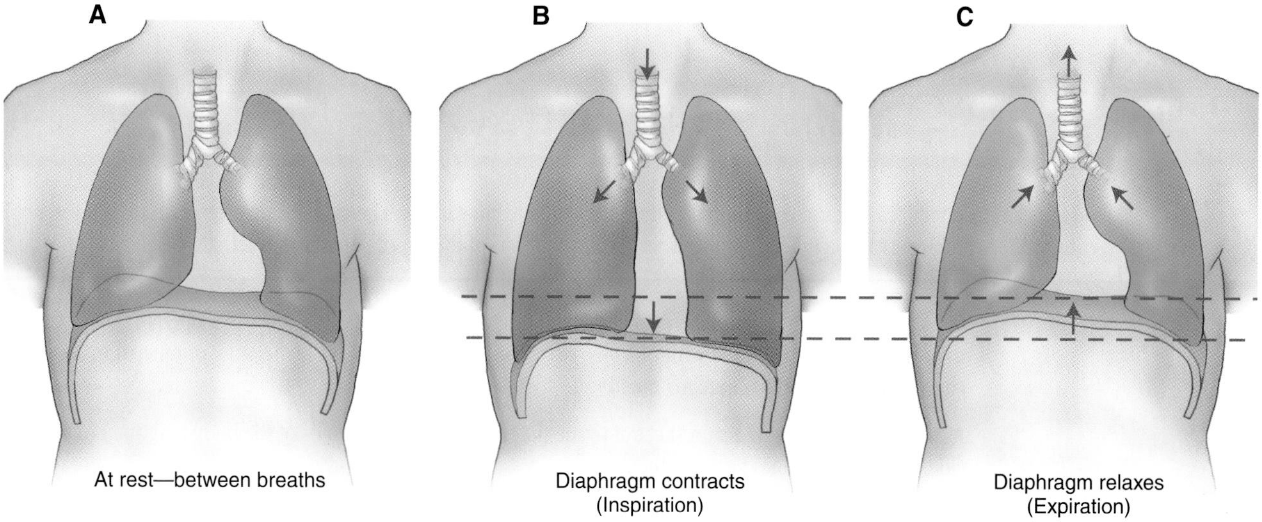

A At rest—between breaths

B Diaphragm contracts (Inspiration)

C Diaphragm relaxes (Expiration)

FIGURE 6-4
Changes in the lungs and diaphragm during respiration. **A,** Diaphragm relaxed, just before inspiration. **B,** Inspiration. The diaphragm contracts, moving downward and increasing the size of the thoracic cavity. Inspiration is also aided by contraction of the intercostal muscles, which are between the ribs. Air moves into the lungs until pressure inside the lungs equals atmospheric pressure. **C,** Expiration. Respiratory muscles relax, and the chest cavity decreases in size as air moves from the lungs out into the atmosphere.

phrenoplegia (fren″o-ple′jə)	**6-24** Learn these word parts: ***pleg(o)*** means paralysis, ***-plegia*** is a suffix meaning paralysis. Paralysis of the diaphragm is _____.
diaphragm	Phreno/ptosis **(fren″op-to′sis)** is a prolapsed or downward displacement of the _____.
	Ptosis **(to′sis)** is a word that means drooping or sagging of an organ or a part. (When ptosis is used as a word, sometimes it means paralytic drooping of the upper eyelid.) When used as a suffix, **-ptosis** means downward displacement or prolapse and does not refer to a specific organ or part. It is added to combining
prolapse	forms to mean sagging or _____.
phrenoptosis	Prolapse of the diaphragm is _____.

❏ SECTION B REVIEW   *S*tructures of the Respiratory Tract

This section review covers frames 6–18 through 6–24. Complete the table by writing either the word part or its meaning in the blank spaces.

Combining Form	Meaning		Suffix	Meaning
1. alveol(o)	_____		8. -plegia	_____
2. bronch(o)	_____		9. -ptosis	_____
3. bronchi(o)	_____			
4. pharyng(o)	_____			
5. pleg(o)	_____			
6. _____	diaphragm or mind			
7. _____	trachea			

(Use Appendix V to check your answers.)

Upper Respiratory Passageways

The upper respiratory tract consists of the nose, the pharynx, and the larynx. The sinuses are often included in the upper passageways. Upper respiratory problems can occur alone or progress to complications of the lower respiratory tract, such as in viral infections.

mucus	**6-25** Air enters the respiratory tract through the nose. Like other structures that open to the outside, the respiratory tract is lined with mucous membrane. Having learned the meaning of muc(o) in an earlier chapter, you know that a mucous membrane secretes _____. A mucous membrane is a thin sheet of tissue that lines cavities or canals of the body that open to the outside. These membranes secrete mucus.
nose pharynx larynx trachea bronchi, bronchioles alveoli	**6-26** Looking back at Figure 6-3, trace the passage of air through the respiratory system by writing the names of respiratory structures in the blanks: Air first enters the body through the _____, where it is warmed, moistened, and filtered. Air then passes to the _____, commonly called the throat. Air then passes over the vocal cords in the _____, commonly called the voice box, before reaching the _____, also known as the windpipe. The trachea divides into two primary _____, which divide further into many _____. Oxygen and carbon dioxide are exchanged within structures called _____.
pertaining to the nose nose nasoseptoplasty (na″zo-sep′to-plas-te) endonasal (en″do-na′zəl)	**6-27** The combining form ***nas(o)*** means nose. The term *nose* includes the external nose, which protrudes from the face, and the nasal cavity. Nas/al (**na′zəl**) means _____. These nares (**na′rēz**), or nostrils, are the external openings of the _____ and are separated by a partition called the nasal septum. Nasal septal reconstruction is the excision and resection of the nasal cartilage, performed to provide an adequate airway by correcting a septal defect. Write a term using nas(o), sept(o), and -plasty that means nasal septal reconstruction: _____. The nares lead into two nasal cavities. Build a word using endo- that means inside (within) the nose: _____.
mouth nose, mouth palate posterior or back	**6-28** Remembering that or(o) means mouth, oral means pertaining to the _____. Both cartilage and bone give structure to the nose. The nasal septum is composed of cartilage. The palate (**pal′ət**) separates the nasal cavity and the oral cavity. The palate, or roof of the mouth, separates the _____ and the _____. The anterior portion of the palate separates the nasal and oral cavities. It consists of bone and the membrane that covers it. Because it contains bone, it is called the hard _____. The soft palate is the fleshy posterior portion of the palate. The uvula (**u′vu-lə**) projects from the soft palate. The soft palate is in the _____ of the mouth.
uvula inflammation of the palate palatoplasty (pal′ə-to-plas″te)	**6-29** The combining form ***palat(o)*** means palate. Palatine (**pal′ə-tīn**) refers to the palate. The pendant, fleshy tissue that hangs from the soft palate, is the palatine _____. Palat/itis (**pal″ə-ti′tis**) is _____. Write a word that means surgical repair (reconstruction) of the palate: _____.

	6-30 The para/nasal (**par″ə-na′sal**) sinuses, which are air-filled cavities in various bones around the nose, surround the nasal cavity and open into it.
sinuses	A sinus is a recess, cavity, or channel. The paranasal sinuses contain air and serve to lighten the bones of the skull. The air-containing cavities connected to the nose are the paranasal _____.
nose	Fluids from the paranasal sinuses are discharged into the _____.
inflammation	Sinus/itis (**si″nə-si′tis**) is _____ of a sinus. During infections and allergies, swelling may block the passages and cause fluid to accumulate in the sinuses. A sinus headache can result from the pressure within the sinuses.
nasal	**6-31** The naso/lacrimal (**na″zo-lak′rĭ-məl**) duct also opens into the nasal cavity. The nasolacrimal duct is a tubular passage that carries fluid (tears) from the eye to the _____ cavity. Now you can understand why the nose fills with fluid when one cries.
nose	Lacrimal pertains to tears. Naso/lacrimal pertains to tears and the _____.
pertaining to smell	The nose has nerve endings that detect many odors. Olfactory (**ol-fak′tə-re**)* pertains to the sense of smell. Olfaction, the sense of smell, is a function of the nose. Olfactory means _____.
nose	**6-32** A polyp (**pol′ip**) is a growth or mass protruding from a mucous membrane. Polyps are usually (but not always) benign. They can grow on almost any mucous membrane, such as the nose, bladder, or rectum. Nasal polyps grow in the _____. (A polyp in the nasal cavity or in the sinuses is called a nasal polyp.)
an instrument for inspecting the nasal cavity	A nasal polyp might be seen by the physician with the help of a nasoscope (**na′zo-skōp**). A naso/scope is _____.
rhinitis (ri-ni′tis)	**6-33** The combining form *rhin(o)* also means nose. Build a word using rhin(o) that means inflammation of the mucous membranes of the nose: _____.
	A sign of rhinitis is coryza† (**ko-ri′zə**), derived from the Greek term *koryza* and meaning a profuse discharge of the mucous membranes of the nose.
nose	The suffix *-rrhea* means flow or discharge. Rhino/rrhea (**ri″no-re′ə**) is discharge from the _____. This is commonly called a runny nose.
surgical repair of the nose	Rhino/plasty (**ri′no-plas″te**) is _____.
nose	**6-34** A rhino/lith (**ri′no-lith**) is a calculus or stone in the _____.
calculus	A calculus (**kal′ku-ləs**) or stone is an abnormal concretion in the body, chiefly occurring in hollow organs or their passages. You may have heard of gallstones or kidney stones. Another name for a stone is a _____.
nasal calculus (stone of the nose)	A calculus (plural is calculi) consists of inorganic substances, such as calcium and phosphate, that crystallize to form a hard mass resembling a pebble. The combining form *lith(o)* means stone or calculus, and the corresponding suffix is *-lith.* A rhino/lith is a _____.
a condition of nasal calculi	**6-35** Lith/iasis (**lĭ thi′ə-sis**) is a condition marked by formation of stones. The suffix *-iasis* means condition. Rhino/lith/iasis is _____.
lithiasis	Write the word that includes -iasis and means a condition characterized by formation of stones: _____.
rhinolithiasis (ri″no-lĭ-thi′ə-sis)	Now write the term that means a condition marked by the presence of nasal calculi: _____.

*(Latin: *olfacere*, to smell.)
†(Greek: *Koryza*.)

origin (or beginning) lithogenesis origin or beginning of cancer	**6-36** The formation or origin of a stone is litho/genesis (**lith″o-gen′ə-sis).** The suffix *-genesis* means origin or beginning. Words that contain -genesis imply _____. It is often impossible to determine the origin of a stone. The origin of a stone is called _____. Carcinogenesis (**kahr″sĭ-no-jen′ə-sis**) is another term that contains -genesis and means _____.
	6-37 The combining form *gen(o)* means origin or beginning; *-gen,* -genic, and *-genous* are suffixes having to do with origin or beginning. They can mean either produced by something or producing. Practice will help you determine which meaning is intended.
carcinogen that which causes cancer carcinolysis (kahr″sĭ-nol′ə-sis)	**6-38** A carcino/gen (**kahr-sin′ə-jen**) is any substance that causes cancer. It has been well documented that the tar in cigarettes is a carcinogen implicated in carcinoma of the lungs. A substance that causes cancer is a _____. Carcino/gen/ic (**kahr″sin-o-jen′ik**) pertains to _____. Destruction of cancer (cells) is _____.
origin of a stone pharynx	**6-39** Litho/genesis is the _____. A rhinolith can interfere with breathing through the nose, making it more comfortable to breathe through the mouth. Regardless of whether air is taken in by the nose or the mouth, it passes to the pharynx, a muscular tube about 13 cm (or 5 inches) long in an adult. The pharynx also functions as part of the digestive system in the swallowing of food. The muscular cavity lying behind the nose and mouth and commonly called the throat is the _____.
pharynx mouth, pharynx	**6-40** Remembering that pharyng(o) means the pharynx, pharyng/eal (**fə-rin′je-əl**) refers to the _____. Oro/pharyngeal (**o″ro-fə-rin′je-əl**), is pertaining to the _____ and _____. (This term also pertains to the oropharynx [o″ro far′inks] [Figure 6-3]).
pharyngitis (far″in-ji′tis) pharyngodynia (fəring″go-din′ e-ə)	**6-41** Build a word that means inflammation of the throat: _____. Sore throat usually accompanies pharyngitis. Sore throat (pharyngeal pain) is _____. This is the same as pharyng/algia (**far″in gal′jə**). Both -dynia and *-algia* mean pain. In many but not all circumstances, both -dynia and -algia are used to write terms for pain in various structures of the body. Tonsill/itis is one reason for a sore throat. The tonsils are located in the oropharynx.
throat (or pharynx) pharyngopathy (far″ing-gop′ə-the) pharyngoplasty (fə-ring′go-plas″te)	**6-42** A pharyngo/scope (**fə-ring′go-skōp**) is an instrument for examining the _____. Write a word that means any disease of the pharynx: _____. Plastic surgery to repair the pharynx is _____.

nose	**6-43** Naso/pharynx (**na′zo-far′inks**) refers to the _____ and throat. The nasopharynx is the upper part of the pharynx and is continuous with the nasal passages.
nose, mouth larynx	In referring to parts of the pharynx, three divisions are recognized (Figure 6-3): the nasopharynx, the oropharynx, and the laryngopharynx [**lə-ring″go-far′ ənks**]). The naso/pharynx is that part of the pharynx that lies behind the _____. The oro/pharynx lies behind the _____. The laryngopharynx is that part of the pharynx that lies near the _____.
behind the nose	**6-44** The auditory tube, formerly called the eustachian (**u-sta′ke-ən**) tube, is a narrow channel connecting the middle ear and the nasopharynx. The opening to the auditory tube is in the nasopharynx. The adenoids are also located in the nasopharynx, which is the part of the pharynx situated _____.
nasopharynx	Naso/pharyng/eal (**na″zo-fə-rin′je-əl**) pertains to the _____.
nasopharyngitis (**na″zo-far″in-ji′tis**)	Inflammation of the nasopharynx is _____.
behind or in the back of the mouth	**6-45** The oropharynx contains the palatine tonsils, which are visible when the mouth is open wide. The oropharynx is situated _____.
larynx	The lowest part of the pharynx is called the laryngopharynx. It is here that the pharynx divides into the larynx and the esophagus. Air passes through the _____, and food passes through the esophagus.
larynx	**6-46** The larynx contains the vocal cords and is also called the voice box. Laryngo/plegia (**lə-ring″ go-ple′jeə**) is paralysis of the _____.
larynx pharynx	Laryngo/pharyng/eal (**lə-ring″go-fə-rin′je-əl**) refers to the _____ and the _____.
laryngitis (**lar″ in-ji′tis**)	**6-47** Build a word that means inflammation of the larynx: _____.
laryngitis	This condition would probably result in temporary loss of voice. Inflammation of the larynx may be caused not only by infectious microorganisms, but also by overuse of the voice, allergies, or irritants. Inflammation of the mucous membrane of the larynx is _____.
larynx	**6-48** A person with laryngitis often suffers only minor discomfort. If the larynx becomes painful, the person has laryng/algia (**lar″in gal′jə**), which is pain of the _____.
	You may be wondering if you could combine laryng(o) with -dynia, which also means pain. Although some people would know what you mean, this term is not generally found in the dictionary.
polyp	**6-49** You learned earlier that a polyp is a tumorlike growth, usually benign, that projects from a mucous membrane. A growth of this type on the vocal cords is called a laryngeal _____.
	The vocal cords consist of a pair of strong bands of elastic tissue with a mouthlike opening through which air passes, creating sound. Observe their structure in Figure 6-5 and the small laryngeal polyp.
	Although painless, laryngeal polyps cause hoarseness. They are generally caused by smoking, allergies, or abuse of the voice, and eliminating the cause often relieves the hoarseness. If the individual smokes, smoking cessation adjuncts may help remove the desire to smoke. Surgery can be performed using direct laryngoscopy if rest does not correct the problem.
examination of the larynx	Laryngo/scopy (**lar″ing-gos′kə-pe**) is _____.
laryngoscope (**lə-ring′gə-skōp**)	Change the suffix in laryngo/scopy to write a term that means the instrument used in this procedure: _____.

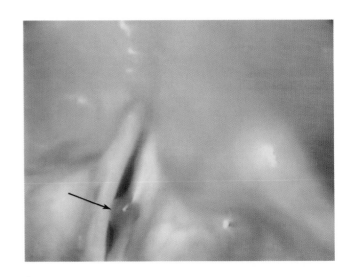

FIGURE 6-5

A laryngeal polyp. This hemorrhagic polyp (arrow) on the vocal cord occurs most commonly in adults who smoke, have many allergies, live in dry climates, or abuse the voice. (From Ignatavicius DD, Workman ML, Mishler MA: *Medical-surgical nursing across the health care continuum,* ed 3, Philadelphia, 1999, WB Saunders.)

laryngectomy (lar"in-jek'tə-me) **laryngospasm** (lə-ring'go-spaz-əm)	**6-50** In laryngeal cancer, surgical removal of the larynx would probably be necessary. Write a word that means excision of the larynx: _____ Spasm of laryngeal muscles is _____.
laryngography (lar"ing-gog'rə-fe) **formation of an opening into the larynx** **laryngoplasty** (lə-ring'go-plas"te) **laryngopathy** (lar"ing-gop'ə-the)	**6-51** X-ray examination of the larynx after application of a radiopaque dye is called _____. Laryngo/stomy (**lar"ing-gos'tə-me**) is _____. Plastic repair of the larynx is _____. Any disease of the larynx is a _____.
glottis	**6-52** The glottis is the vocal apparatus of the larynx. It consists of the vocal cords and the opening between them. The vocal cords are also called vocal folds. These vocal folds are part of the special structure in the larynx called the _____. Muscles open and close the glottis during inspiration and expiration, and they regulate the vocal cords during the production of sound. Muscles also close off a lidlike structure that covers the glottis during swallowing. The lidlike structure, which is composed of cartilage and covers the larynx during the swallowing of food, is called the epiglottis (**ep"ĭ-glot'is**).
above **inflammation**	**6-53** The prefix *epi-* means above or upon. The epi/glottis lies _____ the glottis and closes like a lid during swallowing. Epiglott/itis or epiglottid/itis (**ep"ĭ-glot"ĭ-di'tis**) is _____ of the epiglottis. The combining form *epiglott(o)* means epiglottis. Epiglottides is the plural of epiglottis, hence the term epiglottiditis.

aspiration	**6-54** Aspiration is the drawing in or out as by suction. Foreign bodies may be aspirated into the nose, throat, or lungs on inspiration. Aspiration also refers to the withdrawing of fluid from a cavity by means of suction. Drawing in or out by suction is called _____.
	If one inspires while attempting to swallow, food may be accidentally aspirated into the larynx. Spontaneous coughing is the body's effort to clear the obstructed airway. Respiration stops if complete obstruction of the airway occurs.
epiglottis	In usual situations, food does not enter the larynx, but passes on to the esophagus. Food does not enter the larynx because a lidlike structure, the _____, is closed.
respiration (or breathing)	**6-55** An upper airway obstruction is any significant interruption in the airflow through the nose, mouth, pharynx, or larynx. Laryngoscopy may be helpful in locating and removing the cause of the obstruction. If the cause is not removed, respiratory arrest occurs. Respiratory arrest is cessation of _____.
	Tracheo/stomy (**tra″ke-os′tə-me**) may be necessary in upper airway obstruction. This procedure will be studied along with other terms related to the lower respiratory passages in the next section.

❑ SECTION C REVIEW   𝒰pper Respiratory Passageways

This section review covers frames 6–25 through 6–55. Complete the table by writing either a word part or its meaning in each blank space.

Combining Form	Meaning	Suffix	Meaning
1. epiglott(o)	_____	7. -algia	_____
2. _____	origin	8. -gen, -genous, or -genesis	_____
3. _____	stone	9. -iasis	_____
4. nas(o)		10. -lith	_____
5. _____	palate	11. _____	flow or discharge

Prefix	Meaning
6. epi-	_____

(Use Appendix V to check your answers.)

ℒower Respiratory Passageways

The lower respiratory tract includes the trachea, two primary bronchi and several secondary bronchi, bronchioles, alveolar ducts, and alveoli. The two lungs are composed of millions of alveoli and their related ducts, bronchioles, and bronchi. The lower respiratory tract is a common site of infections, obstructive conditions, and malignancy.

bronchi	**6-56** The lower respiratory tract is a continuation of the upper respiratory tract. The lower respiratory tract begins with the trachea, which is commonly referred to as the windpipe. The trachea branches into the right and left primary _____. Bronchi are lined with cilia, hairlike projections that propel mucus up and away from the lower airway.
bronchioles alveoli	Bronchi branch to become _____, structures that lead to alveolar ducts. At the ends of the ducts are the structures where gas exchange occurs. These structures are called _____.

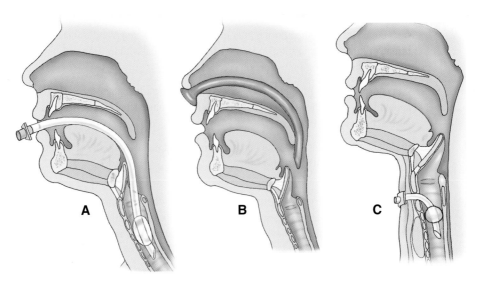

FIGURE 6-6
Comparison of endotracheal intubation and a tracheostomy tube. **A,** Orotracheal intubation for short-term airway management. **B,** Nasotracheal intubation for short-term airway management. **C,** Tracheostomy tube for longer maintenance of the airway.

trachea pertaining to the trachea	**6-57** The dividing point where solid foods are separated from air occurs in the laryngopharynx. Food enters the esophagus, and air passes through the larynx to reach the trachea. You learned earlier that trache(o) means _____. Trache/al (**tra′ke-əl**) means _____.
pertaining to the inside of the trachea	**6-58** Endo/tracheal (**en″do-tra′ke-əl**), abbreviated ET, means _____. In endotracheal intubation, a tube is inserted through the mouth or nose into the trachea to open an airway.
nose	Naso/tracheal (**na″zo-tra′ke-əl**) intubation is insertion of a tube through the _____ into the trachea.
orotracheal (or″o-tra′ke-əl)	Insertion of a tube through the mouth into the trachea is _____ intubation.
trachea, neck	**6-59** Both types of endotracheal intubation are considered to be for short-term use, for example, to provide a patent (**pa′tənt**)* airway when the patient is unable to maintain adequate ventilation. If prolonged airway management is needed, a tracheotomy (**tra″ke-ot′ə-me**) is generally performed. A tracheo/tomy is an incision made into the _____ through the _____ and is done to gain access to the airway.
opening	A tracheo/stomy (**tra″ke-os′tə-me**) is surgical creation of an _____ in the trachea. Although these two terms indicate different procedures, tracheotomy and tracheostomy are often used interchangeably. In addition to long-term artificial airway management, the tracheostomy tube is used in other situations, for example, when an obstruction is present in the upper airway passages. Compare the three types of airway management shown in Figure 6-6.
larynx trachea laryngotracheitis (lə-ring″go-tra″ke-i′tis)	**6-60** Laryngo/trache/al (**lə-ring″go-tra′ke-əl**) means pertaining to the _____ and the _____. Using the previous frame as a guide, build a word that means inflammation of the larynx and trachea: _____.

*(Latin: *patens,* open or unblocked.)

tracheoplasty (tra′ke-o-plas″te)	**6-61** Plastic surgery to repair the trachea is _____.
tracheoscopy (tra″ke-os′kə-pe)	Viewing (inside) the trachea is _____. (Use the combining forms for trachea and examination.)
trachea	**6-62** Tracheo/malacia (tra″ke-o-mə-la′shə) is softening of the _____.
tracheostenosis (tra″ke-o-stə-no′sis)	Now, write a word that means narrowing of the lumen of the trachea: _____.
pain in the trachea	Trache/algia (tra″ke-al′jə) is _____.
bronchitis (brong-ki′tis)	**6-63** Remembering that bronch(o) and bronchi(o) are combining forms for bronchi (singular is bronchus), build a word that means inflammation of the bronchi by combining bronch(o) and -itis: _____.
bronchi lungs bronchogenic (brong-ko-jen′ik)	Broncho/pulmonary (brong″ko-pul′mə-nar″e) pertains to the _____ and the _____. Use bronch(o) to write a term that means originating in a bronchus: _____.
bronchopathy (brong-kop′ə-the) bronchoplasty (brong″ko-plas″te) bronchi	**6-64** Use bronch(o) to write a word that means any disease of the bronchi: _____. Use bronch(o) to write a term that means plastic surgery of a bronchus: _____. Broncho/lith/iasis (brong″ko-lĭ-thi′ə-sis) is a condition in which stones are present in the _____.
lungs	**6-65** Pneumonia (noo-mo′ne-ə), or pneumonitis (noo″mo-ni′tis), means inflammation of the _____. There are many kinds of pneumonia. Most pneumonias are caused by bacteria or viruses. The combining forms *pneumon(o)* and *pneum(o)* mean lungs. (Depending on usage, pneum[o] sometimes means air, as in pneum/atic tires.)
bronchi lungs	Broncho/pneumon/ia (brong″ko-noŏ-mo′ne-ə) involves both the _____ and the _____. Rales (rahlz) are abnormal breathing sounds that may result from bronchopneumonia.
bronchoscope (brong′ko-skōp)	**6-66** Add a suffix to bronch(o) to form a word that means an instrument for viewing the bronchi: _____.
bronchogram (brong′ko-gram) inflammation of the larynx, trachea, and bronchi	A broncho/scopic (brong″ko-skop′ik) examination pertains to broncho/scopy (brong-kos′kə-pe) or direct viewing of the bronchi. Broncho/graphy (brong-kog′rə-fe) involves the use of x-rays after injection of an opaque solution. The film obtained by broncho/graphy is a _____. Laryngo/tracheo/bronch/itis (lə-ring″go-tra″ke-o-brong-ki′tis) is _____.
dilation of the bronchi bronchospasm (brong′ko-spaz″əm)	**6-67** The suffixes *-ectasia* and *-ectasis* mean stretching or dilation. Bronchi/ectasis (brong″ke-ek′tə-sis) means _____. Using bronch(o), write a word that means bronchial spasm: _____. Bronchospasm brings about bronchoconstriction (brong″ko-kən-strik′shən). This can lead to the respiratory sound known as a wheeze (hwēz).
bronchodilator (brong″ko-di-la′tor)	Broncho/dilators are used in asthma and other respiratory conditions that constrict air passages. A bronchodilator expands the bronchi and other air passages. An agent that dilates the bronchi is a _____.

little bronchus	**6-68** The suffix -ole means little or small. Bronchi/oles are branches of the bronchi. Translated literally, bronchi/ole means _____ _____.
bronchioles bronchiolitis (brong″ke-o-li′tis)	Use the combining form **bronchiol(o),** which means bronchioles. Bronchiol/ectasis (**brong″ke-o-lek′tə-sis**) is dilation of the _____. Write a word that means inflammation of the bronchioles: _____.
alveoli bronchus alveoli alveoli	**6-69** At the end of the bronchioles are tiny air sacs called alveoli. Carbon dioxide is exchanged for oxygen in the alveoli. Alveol/ar (**al-ve′ə-lər**) means pertaining to the _____. Broncho/alveolar (**brong″ko-al-ve′ə-lər**) is pertaining to a _____ and _____. The small pockets at the end of the bronchioles where carbon dioxide and oxygen are exchanged between the inspired air and capillary blood are called the _____.
diaphragm	**6-70** The two lungs are composed of millions of alveoli and their related ducts, bronchioles, and bronchi. Examine the chest x-ray in Figure 6-7 and study the relationship of the lungs with other structures in the chest cavity. Normal lungs are highly elastic and fill the chest cavity during inspiration. The lungs press down on the muscular structure called the _____. Locate this structure that contracts and increases the size of the thoracic cavity during inspiration. The air in the lungs appears black in Figure 6-7. Notice also the white appearance of bone (collarbone, breastbone, and ribs). The breasts and other soft tissue appear gray. In looking at the respiratory structures, it is understandable that the trachea and bronchial branches are referred to as the bronchial tree.
lung lungs, thoracic pleura	**6-71** The left lung has two lobes, and the right lung has three lobes (Figure 6-3). A lob/ectomy is an excision of a single lobe. Because other organs, such as the liver and brain, also have lobes, one has to say pulmonary lobectomy, unless it is clear that the lobectomy refers to the _____. The combining form **lob(o)** means lobe. Each lung is surrounded by a membrane called the pleura (**ploor′ə**) (plural is pleurae). One layer of the membrane, the visceral pleura, covers the lung's surface. The other layer, the parietal (**pə-ri′ə-təl**), lines the walls of the thoracic cavity. Visceral* means pertaining to the viscera, the large internal organs enclosed within a body cavity, especially the abdominal cavity. Parietal† pertains to the outer wall of a cavity or organ. Two types of pleura are the visceral pleura and the parietal pleura. The visceral pleura surrounds the _____; the parietal pleura lines the walls of the _____ cavity. Between the two pleurae is a space called the pleural cavity, which contains a thin film of pleural fluid that acts as a lubricant as the lungs expand and contract during respiration. The combining form **pleur(o)** means pleura. Pleur/al (**ploor′əl**) pertains to the _____.
pleural pleural fibrous hydrothorax (hi″dro-thor′aks) pleural	**6-72** Pleural effusion (**ə-fu′zhən**) is a collection of fluid in the _____ cavity. If pleural effusion contains pus, it is called empyema (**em″pi-e′mə**). This condition is an extension of infection from nearby structures. Empyema is when the _____ effusion contains pus. Untreated empyema can lead to fibro/thorax (**fi″bro-thor′aks**) or fibrotic (**fi-brot′ik**) lung disease. The combining form **fibr(o)** means fiber or fibrous (tough, threadlike). Fibro/thorax is a _____ condition of the chest and results in a fusing of the parietal and visceral pleurae. Using fibrothorax as a model, construct a word that means watery chest when translated literally: _____. Hydro/thorax is another way of saying _____ effusion.

*(Latin: *viscus,* internal organs.)
†(Latin: *paries,* wall.)

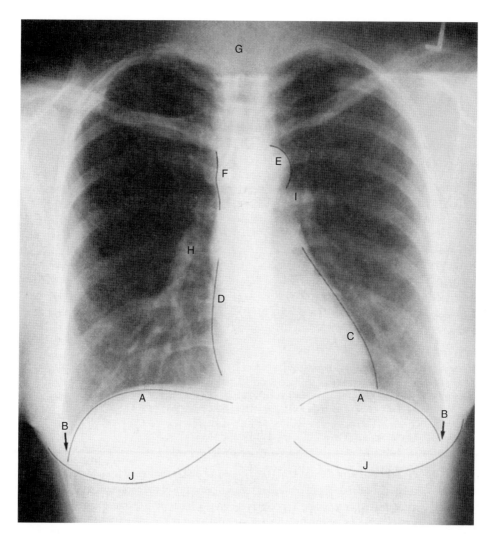

FIGURE 6-7

A normal chest x-ray taken from the posteroanterior view. The backward *L* in the upper right corner is placed on the film to indicate the left side of the chest. The letters *A-J* identify several anatomic structures that can be seen. **A,** Diaphragm; **B,** costophrenic angle, the angle at the bottom of the lung where the diaphragm and the chest wall meet; **C,** left ventricle; **D,** right atrium; **E,** aortic arch; **F,** superior vena cava; **G,** trachea; **H,** right bronchus; **I,** left bronchus; and **J,** shadows produced by the soft tissue of the breasts.(From Polaski AL, Tatro, SE: *Luckmann's core principles and practice of medical-surgical nursing*, Philadelphia, 1996, WB Saunders.)

inflammation of the pleura	**6-73** Pleur/itis (**ploo-ri′tis**) is
	_____.
	Pleurisy (**ploor′ĭ-se**) is another name for pleuritis. Pleurisy may be caused by an infection, injury, or tumor, or it may be a complication of certain lung diseases. A sharp pain on inspiration is characteristic of pleurisy.
pleuritis	Pleurisy is another name for _____.

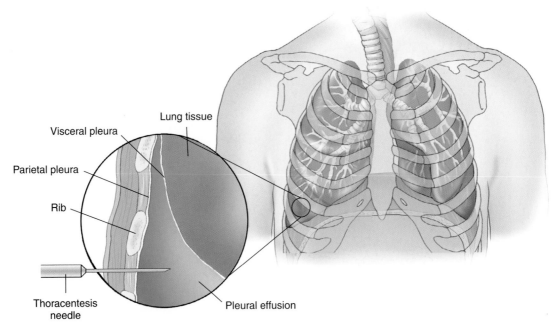

Lung tissue

Visceral pleura

Parietal pleura

Rib

Thoracentesis needle

Pleural effusion

FIGURE 6-8
Insertion of the needle in thoracentesis. The actual site for insertion depends on the location of the effusion and the material that has escaped into the pleural space. Thoracocentesis means the same as thoracentesis, but the latter term is used more often.

6-74 The term *thoracentesis* (**thor″ə-sen-te′sis**) is shortened from the term *thoracocentesis* (**thor″ə-ko-sən-te′sis**). Thora/centesis is surgical puncture of the chest wall and pleural space with a needle to aspirate fluid or to obtain a specimen for biopsy. It has both therapeutic and diagnostic uses. (The term *aspirate** means to withdraw fluid or air from a cavity.)

The suffix -*centesis* means surgical puncture.

surgical puncture

Thora/centesis is _____ _____ of the chest wall and can be used in the treatment of pleural effusion (Figure 6-8).

Thoracentesis is sometimes called pleurocentesis (**ploor″o-sen-te′sis).**

6-75 You have already learned that pulmon(o) means lung; *pulm(o)* also means the lungs.

lungs

Both pulmonary and pulmonic mean pertaining to the _____ or the respiratory system, but pulmonary is more commonly used.

❏ SECTION D REVIEW   *L*ower Respiratory Passageways

This section review covers frames 6–56 through 6–75. Complete the table by writing either a word part or its meaning in each blank space.

Combining Form	Meaning	Combining Form	Meaning	Suffix	Meaning
1. _____	fiber or fibrous	4. pneum(o)	_____	7. -centesis	_____
2. _____	lobe	5. pnemon(o)	_____	8. -ectasia and -ectasis	_____
3. _____	pleura	6. pulm(o)	_____		

(Use Appendix V to check your answers.)

*(Latin: *aspirare*, to breathe upon.)

Diseases and Disorders of the Respiratory System

Disorders of the respiratory system are a major cause of illness and death. Acute or chronic respiratory problems can progress rapidly and become life-threatening emergencies. Chronic lung disease often causes heart disease because of the lungs' functional role in circulation. Cardiovascular disease and lung cancer cause many deaths each year. In this section, we will look at not only respiratory disorders but also the major causes of death in the United States.

resembling fiber, fibrous fibroma or fibroid dissolves fiber fibrous	**6-76** Remembering that fibr(o) means fiber or fibrous, fibr/oid (**fi′broid**) is _____ _____. Fibroid is also used to mean fibr/oma (**fi-bro′mə**), which is a _____ tumor. (In addition, fibroids is a colloquial clinical term for small benign tumors of the uterus. The formal name of this type of fibroid is myoma uteri.) A fibrous tumor is a _____. A fibro/lysin (**fi-brol′ə-sin**) is a substance that _____ _____. If lung tissue becomes fibrous, the lungs cannot function as well as they should. In pulmonary fibro/sis, the lung tissue has become _____.
lungs heart pulmonary difficult breathing upright or sitting up	**6-77** Pulmonary edema is an effusion of fluid into the air spaces and tissue spaces of the _____. Although pulmonary edema may be caused by other things, a major cause is congestive heart failure. In congestive heart failure, the work demanded of the heart is greater than its ability to perform. Decreased output of blood by the left ventricle produces congestion and engorgement of the pulmonary vessels with escape of fluid into pulmonary tissues. Congestive _____ failure can result in a lung disorder, _____ edema. Dyspnea on exertion is one of the earliest symptoms of pulmonary edema. As the condition becomes more advanced, the patient may become orthopneic. Dys/pnea means _____ _____. If a patient becomes ortho/pneic, in what position is the patient most comfortable? _____
pulmonary embolus pulmonary	**6-78** A pulmon/ary embolus (**em′bo ləs**) is an obstruction of the _____ artery or one of its branches. Obstruction of a large pulmonary vessel can cause sudden death. The pulmonary arteries carry blood to the lungs. An embolus (plural is emboli) is a plug, usually part of a thrombus, obstructing a vessel. Write this word, which means a foreign substance brought by the blood to a vessel and resulting in an obstruction: _____. Embolism (**em′bə-liz-əm**) is the sudden blocking of an artery by a clot or foreign material that has been brought to its site of lodgment by the circulating blood. Embol/ism (*embol[o]*, embolus plus -ism, condition) is a general term and does not designate where the embolus has lodged. The obstructed artery in pulmon/ary embolism is a _____ artery.
vessels embolus thrombus	**6-79** Pulmonary angiography is roentgenography of the _____ of the lungs after injection of a contrast medium. Pulmonary angiography is primarily performed on patients with suspected thromboembolic (**throm″bo-em-bo′lik**) disease. Embol/ic pertains to an _____. Thrombo/embolic pertains to a _____ that has become detached from its site of formation and is blocking a blood vessel.

TABLE 6-2 Types of Emboli

TYPE	SOURCES
Thomboemboli	Fragments of a larger thrombus, often within veins of the leg or pelvis; sometimes thrombi form within the heart or, occasionally, within the aorta
Fat emboli	Fractures of long bones; severe burns, trauma to soft tissue; severe fatty liver conditions
Air or gas emboli	May be introduced accidentally during certain surgical procedures; chest injuries; increased atmospheric pressure in underwater diving activities
Miscellaneous:	
Clumps of bacteria or parasites	From infection within the body
Tumor emboli	Cells or, less commonly, small fragments from a malignant tumor find their way into the circulating blood
Amniotic fluid	Escapes into the veins of the uterus, an uncommon complication of pregnancy

blood clot

coronary

excision or removal

6-80 Several types of emboli and their causative factors and consequences are listed in Table 6-2. An embolus may be composed of various substances, but a thrombo/tic embolus is specifically a _____ _____ (thrombus).

Coronary embolism is obstruction of a _____ artery by an embolus. This is a major cause of myocardial infarction. An embol/ectomy (em″bə-lek′tə-me) is _____ of an embolus.

lungs
heart

pneumonectomy (noo″mo-nek′tə-me)
removal of lung tissue
lung
pneumonectomy

blood

blood

6-81 Pneumo/cardi/al (noo″mo-kahr′de-əl) refers to the _____ and _____.

Using pneumon(o), build a word that means removal of a lung: _____.

(The word actually means removal of lung tissue and may involve removal of all or part of the lung.) Pneum/ectomy (noo-mek′tə-me) is also _____.

A total pneumonectomy is removal of an entire _____. If only part of the lung is removed, the surgery is called a partial _____.

Hemo/thorax (he″mo-thor′aks) is _____ in the pleural cavity. Trauma, such as a knife wound, is the most common cause of hemothorax.

Pneumo/thorax (noo″mo-thor′aks) is air or gas in the pleural cavity. Pneumo/hemo/thorax (noo″mo-he″mo-thor′aks) is air and _____ in the pleural cavity. (Both pneumothorax and hemothorax are illustrated in Figure 6-9.)

pleura
lungs

pleura

inflammation of the pleura

6-82 Pleuro/pneumon/ia (ploor″o-noo-mo′ne-ə) involves both the _____ and the _____.

Pleuro/dynia (ploor″o-din′e-əh) is pain of the _____. This could be caused by pleural adhesions, in which the pleural membranes stick together or to the wall of the chest and produce pain on movement or breathing. Adhesion means a sticking together of two surfaces that are normally separated. Pleural adhesion may be associated with pleur/itis, which is _____.

a black condition of the lungs

pneumomelanosis

6-83 Pneumo/melan/osis (noo″mo-mel′ə-no′sis) is _____.

The lungs of a baby are pink. The adult lung darkens, owing to inhalation of dust and soot. If much soot and dust are inhaled, the lung appears black. This abnormal coloration is _____.

(Pneumomelanosis is seen in pneumoconiosis [noo″mo-ko″ne-o′sis], a condition of the respiratory tract resulting from inhalation of dust particles.)

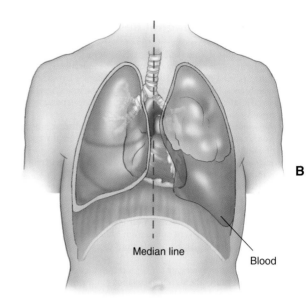

Outside air rushes in due to disruption of chest wall and parietal pleura

Pleural space
Normal lung

A

B

Lung air rushes out due to disruption of visceral pleura

Median line

Median line

Blood

Pneumothorax

Hemothorax

FIGURE 6-9
Two abnormal conditions of the chest cavity. **A,** Pneumothorax is air or gas in the chest cavity. The arrows indicate the two situations that result in pneumothorax. Arrow 1 represents an open chest wound that permits the entrance of air into the pleural space. Arrow 2 represents a tear within the lung, which allows air to enter the pleural space. **B,** Hemothorax, blood in the pleural cavity, below the left lung. The massive hemothorax shown has caused much of the left lung to collapse.

condition dust	**6-84** The combining form ***coni(o)*** means dust. Pneumo/coni/osis is a _____ of the lungs caused by inhalation of _____.
coal	Anthracosis (**an-thrə-ko′sis**), asbestosis (**as″bes-to′sis**), and silicosis (**sil″ĭ-ko′sis**) are forms of pneumoconiosis. The combining form ***anthrac(o)*** means coal. Anthrac/osis is accumulation of carbon deposits in the lungs that can result from breathing smoke or _____ dust.
asbestos	Asbestosis is a form of pneumoconiosis resulting from prolonged exposure to _____.
pneumoconiosis	Silicosis results from inhalation of silica dust. This condition is also a form of _____.
lungs	**6-85** Pneumo/malacia (**noo″mo-mə-la′ shə**) is softening of the _____.
softening of the lungs	Malacia is a morbid softening or softness of a tissue or part. It is derived from the combining form ***malac(o),*** which means softening; ***-malacia*** is a suffix that means softness of a tissue or part. Pneumo/malacia is _____.
lungs	Pneumo/centesis (**noo″mo-sən-te′sis**) is surgical puncture of the _____, usually performed to remove fluids.
respiratory distress	**6-86** Read about additional respiratory diseases and disorders in Table 6-3. Note the two types of respiratory distress syndromes, ARDS in adults and RDS in children. RDS means _____ _____ syndrome.*
	Both ***sym-*** and ***syn-*** mean joined or together. If the letter that follows the prefix is b, m, or p, use sym- as in symbiosis, symmetry, and symphysis; otherwise, use syn-. A syndrome (**sin′drōm**) is a set of signs and symptoms resulting from a common cause or appearing to present a clinical picture of a disease or inherited abnormality.

*Syndrome (Greek: *syn*, together, *dromos*, course).

TABLE 6-3   Additional Respiratory Diseases and Disorders

Adult respiratory distress syndrome (ARDS): A form of acute respiratory failure that is characterized by pulmonary and alveolar edema, dyspnea, and hypoxemia. It is caused by trauma, and the mortality rate is higher than 50%.

Asthma (**az′mə**): Paroxysmal dyspnea accompanied by wheezing. The wheeze is caused by spasm of the bronchi or by swelling of the mucous membranes. Paroxysmal means occurring in a sudden, periodic attack or recurrence of symptoms.

Atelectasis (**at″ə-lek′tə-sis**): Congenital, incomplete expansion of a lung or a portion of a lung, or airlessness of a lung that had once been expanded; usually resulting from trauma.

Chronic obstructive pulmonary disease (COPD): A disease process that decreases the ability of the lungs to perform their ventilatory function. It can result from many disorders such as chronic bronchitis, emphysema, chronic asthma, and chronic bronchiolitis. It is also called chronic obstructive lung disease (COLD).

Cystic fibrosis (**sis′tik fi-bro′sis**): An inherited disease, generally characterized by chronic respiratory infection and disorders of the pancreas and sweat glands.

Emphysema (**em″fə-se′mə**): A chronic, progressive pulmonary disease characterized by destruction of the alveolar walls. The decrease in total alveolar surface area hinders gas exchange between the alveoli and the blood.

Influenza (**in″floo-en′zə**): An acute, highly contagious respiratory infection that is characterized by sudden onset, fever, chills, headache, and muscle ache.

Occupational pulmonary disease: A variety of pulmonary disorders caused by exposure to toxic dust and particulate matter in the workplace. The intensity of the problem ranges from acute, reversible effects to chronic pulmonary disease.

Pertussis (**pər-tus′is**): An acute, infectious disease characterized by a paroxysmal cough, ending in a whooping inspiration. This is commonly called whooping cough.

Respiratory distress syndrome (RDS): A respiratory condition that causes many infant deaths. Clinical signs are usually present at birth. Insufficient surfactant causes the alveoli to collapse. (In the normal lung, surfactant lessens the surface tension and enables the alveoli to function properly.) RDS was formerly known as hyaline membrane disease.

Sudden infant death syndrome (SIDS): The sudden and unexpected death of an apparently healthy infant, and not explained by careful postmortem studies. This is believed by many persons to be caused by respiratory failure such as apnea.

asthma	**6-87** Use the information in Table 6-3 to complete the next four frames. The wheeze, caused by spasm of the bronchial tube or by swelling of the mucous membranes, is characteristic of _____.
stretching	Atelectasis is incomplete expansion of a lung or airlessness of a lung that once functioned. The combining form ***atel(o)*** means imperfect or incomplete, and -ectasis means _____.
fibrosis	An inherited disorder characterized by frequent respiratory infections and disorders of the pancreas and sweat glands is called cystic _____.
emphysema	**6-88** Destruction of the alveolar walls is a major characteristic of _____.
muc(o) **mucolytic** (**mu″ko-lit′ik**)	You have learned that the combining form for mucus is _____. Use this combining form and a suffix to write a word that means destroying or dissolving mucus: _____. *Mucolytic* is a term that also means an agent that destroys or dissolves mucus. An abundance of mucus is produced in certain respiratory disorders, such as emphysema. Mucolytics and bronchodilators are often used in treating these patients to open their breathing passages.
sudden infant	**6-89** SIDS means _____ _____ death syndrome and is believed by many to be caused by respiratory failure.
pertussis	**6-90** The infectious disease that is commonly called whooping cough is _____. This disease is now uncommon in the United States because of widespread vaccination.
influenza	A highly contagious and common respiratory infection that is characterized by fever, chills, headache, and muscle ache is _____. Unlike pertussis vaccine, the influenza virus vaccine is effective for only a short period of time.

inflammation discharge	**6-91** The common cold is a contagious viral infection of the upper respiratory tract. Some of its major characteristics are rhinitis, rhinorrhea, tearing and eye discomfort, and sometimes, low-grade fever. Rhin/itis is _____ of the nasal membranes. Rhino/rrhea is _____ from the nasal membranes. Rest, fluids, analgesics, and decongestants are recommended. Decongestants (de-, away or remove plus L. *congerere,* to pile up) cause vasoconstriction of the nasal membranes, thereby eliminating or reducing swelling or congestion.
against	Antihistamines (**an″tĭ-his′tə-mēnz**) are also used to treat colds and allergies. Antihistamines act _____ histamine to reduce its effects. Histamine brings about many of the symptoms that we recognize as the common cold.
lungs	**6-92** Tuberculosis (**too-ber″ku-lo′sis**) (TB) is an infectious disease that often is chronic and commonly affects the lungs, although it may occur in other parts of the body. Pulmonary tuberculosis affects the _____.

Resistance to tuberculosis depends a great deal on a person's general health. Early symptoms of tuberculosis (loss of energy, appetite, and weight) may go unnoticed. Fever, night sweats, and spitting up of bloody or purulent sputum may not occur until a year or more after the initial exposure to the disease. The disease is named after the tubercles (**too′bər-kəlz**) that are small round nodules produced in the lungs by the infective bacteria. |
| against

out

hemoptysis (he-mop′tĭ-sis) | **6-93** Liquefaction of the tubercles not only results in tubercular cavities in the lungs, but can also cause the production of a large quantity of highly infectious sputum that is raised when the infected person coughs. Anti/tussive (**an″tĭ-tus′iv**) means _____ coughing. In other words, antitussive (anti-, against plus Latin: *tussis,* cough) means preventing or relieving coughing, or an agent that does so.

To ex/pectorate (**ek-spek′tə-rāt**) is to cough up and spit _____ material from the lungs and air passages. (The material coughed up from the lungs is sputum.)

Blood-stained sputum is often produced in tuberculosis. Hemo/ptysis is the spitting of blood or blood-stained sputum. The suffix *-ptysis* means spitting. Spitting of blood is _____. |
| heart cancer | **6-94** Examine Table 6-4. The leading cause of death in the United States is _____ disease. What is the second leading cause of death? _____

About 55% of deaths in the United States are caused by heart disease or cancer. You studied many cardiovascular diseases and disorders in the previous chapter, and the next several frames focus on the second leading cause of death, cancer.

Although cancer is sometimes regarded as a disease of older individuals, it is also the second leading cause of death among children aged 1 to 14 years in the United States, with accidents being the most frequent cause of death. |
| localized

black tumor | **6-95** Most skin cancers (basal and squamous cell) and most in situ cancers are not included in cancer predictions and statistics about cancer deaths. Basal and squamous cell cancers are common types of skin cancer that are rarely invasive. In other words, they rarely spread to other organs. *In situ* is Latin and means localized and not invading the surrounding tissue. A word that means in situ is

_____.

Examine Figure 6-10. Note that most skin cancers and in situ cancers are not included. One type of skin cancer that is included is malignant melanoma. Translated literally, melan/oma means a

_____ _____. It is a malignant, darkly pigmented mole or tumor of the skin. |

TABLE 6-4 Leading Causes of Death in the United States, 1996

TOTAL NUMBER OF DEATHS IN THE UNITED STATES IN 1996: 2,314,690

Number of deaths caused by heart disease 733,361
Number of deaths caused by cancer 539,533

RANK	CAUSE OF DEATH	PERCENTAGE OF TOTAL DEATHS
1	Heart diseases	31.7
2	Cancer	23.3
3	Stroke	7.0
4	Chronic obstructive lung diseases	4.6
5	Accidents	4.1
6	Pneumonia and influenza	3.6
7	Diabetes	2.7
8	Suicide	1.3
9	HIV/AIDS	1.3
10	Chronic liver disease and cirrhosis	1.1
	Other and ill-defined	19.3

Calculated percent of deaths in the United States, age-adjusted to the 1970 U.S. standard population. From National Vital Statistic Records, Vol 47, No. 9: Vital Statistics of the United States, 1999, Washington, DC, Public Health Service, 1999.

---

malignant (or malignancy)
metastatic (or metastasis)

6-96 Remembering that mal- means bad, malignant (mə-lig′nənt) means tending to become worse and to cause death. When describing cancer, a malignant tumor is one that is invasive or metastatic (met″ə-stat′ik). The prefix *meta-* means after, change, or next in a series; the suffix *-stasis* means stopping or controlling. Metastasis (mə-tas′tə-sis) is the transfer of cancer from one organ or part of the body to another. One could translate meta/stasis as a change in the state, or control of cancer, and the cancer would be described as meta/static. In summary, a term that begins with mal- that is associated with cancer is _____.

A second closely associated term that begins with meta- is _____.

---

prostate

lung and bronchus

breast
lung and bronchus

6-97 Look at the estimated new cancer cases for the year 2000 in Figure 6-10. Look first at new cancer cases in American males. The _____ is the site of greatest cancer incidence in males. But which type of cancer causes the greatest number of male deaths?
_____ and _____

In females, what is overwhelmingly the site of the greatest number of new cancer cases?
_____ What type of cancer causes the greatest number of female deaths?
_____ and _____

---

cigarettes (or smoking)

6-98 Significant decreases in mortality from lung and bronchial cancer have occurred only among males. Rates among females have recently begun to slow and may be stabilizing. Lung cancer remains a highly lethal disease, although significant improvements in treatment have occurred in the last decade. The most important cause of lung cancer is tobacco smoking.

Besides cigarettes, exposure to airborne asbestos, uranium, radon, and high doses of ionizing radiation has been linked to increased incidence of lung cancer, according to the American Cancer Society. However, the greatest cause of lung cancer is _____.

Cigarette smoking increases the risk of lung cancer more than the risk of cancer at any other site, but cigarette smoking—as well as pipe smoking—also multiplies the risk of cancer of the lip, mouth, tongue, and pharynx.

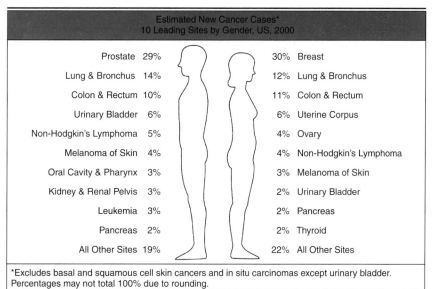

Estimated New Cancer Cases*
10 Leading Sites by Gender, US, 2000

Prostate 29%		30% Breast
Lung & Bronchus 14%		12% Lung & Bronchus
Colon & Rectum 10%		11% Colon & Rectum
Urinary Bladder 6%		6% Uterine Corpus
Non-Hodgkin's Lymphoma 5%		4% Ovary
Melanoma of Skin 4%		4% Non-Hodgkin's Lymphoma
Oral Cavity & Pharynx 3%		3% Melanoma of Skin
Kidney & Renal Pelvis 3%		2% Urinary Bladder
Leukemia 3%		2% Pancreas
Pancreas 2%		2% Thyroid
All Other Sites 19%		22% All Other Sites

*Excludes basal and squamous cell skin cancers and in situ carcinomas except urinary bladder. Percentages may not total 100% due to rounding.

Estimated Cancer Deaths*
10 Leading Sites by Gender, US, 2000

Lung & Bronchus 31%		25% Lung & Bronchus
Prostate 11%		15% Breast
Colon & Rectum 10%		11% Colon & Rectum
Pancreas 5%		5% Pancreas
Non-Hodgkin's Lymphoma 5%		5% Ovary
Leukemia 4%		5% Non-Hodgkins Lymphoma
Esophagus 3%		4% Leukemia
Liver & Intrahepatic Bile Duct 3%		2% Uterine Corpus
Urinary Bladder 3%		2% Brain & Other Nervous System
Stomach 3%		2% Stomach†
		2% Multiple Myeloma†
All Other Sites 19%		21% All Other Sites

*Excludes in situ carcinomas except urinary bladder.
†These two cancers both received a ranking of 10; they have the same projected number of deaths and contribute the same percentage. Percentages may not total 100% due to rounding.

FIGURE 6-10
Cancer incidence and deaths by site and sex, estimates for year 2000 for the United States. (From CA: *A Cancer Journal for Clinicians,* Vol 50, No 1, American Cancer Society.)

6-99 Many malignant lesions are curable if detected in the early stage. Treatment selection depends on the site, stage of the cancer, and unique characteristics of the individual. Some anticancer treatments include surgery, irradiation, and chemotherapy with antineoplastic agents.

against

Anti/cancer means acting _____ cancer.

A neoplasm (**ne′o-plaz-em**) means any abnormal growth, benign or malignant. The term *neo/plasm* is derived from *neo-,* meaning new, and *-plasm,* meaning formation. (You will study neo- in a later chapter.)

neoplasms

An anti/neoplas/tic is a treatment that acts against _____. These treatments are designed to kill or prevent the spread of cancer cells.

Irradiation uses radiant energy such as x-ray and radioactive substances to treat cancer.

thoracotomy	**6-100** Lung and bronchial cancer cause more adult cancer deaths than any other type of cancer. A pneumonectomy, either partial or complete, is one means of treating lung cancer. Removal of a lung requires an open surgery that will provide full access to structures in the chest cavity. Write a term that means a surgical incision into the chest: _____. Many diagnostic tools are available for diagnosing diseases and disorders of the respiratory tract. Radiography, angiography, and tomography give the physician a great deal of information that is not available by direct examination.
	6-101 The act of listening for sounds within the body, generally aided by the use of a stethoscope, is called auscultation* (**aws″kəl-ta′shən**). By placing the stethoscope on the chest and back, one can listen to the lungs during respiration. Wheezing and other abnormal sounds can often be detected in this manner. One such abnormal sound is a crackle (**krak′əl**), which is characterized by discontinuous cracking, popping, or bubbling noises. Percussion (**pər-kŭ′shən**) is the act of striking a part of the body with short, sharp blows. It is used to assess the condition of underlying tissue by the sound obtained. Tapping on the chest wall between the ribs produces various sounds that are meaningful to the experienced person. This means of diagnosing
percussion	the condition of underlying tissue is called _____.
decreased **pulse, blood pressure** **oximetry** (ok-sim′ə-tre)	**6-102** Hyp/ox/ia is _____ oxygen at the cellular level. It is characterized by tachycardia, hypertension, vasoconstriction, dizziness, and mental confusion. The first two characteristics mean that both the _____ and the _____ _____ are increased. A device that provides an easy means of measuring oxygen in the blood is called a pulse oxi/meter (**ok-sim′ə-tər**). Write the name of the process in which a device is used to measure oxygen in the blood: _____.
hyperoxemia (hi″pər-ok-se′ me-ə)	**6-103** Oximetry is shown in Figure 6-11. The test evaluates arterial oxygen saturation (SaO_2). Normal values of 95% to 99% SaO_2 in adults mean that the blood hemoglobin is 95% to 99% saturated with oxygen. Oxygen is administered in hypoxic patients to increase the amount of oxygen in circulating blood. It is also administered during anesthesia, since oxygen functions as a carrier gas for the delivery of anesthetic agents to the tissues of the body. An overdose of oxygen can have toxic effects, which include respiratory depression and damage to the lungs. Using hyp/ox/emia as a model, write a word that means increased oxygen content of the blood: _____.
condition **a condition without oxygen**	**6-104** The suffix *-ia* means condition. You have already seen it used to form several nouns. For example, pneumon/ia is a particular _____ of the lungs. An/ox/ia is _____. Anoxia (**ə-nok′se-ə**) means an absence or deficiency of oxygen in body tissues below the level needed for proper functioning. Anoxia is more severe than hypoxia, but both mean oxygen deficiency.
absence of voice **aphonia**	**6-105** The remaining frames of this section deal with various disorders that may affect the respiratory tract. A/phonia (**a-fo′ne-ə**) is inability to produce speech sounds from the larynx. The combining form *phon(o)* means voice. A tele/phone enables us to hear another person's voice. A/phon/ia is _____. Laryngitis may result in absence of voice, which is _____.
difficult (weak) voice **phonic** (fon′ik)	**6-106** Dys/phonia (**dis-fo′ne-ə**) means _____ _____. Dysphonia is not related to the ability to pronounce words. It is the same as hoarseness and may precede aphonia. Write a word that means pertaining to the voice, using the suffix *-ic:* _____.

*(Latin: *auscultare*, to listen.)

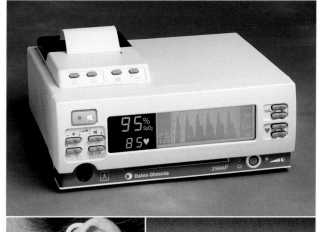

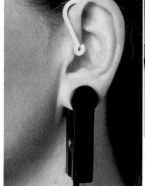

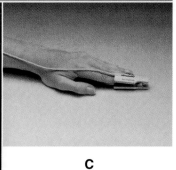

C

FIGURE 6-11
Oximetry, noninvasive monitoring of oxygen saturation. **A,** The oximeter shows a reading of SaO₂% = 95. **B,** The earlobe is a common site for measurement during exercise. **C,** The finger probe is most frequently used for stationary measurements. (Courtesy of Ohmeda, Boulder, CO.)

difficult speech	**6-107** The combining form *phas(o)* means speech. Dys/phas/ia is _____ _____. Dysphasia (**dis-fa′zhə**) is impairment of speech. There is a lack of coordination and an inability to arrange words in their proper order. This problem results from a brain lesion.
dysphasia	Difficulty in speech caused by a brain lesion is _____.
absence of speech	**6-108** A/phasia (ə-fa′zhə) is _____.
aphasic (ə-fa′zik)	Aphasia is an inability to communicate through speech, writing, or signs owing to dysfunction of the brain. A person who has aphasia is said to be _____ (change aphasia to an adjective).
tachyphasia (tak″ĭ-fa′zhə) bradyphasia (brad″ĭ-fa′zhə)	**6-109** Using aphasia as a guide, write a word for fast speech: _____; for slow speech: _____.
speech voice	Phas(o) is used when one is referring to _____; phon(o) is used when one is referring to the _____.
formation or development	**6-110** The combining form *plas(o)* means formation or development, and the suffix -plasia is derived from plas(o); *-plasia* means formation or development. A/plasia (ə-pla′zhə) means absence of _____.
formation or development	Aplasia of the lung is incomplete _____ of the lung. You have studied many diseases and disorders of the respiratory structures. Many new word parts were introduced and will be included in the following review.

❑ SECTION E REVIEW 𝒟iseases and Disorders of the Respiratory System

This section review covers frames 6–76 through 6–110. Complete the table by writing the appropriate word part in each blank.

Combining Form	Meaning	Prefix	Meaning
1. _____	coal	9. _____	change; next, as in a series
2. _____	imperfect or incomplete	10. _____	joined or together
3. _____	dust	**Suffix**	**Meaning**
4. _____	embolus	11. _____	abnormal softness
5. _____	soft or softening	12. _____	formation or development
6. _____	speech	13. _____	spitting
7. _____	voice	14. _____	stopping or controlling
8. _____	formation or development		

(Use Appendix V to check your answers.)

𝒯erminology Challenge

This section challenges you to read, write, and understand new terms or concepts about the respiratory system. At times, you will use unfamiliar word parts. It is important to remember the new terms introduced in this section.

tracheotome (tra′ke-o-tōm)	**6-111** Remembering that -tome means an instrument that is used for cutting, write the name of the instrument used to incise the trachea: _____. Ostomy is a general term for an operation in which an artificial opening is formed. A tracheostomy may be temporary or permanent, but in either case, an artificial opening has been created. A stoma (sto′mə) is a mouthlike opening, particularly one that is kept open for drainage or other purposes. Sometimes a person has a stoma at the base of the neck. Surgical creation of this type of opening into the trachea is called a tracheostomy. A general term for a mouthlike opening is a
stoma	_____.
tracheorrhagia (tra″ke-o-ra′jə)	**6-112** An injury to the trachea can result in tracheal hemorrhage. Using the suffix -rrhagia, which means hemorrhage, write a term that means tracheal hemorrhage: _____. Nosebleed has many causes, including irritation of the nasal membranes, fragility of these membranes, violent sneezing, trauma, hypertension, vitamin K deficiency, or particularly in children, picking the nose. Rhinorrhagia (ri-no-ra′je-ə) means profuse bleeding from the nose. Literal translation of rhino/rrhagia is
hemorrhage	_____ from the nose.
paralysis of the larynx **pharynx** **pyothorax**	**6-113** Laryngo/plegia (lə-ring″go-ple′jeə) is _____, actually of the laryngeal muscles. Pharyngo/myc/osis (fə-ring″go-mi-ko′sis) is a fungal condition of the _____. (The combining form myc[o] means fungus and will be studied in the next chapter.) Pyo/thorax (pi″o-tho′raks) is accumulation of pus in the chest cavity. The combining form py(o) means pus. Write this term that means accumulation of pus in the chest cavity: _____.

6-114 The term *stridor** means an abnormal high-pitched musical sound caused by an obstruction in the trachea or larynx, most often heard during inspiration. It is sometimes described as the sound of wind blowing.

The barking cough of croup (**kroop**) is often accompanied by difficulty in breathing. Croup is an acute viral infection of the upper and lower respiratory tract that occurs primarily in infants and young children.

Write the term that means difficult breathing: _____.
Use the prefix *eu-,* which means normal, to write a term that means normal breathing: _____.

dyspnea
eupnea
(ūp-neʹə)

6-115 Several prefixes, some of which will be covered more extensively in later chapters, are used to indicate direction or position. You are now able to write or recognize the meaning of several new terms. Pulmonary means pertaining to the lungs. Outside, or not connected with, the lungs is _____.

Use -al to write a word that means outside the pleural cavity: _____.

extrapulmonary
(eks"trə-pulʹmo-nar"e)

extrapleural
(eks"trə-ploorʹəl)

interalveolar
(in"tər-al-veʹo-lər)

Alveolar means pertaining to the alveoli. Write a word that means between alveoli: _____.

6-116 Use these prefixes to write and understand new terms:
Prefix   Meaning
retro-   behind or backward
sub-   below or under
supra-   above or beyond

Sub/pulmonary (səb-pulʹmo-nar"e) means _____.

Sub/phrenic (səb-frenʹik) is located _____.
Write a term that means behind the nose: _____.

Write a term that means above the nose: _____.

below the lung
beneath the
diaphragm
retronasal
(ret"ro-naʹzəl)
supranasal
(soo"prə-naʹzəl)

6-117 When translated literally, hyper/algia (hi-pər-alʹjə) means _____ pain. It means excessive sensitivity to pain and means the same as hyperesthesia (hi"pər-es-theʹzhə).

excessive

*(Latin: *stridor,* harsh sound.)

In the next chapters, you will practice using the less familiar word parts in this section. For now, be able to read and write the new terms. There is no review for this section.
Study the following list of selected abbreviations. Then read through the Chapter Pharmacology section and be sure you understand the effects and uses of the drug classes that are presented. When you are finished, work the Chapter Review. After completing the exercises, check your answers with the solutions in Appendix V.
You will find these items presented after the Chapter Review:
• Listing of Medical Terms
• Enhancing Spanish Communication

Selected Abbreviations

AFB	acid-fast bacillus (some cause tuberculosis)		pH	potential hydrogen
ARDS	adult respiratory distress syndrome		R	respiration
CAL	chronic airflow limitation		RDS	respiratory distress syndrome
COLD	chronic obstructive lung disease		RLL	right lower lobe
COPD	chronic obstructive pulmonary disease		RUL	right upper lobe
CPR	cardiopulmonary resuscitation		SaO_2	arterial oxygen saturation
CXR	chest x-ray		SIDS	suddent infant death syndrome
ET	endotracheal		SOB	shortness of breath
IRDS	infant respiratory distress syndrome		TB	tuberculosis
LLL	left lower lobe		TTO	transtracheal oxygen
LUL	left upper lobe		URI	upper respiratory infection
PaO_2	partial pressure of arterial oxygen		VC	vital capacity
PFT	pulmonary function test			

Chapter Pharmacology

Class	Effects and Uses
Antiasthmatic Drugs/Bronchodilators	**Used to Treat Asthma, Relax the Bronchioles to Improve Respiration**
salmeterol (Serevent)	Used by inhalation
terbutaline (Brethaire)	Used in asthma and bronchospasm
albuterol (Proventil)	Used in asthma and bronchospasm
metaproterenol (Alupent)	Used for asthma and bronchospasm
epinephrine (Primatene Mist)	Used for temporary relief of shortness of breath, wheezing
theophylline (Elixophyllin)	Used in bronchial asthma
aminophylline	Used in bronchial asthma
zileuton (Zyflo)	Used in adults and children 12 years of age or older
montelukast (Singulair)	Used in adults and children 6 years or older
Corticosteroids	**Have Potent Antiinflammatory Activity**
beclomethasone (Beclovent)	For asthma patients in need of a corticosteroid
triamcinolone (Azmacort)	Prophylactic therapy for patients requiring systemic corticosteroids
fluticasone (Flovent)	Prophylactic therapy for patients requiring systemic corticosteroids
Anticholinergics	**Dilate the Bronchi and Bronchioles**
ipratropium (Atrovent)	Used to treat bronchospasm associated with COPD
Miscellaneous	
cromolyn (Nasalcrom)	Prophylactic treatment of bronchial asthma
nedocromil (Tilade)	Maintenance therapy for mild to moderate bronchial asthma
Anti–cystic Fibrosis Agents	**Have Pulmonary Mucolytic Activity**
acetylcysteine (Mucomyst)	Treats pulmonary complications of cystic fibrosis

Chapter Pharmacology—cont'd

Class	Effects and Uses
Antihistamines	**Oppose the Action of Histamine**
diphenhydramine (Benadryl)	Used in hypersensitivity reactions
promethazine (Phenergan)	Used in hypersensitivity reactions and for motion sickness
hydroxyzine (Atarax)	Used for pruritis
loratadine (Claritin)	Used in allergic rhinitis
fexofenadine (Allegra)	Used for allergic rhinitis
Antitussives	**Suppress Coughing**
Narcotic	
codeine derivatives	The dose is normally lower than that to relieve pain
Nonnarcotic	
dextromethorphan (Robitussin)	Makes nonproductive cough more productive, thus reducing frequency of coughing
benzonatate (Tessalon)	Reduces cough reflex
Expectorants	
guaifenesin	Used to remove excess mucus from respiratory tract
Smoking Cessation Adjuncts	**To Encourage Abstinence from Smoking**
nicotine polacrilex (Nicorette)	Nicotine-containing chewing gum

CHAPTER REVIEW 6

▶ BASIC UNDERSTANDING

REVIEWING WORD PARTS
I. Write a word (prefix, suffix, or combining form) for each clue.

CROSSWORD PUZZLE 6

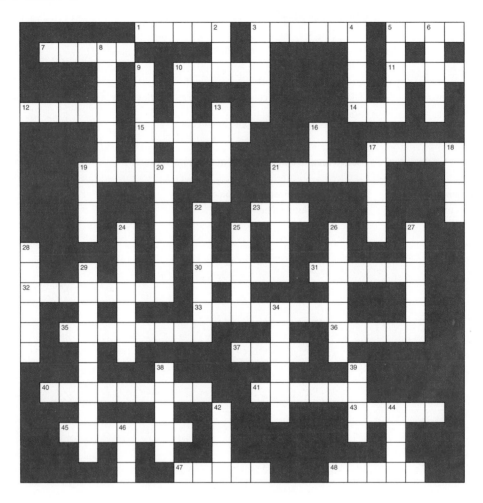

Across

1 stone
3 spitting
5 many
7 lungs
10 acid
11 against
12 discharge
14 muscle
15 stopping
17 blue
19 palate
21 pleura
23 mouth
30 nose
31 lungs
32 pharynx
33 surgical puncture
35 coal
36 condition
37 lobe
40 epiglottis
41 paralysis
43 to breathe
45 alveoli
47 slow
48 cramp

Down

2 oxygen
3 voice
4 twitching
5 speech
6 capable of destroying
8 softness
9 development
10 alkaline
13 fiber
16 small
17 dust
18 condition
19 breathing
20 trachea
21 diaphragm
22 chest
24 bronchi
25 process
26 origin
27 prolapse
28 carbon dioxide
29 bronchioles
34 embolus
38 imperfect
39 nose
42 change
44 inflammation
46 upon

MATCHING

II. Match the following structures with their characteristics or functions (A-G):

_____ 1. alveolus
_____ 2. bronchus

_____ 3. diaphragm
_____ 4. larynx

A. a branch of the trachea
B. a muscular partition that
     facilitates breathing
C. commonly called the windpipe
D. connected with the paranasal
     sinuses

_____ 5. nose
_____ 6. pharynx
_____ 7. trachea

E. contains the palatine tonsils
F. contains the vocal cords
G. where oxygen and carbon
     dioxide exchange occurs

III. Match diseases or disorders in the left column (1–6) with their characteristics in the right column (A–H):

_____ 1. anthracosis
_____ 2. atelectasis
_____ 3. COPD
_____ 4. cystic fibrosis
_____ 5. emphysema
_____ 6. asthma

A. Pulmonary and alveolar edema, dsypnea, and hypoxia
B. Congenital, incomplete expansion of a lung or a portion of a lung
C. Can result from many disorders such as chronic bronchitis, emphysema, chronic asthma
D. Paroxysmal cough, ending in a whooping inspiration
E. Paroxysmal dyspnea accompanied by wheezing
F. Chronic respiratory infection and disorders of the pancreas and sweat glands
G. Destruction of the alveolar walls that leads to hindered gas exchange between the alveoli and the blood
H. Accumulation of carbon deposits in the lungs

LABELING

IV. Label structures in the diagram with the corresponding combining form. The first one is done as an example. Note that 2 and 6 have two answers.

1. sin(o)

2. (2CF's)

3.

4.

5.

6. (2CF's)

7.

8.

9.

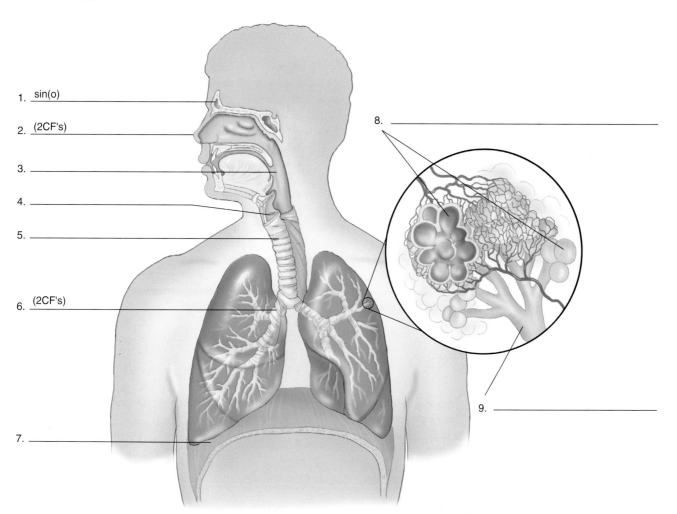

SEQUENCING

V. Number the following structures to show the sequence of passage of air from the nose to the lungs. The first one is done as an example.

nasal cavity   __1__   bronchi   _____   larynx   _____   pharynx   _____
trachea   _____   alveoli   _____   bronchioles   _____

LISTING

VI. Name 5 functions of the respiratory system.

1. _____   4. _____
2. _____   5. _____
3. _____

MULTIPLE CHOICE

VII. Choose one answer (A–D) for each of the following multiple choice questions:

1. Which of the following activities is the respiratory system's greatest contribution to the acid-base balance?
   A. expelling of CO_2
   B. helping maintain body temperature
   C. regulating water loss
   D. taking in PaO_2

2. What does phrenitis mean?
   A. inflamed diaphragm
   B. paralyzed diaphragm
   C. inflamed chest
   D. sagging chest

3. What does expectoration mean?
   A. a falling away of tissue in scales or layers
   B. hollowing or digging out
   C. coughing up and spitting out sputum
   D. expelling air from the lungs

4. Which term means occurring in a sudden, periodic attack or recurrence of symptoms?
   A. atelectasis
   B. asphyxiation
   C. pertussis
   D. paroxysmal

5. What does apnea mean?
   A. increased breathing
   B. labored or difficult breathing
   C. absence of breathing
   D. breathing is possible only in an upright position

6. What is the serous membrane that lines the walls of the thoracic cavity?
   A. visceral pleura
   B. parietal pleura
   C. rhinorrhea
   D. silicosis

7. What does dyspnea mean?
   A. increased breathing
   B. labored or difficult breathing
   C. absence of breathing
   D. breathing is possible only in an upright position

8. What is bradyphasia?
   A. fast speech
   B. slow speech
   C. difficult speech
   D. absence of speech

9. Which of the following is an acute infectious disease characterized by cough, ending in a whooping inspiration?
   A. pertussis
   B. paroxysmal
   C. chronic obstructive lung disease
   D. respiratory distress syndrome

10. Which term means the drawing of air into the lungs?
    A. pneumomalacia
    B. orthopnea
    C. inspiration
    D. hypoxia

11. What is the term for loss of acid by the body, such as may occur in hyperventilation?
    A. acidosis
    B. alkalosis
    C. acid-base balance
    D. acid-base compensation

12. What is the name of the instrument that measures the amount of air taken into and expelled from the lungs?
    A. stethoscope
    B. pneumoscope
    C. cardiometer
    D. spirometer

13. Which of the following is *not* meant by the word *ptosis*?
    A. surgical puncture
    B. sagging
    C. downward displacement
    D. prolapse

14. What is effusion of fluid into the air spaces and tissue spaces of the lungs called?
    A. pleuropneumonia
    B. pneumonitis
    C. pulmonary edema
    D. pulmonary insufficiency

15. What is another name for pneumonia?
    A. pulmonary edema
    B. pulmonary insufficiency
    C. congestive heart
    D. pneumonitis

WRITING TERMS

VIII. Write a term for each of the following:

1. below normal carbon dioxide   _____
2. excision of the larynx   _____
3. fibrous condition of the chest   _____
4. inflammation of the bronchioles   _____
5. nasal septal reconstruction   _____
6. origin of cancer   _____
7. pertaining to the alveoli   _____
8. pertaining to the pharynx   _____

9. plastic surgery of a bronchus   _____
10. prolapse of the diaphragm   _____
11. rapid respiration   _____
12. removal of an embolus   _____
13. runny nose   _____
14. softening of the lungs   _____
15. surgical repair of the palate   _____

▶ GREATER COMPREHENSION

SPELLING

IX. Circle all incorrectly spelled terms and write their correct spelling:

acapnia   awscultation   bronchiolectasis   cardiodiaphragmatic   hemoptusis

INTERPRETING ABBREVIATIONS

X. Write the meaning of these abbreviations:

1. ET _____
2. PFT _____
3. RLL _____

4. TTO _____
5. URI _____

CASE STUDY

XI. Choose A, B, C, or D for questions 1 through 5 after reading the summary about this patient.

I.A., female, 20 years of age	
Sx	Patient complains of pharyngodynia, cough, fever, and muscular aches and pains.
PE	T 102.2
	BP 135/80 P 95
	Enlarged and inflamed tonsils. No other significant findings. No known allergies.
Dx	Influenza
Rx	Bed rest
	Drink fluids
	Amoxicillin 250 mg, po 1 capsule q8h for 10 days
	Acetaminophen 500 mg, po 2 tablets t.i.d.

1. Pharyngodynia means
   A. absence of voice
   B. congenital malformation of the pharynx
   C. sore throat
   D. weak voice

2. The abbreviation T means
   A. tablet
   B. temperature
   C. tetanus
   D. thyroxine

3. The disease that was diagnosed is
   A. caused by a virus
   B. chronic
   C. congenital
   D. not contagious

4. How often is the prescription for amoxicillin to be taken?
   A. eight times a day
   B. every four hours
   C. every eight hours
   D. four times a day

5. How often is acetaminophen to be taken?
   A. once a day
   B. twice a day
   C. three times a day
   D. four times a day

PRONUNCIATION

XII. The pronunciation is shown for several medical words. Indicate which syllable has the primary accent by marking it with an ′.

1. asphyxia (**as fik se ə**)
2. pneumomalacia (**noo mo mə la shə**)
3. pulmonic (**pəl mon ik**)

4. rhinolithiasis (**ri no lĭ thi ə sis**)
5. spirometer (**spi rom ə tər**)

CATEGORIZING TERMS

XIII. In each of the following words, categorize the term by writing A, D, R, S, or T to indicate anatomical, diagnostic, radiological, surgical, or therapeutic. Number four is done as an example.

Category

1. acidosis _____
2. apnea _____
3. bronchography _____
4. coryza ___D___
5. decongestant _____

Category

6. laryngoplasty _____
7. oximeter _____
8. palate _____
9. thoracotomy _____
10. uvula _____

DRUG CLASSES

XIV. Match the drug classes in the left column with their effects or uses by choosing A, B, C, or D.

_____ 1. antihistamines   **A.** divided into H_1 and H_2 blockers
_____ 2. antitussives   **B.** eliminate or reduce swelling
_____ 3. bronchodilators   **C.** relax the contraction of smooth muscle of bronchioles
_____ 4. decongestants   **D.** suppress coughing

(Check your answers with the solutions in Appendix V.)

Listing of Medical Terms

acapnia	aphasia	bronchiolectasis	calculus
acid-base balance	aphasic	bronchiolitis	cannula
acidemia	aphonia	bronchitis	carcinogen
acidosis	aplasia	bronchoalveolar	carcinogenesis
acute	apnea	bronchoconstriction	carcinogenic
alkalemia	asbestosis	bronchodilator	carcinolysis
alkaline	asphyxia	bronchogenic	cardiopulmonary
alkalosis	asphyxiation	bronchogram	resuscitation
alveolar	aspiration	bronchography	chronic
alveolus	asthma	broncholithiasis	congestive heart failure
anoxia	asthmatic	bronchopathy	corticosteroid
anthracosis	atelectasis	bronchoplasty	coryza
antiasthmatic	auditory tube	bronchopneumonia	crackle
anticancer	auscultation	bronchopulmonary	croup
anticholinergic	bradyphasia	bronchoscope	cystic fibrosis
anti–cystic fibrosis	bradypnea	bronchoscopic	decongestant
antihistamine	bronchi	bronchoscopy	diaphragm
antineoplastic	bronchiectasis	bronchospasm	dysphasia
antitussive	bronchiole	bronchus	dysphonia

Listing of Medical Terms—cont'd

dyspnea
embolectomy
embolism
embolus
emphysema
empyema
endonasal
endotracheal intubation
epiglottiditis
epiglottis
epiglottitis
eupnea
eustachian tube
exhalation
expectorant
expectorate
expectoration
expiration
extrapleural
extrapulmonary
fibroid
fibrolysin
fibroma
fibrothorax
glottis
hemoptysis
hemothorax
hydrothorax
hyperalgia
hypercapnia
hyperesthesia
hyperoxemia
hyperpnea
hyperventilation
hypocapnia
hypopharynx
hypoxemia
hypoxia
influenza
inhalation
inspiration
interalveolar
lacrimal
laryngalgia
laryngeal
laryngectomy
laryngitis
laryngography
larngopathy

laryngopharyngeal
laryngopharynx
laryngoplasty
laryngoplegia
laryngoscope
laryngoscopy
laryngospasm
laryngostomy
laryngotracheal
laryngotracheitis
laryngotracheobronchitis
larynx
lithiasis
lithogenesis
lobectomy
malignant
mediastinum
melanoma
metastasis
metastatic
mucolytic
mucus
nares
nasal polyp
nasolacrimal duct
nasopharyngeal
nasopharyngitis
nasopharynx
nasoscope
nasoseptoplasty
nasotracheal intubation
neoplasm
olfactory
oropharyngeal
oropharynx
orotracheal intubation
orthopnea
ostomy
oximeter
oximetry
palate
palatine tonsil
palatitis
palatoplasty
paranasal sinus
parietal pleura
patent
percussion
pertussis

pharyngalgia
pharyngeal
pharyngitis
pharyngodynia
pharyngomycosis
pharyngopathy
pharyngoplasty
pharyngoscope
pharynx
phonic
phrenic
phrenitis
phrenodynia
phrenoplegia
phrenoptosis
pleura
pleural cavity
pleural effusion
pleurisy
pleuritis
pleurocentesis
pleurodynia
pleuropneumonia
pneumectomy
pneumocardial
pneumocentesis
pneumoconiosis
pneumohemothorax
pneumomalacia
pneumomelanosis
pneumonectomy
pneumonia
pneumonic
pneumonitis
pneumothorax
polyp
ptosis
pulmonary angiography
pulmonary edema
pulmonary embolus
pulmonary fibrosis
pulmonary lobectomy
pulmonic
pyothorax
rale
respiration
respiratory
retronasal
rhinitis

rhinolith
rhinolithiasis
rhinoplasty
rhinorrhagia
rhinorrhea
silicosis
sinusitis
smoking cessation adjuncts
spirometer
spirometry
sputum
stoma
stridor
subphrenic
subpulmonary
supranasal
syndrome
tachyphasia
tachypnea
thoracentesis
thoracic paracentesis
thoracocentesis
thoracopathy
thoracoplasty
thoracotomy
thorax
thromboembolic
tonsillitis
tracheal
trachealgia
tracheomalacia
tracheoplasty
tracheorrhagia
tracheoscopy
tracheostenosis
tracheostomy
tracheotome
tracheotomy
transtracheal
tubercle
tuberculosis
uvula
ventilation
visceral pleura
vital capacity
wheeze

Español ## Enhancing Spanish Communication

English	Spanish (pronunciation)
acidity	acidez (ah-se-DES)
acute	agudo (ah-GOO-do)
asphyxia	asfixia (as-FEEC-se-ah)
asthma	asma (AHS-mah)
benign	benigno (bay-NEEG-no)
breathe	alentar (ah-len-TAR), respirar (res-pe-RAR)
breathing	respiración (res-pe-rah-se-ON)
calculus	cálculo (CAHL-coo-lo)
cancer	cáncer (CAHN-ser)
chest	pecho (PAY-cho)
chronic	crónico (CRO-ne-co)
cough	tos (tos)
diaphragm	diafragma (de-ah-FRAHG-mah)
edema	hidropesía (e-dro-pay-SEE-ah)
erect, straight	derecho (day-RAY-cho)
fiber	fibra (FEE-brah)
imperfect	imperfecto (im-per-FEC-to)
influenza	gripe (GREE-pay)
lobe	lóbulo (LO-boo-lo)

English	Spanish (pronunciation)
lung	pulmón (pool-MON)
malignant	maligno (mah-LEEG-no)
membrane	membrana (mem-BRAH-nah)
nose	nariz (nah-REES)
nostril	orificio de la nariz (or-e-FEE-se-o day lah nah-REES)
obstruction	obstrucción (obs-trooc-se-ON)
pain	dolor (do-LOR)
paralysis	parálisis (pah-RAH-le-sis)
pneumonia	neumonía (nay-oo-mo-NEE-ah), pulmonía (pool-mo-NEE-ah)
respiration	respiración (res-pe-rah-se-ON)
stone	cálculo (CAHL-coo-lo)
symptom	síntoma (SEEN-to-mah)
throat	garganta (gar-GAHN-tah)
tonsil	tonsila (ton-SEE-lah), amígdala (ah-MEEG-dah-lah)
trachea	tráquea (TRAH-kay-ah)
voice	voz (vos)

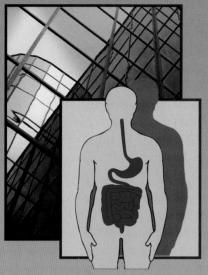

Digestive System

7

Outline

Principal Word Parts

COMBINING FORMS

amyl(o)	starch
an(o)	anus
append(o), appendic(o)	appendix
bil(i)	bile
cec(o)	cecum
cheil(o)	lip
chol(e)	bile or gall
cholecyst(o)	gallbladder
choledoch(o)	common bile duct
col(o), colon(o)	colon; large intestine
cyst(o)	bladder or sac
dent(i), dent(o), odont(o)	teeth
dips(o)	thirst
diverticul(o)	diverticula
duoden(o)	duodenum
enter(o)	intestines; small intestine
esophag(o)	esophagus
fruct(o)	fruit
fung(i)	fungus
gastr(o)	stomach
gingiv(o)	gums
gloss(o), lingu(o)	tongue
glyc(o)	sugar
hepat(o)	liver
ile(o)	ileum
intestin(o)	intestines
jejun(o)	jejunum
lact(o)	milk
lip(o)	fats
mandibul(o)	mandible
maxill(o)	maxilla
myc(o)	fungus
or(o), stomat(o)	mouth
pancreat(o)	pancreas
pex(o)	surgical fixation
pharyng(o)	pharynx
proct(o)	anus, rectum
prote(o)	protein
py(o)	pus
pylor(o)	pylorus
rect(o)	rectum
sial(o)	saliva, salivary glands
sialaden(o)	salivary gland
sigmoid(o)	sigmoid colon
top(o)	place or position
vag(o)	vagus nerve
vir(o), virus(o)	virus

PREFIXES

eu-	normal, well, or good	-clysis	irrigation or washing out
exo-	outside or outward	-emesis	vomiting
mal-	bad	-id	structure; having the shape of
par-, para-	near, beside, or abnormal	-ose	sugar
sub-	below or under	-pepsia	digestion
		-pexy	surgical fixation
SUFFIXES		-phage	eat or swallow
		-phagia	eating or swallowing
-ase	enzyme	-stalsis	contraction
-cele	hernia		

Learning Goals

▶ **BASIC UNDERSTANDING**

In this chapter, you will learn to do the following:

1. Describe the structures and functions of the digestive system and define terms associated with these structures.
2. Demonstrate an understanding of the five functions of the digestive system.
3. Recognize the three classes of nutrients and their functions, and identify glucose as the major source of cellular energy.
4. Identify the role of the salivary glands, the liver, the gallbladder, and the pancreas in digestion and absorption.
5. Write the meaning of the word parts associated with the digestive system and use them to build and analyze terms.

▶ **GREATER COMPREHENSION**

6. Spell the terms accurately.
7. Pronounce the terms correctly.
8. Differentiate terms as being related to diagnosis, anatomy, surgery, therapy, or radiology.
9. Write the meaning of the abbreviations.
10. Identify the effects or uses of the drug classes presented in this chapter.

Digestive System and Nutrition

The primary function of the digestive system is to provide the body with water, nutrients, and minerals. It does this by breaking down food until nutrient molecules are small enough to be absorbed. Waste materials are eliminated. Nutrition is the sum of the processes involved in the taking in, digestion, absorption, and use of food substances by the body. The first three processes occur in the digestive system. After the nutrients are absorbed, they are available to all of the body cells for metabolism.

	7-1 The digestive system is composed of the organs, structures, and glands of the digestive tube of the body, through which food passes from the mouth to the esophagus, stomach, intestines, and anus (a′nəs).
	It is known by many names, including the digestive tract, the alimentary (al″e-men′tər-e) tract, and the gastrointestinal (gas″tro in tes′tĭ nəl) or GI system. The combining form ***intestin(o)*** means intestine.
intestines	Gastro/intestin/al refers to the stomach and the _____.

mouth	**7-2** In humans, ingestion (**in jes′chən**) is orally taking substances into the body. Ingestion means swallowing the substances or, in other words, the substance is taken into the body through the _____.
eats	The terms *ingest* (verb) and *ingestion* (noun) are also used to describe the activity of phago/cytic cells. You have learned that phag(o) means to eat or ingest. A phago/cyte (**fag′o-sīt**) is a cell that _____ something else. The suffix **-*phage*** means to eat or swallow, and in the term macro/phage, -phage is used to designate the cell that eats or ingests something else. Phage is also a term that means a bacterio/phage, which is a virus that destroys certain bacteria. Combine phag(o) and -ia,
-phagia	which means condition: _____.
	The suffix **-*phagia*** means eating or swallowing.
eating	**7-3** A/phag/ia (**ə-fa′jə**) is absence of _____. In aphagia it is not possible to swallow. This differs from anorexia nervosa, which was discussed in Chapter 2. An/orexia means _____
absence	or lack of appetite. Anorexia nervosa is a disorder characterized by self-imposed starvation and is usually associated with psychologic stress or conflict.
dysphagia (dis-fa′je-ə)	**7-4** Using aphagia as a model, build a word that means difficult eating: _____. Canker sores on the mouth could cause dysphagia.
excessive	Poly/phag/ia (**pol″e-fa′jə**) means _____ eating, which in actuality means excessive hunger. (Some interpretation is needed, since poly- means many.) Excessive eating over a long period of time generally leads to weight gain as a result of taking in more calories than the number needed for normal body metabolism. The amount of fuel or energy in food is measured in calories.
obesity (o-bē′sĭ-te)	Obesity is an abnormal increase in the proportion of fat cells of the body, and a person is regarded as medically obese if he or she is 20% above desirable body weight for the person's age, sex, height, and body build. An abnormal increase in the proportion of fat cells of the body is called _____.
outside origin	Exo/gen/ous (**ek-soj′ə-nəs**) obesity is caused by a greater caloric intake than that needed to meet the metabolic needs of the body. Endo/gen/ous (**en-doj′ə-nəs**) obesity originates from within the body, as one would see in hormonal disorders such as uncontrolled diabetes. The prefix **exo-** means outside or outward. Breaking exo/gen/ous into its component parts, exo- means _____, gen(o) means _____, and -ous means pertaining to.
bad or poor	**7-5** If something interferes with eating or the digestion of food, body cells will not have needed nutrients. Mal/nutrition results. The prefix **mal-** means bad. Mal/nutrition is _____ nutrition.
	Mal/absorption is improper absorption of nutrients into the bloodstream from the intestines. This will eventually result in malnutrition.
excessive vomiting	**7-6** Excessive vomiting, unless treated with an anti/emetic, can also lead to malnutrition. Emesis (**em′ə-sis**) means vomiting, as does the suffix **-*emesis*.** Hyper/emesis (**hi″pər-em′ə-sis**) is _____ _____.
	Self-induced vomiting sometimes occurs in bulimia (**bu-lim′e-əh**). The derivation of the term *bulimia* from Greek is *bous,* ox, and *limos,* hunger. This disorder occurs predominantly in females and is characterized by episodes of binge eating that continue until terminated by abdominal pain, sleep, self-induced vomiting, or purging with laxatives.
vomiting blood	Hemat/emesis (**he″mə-tem′ə-sis**) is _____ _____.

	7-7 Thirst is the desire for fluid, especially for water. Not only does water serve to transport food in the digestive tract, but it is also the principal medium in which chemical reactions occur.
	The combining form ***dips(o)*** means thirst. Poly/dips/ia (**pol″e-dip′se-ə**) is excessive _____.
thirst **absence of thirst**	A/dips/ia (**ə-dip′se-ə**) is _____.
digestive	**7-8** The alimentary tract is also referred to as the _____ tract.
alimentation	Alimentation (**al″ə-men-ta′shən**) is the process of providing nourishment, or nutrition,* for the body. The role of the digestive system in nutrition is taking in, digesting, and absorbing nutrients from food. Providing nutrition for the body is called _____.
	Good nutrition is essential for metabolism (**mə-tab′ə-liz″əm**), the processes that occur after absorption and bring about growth, repair, and maintenance of the body. A balanced diet is one that is adequate in energy-providing substances (carbohydrates and fats), tissue-building compounds (proteins), inorganic chemicals (water and mineral salts), vitamins, and certain substances, such as bulk for promoting movement of the contents of the digestive tract. The recommended dietary allowances (RDAs) are the levels of daily intake of essential nutrients that are considered adequate to meet nutritional needs. The abbreviation
recommended dietary allowances	RDAs means _____.
	7-9 Carbohydrates, fats, and proteins are the three major classes of nutrients. Carbohydrates, the basic source of energy for human cells, include starches and sugars.
	The combining form ***glyc(o)*** means sugar. Glyco/lysis (**gli-kol′ĭ-sis**) is the breaking down of
sugar	_____.
above the normal amount of sugar in the blood	Hyper/glyc/emia (**hi″pər-gli-se′me-ə**) is _____.
less than the normal amount of sugar in the blood	Hypo/glyc/emia (**hi″po-gli-se′me-ə**) is _____.
	7-10 The suffix ***-ose*** means sugar. Glucose (**gloo′kōs**) is the most important carbohydrate in body metabolism. The concentration of glucose in the blood in healthy individuals is maintained at a fairly constant level. Someone who says "glycemia" is almost always referring to the presence of what sugar in the
glucose	blood? _____
lactose	The combining form ***lact(o)*** means milk. Form a new word that means milk sugar: _____.
fructose	Use ***fruct(o)*** plus the suffix for sugar to write the name of fruit sugar: _____.
	7-11 Starches, a second type of carbohydrate, break down easily and are eventually reduced to glucose before being absorbed into the blood. The combining form ***amyl(o)*** means starch. Amylo/lysis
destruction of starch	(**am″ə-lol′ə-sis**) is _____.
	Amylolysis is the breaking down (digestion) of starch.

*Nutrition (Latin: *nutriens,* food that nourishes).

7-12 Fats, also called lipids, serve as an energy reserve. Having about twice as many calories per gram as carbohydrates and proteins, fats are well suited for storage of unused calories. The combining form *lip(o)* means fats. Although lipids also include steroids, waxes, and fatty acids, lip(o) usually refers to fats.

fats

Lip/oid (**lip′oid**) means resembling _____.

lipopenia
(lip″o-pe′ne-ə)

Write a word that means a deficiency of fats: _____.

**increased amount
of fat in the blood**

Hyper/lip/emia (**hi″pər-li-pe′me-ə**) is

_____.

Sometimes the combining form *lip(o)* is not used, and hyperlipidemia is used to mean an increased amount of fat in the blood.

protein

7-13 The combining form ***prote(o)*** means protein. Prote/uria (**pro″te-u′re-ə**) is _____ in the urine. This is generally called proteinuria (**pro″te-nu′re-ə**) rather than proteuria. Protein in the urine is almost always an abnormal condition.

protein

Proteo/lysis (**pro″te-ol′ĭ-sis**) is breaking down (destruction, digestion) of _____. Proteolysis is necessary for digestion. Proteins must be chemically broken down before they can be absorbed.

7-14 Enzymes act upon food substances, causing them to break down into simpler compounds. The suffix ***-ase*** means enzyme. Enzymes are usually named by adding "ase" to the combining form of the substance on which they act. For example, lip/ase breaks down lipids.

Write the name of the enzyme that breaks down the following:

proteinase
(pro′tēn-ās) or
protease (pro′te-ās)
lactase
sucrase

Substance	Effective Enzyme
lipid	lipase (**li′pās**)
protein	_____
lactose	_____
sucrose	_____

amylase (am′ĭ-lās)
**an enzyme that
breaks down starch**

Form a new word by joining amyl(o) and -ase: _____.

The new word means _____.

7-15 The suffix ***-pepsia*** refers to digestion. Dys/pepsia (**dis-pep′se-ə**) means bad or

difficult digestion

_____ _____.

bradypepsia
(brad″e-pep′se-ə)

Write a word that means slow digestion: _____.

eupepsia
(u-pep′se-ə)

The prefix ***eu-*** means normal, well, or good. Build a word that means normal or good digestion:

_____.

nutrients or nutrition	**7-16** You learned earlier that alimentation is the process of providing _____ for the body.
excessive nutrition	Translated literally, hyper/alimentation means _____ _____.
	Hyperalimentation is overfeeding, or the ingestion or administration of an amount of nutrients that exceeds the demands of the body. Overfeeding on one's own leads to obesity. Build a word using an-, -orexia, and -ant, which means a drug or other agent that lessens the appetite: _____.
anorexiant (an"o-rek′se-ənt)	Total parenteral nutrition (TPN), the administration of all nutrition through an indwelling catheter into the vena cava, is also called hyperalimentation.
	Patients who can digest and absorb nutrients but need nutritional support may receive enteral nutrition. Enteral nutrition is the provision of nutrients to the alimentary tract through a feeding tube, usually into the stomach. You will learn in the next section that enter(o) means either intestine or small intestine. Enter/al (en′tər-əl) means within or via the small intestine. Par/enteral (pə-ren′tər-əl) means not through the alimentary tract but through some other route; in other words, by injection. The prefixes *par-* and *para-* mean near, beside, or abnormal. TPN is the abbreviation for total _____
parenteral nutrition	_____.

❏ SECTION A REVIEW   𝒟igestive System and Nutrition

This section review covers frames 7–1 through 7–16. Complete the table by writing a word part or its meaning in each blank.

Combining Form	Meaning	Suffix	Meaning
1. amyl(o)	_____	13. _____	enzyme
2. dips(o)	_____	14. -emesis	_____
3. _____	fruit	15. _____	sugar
4. _____	sugar	16. _____	digestion
5. intestin(o)	_____	17. -phage	_____
6. lact(o)	_____	18. -phagia	_____
7. lip(o)	_____		
8. prote(o)	_____		

Prefix	Meaning
9. eu-	_____
10. exo-	_____
11. mal-	_____
12. par-, para-	_____

(Use Appendix V to check your answers.)

Structures of the Digestive Tract

The digestive tract is a muscular tube, lined with mucous membrane, that extends from the mouth to the anus. Its accessory organs are the salivary glands, the liver, the gallbladder, and the pancreas.

7-17 The digestive tract and its accessory organs make up the digestive system. The digestive tract, beginning at the mouth and ending at the anus, is basically a long, muscular tube. Its accessory organs (salivary glands, liver, gallbladder, and pancreas) secrete fluids that aid in digestion and absorption of nutrients. Label the structures in Figure 7-1 as you read the following information.

Digestion begins in the mouth (1). The teeth grind and chew the food before it is swallowed. The mass of chewed food is called a bolus.

The pharynx (2) passes the bolus to the esophagus (3), which leads to the stomach (4), where food is churned and broken down chemically and mechanically.

The liquid mass, called chyme, is passed to the small intestine, where digestion continues and absorption of nutrients occurs. The three parts of the small intestine are shown: duodenum (5), jejunum (6), and ileum (7).

Undigested food passes to the large intestine (8), where much of the water is absorbed. It is stored in the rectum until it is eliminated through the anus (9).

7-18 The role of the digestive system in nutrition is achieved by several activities that begin with ingestion. You saw earlier that ingestion is the way in which the body takes in nutrients.

digestion

The second activity, digestion, is the conversion of food into substances that can eventually be absorbed by cells. The two types of digestion are mechanical and chemical digestion. Mechanical digestion begins in the mouth with chewing, and continues with churning actions in the stomach. Through chemical digestion, carbohydrates, proteins, and fats are transformed into smaller molecules. The accessory organs contribute digestive fluids to aid this process. The second activity of nutrition, called _____, consists of both mechanical and chemical processes that break down the food.

7-19 The third activity consists of various movements of the food particles, both along the digestive tract and by mixing of food particles with enzymes and other fluids. All of these movements are brought about by the contractions of smooth muscles of the digestive system. The third stage, in which food is moved along or mixed with fluids, is called _____.

movements

around

The movement of food particles through the digestive tract is called peristalsis (per″ĭ-stal′sis). You learned earlier that peri- means _____. The suffix -*stalsis* means contraction. The presence of food in the digestive tube stimulates a coordinated, rhythmic muscular contraction called peristalsis.

7-20 The fourth activity is absorption, the process in which the digested food molecules pass through the lining of the small intestine into the blood or lymph capillaries. This passage of the simple molecules from the lining of the small intestine into the blood or lymph is called _____.

absorption

7-21 The fifth activity, called elimination, is removal of undigested food particles (waste). Wastes are excreted (eliminated) through the anus in the form of feces. This fifth function of the digestive system is called _____. The five activities, representing the functions of the digestive system, are summarized in Table 7-1.

elimination

The elimination of undigested food particles is only one type of elimination of body wastes. In the previous chapter, you studied the elimination of another waste product, carbon dioxide.

TABLE 7-1 Functions of the Digestive System*

- Ingestion: eating food
- Digestion: mechanically and chemically breaking down food
- Peristaltic movements: moving food along the digestive tract and mixing it
- Absorption: passage of simple nutrient molecules from the small intestine to the blood or lymph
- Elimination: removal of wastes

*Some anatomy books list only the functions of digestion, absorption, and elimination.

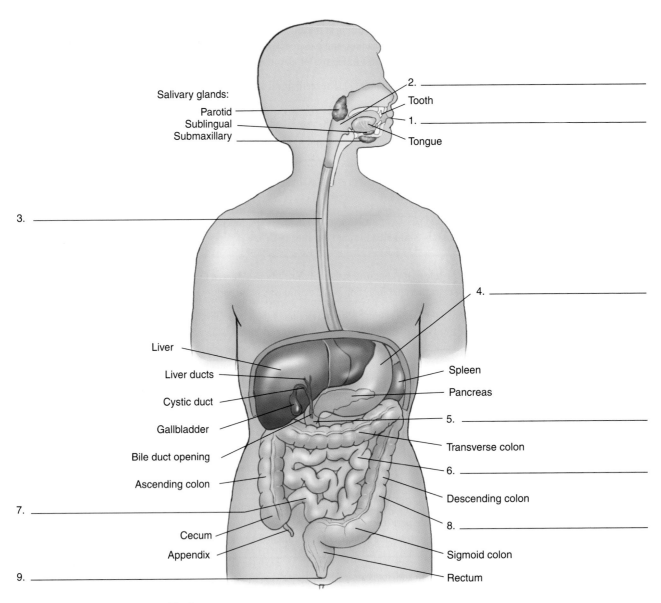

Salivary glands:
    Parotid
    Sublingual
    Submaxillary

2. _____
Tooth
1. _____
Tongue

3. _____

4. _____

Liver
Liver ducts
Cystic duct
Gallbladder
Bile duct opening
Ascending colon

Spleen
Pancreas
5. _____
Transverse colon
6. _____
Descending colon

7. _____
Cecum
Appendix
9. _____

8. _____
Sigmoid colon
Rectum

FIGURE 7-1

Structures of the digestive system. The alimentary tract, beginning at the mouth and ending at the anus, is basically a long, muscular tube. Several accessory organs (salivary glands, liver, gallbladder, and pancreas) are also shown. Digestion begins in the mouth. The teeth grind and chew the food before it is swallowed. The mass of chewed food is called a bolus. The pharynx passes the bolus to the esophagus, which leads to the stomach, where food is churned and broken down chemically and mechanically. The liquid mass, called chyme, is passed to the small intestine, where digestion continues and absorption of nutrients occurs. The three parts of the small intestine are shown: duodenum, jejunum, and ileum. Undigested food passes to the large intestine, where much of the water is absorbed. It is then excreted from the anus, the opening of the rectum on the body surface.

7-22 Look again at the structures you labeled in Figure 7-1. These structures make up the muscular tube portion of the digestion tract. Several accessory organs are also shown. The salivary glands, the liver, the gallbladder, and the pancreas are the accessory organs of the digestive system.

You already know the combining forms for some of the structures you labeled. Write the name of the structure associated with these combining forms:

mouth — or(o) _____

pharynx — pharyng(o) _____

intestine — intestin(o) _____

7-23 A second combining form that means mouth is **stomat(o).** In general, or(o) is used in terms that describe the mouth as a structure, and stomat(o) is used to write other terms, such as diagnostic and surgical terms. Pharyngeal means pertaining to the pharynx. Using a combining form for mouth plus pharyngeal, write a term that means pertaining to the mouth and pharynx: _____.

oropharyngeal

Oropharyngeal also means pertaining to the oropharynx.

Decide which combining form to use to write a word that means any disease of the mouth: _____.

stomatopathy (sto″mə-top′ə-the)

7-24 Use **esophag(o)** to write terms about the esophagus. Esophag/eal means pertaining to the _____.

esophagus

The esophagus is a long muscular canal that extends from the pharynx to the stomach. The combining form **gastr(o)** means stomach. Using -ic, write a word that means pertaining to the stomach: _____.

gastric (gas′trik)

7-25 You already know that intestin(o) means intestine. A second combining form that means intestine is **enter(o),** but it sometimes is used to mean specifically the small intestine. Intestin/al means _____.

pertaining to the intestines

Gastro/intestinal means pertaining to the _____ and intestines.

stomach

Most medical words concerning the intestines are formed using enter(o). Enter/ic means pertaining to the small intestine. Enter/al means within, by way of, or pertaining to the small intestine. Enter/al feeding introduces food into the gastrointestinal tract (usually the stomach). Practice will help you remember which meaning is intended.

7-26 The combining form **col(o)** means the large intestine. This combining form can also mean the colon, the structure that comprises most of the large intestine and where much of the water is absorbed as the wastes are moved along to the rectum. Col/itis is _____ of the large intestine.

inflammation

small intestines

Entero/col/itis is inflammation involving both the large and _____ _____.

7-27 The rectum (rek′təm) is the lower part of the large intestine. The anus (a′nəs) is the outlet of the rectum, and it lies in the fold between the buttocks. The anal canal is about 4 cm long. Solid wastes are eliminated via the anus. The combining form **an(o)** means anus. An/al means _____.

pertaining to the anus

mucus **mucous** (mu′kəs) **mucosa** (mu-ko′sə) resembling mucus	**7-28** The digestive tract is lined with a mucous membrane, which secretes mucus for lubrication. Mucus is the slippery material produced by mucous membranes. Several words using the combining form muc(o) are similar. The noun that means a slick material in the digestive tract that provides lubrication is _____. The adjective that one uses to describe a membrane that secretes mucus is _____. A mucosa is the same as a mucous membrane. The digestive tract is lined with a mucous membrane, or a _____. Muc/oid means _____ _____.

❑ SECTION B REVIEW   𝒮tructures of the Digestive Tract

This section review covers frames 7–17 through 7–28. Complete the table by writing a word part or its meaning in each blank.

Combining Form	Meaning	Combining Form	Meaning
1. an(o)	_____	6. stomat(o)	_____
2. col(o)	_____	**Suffix**	**Meaning**
3. enter(o)	_____	7. -stalsis	_____
4. _____	esophagus		
5. _____	stomach		

(Use Appendix V to check your answers.)

𝒪ral Cavity

The oral cavity is the beginning of the digestive tract. It contains many structures that hold the food in place and facilitate chewing. Salivary glands, which are accessory organs of digestion, secrete saliva into the oral cavity.

inflammation of the mouth stomatodynia (sto″mə-to-din′e-ə) mouth	**7-29** The oral cavity, or mouth, is the beginning of the digestive tract. The combining form *stomat(o)* means mouth. Stomat/itis (sto″mə-ti′tis) is _____. If one has stomatitis, eating is difficult because the mouth is painful. Build a word using -dynia that means painful mouth: _____. A familiar cause of stomatodynia is canker (**kang′ kər**) sores. The term *canker* has several definitions, but when associated with humans, it means an ulcer (**ul′sər**), particularly on the mouth and lips. Ulcers are defined, craterlike lesions. Canker sores are often called cold sores or fever blisters. Do not confuse stomat(o) with stomach. The combining form for stomach is *gastr(o)*. Stomat/o means _____.
mouth fungal condition stomatomycosis surgical repair of the mouth	**7-30** Stomato/mycosis (sto″mə-to-mi-ko′sis) is a fungal condition of the _____. The combining form *myc(o)* means fungus. Myc/osis is a _____ _____. Fung/al (**fun′gəl**) means pertaining to a fungus and uses the combining form *fung(i),* which means fungus. Most words that pertain to a fungus, however, use the combining form *myc(o)*. Any fungal disease of the mouth is _____. Stomato/plasty (sto′mə-to-plas″te) is _____.

lip surgical repair of the lips and mouth lips	**7-31** Use *cheil(o)* to write terms about the lip. Cheilo/plasty (ki′lo-plas″te) is surgical repair of the _____. Cheilo/stomato/plasty (ki″lo-sto-mat′o-plas″te) is _____. Cheil/osis (ki-lo′sis) is a condition of the _____. In cheilosis there is splitting of the lips and angles of the mouth. Cheilosis is a characteristic of riboflavin deficiency in the diet.
cheilitis (ki-li′tis) inflammation of the lip mouth	**7-32** Inflammation of the lip is _____. Cheilitis often produces pain when one attempts to eat. Cheilitis and other abnormal conditions of mouth structures can result in poor nutrition. Cheil/itis is _____. Gingivo/stomat/itis (jin″jĭ-vo-sto″mə-ti′tis) is inflammation of the gums and _____.
gums gingiva	**7-33** From the previous frame, you see that *gingiv(o)* is a combining form that means the gums. Gingiv/al (jin′jĭ-vəl) pertains to the _____. Another name for the gum is gingiva. The mucous membrane that provides support for the teeth is the gum. Another name for the gum is _____.
gingivitis (jin″jĭ-vi′tis) painful gums	**7-34** Inflammation of the gum is _____. Gingiv/algia (jin″jĭ-val′jə) is _____ _____.
excision of the gums gingivectomy	**7-35** Gingiv/ectomy (jin″gĭ-vek′tə-me) is _____. Gingivectomy is surgical removal of all loose and diseased gum tissue. Excision of the gum is _____.
gums glossopathy (glos-op′ə-the)	**7-36** Gingivo/gloss/itis (jin″jĭ-vo-glos-i′tis) is inflammation of the tongue and _____. Using *gloss(o)* to mean tongue, any disease of the tongue is a _____.
cancerous tumor excision of all or a portion of the tongue	**7-37** A gloss/ectomy (glos-ek′tə-me) is often done in cases of carcinoma of the tongue. What is carcinoma? _____ _____ A gloss/ectomy is _____.
tongue throat (or pharynx) glossitis (glos-si′tis) glossoplegia (glos-o-ple′je-ə) glossoplasty (glos′o-plas″te)	**7-38** Gloss/pharyng/eal (glos″o-fə-rin′je-əl) refers to the _____ and the _____. Write words for the following: Inflammation of the tongue: _____. Paralysis of the tongue: _____. Surgical repair of the tongue: _____.
pertaining to the tongue tongue hypoglossal	**7-39** Gloss/al (glos′əl) means _____. Hypo/glossal (hi″po-glos′əl) means under the _____. Some medications are designed to be placed under the tongue, where they dissolve. Beneath or under the tongue is _____.

tongue gloss(o) lingu(o)	**7-40** Most words involving the tongue use the combining form *gloss(o)*. Some words use **lingu(o)**, which also means tongue. Lingu/al (**ling′gwəl**) pertains to the _____. Two combining forms you have learned, both meaning tongue, are _____ and _____.
teeth dental	**7-41** You have already learned that dent(o) means teeth. Dent/al pertains to the _____. A dental hygienist is one whose primary concern is maintenance of dental health and prevention of oral disease. Dental hygienists work with dentists, and one of their major tasks is cleaning teeth. Those concerned with the maintenance of dental health and prevention of oral disease are _____ hygienists.
teeth between the teeth	**7-42** Remembering that inter- means between, inter/dental (**in″tər-den′təl**) means between the _____. An interdental cavity occurs where? _____
painful tooth or toothache denture	**7-43** What is dent/algia (**den-tal′jə**)? _____. The "dent" in denture refers to teeth. A dent/ure (**den′chər**) refers to a set of teeth, either natural or artificial, but is ordinarily used to designate artificial ones. A replacement for one's natural teeth is an artificial _____.
teeth, tongue teeth dental	**7-44** Another combining form for teeth is **dent(i)**. Denti/lingual (**den″tĭ-ling′wəl**) pertains to the _____ and the _____. A denti/frice* (**den′tĭ-fris**) is a substance used to clean and polish the _____. Caries† (**kar′ēz**) means decay. Cavities in teeth are _____ caries.
teeth	**7-45** Dentistry is the art and science of diagnosing, preventing, and treating diseases and disorders of the teeth and surrounding structures of the oral cavity. There are several dental specialties, each requiring additional training after graduating from dental school. Remembering that odont(o) also means teeth, orth/odont/ics is concerned with irregularities of _____ and associated facial problems.
inflammation of the tooth pulp inside the tooth endodontium	**7-46** The soft tissue inside the tooth is the dental pulp, also called the endodontium (**en″do-don′she-əm**). Endodont/itis (**en″do-don-ti′tis**) is _____. When the word *endodontium* is broken down into its component parts, we see that its parts mean _____. For this reason, tooth pulp is given the name _____.
around inflammation of the periodontium	**7-47** The tissue investing and supporting the teeth is peri/odont/ium (**per″e-o-don′she-əm**). You learned that peri- means around, so peri/odont/ium is the tissue _____ the teeth. Peri/odont/al (**per″e-o-don′təl**) means around a tooth, or pertaining to the periodontium. Peri/odont/itis (**per″e-o-don-ti′tis**) is _____.

*Denti/frice (Latin: *fricare,* to rub).
†Caries (Latin: *decay*).

periodontics (per"e-o-don'tiks)	**7-48** A peri/odont/ist (per"e-o-don' tist) specializes in the study and treatment of the periodontium. What is the specialty of a periodontist? _____
flow or discharge	Periodontal disease is also known as pyorrhea (pi"o-re'ə). Pyo/rrhea means _____ of pus. The combining form *py(o)* means pus.
gums	Pyorrhea is an inflammation of the gingiva and the periodontal ligament, the fibrous connective tissue that anchors the tooth to the base. Gingiva is the _____.

7-49 The primary or deciduous teeth, often called "baby teeth," begin to fall out and to be replaced with permanent teeth when the child is about 6 years of age. The wisdom teeth are the last teeth to erupt, generally between 17 and 25 years of age.

There are 32 permanent teeth in a full set. The mouth has an upper and a lower dental arch, the curving shape formed by the arrangement of a normal set of teeth in the jaw. A complete set has 16 teeth in each dental arch. Observe the dental arch in Figure 7-2, A. The eight teeth on each side of the dental arch make up a quadrant. Label the teeth in a quadrant as you read the information that follows.

There are two incisors (in-si'zorz) (1), one cuspid (kus'pid) (2), two bicuspids (3), and three molars (4). Anterior teeth generally fall out and are replaced sooner than posterior ones. The last molar, which is posterior to all other teeth, is known as the wisdom tooth.

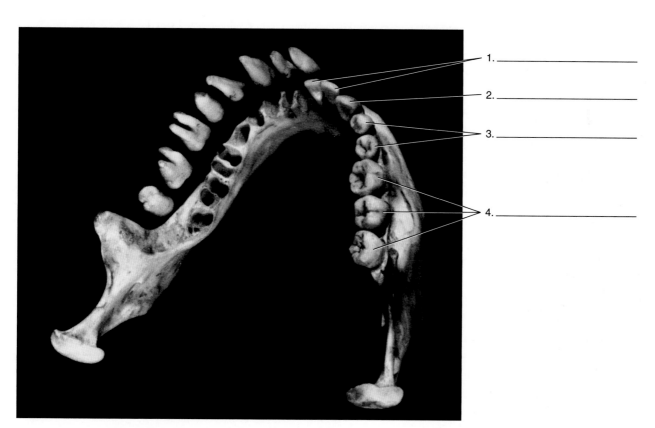

1. _____
2. _____
3. _____
4. _____

FIGURE 7-2
Designations of permanent teeth. **A,** Teeth of the lower jaw (mandibular arch). The teeth are shown on the right side and are removed on the left side to demonstrate the roots. (**A,** Adapted from Liebgott B: *The anatomical basis of dentistry,* 1982, Mosby.)

Continued

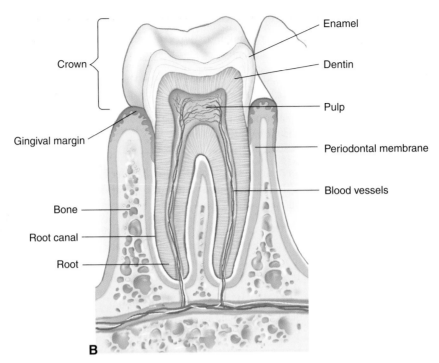

Enamel
Dentin
Pulp
Periodontal membrane
Blood vessels
Crown
Gingival margin
Bone
Root canal
Root

B

FIGURE 7-2, cont'd

B, Section of a molar tooth. All teeth follow a basic plan, consisting of two basic parts: the crown and the root or roots (embedded in the bony socket). The central cavity contains the root canal and tooth pulp, which are richly supplied with blood and lymph vessels, as well as nerves. The chief substance of the tooth, dentin, is similar to bone but harder and more compact. Dentin is covered by enamel on the crown. Enamel is the hardest substance in the body and is composed mainly of calcium phosphate. The cementum is a bonelike connective tissue that provides support to the tooth.

crown	**7-50** The structure of a molar is shown in Figure 7-2, *B*. All teeth consist of two basic parts: the crown and the root or roots (embedded in the bony socket). A socket is a hollow or depression into which another part fits, in this case, the tooth. The part that projects above the gum is the _____. The exposed part of the crown is covered by enamel, the hardest substance in the body. The central cavity contains the root canal and tooth pulp.
decay **pulp**	**7-51** The teeth and adjacent tissues are subject to many diseases and disorders. To a large extent, the mouth is examined for oral cancer during a routine dental examination. An almost universal affliction is dental caries, which means tooth _____. Neglected caries, over a period of time, invade and inflame pulpal tissues. End/odont/itis means inflammation of the endodontium, or the tooth _____. An impacted tooth is one that is unable to erupt because of adjacent teeth or mal/position of the tooth.
straighten **maxillary** (mak'sĭlar″e) **lower**	**7-52** Mal/occlusion, or improper bite, is abnormal contact of the teeth of the upper jaw, the maxilla (**mak-sil′ə**), with the teeth of the lower jaw, the mandible (**man′dĭ-bəl**). Ortho/dontic braces are used to move the teeth into alignment, in other words to _____ the teeth. Using *maxill(o)*, meaning maxilla, and -ary, write an adjective that means pertaining to the maxilla: _____. The combining form *mandibul(o)* means mandible. Mandibul/ar means pertaining to the mandible, or the _____ jaw.

temporo-mandibular (tem″pə-ro-mən-dibʹu-lər)	**7-53** TMJ syndrome is an abnormal condition that interferes with eating and is believed to be caused by a defective or dislocated temporo/mandibular joint (TMJ) in the jaw. It is characterized by facial pain and clicking sounds while chewing. The temporomandibular joint connects the lower jaw bone to the temporal bone of the skull. Malocclusion, ill-fitting dentures, and a variety of conditions can cause TMJ syndrome. TMJ refers to the _____ joint.
	7-54 The oral cavity is the gateway to the digestive tract. The mouth tastes what we consume and performs other functions of digestion by mixing the food with saliva, chewing, and voluntarily swallowing it.

❑ SECTION C REVIEW 𝒪ral Cavity

This section review covers frames 7–29 through 7–54. Complete the table by writing a word part or its meaning in each blank.

Combining Form	Meaning	Combining Form	Meaning
1. cheil(o)	_____	6. lingu(o)	_____
2. dent(i)	_____	7. mandibul(o)	_____
3. fung(i)	_____	8. myc(o)	_____
4. _____	gums	9. maxill(o)	_____
5. gloss(o)	_____	10. py(o)	_____

(Use Appendix V to check your answers.)

SECTION D

𝓔sophagus and Stomach

The esophagus is a muscular canal, about 24 cm (about 9.5 inches) long, extending from the pharynx to the stomach. The esophagus secretes mucus to facilitate the movement of food into the stomach, which also is lined with mucous membrane. Food is broken down both mechanically and chemically in the stomach.

| pertaining to the esophagus

sphincter
stomach	**7-55** Food that is swallowed passes from the mouth to the pharynx and the esophagus. Both the pharynx and the esophagus are muscular structures that move food along on its way to the stomach. Upper and lower esophag/eal sphincters control the movement of food into and out of the esophagus. A sphincter* (**sfingkʹtər**) consists of circular muscle that constricts a passage or closes a natural opening in the body. Esophag/eal means _____. The circular esophageal muscle that controls movement of food from the pharynx into the esophagus is called the upper esophageal _____. The lower esophageal sphincter controls the movement of food into the _____. This sphincter is also called the cardiac sphincter because the name of the portion of the stomach near the upper opening is the cardiac region. The region was so named because of its proximity to the heart.
tracheoesophageal (tra″ke-o-e-sofʹə-je-əl)

esophagitis (ə-sof″ə-jiʹtis)

pain | **7-56** Place a combining form before esophageal to write a word that means pertaining to the windpipe and esophagus: _____. Inflammation of the esophagus is _____. Esophago/dynia (**ə-sofʹə-go-dinʹe-ə**) is _____ of the esophagus. |

*Sphincter (Greek sphinkter, that which binds tight).

7-57 Fluoroscopy (**floo-ros´kə-pe**) permits both structural and functional visualization of internal body structures and is used frequently when testing the digestive tract and several other body systems. Using contrast media, the motion of a body part can be viewed, and the image can be recorded on film if so desired. The permanent record is called a photo/fluoro/gram (**fo″to-floor´o-gram**). The procedure that shows motion of a body part is called _____.

fluoroscopy

An esophagram (**ə-sof´ə-gram**) (or esophagogram [**ə-sof´ə-go-gram**]) is an x-ray of the esophagus taken while the patient swallows a barium solution and thus is called a barium swallow. Being careful with the spelling, write the term that is a shortened version of esophagogram: _____.

esophagram

esophagus

7-58 Esophag/ectasia (**ə-sof´ə-jek-ta´shə**) is dilation or stretching of the _____.

esophagus
stomach

Esophago/gastro/scopy (**ə-sof″ə-go-gas-tros´kə-pe**) refers to examination of the _____ and the _____.

esophagomalacia (**ə-sof″ə-go-mə-la´shə**)

Using -malacia, write a word that means a morbid softening of the esophagus: _____.

esophagoptosis (**ə-sof″ə-gop-to´sis**)

Using -ptosis, write a word that means prolapse of the esophagus: _____.

7-59 Examine Figure 7-3, *A*, to learn more about the structure of the stomach. Regions of the stomach are the cardiac region, the fundus (**fun´dəs**), the body, and the pyloric (**pi-lor´ik**) region.

The cardiac region lies near the upper opening from the esophagus. The round and most superior region of the stomach is called the _____.

fundus

The main portion of the stomach is called the body. As the body of the stomach approaches the lower opening, it narrows and is called the _____ region.

pyloric

The combining form *pylor(o)* means pylorus. The pylorus is the distal opening of the stomach through which the stomach contents are emptied into the duodenum, the first part of the small intestine. Pylorus is variously used to mean the pyloric region of the stomach. Within these frames, pylor(o) refers to the opening.

7-60 Look again at Figure 7-3, *B*. The mucosa that lines the stomach is arranged in temporary folds called _____. Ruga (singular of rugae) means ridge, wrinkle, or fold. The rugae, most apparent when the stomach is empty, allow the stomach to expand as it fills.

rugae (**roo´je**)

The outer layer of the stomach is called _____. This type of visceral peritoneum holds the stomach in position by its folding back on and over the structure.

serosa (**ser-o´sə**)

Three muscle layers are present in the stomach, rather than two, which are found in other structures of the digestive tract.

7-61 You learned that gastr(o) means stomach.

pertaining to the stomach

Gastr/ic (**gas´trik**) means _____.

gastric

Cancer of the stomach is _____ carcinoma.

endogastric (**en″do-gas´trik**)

Place a prefix before gastric to write a word that means pertaining to the inside (interior) of the stomach: _____.

pain of the stomach or stomachache

You should be able to recognize the meaning of many words in which gastr(o) is used. Gastr/algia (**gas-tral´jə**) is _____.

pertaining to the diaphragm and stomach

Phreno/gastric (**fren″o-gas´trik**) means

_____.

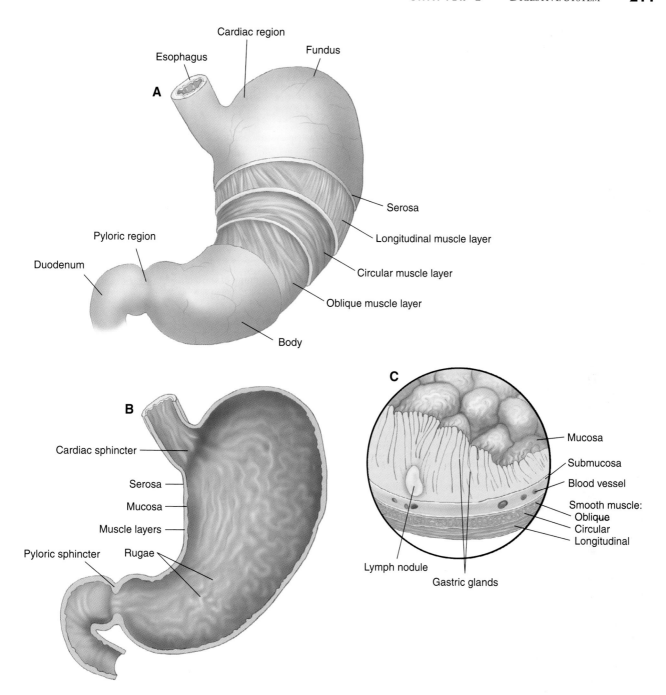

FIGURE 7-3

Features of the stomach. **A,** External view: The stomach is composed of the cardiac region, a fundus or round part, a body or middle portion, and a pyloric portion, which is the small distal end. The stomach has a serous coat (serosa) and three muscular layers. **B,** Internal view: The cardiac sphincter guards the opening of the esophagus into the stomach and prevents backflow of material into the esophagus. The stomach ends with the pyloric sphincter, which regulates outflow. The lining of the stomach, the mucosa, is arranged in temporary folds called rugae (visible in the empty stomach), which allow expansion as the stomach fills. **C,** Structure of the stomach wall: Longitudinal, circular, and oblique smooth muscle lie just beneath the serosa. All stomach layers are richly supplied with blood vessels and nerves. Gastric glands secrete gastric juice through gastric pits, tiny holes in the mucosa.

enlargement of the stomach	**7-62** Megalo/gastr/ia (**meg″ə-lo-gas′tre-ə**) is _____.
	(This is commonly called gastric hypertrophy.)
gastromegaly (gas″tro-meg′ə-le)	You learned earlier that *-megaly* is a suffix that means large. Form another word that means large stomach by using -megaly: _____.
	Some prominent signs and symptoms of gastric dysfunction are pain, excessive belching, flatulence, nausea, vomiting, blood in the stool, and diarrhea. Belching is the expelling of air or gas through the mouth or nose. Flatulence is excessive gas in the stomach or intestines. Diarrhea is frequent passage of unformed watery bowel movements, often accompanied by cramping. Anti/spasmodics are given to relieve the cramping, as well as the diarrhea.
stretching of the stomach	**7-63** Gastr/ectasis (**gas-trek′tə-sis**) or gastr/ectasia (**gas-trek-ta′zhə**) is _____.
gastromalacia (gas″tro-mə-la′shə)	Using -malacia, write a word that means a morbid softening of the stomach: _____.
gastroplasty (gas′tro-plas″te)	Write a word that means surgical repair of the stomach: _____.
stomach lungs	Gastro/pulmon/ary (**gas″tro-pul′mo-nar-e**) pertains to the _____ and the _____.
	7-64 Add various suffixes to gastr(o) to form words.
gastritis (gas-tri′tis)	Inflammation of the stomach: _____
gastropathy (gas-trop′ə-the)	Any disease of the stomach: _____
gastroscope (gas′tro-skōp)	Instrument to view (inside) the stomach: _____
gastrostomy (gas-tros′tə-me)	Use -stomy to write a word that means making an artificial opening into the stomach: _____.
	Sometimes long-term enteral nutrition via a feeding tube is done when the patient can digest and absorb food but cannot swallow.
esophagogastros-tomy (ə-sof″ə-go-gas-tros′tə-me)	Trauma or a tumor in the cardiac region of the stomach sometimes makes it necessary to create a new opening between the esophagus and stomach. Write this term by combining esophag(o), gastr(o), and the suffix for creating a new opening: _____.
gastralgia **gastrodynia** (gas″tro-din′e-ə)	Two words that mean stomachache or pain of the stomach are _____ and _____.
	7-65 The combining form *pex(o)* means surgical fixation (fastening an organ or part into a stable and permanent position by means of surgery). The combining form for surgical fixation is _____; -**pexy** is a suffix that means surgical fixation.
pex(o) **stomach**	Gastro/pexy (**gas′tro-pek″se**) is surgical fixation of the _____. Gastropexy involves suturing (sewing) the stomach to the abdominal walls for correction of displacement. Downward displacement or prolapse is indicated by the suffix *-ptosis*. Write a word that means stomach prolapse: _____.
gastroptosis (gas″trop-to′sis)	
suture	Suture (**soo′chər**) has many meanings. These are the seam or line of union formed by surgical stitches, to unite by stitching, and the material used to stitch parts of the body together. Write this word that has many meanings, among them "the material used for surgical sewing": _____.

suture	**7-66** An important feature of suture material is whether it is absorbable or nonabsorbable. Absorbable _____ is gradually dissolved by body tissue. Catgut is one of the best examples of absorbable suture material.
nonabsorbable	Nonabsorbable suture is either left in the body, where it becomes embedded in scar tissue, or removed when healing is complete. Silk, cotton, and certain synthetic materials are not absorbed by the body and are examples of _____ sutures.
approximate (ə-prok′sĭ-māt″)	**7-67** Approximate means to bring close together by suture or other means. The act of bringing closer together is approximation. Tissue approximation can be accomplished with materials other than suture, such as tape, clips, and staples. In some instances, special adhesives that bond almost instantly can be sprayed on a wound to _____ the skin, thus eliminating the need for stitches.
peritoneum inflamed peritonitis	**7-68** The membrane that lines the walls of the abdominal and pelvic cavities and covers certain organs is called peritoneum. Peritoneum that lines the walls of the cavities is parietal peritoneum; that which invests certain organs is called visceral _____. Periton/itis occurs when the peritoneum becomes _____. (The noted magician Houdini died of peritonitis caused by a perforated appendix.) Peritonitis may be caused by inflammation of abdominal organs; by perforation of one of these organs, such as the gallbladder; or by internal bleeding. Infection can spread from abdominal organs to the peritoneum, causing _____.
stomach stomach	**7-69** Gastro/cele (**gas′tro-sēl**) is a hernia of the _____. A hernia (**hәr′ne-ә**) is a protrusion of an organ or part of it through the wall of the cavity that contains the organ. A weak spot or other abnormal opening in the body wall allows part of the organ to bulge through it. Notice that *-cele* means hernia. You now know that gastrocele is a hernia of the _____.
umbilical incisional femoral (fem′or-әl) inguinal (ing′gwĭ-nәl)	**7-70** A hernia can occur through any weakness or defect in the peritoneum that lines the abdominal or pelvic cavities. Principal sites of such weaknesses are the inguinal (groin) and femoral (thigh) canals, the navel, and old surgical scars. Four common types of hernias are shown in Figure 7-4. Read the information that accompanies the illustration and write answers in the blanks. A hernia that results from a weakness in the abdominal wall around the umbilicus is an _____ hernia. A hernia that occurs through inadequately healed surgery is an _____ hernia. The type of hernia that occurs if a loop of intestine descends through the femoral canal into the groin is a _____ hernia. A direct or indirect hernia that occurs in the groin is an _____ hernia.
hernias	**7-71** One type of gastrocele is a hiatus (**hi-a′tәs**) or hiatal (**hi-a′tәl**) hernia. In a hiatal hernia, there is protrusion of a structure through the opening in the diaphragm that allows passage for the esophagus. Often the structure protruding through the esophageal opening in the diaphragm is part of the stomach. These types of hernias are called hiatal _____. Figure 7-5 shows two types of hiatal hernias.

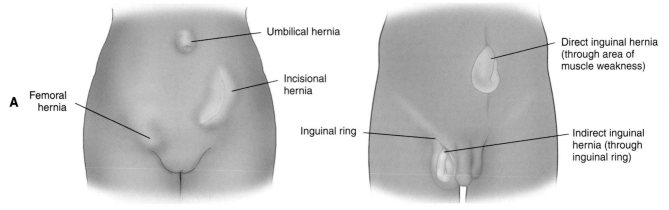

FIGURE 7-4

Common types of abdominal hernias. **A,** Umbilical hernias result from a weakness in the abdominal wall around the umbilicus. An incisional hernia is herniation through inadequately healed surgery. In a femoral hernia, a loop of intestine descends through the femoral canal into the groin. **B,** Inguinal hernias are of two types. A direct hernia occurs through an area of weakness in the abdominal wall. In an indirect hernia, a loop of intestine descends through the inguinal canal, an opening in the abdominal wall for passage of the spermatic cord in males and a ligament of the uterus in females.

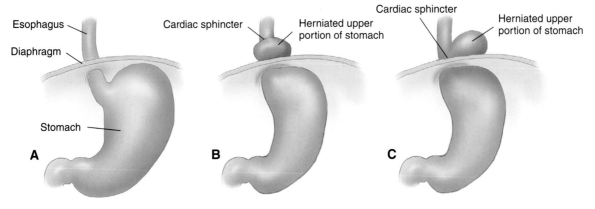

FIGURE 7-5

The normal position of the stomach versus two types of hiatal hernias. **A,** Normal position of the stomach **B,** The sliding type of hiatal hernia accounts for 85% to 90% of hiatal hernias. The upper portion of the stomach slides up and down through the opening in the diaphragm. **C,** The rolling type of hiatal hernia accounts for 10% to 15% of hiatal hernias. The upper portion of the stomach is found alongside the esophagus above the diaphragm.

stomach
esophagus
inflammation

7-72 As much as 40% of the population may have hiatal hernia, but most experience few, if any, symptoms. The major symptom experienced is gastro/esophag/eal reflux, the backflow of the acid contents of the stomach into the esophagus. Diagnosis is generally confirmed by radiology, and surgery is seldom necessary.

Gastroesophageal reflux disease (GERD) is a dysfunction that involves a backflow of the contents of the _____ into the _____. The cause is often a weak cardiac sphincter. Repeated episodes of reflux can result in esophagitis, which is _____ of the esophagus, stricture (narrowing) of the esophagus, or an esophageal ulcer. Treatment of the disorder in its early stages is elevation of the head of the bed, avoidance of acid-stimulating foods, and use of ant/acids or antiulcer medications that block either histamine (H_2 receptor antagonists) or gastric acid.

counteracts acidity	**7-73** An ant/acid (**ant-as′id**) is an agent that _____ _____. (Note the omission of the "i" in antacid.) Antacids are also used to counteract hyperacidity. Hyper/acidity (**hi″pər-ə-sid′ĭ-te**) means _____ acid. Gastric hyperacidity, excessive acid in the stomach, may lead to ulcers.
excessive	
esophagus stomach	If either the stomach or the esophagus becomes diseased near the cardiac sphincter, an esophagogastro-plasty (**ə-sof″ə-go-gas′tro-plas″te**) may be performed. This new term means surgical repair of the _____ and the _____.
duodenum	**7-74** An ulcer (**ul′sər**) is an open sore or lesion of the skin or mucous membrane produced by slough-ing of inflamed tissue. Most ulcers of the mucous membrane of the stomach, esophagus, or duodenum are caused by a particular bacterium and can be treated with antibiotics. Medications can also cause ulcers. An ulcer of the esophagus, stomach, or duodenum aggravated by the gastric juice is a peptic ulcer. A duo-denal ulcer is one that occurs in the _____.
removal of part of the stomach	Treatment of peptic ulcer can include any of the following: antibiotic, change of a suspected medication, dietary management, and antacids to counteract the acidic gastric contents. People who do not respond to medical treatment or who develop complications (perforation or hemorrhage) may require partial gastr/ectomy (**gas-trek′tə-me**), which is _____.
incision of the vagus nerve	**7-75** Gastric secretions are controlled by the vagus (**va′gəs**) nerve, the tenth cranial nerve. The combining form ***vag/o*** refers to the vagus nerve. Vago/tomy (**va-got′ə-me**) is _____.
	Vagotomy may be done in such a way that the branches supplying the acid-secreting glands of the stomach are severed without disturbing those branches that supply other abdominal structures.
gastric	**7-76** Lavage (**lah-vahzh′**) is irrigation or washing out of an organ, such as the stomach or bowel. Washing out of the stomach is _____ lavage.
	You will learn a suffix that means irrigation or washing out; however, it is generally not used in describing the procedure performed on the stomach. Gastric lavage may be performed to remove irritants or toxic substances before or after surgery on the stomach and before gastroscopy.
small intestine	**7-77** After food has been broken down by mechanical and chemical actions, it moves from the stomach to the small intestine by way of an opening at the lower end of the stomach. This opening is the pylorus, which is closed most of the time but opens at intervals to allow food to enter the _____ _____.
pyloric pylorostenosis (pi-lor″o-stə-no′sis) pyloroplasty (pi-lor′o-plas″te)	The _____ sphincter is a muscle that regulates the outflow of churned food from the stom-ach. Pyloric stenosis is narrowing of the pyloric orifice. Using pylor(o), write a word that means pyloric stenosis: _____.
	Pyloric stenosis may be relieved by surgical repair of the pylorus, called _____.
incision of the pylorus	**7-78** Pyloro/tomy (**pi″lor-ot′o-me**) is _____.
incision	Pylorotomy is often called pyloromyotomy (**pi-lor″o-mi-ot′ə-me**), which means _____ of the muscles of the pylorus.
pyloroscopy (pi″lor-os′kə-pe)	**7-79** Visual inspection of the pylorus is _____. Pyloroscopy may be accomplished by flu-oroscopic methods. Fluoroscopy enables the radiologist to see internal parts of the body in motion. Spot films are usually taken during fluoroscopy to provide a permanent record.
	The stomach is a temporary reservoir for food and is the first major site of digestion. After digestion, the stomach gradually feeds liquefied food (chyme) into the small intestine.

❑ SECTION D REVIEW   *Esophagus and Stomach*

This section review covers frames 7–55 through 7–79. Complete the table by writing a word part or its meaning in each blank.

Combining Form	Meaning	Suffix	Meaning
1. _____	pylorus	4. _____	hernia
2. _____	vagus nerve	5. _____	surgical fixation
3. pex(o)	_____		

(Use Appendix V to check your answers.)

SECTION E

Intestines

The intestine, sometimes referred to as the lower digestive tract, is the portion of the alimentary tract that extends from the pylorus to the anus. It is divided into the small intestine and large intestine. The adult small intestine is 6 to 7 meters (about 20 to 23 feet) long. The large intestine is so named because it is larger in diameter than the small intestine, but is less than one fourth as long. Assessment and treatment of these structures has been greatly facilitated by technological advances, especially in endoscopy and radiology.

stomach	**7-80** The intestines make up the lower digestive tract; however, disorders of the duodenum (first part of the small intestine) are sometimes included in disorders of the upper digestive tract. Extending from the pyloric opening to the anus, the intestinal tract (bowel) is about 7.5 to 8.5 meters (24.5 to 28 feet) long. The small intestine comprises more than three fourths the length of the intestines. The pylorus is the opening between the _____ and the first part of the small intestine.
digestion **absorption**	**7-81** The small intestine finishes the process of digestion, absorbs the nutrients, and passes the residue on to the large intestine. In other words, the small intestine is responsible for two successive processes, _____ and _____, before passing the residue to the large intestine.
stomach and intestines and associated diseases **gastroenteritis** (gas″tro-en″tər-i′tis)	**7-82** The combining form *enter(o)* means intestines, sometimes referring to the small intestine only. Gastro/entero/logy is the study of the _____. Using the preceding frame as a reference, build a word that means inflammation of the stomach and intestines: _____.
loss of appetite **water** **viral**	**7-83** Gastroenteritis occurs in several gastrointestinal disorders. Symptoms are anorexia, nausea, vomiting, abdominal discomfort, diarrhea, and depending on the cause, fever. Anorexia is _____. Diarrhea is the frequent passage of loose, watery stools (feces). The stool may also contain blood, mucus, pus, or excessive amounts of fat. Untreated severe diarrhea may lead to rapid dehydration. Dehydration is excessive loss of _____ from body tissues. Control of diarrhea may be achieved with antidiarrheal medication and a diet limited to clear fluids. Intestinal flu is a viral gastroenteritis. The combining forms *vir(o)* and *virus(o)* mean virus,* a minute microorganism much smaller than a bacterium that can replicate only within host cells. The word that means pertaining to a virus is _____.

*Virus (Latin: poison).

intestines	**7-84** Entero/stasis (**en″tər-o-sta′sis**) is the stopping of food in its passage through the _____. When enterostasis occurs, there is a delay or a stopping of the movement of food in the intestinal tract.
stopping, controlling	You learned that -*stasis* means stopping or controlling. As a word, stasis is used to mean stagnation of the normal flow of fluids, as of the blood or urine or of the intestinal mechanism. The suffix -*stasis* means _____ or _____.
stopping	**7-85** Chole/stasis (**ko″le-sta′sis**) is _____ the flow of bile. Bile is produced by the liver, stored in the gallbladder, and transported to the small intestine when needed for digestion. Anything that interferes with the flow of bile interferes with digestion. Cholestasis is stoppage or suppression of bile flow.
enterostasis	The stoppage of food in its passage through the intestine is _____. Contractions occur involuntarily to move the contents of the stomach and intestines onward.
enteritis (en″tər-i′tis)	**7-86** Write a word that means inflammation of the intestine, especially the small intestine: _____.
intestinal pain	Entero/dynia (**en″tər-o-din′e-ə**) is _____ _____.
enteroclysis (en″tər-ok′lə-sis)	You know that lavage means the irrigation of an organ. The suffix **-clysis** means irrigation or washing out of an organ. Write a term that means intestinal irrigation by combining enter(o) and -clysis: _____.
fluoroscope	**7-87** Fluoroscopy is a radiologic technique that provides immediate serial images that are invaluable in assessing the function of internal organs, especially those of the gastrointestinal system. The instrument used in fluoro/scopy is a _____. A contrast medium is a radiopaque substance that makes internal organs more visible in radiographic imaging.
gastrointestinal	**7-88** The designations of the "upper gastrointestinal (GI) tract" and the "lower gastrointestinal (GI) tract" apply mainly to radiographic or fluoroscopic views after use of a barium sulfate solution, a contrast medium. The digestive structures from the esophagus to and including the duodenum are studied in an upper GI series. Upper GI means upper _____.
upper	In an upper GI, the patient drinks barium sulfate. X-ray films are taken as the barium passes through the esophagus, stomach, and small intestine. The barium meal is used for an _____ GI study.
lower	The large intestine is studied with a barium enema, or _____ GI study.
	Structural and functional abnormalities can be seen in a GI series. For example, the emptying time of the stomach can be determined, and structural defects of the pylorus and other parts of the GI tract can be observed. Computed tomography, ultrasound, and nuclear imaging using radioactive chemicals give additional information to help locate the nature and extent of problems of the GI tract.
	7-89 The small intestine consists of three parts: the duodenum (**doo″o-de′nəm**), the jejunum (**jə-joo′nəm**), and the ileum (**il′e-əm**). The structure of the small intestine is shown in Figure 7-6.
mucosa villi (vil′i)*	Study the layers of the wall of the small intestine to write answers in these blanks. The innermost membrane is called the _____. Both the mucosa and submucosa have many folds and fingerlike projections called _____. Both of these features increase the surface area of the mucosa. In addition, the villi function to absorb nutrients.
serosa	There are two layers of muscle and an outer membrane called the _____.

*Villus, pl. villi (Latin: tuft of hair).

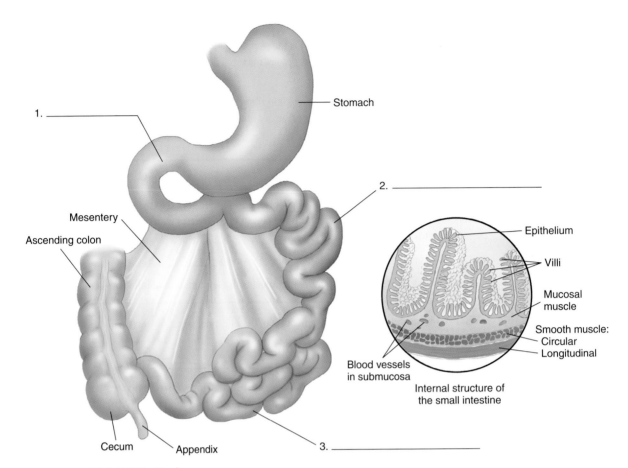

FIGURE 7-6

Characteristics of the small intestine. Label the three parts of the small intestine (1 to 3) as you read. The first portion, the duodenum (1) begins at the pyloric sphincter and is the shorter section. The second portion is the jejunum (2), which is continuous with the third portion, the ileum (3). The ileum is the longest of the three parts of the small intestine. Note that the small intestine decreases in diameter from beginning at the duodenum to its ending, at the ileum. The internal structure is similar throughout its length. The wall *(inset)* has an inner lining of mucosa, two layers of muscle, and an outer layer of serosa.

duodenum **duodenitis** (doo″o-də-ni′tis) **duodenotomy** (doo″o-də-not′ə-me)	**7-90** The duodenum is short, less than a foot long. The combining form **duoden(o)** means duodenum. Duoden/al (**doo″o-dē′nəl**) means pertaining to the _____. Inflammation of the duodenum is _____. An incision of the duodenum is a _____.
duodenostomy (doo″o-də-nos′tə-me) **stomach and duodenum** **cancer of the duodenum** **duodenography** (doo″o-də-nog′rə-fe)	**7-91** Formation of a new opening into the duodenum is a _____. Gastro/duoden/itis (**gas″tro-doo-ad″ə-ni′tis**) is inflammation of the _____. Duodenal carcinoma is _____. Write a word that means taking x-rays of the duodenum: _____.

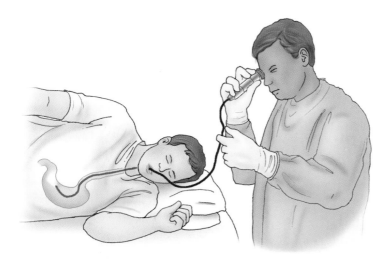

FIGURE 7-7
Upper GI endoscopy. If the focus of the examination is the esophagus, the procedure is called esophagoscopy. If the stomach is the focus, the procedure is called gastroscopy.

inside **viewing**	**7-92** Endoscopy (**en-dos′ko-pe**) is direct visualization of the interior of organs and cavities using a flexible fiberoptic endoscope. Fiberoptic materials are flexible glass or plastic fibers that transmit light and permit visual images around corners. The word part *endo-* means _____, and *-scopy* means _____.
duodenoscopy (doo″o-də-nos′ kə-pe) **duodenoscope** (doo″o-de′no-skōp)	Write a word that means endoscopic examination of the duodenum: _____ (literally, inspection of the duodenum). An instrument used to inspect the duodenum is called a fiberoptic _____.
esophagus, **stomach, and** **duodenum** **gastroscopy** (gas-tros′kə-pe)	**7-93** In an esophago/gastro/duodeno/scopy (ə-sof″ə-go-gas″tro-doo″od-ə-nos′kə-pe), what structures are examined? _____ This is also called an upper GI endoscopy (Figure 7-7). If the esophagus is the focus of the examination, the procedure is called esophagoscopy (ə-sof″ə-gos′ko pe). If the stomach is the focus, the procedure is called _____.
jejunum **stomach, jejunum**	**7-94** The part of the small intestine below the duodenum is the jejunum. It is about 2.4 meters (8 feet) long and joins the ileum, which is the twisted end of the small intestine. The combining form *jejun(o)* means jejunum. Jejuno/tomy (jə″joo-not′ə-me) is surgical incision of the _____. Gastro/jejuno/stomy (gas″tro-jə-joo-nos′tə-me) is surgical formation of a new opening between the _____ and the _____.
	7-95 Anastomosis* (ə-nas′tə-mo′sis) is a natural opening between two vessels, or it may be created by surgical, traumatic, or pathological means between two normally distinct organs or spaces. The communication (union) itself is also called an anastomosis. The verb that is used to indicate the structures that are joined is *anastomose* (ə-nas′-tə-mōs). Study the three types of surgical anastomoses of the gastrointestinal tract in Figure 7-8.

*Anastomose (Greek: *anastomoien*, to provide a mouth).

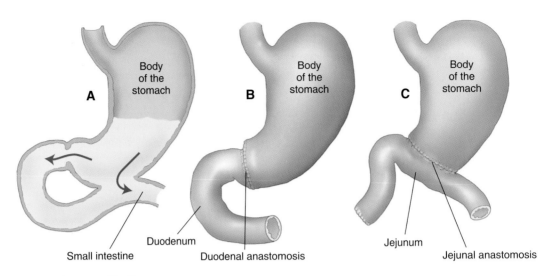

FIGURE 7-8
Three types of surgical anastamoses. **A,** Gastroenterostomy. A passage is created between the stomach and some part of the small intestine, often the jejunum. **B,** Gastroduodenostomy. The lower portion of the stomach is removed, and the remainder is anastomosed to the duodenum. **C,** Gastrojejunostomy. The lower portion of the stomach is removed and the remainder is anastomosed to the jejunum. The remaining duodenal stump is closed.

small intestine	**7-96** Read the information in Figure 7-8 and write answers in these blanks. The gastro/entero/stomy (**gas″tro-en-tǝr-os′tǝ-me**) is the simpler of these three anastomoses. In a gastro/entero/stomy, the body of the stomach is joined with some part of the _____ _____.
duodenum	In the two other types of anastomoses, the lower portion of the stomach is removed before it is anastomosed to another structure. In a gastro/duodeno/stomy (**gas″tro-doo″o-dǝ-nos′tǝ-me**), the stomach is joined with the _____. This is also called a gastroduodenal (**gas″tro-doo″o-de′nǝl**) anastomosis.
gastrojejunostomy (gas″tro-jǝ-joo-nos′tǝ-me)	Write the term for the type of anastomosis that joins the stomach with the jejunum: _____.
stomach	**7-97** When the lower portion of the stomach is removed in either a gastroduodenostomy or a gastrojejunostomy, a partial gastrectomy is performed before anastomosing the two structures. Gastr/ectomy means surgical excision of all, or part, of the _____.
cancer	A total gastrectomy, with anastomosis of the esophagus to the jejunum, is the principal medical intervention for extensive gastric cancer. Gastr/ic carcinoma is _____ of the stomach.
esophagojejunostomy (ǝ-sof-ǝ-go-je″joo-nos′tǝ-me)	Beginning with the proximal organ (that nearest the place where nutrition begins), build a term that means surgical anastomosis of the esophagus to the jejunum: _____.
esophagoduodenostomy (ǝ-sof″ǝ-go-doo″o-de-nos′tǝ-me)	Write a word that means an anastomosis between the esophagus and the duodenum: _____.
jejunum, ileum	**7-98** Use *ile(o)* to write terms about the ileum. Jejuno/ileo/stomy (**jǝ-joo″no-il″e os′tǝ-me**) is formation of an opening between the _____ and the _____.

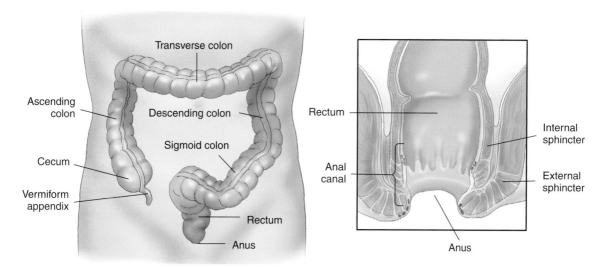

FIGURE 7-9
Features of the large intestine. The colon is anatomically divided into four parts. The first part rises upward and is called the ascending colon. The transverse colon is the part that crosses the abdomen. The colon then descends on the left side of the abdomen and thus is called the descending colon. The last part is S-shaped and is called the sigmoid colon.

ileostomy (il″e-os′tə-me)	**7-99** If the large intestine must be removed, a new opening is made into the ileum through the abdominal wall. Fecal material drains into a bag worn on the abdomen. Formation of an opening into the ileum is _____.
ileitis (il″e-i′tis)	Inflammation of the ileum is _____.
large intestine	**7-100** The large intestine is much broader and shorter than the small intestine. The large intestine is only about 1.5 meters (5 feet) long. The combining form *col(o)* and ***colon(o)*** mean the colon (ko′lon), or the large intestine. Colon means the _____ _____.
colitis (ko-li′tis)	Using col(o), write a word for inflammation of the colon: _____.
	Unless instructed otherwise, use col(o) in the next few frames to write words pertaining to the colon.
stomach, small intestine, and colon	**7-101** Gastro/entero/col/itis (**gas″tro-en″tər-o-ko-li′tis**) is inflammation of the _____.
colon	Col/ectasia (**ko″lek-ta′zhə**) is stretching of the _____.
irrigation	Colo/clysis is _____ of the colon (large intestine). An enema is one example of coloclysis (**ko″lo-kli′sis**).
coloptosis (ko″lop-to′sis)	**7-102** Downward displacement or prolapse of the large intestine is _____.
colon	When coloptosis occurs, the intestine must be sutured to the abdominal wall to correct the problem. This surgical procedure, colo/pexy (**ko′lo-pek″se**), is surgical fixation of the _____.
pertaining to the large intestine	**7-103** Colic (**kol′ik**) means _____.
	Colic also means spasm in any hollow or tubular soft organ accompanied by pain. You may be most familiar with infantile colic, which is colic occurring in infants, principally during the first few months.
	The large intestine is shown in Figure 7-9. It is composed of the cecum, colon, rectum, and anal canal. Use the diagram, if necessary, to work the next frame.

sigmoid colon	**7-104** Different parts of the colon are designated as ascending, transverse, descending, and the sigmoid (**sig′moid**) colon. The last part of the colon is the _____ colon. Colo/scopy (**ko-los′ko-pe**) is visual examination of the _____ by using a sigmoidoscope (**sig-moi′do-skōp**). This is also called flexible sigmoidoscopy (**sig″moi-dos′kə-pe**) or colonoscopy. The combining form *sigmoid(o)* means the sigmoid colon.
colectomy (ko-lek′tə-me) **colon**	**7-105** Write a word that means excision of all, or a part, of the colon: _____. A colo/stomy (**kə-los′tə-me**) is generally performed after partial colectomy. A colostomy is surgical creation of an artificial anus on the abdominal wall by drawing the colon out to the surface or, in other words, creating an artificial opening from the _____ on the abdominal surface. If all of the colon is removed, an ileostomy is necessary. An ileo/stomy is forming an ileal stoma onto the surface of the abdomen.
cecum, ileum **ileum** **cecum**	**7-106** The cecum (**se′kəm**) forms the first portion of the large intestine and is located just below the ileum. The combining form *cec(o)* means cecum. Ceco/ileo/stomy (**se″ko-il″e-os′tə-me**) is formation of a new opening between the _____ and the _____. The ileo/cecal (**il″e-o-se′kəl**) valve is located between the _____ and the _____.
appendix **inflammation of the appendix**	**7-107** The appendix is a wormlike structure that opens into the cecum. An appendix simply means an appendage, but its most common usage is in referring to the vermiform appendix just described. The combining forms *append(o)* and *appendic(o)* both mean appendix. You have heard of an append/ectomy, which is removal of the _____. Appendic/itis (**ə-pen″dĭ-si′tis**) is _____.
col(o), colon(o) **colon, rectum**	**7-108** The colon makes up most of the 5 feet of large intestine, and when one speaks of the colon, one is usually referring to the large intestine in general. The colon is actually that part of the large intestine that extends from the end of the cecum to the beginning of the rectum. Two combining forms that you learned for colon or large intestine are _____ and _____. The lower part of the large intestine is the rectum, which terminates in a narrow anal canal. This canal in turn opens to the exterior at the anus. Feces is body waste that is discharged from the bowels by way of the anus. Feces is also called stool, or fecal material. The combining form *rect(o)* means rectum. Colo/rectal (**ko″lo-rek′tal**) means pertaining to or affecting the _____ and the _____. In this term, col(o) refers specifically to that part of the large intestine recognized as the colon.
inflammation **diverticulum** **diverticulosis** **diverticulectomy (di″vər-tik″u-lek′ tə-me)**	**7-109** A diverticulum (**di″vər-tik′u-ləm**) (plural is diverticula) is a pouchlike herniation through the muscular wall of a tubular organ. A diverticulum is most commonly present in the colon but also can occur in the stomach or small intestine. The combining form *diverticul(o)* refers to diverticula; therefore colonic diverticul/itis (**di″vər-tik″u-li′tis**) is _____ of a _____ of the colon. If diverticula are present in the colon without inflammation or symptoms, it is called diverticulosis (**di″vər-tik″u-lo′sis**). Build this word by combining -osis with the word part for diverticula: _____. Write a word that means excision of a diverticulum: _____.

rectum	**7-110** A recto/cele (**rek′to-sēl**) is a herniation of the _____. (A rectocele is hernial protrusion of part of the rectum into the vagina.)
rectoscope (rek′to-skōp)	Write the word for a tubular instrument with illumination that is used for inspecting the rectum, by writing rect(o) and a suffix for an instrument for viewing: _____.
rectoscopy (rek-tos′kə-pe)	The process in which a rectoscope is used is _____. This procedure is more commonly called proctoscopy, and the instrument is called a proctoscope. The combining form **proct(o)** means anus or rectum.
rectoplasty (rek′to-plas″te)	**7-111** Surgical repair of the rectum is _____.
proct(o), rect(o) **rectum** **anus**	**7-112** The combining form *proct(o)* refers to the anus (**a′nəs**) or rectum. You have now learned two combining forms for rectum: _____ and _____. A procto/logist (**prok-tol′ə-jist**) studies diseases of the _____ and the _____ as well as the colon.
pain **proctodynia** (prok″to-din′e-ə)	**7-113** Proct/algia (**prok-tal′jə**) is _____ in the rectum or in the area of the anus. Another word using proct(o) that means pain in the rectum or about the anus is _____.
proctoplasty (prok′to-plas″te) **paralysis of the rectum** **enteroplegia** (en″tər-o-ple′jə)	**7-114** Using proct(o), write a word that means surgical repair of the rectum: _____. Remember that -plegia is a suffix that means paralysis. Procto/plegia (**prok″to-ple′jə**) is _____. Write a word that means paralysis of the small intestine: _____.
colon **rectum** **rectum**	**7-115** Colo/proct/itis (**ko″lo-prok-ti′tis**) is inflammation of the _____ and _____. Recto/rrhaphy (**rek-tor′ə-fe**) is suture of the rectum for the purpose of repair. Procto/rrhaphy (**prok-tor′ə-fe**) is also suture of the _____.
rectum **surgical fixation** **colopexy**	**7-116** Procto/ptosis (**prok″top-to′sis**) is prolapse of the _____. This can be remedied by procto/pexy (**prok′to-pek″se**). Procto/pexy is _____ _____ of the rectum. Surgical fixation of the large intestine is _____.
anus **anus**	**7-117** Remember that *an(o)* also refers to the anus. Most medical terms that refer to the anus use proct(o), but you need to remember that an(o) also means anus. An/al (**a′nəl**) refers to the _____, as in the phrases "anal opening" or "anal canal." Abnormal passages between internal organs or abnormal communications leading from internal organs to the body surface are called fistulas.* An anal fistula (**fis′tu-lə**) is an abnormal opening near the _____.

*Fistula (Latin: pipe).

A

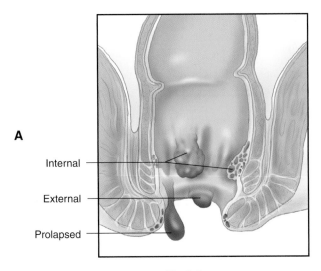

Internal

External

Prolapsed

B

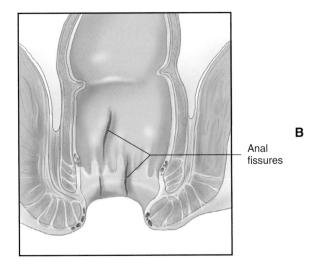

Anal
fissures

FIGURE 7-10
Two disorders of the anorectal area. **A,** Hemorrhoids. Three types of hemorrhoids are shown: internal, external, and prolapsed. Internal hemorrhoids lie above the anal sphincter and cannot be seen on inspection of the anal area. External hemorrhoids lie below the anal sphincter and can be seen on inspection of the anal region. Hemorrhoids that enlarge, fall down, and protrude through the anus are called prolapsed hemorrhoids. **B,** Anal fissures. An ulceration or tear of the lining of the anal canal may be caused by excessive tissue stretching. These tears are very tender and tend to reopen when stool is passed.

removal of hemorrhoids	**7-118** Hemorrhoids are masses of dilated veins of the anal canal that are varicose and lie just inside or outside the rectum. Several types are shown in Figure 7-10. They are often accompanied by pain, itching, and bleeding. If symptoms are too severe, a hemorrhoidectomy may be performed. A hemorrhoid/ectomy (**hem″ə-roid-ek′tə-me**) is _____.
colon	Piles is a synonym for hemorrhoids. This condition is aggravated by constipation, a term meaning colon/ic stasis. In colonic stasis, there is a stagnation of the normal flow of contents of the _____.
pain	**7-119** Nonsurgical management of hemorrhoids is aimed at reducing symptoms without surgery and decreasing the likelihood that the symptoms reoccur. Topical anesthetics, application of cold packs, and soaks are used to alleviate hemorrhoid/al pain. The combining form **top(o)** means place. Topi/cal means pertaining to a particular place on the surface area. A topical anesthetic is applied to a certain area of the skin and affects only that area. The purpose of a topical an/esthetic is to alleviate _____ on a particular area of the skin.
	Constipation, straining to defecate (**def′ə-kāt**), and prolonged sitting contribute to the development of hemorrhoids. Defecation (**def″ə-ka′shən**) is the elimination of feces from the rectum. Exercise, diets high in fiber and fluids, plus stool softeners used on a temporary basis are generally recommended for constipation.
fissure	**7-120** In addition to the diseases and disorders that have been discussed, some additional ones are included in Table 7-2. Read the information in the table, and complete the blanks in the next few frames.
	A fissure* (**fish′ər**) is a cleft or a groove or a cracklike lesion of the skin. A painful linear ulceration or tear at the anal opening is called an anal _____.

*Fissure (Latin: *fissura*, to split).

TABLE 7-2 Additional Diseases or Disorders of the Digestive System

Anal fissure (**fish′ər**): A linear ulcer on the margin of the anus. Fissure is a general term for a cleft or groove in an organ
Anorexia nervosa: A disorder characterized by a prolonged refusal to eat, resulting in emaciation, absence of menstruation, emotional disturbance concerning body image, and fear of becoming obese
Bulimia (**bu-lim′e-ə**) An emotional disorder characterized by binge eating and often terminating in self-induced vomiting
Crohn's disease: A chronic inflammatory disease of the gastrointestinal tract, generally affecting the ileum and of unknown origin. Complications include intestinal obstruction and abscess formation, with a high degree of recurrence after treatment
Fecal impaction (**im-pak′shən**): A collection of hardened feces in the rectum or sigmoid colon that the person is unable to expel
Food poisoning: A group of illnesses, varying in severity from mild to life-threatening, resulting from ingestion of contaminated foods or food that is inherently poisonous
Irritable bowel syndrome: A chronic, noninflammatory disease characterized by abdominal pain, altered bowel habits consisting of diarrhea or constipation or both, and no pathologic change. Called also spastic or irritable colon
Malabsorption syndrome: A group of disorders in which there is subnormal absorption of dietary constituents and thus excessive loss of nonabsorbed substances in the bowel
Obesity: An abnormal amount of fat in the body. This term is usually not employed unless the individual is at least 20% to 30% over average weight for his or her age, sex, and height
Ulcerative (**ul′sər-a″tiv**) *colitis:* Chronic ulceration of the mucosa of the colon. It produces diarrhea, loss of weight, and sometimes anemia

Crohn's	**7-121** A chronic inflammatory bowel disease (IBD) that has a proper name is _____ disease.
impaction	An accumulation of hardened feces in the rectum or sigmoid colon that the individual cannot expel is _____.
food poisoning	Mushroom poisoning and shellfish poisoning are examples of a large group of illnesses called _____ _____.
irritable bowel	Another name for irritable colon is _____ _____ syndrome, abbreviated IBS.
ulcerative	Chronic ulceration of the colon is _____ colitis.
anorexia	**7-122** You learned that a disorder (probably psychological) characterized by a prolonged refusal to eat, resulting in emaciation, is called _____ nervosa. Emaciation (**e-ma″she-a′shən**) is excessive leanness caused by disease or lack of nutrition.
bulimia	An emotional disorder characterized by insatiable craving for food, often resulting in binge eating and often followed by purging, is _____. It differs from anorexia nervosa, in which bulimic episodes may occur, in that there is no extreme weight loss in bulimia.
malabsorption	**7-123** Subnormal absorption of dietary constituents is _____ syndrome.
obesity	An abnormally large amount of fat in the body is _____.
	7-124 Structural features of both the small intestine and large intestine are well suited for their role in the digestive system. As you studied earlier, the small intestine is responsible for further digestion of the chyme and absorption of nutrients. The functions of the large intestine are summarized in Table 7-3. Read the information in the table and complete these blanks:
water	While moving wastes along its length, the large intestine absorbs _____, sodium, and chloride. The large intestine is capable of absorbing 90% of the water and sodium it receives.
mucus	The large intestine secretes _____, which binds fecal particles into a formed mass and lubricates the mucosa.
vitamins	Bacteria in the large intestine are responsible for the production of several _____.
expelling	The last function described is defecation, which means the act of _____ feces from the body.

TABLE 7-3 Functions of the Large Intestine

- *Churning and peristalsis:* moving residue through the large intestine
- *Secretion of mucus:* binds fecal particles into a formed mass, protects the mucosa, lubricates
- *Absorption of water, sodium, and chloride:* reduces the volume of residue and helps maintain fluid and electrolyte balance
- *Vitamin synthesis:* bacteria synthesize vitamin K and several other vitamins
- *Formation of feces:* solid waste includes food residues and dead cells
- *Defecation:* expelling feces from the body

❏ SECTION E REVIEW *Intestines*

This section review covers frames 7–80 through 7–124. Complete the table by writing a word part or its meaning in each blank.

Combining Form	Meaning	Combining Form	Meaning
1. append(o), appendic(o)	_____	10. _____	sigmoid colon
2. _____	cecum	11. top(o)	_____
3. colon(o)	_____	12. vir(o)	_____
4. _____	diverticula	13. virus(o)	_____
5. duoden(o)	_____	**Suffix**	**Meaning**
6. ile(o)	_____	14. _____	irrigation or washing out
7. _____	jejunum		
8. _____	anus or rectum		
9. rect(o)	_____		

(Use Appendix V to check your answers.)

Accessory Organs of Digestion

Several organs are considered to be accessory organs to the digestive system because they produce substances that are needed for proper digestion and absorption of nutrients. The liver, gallbladder, pancreas, and salivary glands are accessory organs of digestion. These organs lie outside the digestive tract, yet produce or store secretions that aid in the chemical breakdown of food. The secretions are released into the digestive tract through ducts.

	7-125 The accessory organs of digestion are the liver, the gallbladder, the pancreas, and the salivary glands. The salivary glands are located in the oral cavity. Look back at Figure 7-1. The three pairs of salivary glands shown are the parotid, submaxillary, and sublingual glands. The parotids are the largest salivary glands and are located below and in front of each ear.
	Remembering that *par-* and *para-* mean near, beside, or abnormal, par/ot/id (pə-rot′id) means near the ear. The suffix *-id* means either having the shape of or a structure. The salivary gland located near the ear
parotid	is the _____ gland.
parotid	**7-126** Parot/itis (par″o-ti′tis) is inflammation of the _____ gland. Epidemic parotitis is another name for mumps, a contagious viral disease. Mumps chiefly involves the salivary glands, most
near	often the parotids. The parotid gland is a salivary gland located _____ the ear.

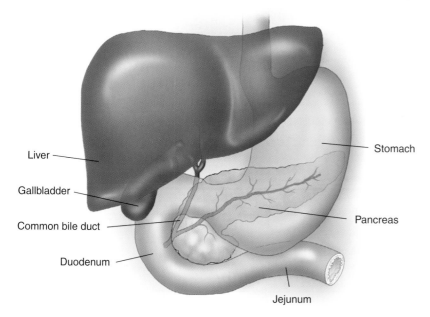

Liver

Gallbladder

Common bile duct

Duodenum

Jejunum

Stomach

Pancreas

FIGURE 7-11
The liver, gallbladder, and pancreas are accessory digestive organs. The liver and pancreas have additional functions as well. More than 500 functions of the liver have been identified. The formation and excretion of bile for digestion of fats is one of its most commonly known activities. Bile is stored in the gallbladder and released when fats are ingested. The pancreas secretes many substances, including digestive enzymes and insulin.

beneath	**7-127** Submaxillary (sǝb-mak″sĭ-lar′e) means below the maxilla, the upper jaw bone. The prefix **sub-** means below or under. You need to remember, however, that the submaxillary gland is located beneath the mandible, the lower jaw bone, rather than beneath the maxilla, as the name implies. The sub/maxillary gland is located _____ the mandible.
under the tongue	Sub/lingu/al (sǝb-**ling′gwǝl**) means under the tongue. The sublingual glands are salivary glands that are located where? _____
under the tongue	Sub/gloss/al (sǝb-glos′ǝl) also means under the tongue. Sublingual and subglossal both mean _____.
starch	**7-128** Saliva produced by the salivary glands moistens the mouth parts as well as the food, making it easier to swallow. In addition, saliva contains amylase, which begins digestion of _____ in the mouth.
sialography (si″ǝ-log′rǝ-fe)	The combining form **sial(o)** means saliva or the salivary glands. Write a word that means taking an x-ray of the ducts of the salivary glands (literally, radiography of the salivary glands): _____.
salivary **sialolith** (si-al′o-lith)	Sialography is accomplished by injecting radiopaque substances into the _____ ducts. Sometimes sialography demonstrates the presence of calculi in the salivary ducts. Write a word that means salivary calculus: _____.
sialitis (si″ǝ-li′tis) **sialadenitis** (si″ǝl-ad″ǝ-ni′tis)	Another combining form, **sialaden(o),** means salivary gland also; however, it is used less frequently than sial(o). Write two terms that mean inflammation of a salivary gland: _____ and _____.
	7-129 Food does not pass through the accessory organs of digestion as it does with the other digestive structures. The accessory organs have secretions that are conveyed to the digestive tract by ducts. The liver, gallbladder, and pancreas are located near the other digestive structures within the abdominal cavity. See these structures in Figure 7-11.
inflammation of the liver	The liver is essential for the maintenance of life. It is the largest organ in the body. The combining form **hepat(o)** means the liver. Hepat/itis (hep″ǝ-ti′tis) is _____.
	Hepatitis may result from bacterial or viral infections or other causes, such as medications, toxins, or alcohol. Hepatitis A, hepatitis B, and hepatitis C are caused by the hepatitis A virus (HAV), hepatitis B virus (HBV), and hepatitis C virus (HCV), respectively. There are also other types of hepatitis. Hepatitis B immune globulin (HBIG) provides short-term protection against the hepatitis B virus.

TABLE 7-4 Major Functions of the Liver

- Production of bile and bile salts
- Involvement in blood glucose regulation (stores glucose in the form of glycogen, converts it as needed)
- Lipid metabolism
- Synthesis of plasma proteins
- Storage of iron and vitamins A, B_{12}, D, E, and K
- Detoxification (breaks down toxic compounds)
- Excretion of hormones, cholesterol, and bile pigments from the breakdown of hemoglobin
- Filtering of the blood

pertaining to the liver	**7-130** Hepat/ic (hə-pat′ik) means _____.
hepatocyte (hep′ə-to-sīt)	Write a word that means liver cell: _____. The term you just wrote means the functional cell of the liver.
hepatolith (hep′ə-to-lith″) liver	**7-131** Production of bile is a major function of the liver. The bile is then transported to the gallbladder for storage. The major functions of the liver are listed in Table 7-4. Form a new word by combining word parts for liver and stone: _____. (This is actually a gallstone that is located in the liver. You will study more about gallstones shortly and will learn new terms, but do not be confused. Remember that the term *hepatolith* refers to a gallstone located in the _____.)
hepatoma (hep″ə-to′mə) carcinoma	**7-132** A tumor of the liver is a _____. This term is usually reserved for a specific type of primary liver carcinoma. Tumors of the liver may be benign or malignant. Cancer of the liver is called hepatic _____. Malignancy in the liver that is spread from another source is many times more frequent than primary tumor of the liver.
liver, spleen **hepatopathy** (hep″ə-top′ə-the)	**7-133** Hepato/spleno/megaly (hep″ə-to-sple″no-meg′ə-le) is enlargement of the _____ and the _____. The combining form for spleen is splen(o). Any disease of the liver is a _____.
hepatotomy (hep″ə-tot′ə-me) **hepatectomy** (hep″ə-tek′tə-me)	**7-134** Surgical incision of the liver is _____. Excision of part of the liver is _____. The liver is one of the most vital internal organs and is necessary for life. Hepatectomy is generally removal of part of the liver. The entire liver may be removed if a liver transplant is available.
liver	**7-135** Cirrhosis (sĭ-ro′sis) is a chronic liver disease that is characterized by degeneration of liver cells with eventual increased resistance to flow of blood through the liver. Cirrhosis is a disease of what organ? _____ Alcoholic cirrhosis occurs in approximately 20% of chronic alcoholics. In addition to alcohol, nutritional deficiencies, poisons, or previous hepatitis can lead to cirrhosis.
liver	**7-136** Bile aids in the digestion of fats. In certain liver diseases, or in any situation in which the flow of bile is obstructed, a condition called jaundice (jawn′dis) may result. Jaundice is a yellow discoloration of the skin, whites of the eyes, mucous membranes, and body fluids, caused by greater than normal amounts of bilirubin in the blood. Bilirubin is the yellow-orange pigment of bile. Hemolytic anemias can also cause jaundice, but _____ disease is a leading cause of jaundice.

liver	**7-137** Hepato/lytic (**hep″ə-to-lit′ik**) means destructive to the _____. (The term hepatolytic is less common than hepatotoxic [**hep″ə-to-tok′sik**], which means essentially the same thing.)
enlarged liver	Hepato/megaly (**hep″ə-to-meg′ə-le**) is _____ _____.
biliary	**7-138** The combining form ***chol(e)*** refers to bile or gall; **bil(i)** also means bile but is used far less frequently than chol(e) to build terms. Biliary (**bil′e-ar-e**) means pertaining to bile. The organs and ducts that participate in the secretion, storage, and delivery of bile make up the _____ tract.
bile	**7-139** Bile leaves the liver by the hepatic duct and is taken to the gallbladder for storage until it is needed. Chol/angitis is inflammation of a _____ vessel, or duct. (Note that the "e" is dropped from chol[e] when it is combined with angi[o].)
cholangiography (ko-lan″je-og′rə-fe)	Using cholangitis (**ko″lan-ji′tis**) as a model, write a word that means radiology of the bile ducts: _____.
vein	**7-140** Intravenous cholangiography is radiography of the major bile ducts and is useful in demonstrating gallstones and tumors. Contrast medium is used to render the bile ducts opaque to x-rays. Because it is called an intravenous cholangiogram (IVC), we know the contrast medium is injected into the _____.
across the liver	Sometimes IVC is not recommended or does not yield satisfactory results, so trans/hepatic cholangiography is done. Trans/hepatic literally means _____.
transhepatic	In transhepatic cholangiography, a needle is placed in the liver to puncture a bile duct, and contrast medium is injected. An alternative to IVC is _____ cholangiography.
within	**7-141** One type of cholangiography is performed during surgery, after the gallbladder has been removed. This radiographic procedure is called intraoperative cholangiography. You learned earlier that intra- means _____. This prefix in intra/operative refers to the time during which the patient is in surgery.
intraoperative	Intraoperative cholangiography is performed by injecting contrast medium through a catheter placed in the common bile duct. This allows residual stones in the bile ducts to be seen. This type of angiography is called _____ cholangiography.
gallstones cholelith	**7-142** Chole/lith/iasis (**ko″le-lĭ-thi′ə-sis**) is the presence of _____. Another name for a gallstone is _____.
lithotripsy	**7-143** Extracorporeal shock wave lithotripsy (**lith′o-trip″se**) is a noninvasive procedure that is used in the treatment of gallstones in certain situations. (See Figure 7-12.) You have not yet studied the suffix ***-tripsy,*** which means surgical crushing, and will do so in the next chapter. For now, remember that an alternative to conventional surgery to remove gallstones is extracorporeal shock wave _____.
lithotriptor	Biliary lithotripsy uses a computer and an ultrasound monitor, with the patient positioned over a shock wave generator (lithotriptor) by means of a table that moves upward and downward, forward and backward, and side to side. Particles slough off the gallstone as the lithotriptor is fired, and the particles pass through the biliary ducts and are eliminated. This noninvasive procedure is useful in certain cases and is an alternative to cholecystectomy. The name of the shock wave generator in biliary lithotripsy is a _____.

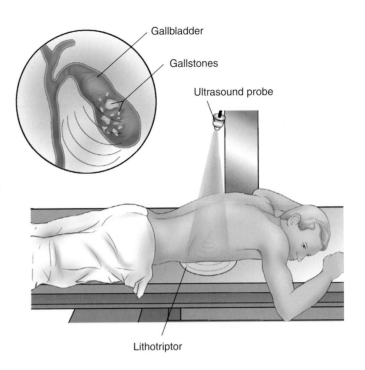

FIGURE 7-12
Biliary lithotripsy. The gallbladder is positioned over the lithotriptor, then the lithotriptor is fired and particles slough off the gallstones until they are fragmented and can pass through the biliary ducts.

cholecyst **cholecystitis** (ko″le-sis-ti′tis)	**7-144** The combining form *cyst(o)* means a bladder or sac. Combine chol(e) and cyst to write the scientific name of the gallbladder: _____. This word part is seldom seen alone, but *cholecyst(o)* frequently forms part of a term that refers to the gallbladder (GB). Inflammation of the gallbladder is _____.
making a record of the gallbladder **mouth** **cholecystogram**	**7-145** Chole/cysto/graphy (ko″le-sis-tog′rə-fe) is _____. Cholecystography is accomplished by rendering the gallbladder and ducts opaque with contrast medium. In an oral cholecystogram (ko″le-sis′to-gram), the patient is given a contrast agent in tablet form to be taken by _____. For this reason it is called an oral _____ (the record of the gallbladder that is produced, abbreviated OCG). Examine the appearance of several gallstones in Figure 7-13. Oral cholecystograms were the principal method for investigating the presence of gallstones until the advent of ultrasound.
cholecystectomy (ko″le-sis-tek′tə-me) **abdominal wall** **gallbladder** **stomach**	**7-146** Surgical removal of the gallbladder is a _____. The gallbladder stores bile but is not essential for life, since bile is produced continuously. Sometimes a cholecystectomy is done to remove gallstones. You will later study that *lapar(o)* means abdominal wall. Laparo/scopic cholecystectomy, removal of the gallbladder through a small incision in the _____ _____, is performed more often than the traditional, open cholecystectomy. Laparoscopic cholecystectomy is commonly done as an outpatient surgery. The gallbladder is excised with laser and removed through the small opening. Cholecysto/gastric (ko″le-sis″to-gas′trik) pertains to the _____ and the _____.

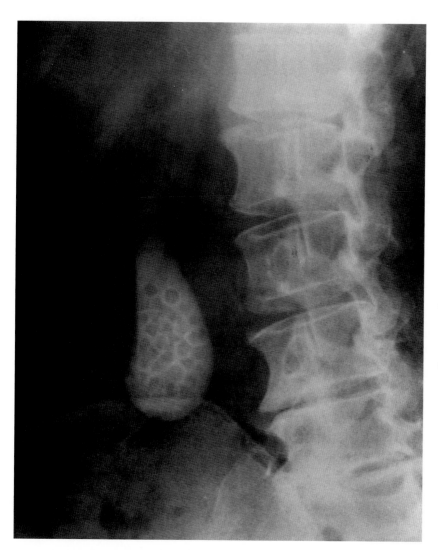

FIGURE 7-13
Oral cholecystogram. Numerous gallstones are evident on this cholecystogram. In oral cholecystography, radiography of the gallbladder is obtained 12 to 15 hours after ingestion of contrast medium. Because nausea, vomiting, and diarrhea are fairly common with this means of diagnosing biliary disease, it has been largely replaced by ultrasound. (From Carlson K, Eisenstat S: *Primary care of women*, 1995, Mosby.)

cholecystostomy (ko″le-sis-tos′tə-me)	**7-147** Write a term that has a literal translation of forming a new opening into the gallbladder: _____. This new term means surgical formation of an opening into the gallbladder for the purpose of drainage or removal of stones.
abdominal wall	Laparo/cholecysto/tomy (**lap″ə-ro-ko″le-sis-tot′ə-me**) means incision into the gallbladder through the _____ _____.
common bile duct **choledochitis** (kol″ə-do-ki′tis)	**7-148** A few words contain the combining form ***choledoch(o),*** which means the common bile duct. Choledoch/al (**ko-led′ə-kəl**) means pertaining to the _____. Inflammation of the common bile duct is _____.

TABLE 7-5 **Important Signs/Symptoms of Uncontrolled or Untreated Diabetes Mellitus**

SYMPTOM	CAUSE
Polyuria	Excretion of sugar in urine causes an increased volume of water to be excreted
Polydipsia	Dehydration, resulting from polyuria, leads to thirst
Weight loss (despite good appetite)	Glucose cannot be used properly because of insufficient insulin. In absence of available glucose, fats are broken down and used for cellular energy
Polyphagia	Tissue wasting causes starvation and results in hunger

---

choledocholithiasis (ko-led″ə-ko-lĭ-thi′ə-sis)

7-149 The presence of a calculus in the common bile duct is _____.

choledochoplasty (ko-led″ə-ko-plas′te)

Surgical repair of this duct is _____.

opening

Choledochostomy (ko-led″ə-kos′tə-me) is surgical formation of an _____ into the common bile duct through the abdominal wall. This is commonly done for temporary drainage of the duct after cholecystectomy.

common bile duct and the duodenum

Choledocho/duodeno/stomy (ko-led″o-ko-doo″o-də-nos′tə-me) is surgical formation of a new opening between the _____.

pertaining to the pancreas

7-150 The pancreas has both digestive and hormonal functions. The combining form *pancreat(o)* means pancreas. Pancreat/ic (pan″kre-at′ik) means _____.

Pancreatic juice plays an important role in the digestion of all classes of food. Pancreatic juice contains lipase, amylase, maltase, and several other enzymes that are essential to normal digestion. The pancreas also produces hormones (including insulin) that play a primary role in regulation of carbohydrate metabolism.

increased sugar in the blood

7-151 The pancreas releases insulin (in′sə-lin) into the blood stream. Insulin is essential for the proper use of sugar in the body. If the pancreas does not produce enough insulin, diabetes mellitus (di″ə-be′tēz mel′lə-təs) results. One sign of diabetes is hyper/glyc/emia, which means _____.

7-152 Although there is more than enough sugar present in the blood, the diabetic person cannot use the sugar properly without insulin. Four important symptoms of diabetes mellitus are explained in Table 7-5.

Sometimes the pancreas produces too much insulin. If too much insulin is produced, there will be less than the normal amount of sugar in the blood. Write a word that means less than the normal amount of sugar in the blood: _____.

hypoglycemia

pancreatolith (pan″kre-at′o-lith)

7-153 Remembering that the combining form for pancreas is pancreat(o), write a word that means a pancreatic stone: _____.

removal of pancreatic stones

Pancreato/lith/ectomy (pan″kre-ə-to-lĭ-thek′tə-me) is _____.

pancreatitis (pan″kre-ə-ti′tis)

Inflammation of the pancreas is _____.

pancreatography	**7-154** Pancreato/graphy (**pan″kre-ə-tog′rə-fe**) is performed during surgery by injecting the pancreatic duct with a contrast medium, which makes the vessels visible on x-ray. This procedure is _____ (recording of the pancreas).
bile ducts	Chol/angio/pancreato/graphy (**ko-lan″je-o-pan-kre-ə-tog′rə-fe**) is the radiographic study of the pancreas and of the _____ _____.
pancreatolysis (pan″kre-ə-tol′ĭ-sis) pancreatopathy (pan″kre-ə-top′ə-the)	**7-155** Destruction of pancreatic tissue is _____. Write a word that means any disease of the pancreas: _____.
pancreatectomy (pan″kre-ə-tek′tə-me) incision of the pancreas	**7-156** Removal of the pancreas is _____. Pancreato/tomy (**pan″kre-ə-tot′ə-me**) is _____.

7-157 Pancreat/ic carcinoma is one of the most deadly neoplasms. Though uncommon, its incidence is increasing in industrialized parts of the world. Few persons with pancreatic carcinoma live more than a year after diagnosis.

The pancreas, like the other accessory digestive organs, secretes enzymes that break down food substances in preparation for absorption and transport to all of the body tissues.

❑ SECTION F REVIEW   𝒜ccesory Organs of Digestion

This section review covers frames 7–125 through 7–157. Complete the table by writing a word part or its meaning in each blank.

Combining Form	Meaning	Prefix	Meaning
1. bil(i)	_____	10. sub-	_____
2. chol(e)	_____	**Suffix**	**Meaning**
3. cholecyst(o)	_____	11. -id	_____
4. _____	common bile duct		
5. _____	bladder or sac		
6. hepat(o)	_____		
7. _____	pancreas		
8. sial(o)	_____		
9. sialaden(o)	_____		

(Use Appendix V to check your answers.)

Terminology Challenge

This section challenges you to read, write, and understand new terms or concepts about the digestive system. At times, you will use less familiar word parts that are covered more extensively in other chapters. It is important to remember the new terms introduced in this section.

fistula trachea, esophagus gastric opening (or passage)	**7-158** You learned that an abnormal communication between two internal organs or one that leads from an internal organ to the body surface is called a _____. Abnormal passages can occur between almost any adjacent structures. A tracheo/esophageal fistula is an abnormal communication between the _____ and the _____. Any abnormal passage communicating with the stomach is called a _____ fistula. Surgical repair is needed to correct a fistula. In repairing a fistula, the abnormal _____ is closed.
abdominal wall laparogastrotomy (**lap″ə-ro-gas-trot′ə-me**) laparohepatotomy (**lap″ə-ro-hep″ə-tot′ə-me**)	**7-159** Many words that begin with lapar(o), meaning abdominal wall, have implied meanings. For example, laparo/colo/tomy (**lap″ə-ro-ko-lot′ə-me**) is incision of the colon through the abdominal wall. Laparo/colo/stomy (**lap″ə-ro-ko-los′tə-me**) is forming a permanent opening into the colon by incision of the _____ _____. Incision of the stomach through the abdominal wall is _____. Incision of the liver through the abdominal wall is _____. Both laparocystotomy (**lap″ə-ro-sis-tot′o-me**) and laparocystectomy (**lap″ə-ro-sis-tek′tə-me**) mean removal of a cyst by incision of the abdominal wall.
rectum stomach lip tongue	**7-160** In rectoplasty, suture of the rectum is necessary to repair it. The suffix that means suture is -rrhaphy. Recto/rrhapy (**rek-tor′ə-fe**) is suture of the _____. Gastro/rrhaphy (**gas-tror′ə-fe**) is suture of the _____. Cheilo/rrhaphy (**ki-lor′ə-fe**) is suture of the _____. Glosso/rrhaphy (**glos-or′ə-fe**) is suture of the _____.
tongue	**7-161** Glossopyrosis (**glos″o-pi-ro′sis**) is an abnormal sensation of pain, burning, and stinging of the tongue without apparent lesions or cause. The combining form pyr(o), which means fire, in glosso/pyr/osis refers to the stinging sensation of the _____.
rectum stomatorrhagia (**sto″mə-to-ra′jə**)	**7-162** Procto/rrhagia (**prok″to-ra′jə**) is hemorrhage from the _____. The suffix -rrhagia means hemorrhage. Use stomat(o) to write a term that means hemorrhage from the mouth: _____.
intestine	**7-163** You learned that mal- means bad. Mal/aise (**mah-lāz′**) is a general feeling of ill health. Malaise is a feeling of body weakness, distress, or discomfort. Many disturbances of the digestive system and other disorders can give a feeling of malaise. Remembering that dys- is another prefix that means bad or difficult, dysentery (**dis′ən-ter″e**) is inflammation of the intestine, especially of the colon, that may be caused by chemical irritants or microorganisms. It is characterized by abdominal pain and frequent and bloody stools. Literal translation of dys/enter/y is a bad condition of the _____.

near, beside abnormal	**7-164** It is not always easy to determine the meaning of words that use par- or para-. Remember that par- and para- mean _____, _____, or _____.
beside (or near)	Para/appendic/itis (**par″ə-ə-pen″dĭ-si′tis**) is inflammation of tissue _____ the appendix.
beside the colon	Para/col/itis (**par″ə-ko-li′tis**) is inflammation of tissue _____.
	Paracolitis is inflammation of the outer coat of the colon.
parasplenic (**par″ə-sple′nik**)	If splenic pertains to the spleen, write a word that means beside the spleen: _____.
	7-165 Tumors, also called neoplasms, are common occurrences in digestive structures. Neoplasms are either benign or malignant. Sometimes a neoplasm is classified as pre/cancerous, meaning a tumor that is likely to develop into a malignant one.
neoplasm neoplastic (**ne″o-plas′tik**)	Neoplasia (**ne″o-pla′zhə**) is the formation of a _____. It is the progressive multiplication of cells under conditions that would not cause multiplication of normal cells. Think of an adjective that pertains to neoplasia and then write it: _____. (If you answered this correctly, you have begun to think about medical vocabulary, rather than just memorizing words!)
large teeth	**7-166** Macrodontia (**mak″ro-don′shə**) is the term that results when one combines macro-, odont(o), and -ia. (One "o" is omitted to prevent "oo.") Macrodontia means _____ _____. An interesting aspect of macrodontia is that all of the teeth may be affected or only two symmetric teeth.
without teeth	Look at another term: an/odont/ia. Translated literally, anodontia (**an″o-don′shə**) means a condition in which a person is _____ _____. Andontia is a disturbance in dental development in which a person lacks either primary or permanent teeth. It may involve only one or all of the teeth and tends to be hereditary.
against toothache	Anti/odont/algic (**an″tĭ-o-don-tal′jik**) means _____ _____. In other words, antidontalgic means relieving a toothache.
extrahepatic (**eks″trə-hə-pat′ik**)	**7-167** Several prefixes are added to terms to describe locations relative to various structures. Remembering that extra- means outside, write a term that means situated or occurring outside the liver: _____.
above	Supra/hepatic (**soo″prə-hə-pat′ik**) means above the liver. The prefix *supra-* means above or beyond. In supra/hepatic, supra- means _____.
behind the esophagus	The prefix *post-* means after or behind. Post/esophag/eal (**pōst-ə-sof″ə-je′əl**) means situated where? _____.
behind	Another prefix, retro-, means behind or backwards. Retro/cecal (**ret″ro-se′kəl**) means _____ the cecum, the first part of the large intestine.
retroperitoneal (**re″tro-per′ ĭ to-ne′əl**)	Using retrocecal as a model, write a word that means behind the peritoneum: _____.
behind	Retro/colic (**ret″ro-kol′ik**) means _____ the colon.

around peri/tonsill/ar (per″ĭ-ton′sĭ-lər)	**7-168** Remembering that peri- means around, the literal translation of peri/col/ic pertains to _____ the colon. Pericolic means pertaining to the tissue around the colon. In this frame, "the tissues around the structure" are implied. Write a term that means pertaining to the tissue around a tonsil: _____.
pericolitis (per″ĭko-li′tis)	Knowing that colitis is inflammation of the colon, write a term that means inflammation of tissue around the colon: _____.
	Write terms that mean inflammation of the tissue around these structures:
perihepatitis (per″e-hep″ə-ti′tis)	the liver _____
periappendicitis (per″e-ə-pen″dĭ′-si′tis)	the appendix _____
peripancreatitis (per″ĭ-pan″kre-ə-ti′tis)	the pancreas _____

You will practice using the less familiar word parts in this section in other chapters of this book. For now, be able to read and write the new terms. There is no review for this section.

Study the following list of selected abbreviations and then read through the Chapter Pharmacology section and be sure you understand the effects and uses of the drug classes that are presented. When you are finished, work the Chapter Review. After completing the exercises, check your answers with the solutions in Appendix V.

You will find these items presented after the Chapter Review:

• Listing of Medical Terms
• Enhancing Spanish Communication

Selected Abbreviations

(Many abbreviations concerning the digestive system, particularly those related to dosage and time, were presented in the list of abbreviations in Chapter 2.)

ALP	alkaline phosphatase (liver function test)
BaE	barium enema
GA	gastric analysis
GB	gallbladder
GERD	gastric esophageal reflux disease
GI	gastrointestinal
IBD	inflammatory bowel disease
IC	irritable colon
IVC	intravenous cholangiogram
NG tube	nasogastric tube

NPO	nothing by mouth (*nulla per os*)
OCG	oral cholangiogram
PP	after meals (postprandial)
PU	peptic ulcer
RDAs	recommended dietary allowances
SGOT	enzyme test of heart and liver function
SGPT	enzyme test of liver function
TPN	total parenteral nutrition
UGI	upper gastrointestinal
US	ultrasound

Chapter Pharmacology

Drug Class	Effects and Uses
Anorexiants	**Appetite Suppression**
benzphetamine (Didrex)	Used for short-term treatment of exogenous obesity
dextroamphetamine (Dexedrine)	Used for short-term treatment of exogenous obesity
phenteramine (Adipex-P)	Used for short-term treatment of exogenous obesity
sibutramine (Meridia)	Used for short-term treatment of exogenous obesity
phenylpropolamine (Dexatrim)	Used for short-term treatment of exogenous obesity
orlistat (Xenical)	A lipase inhibitor
Anticanker Sore Drugs	**Relief of Minor Oral Inflammation of Canker Sores**
carbamide peroxide (Gly-Oxide)	Local oral hygiene preparation
benzocaine (Tanac)	A topical local anesthetic
Antidiabetic Drugs	**Used to Treat Diabetes**
Sulfonylureas	*Adjunct to diet and exercise for type II diabetes (NIDDM)*
chlorpropramide (Diabinese)	Adjunct to diet and exercise for type II diabetes (NIDDM)
tolazamide (Tolinase)	Adjunct to diet and exercise for type II diabetes (NIDDM)
glipizide (Glucotrol)	Adjunct to diet and exercise for type II diabetes (NIDDM)
glyburide (DiaBeta)	Adjunct to diet and exercise for type II diabetes (NIDDM)
Biguanides	*Adjunct to diet and exercise for type II diabetes (NIDDM)*
metformin (Glucophage)	Adjunct to diet and exercise for type II diabetes (NIDDM)
Thiazolidinediones	*Adjunct to diet and exercise for type II diabetes (NIDDM)*
troglitazone (Rezulin)	Adjunct to diet and exercise for type II diabetes (NIDDM)
rosiglitazone (Avandia)	Adjunct to diet and exercise for type II diabetes (NIDDM)
Insulins	*Used for type I diabetes mellitus (IDDM). See Chapter 13 pharmacology section.*
Antidiarrheal Drugs	**Relieve Symptoms of Diarrhea**
diphenoxylate (Lomotil)	Used to treat diarrhea
loperamide (Imodium)	Used to treat diarrhea
Antiemetics	**Prevent or Alleviate Nausea and Vomiting**
cyclizine (Marezine)	Used to prevent motion sickness
dimenhydrinate (Dramamine)	Used to prevent motion sickness
meclizine (Antivert)	Used to prevent motion sickness
prochlorperazine (Compazine)	Used to control nausea and vomiting
trimethobenzamide (Tigan)	
Antispasmodics	**Prevent Cramping of Smooth Muscle of GI Tract, Urinary Tract, and Uterus**
dicyclomine (Bentyl)	Decreases motility of gastrointestinal tract
Antiulcer Drugs	**Prevent or Alleviate Symptoms of Ulcers**
Antibiotic combinations	Eliminate *H. pylori* infections
metronidazole, tetracycline, and bismuth subsalicylate	Used to treat *H. pylori* infections

Chapter Pharmacology—cont'd

Drug Class	Effects and Uses
H₂ Antagonists	*Competitive blockers of histamine at H₂ site*
cimetidine (Tagamet)	Competitive blockers of histamine at H_2 site
famotidine (Pepcid)	Competitive blockers of histamine at H_2 site
ranitidine (Zantac)	Competitive blockers of histamine at H_2 site
sucralfate (Carafate)	Competitive blockers of histamine at H_2 site
Proton pump inhibitors	*Block final step of gastric acid production*
omeprazole (Prilosec)	Blocks final step of gastric acid production
lansoprazole (Prevacid)	Blocks final step of gastric acid production
Antiflatulents	**Relieve or Prevent Excessive Gas in the Stomach and Intestinal Tract**
simethicone (Gas-X)	Prevents formation of gas pockets
Miscellaneous	**Action May Be Topical Rather Than Systemic**
mesalamine (Asacol)	Used in ulcerative colitis
Laxatives	**Promote Bowel Evacuation**
Saline types	*Attract and retain water in intestinal tract*
milk of magnesia	Increases pressure in the intestinal tract
epsom salts	Increases pressure in the intestinal tract
Stimulants	*Stimulate intestinal mucosa*
cascara sagrada	Stimulates intestinal mucosa
sennoside (Ex-Lax)	Stimulates intestinal mucosa
senna (Senokot)	Stimulates intestinal mucosa
castor oil	Stimulates intestinal mucosa
bisacodyl (Dulcolax)	Stimulates intestinal mucosa
Bulk-Producing	Holds water in the stool
psyllium (Metamucil)	
Emollient	
mineral oil	Lubricates and softens tissue
Fecal softeners	
docusate (Kasof/Colace)	Facilitates action of fat and water to soften the stool

CHAPTER REVIEW 7

▶ **BASIC UNDERSTANDING**

REVIEWING WORD PARTS

I. Write a word (prefix, suffix, or combining form) for each clue.

CROSSWORD PUZZLE 7

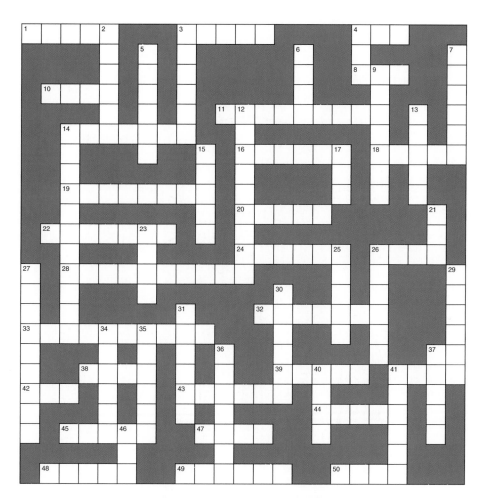

Across

1 eat or swallow
3 fungus
4 bad
8 sugar
10 hernia
11 mandible
14 duodenum
16 digestion
18 starch
19 esophagus
20 thirst
22 contraction
24 irrigation
26 many
28 gallbladder
32 maxilla
33 common bile duct
37 inside
38 cecum
39 rectum
41 surgical fixation
42 anus
43 tongue
44 milk
45 bladder
47 fats
48 capable of destroying
49 tongue
50 fungus

Down

2 small intestine
3 fruit
4 muscle
5 protein
6 bile
7 liver
9 mouth
12 appendix
13 sugar
14 diverticulum
15 bile
17 enzyme
21 pertaining to
23 ileum
25 saliva
26 pylorus
27 pancreas
29 jejunum
30 stomach
31 lip
34 vomiting
35 teeth
36 gum
37 outside
40 large intestine
41 anus or rectum
46 pertaining to

MATCHING

II. Match the processes of achieving nutrition in the left column with their descriptions in the right column.

_____ 1. ingestion	**A.** eating food
_____ 2. digestion	**B.** mechanically and chemically breaking down food
_____ 3. movements	**C.** passage of nutrient molecules into blood or lymph
_____ 4. absorption	**D.** removal of wastes
_____ 5. elimination	**E.** transporting food along the digestive tract and mixing it

III. Match terms on the left with meanings on the right.

_____ 1. caries	**A.** abnormal opening
_____ 2. fissure	**B.** cleft or groove
_____ 3. fistula	**C.** decay
_____ 4. hernia	**D.** irrigation of an organ
_____ 5. lavage	**E.** lining of the abdominal and pelvic cavities
_____ 6. mucosa	**F.** lining of the digestive tract
_____ 7. peritoneum	**G.** open sore or lesion
_____ 8. ulcer	**H.** protrusion of an organ through the wall of a cavity

LABELING

IV. Label the structures (1 through 13) in the diagram with the corresponding combining form. (Write two combining forms for 2 and 6.)

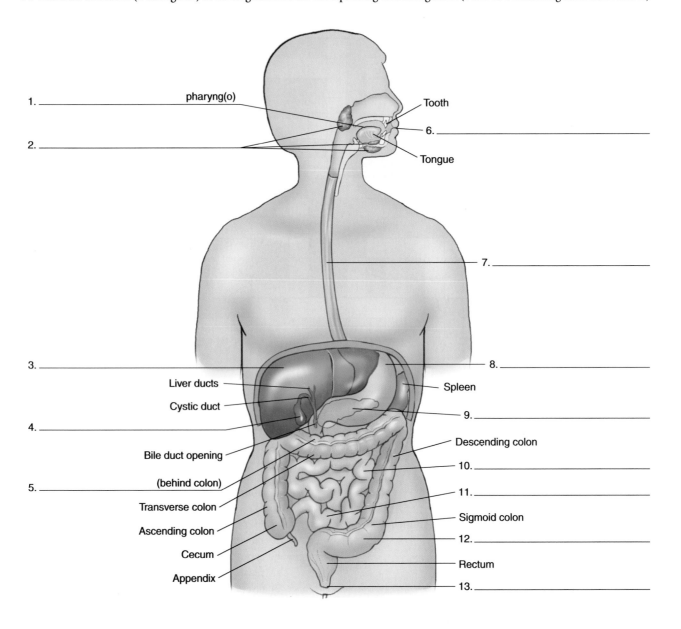

LABELING

V. Label 1 through 4 with the types of teeth.

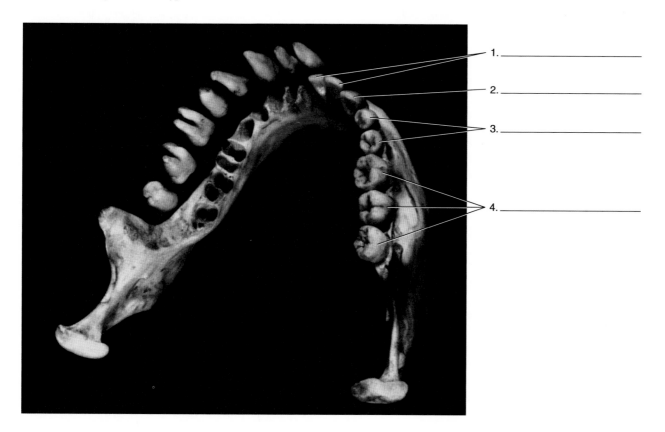

1. _____

2. _____

3. _____

4. _____

MULTIPLE CHOICE

VI. Select one answer (A-D) for each of the following multiple choice questions:

1. What is another name for the gastrointestinal system?
   A. alimentary tract
   B. peritoneal tract
   C. cardiogastric system
   D. gastrourinary system

2. Which statement is true of the cecum?
   A. part of the small intestine
   B. part of the large intestine
   C. part of the esophagus
   D. none of the above

3. Which of the following is *not* a surgical procedure?
   A. gastroenteritis
   B. gastroduodenostomy
   C. jejunotomy
   D. hepatectomy

4. What is the name of the procedure that is used to correct coloptosis?
   A. coloscopy
   B. colectasia
   C. colopexy
   D. colopathy

5. Which of the following is a type of gastrocele?
   A. caries
   B. cholelith
   C. anorexia nervosa
   D. hiatal hernia

6. Which of the following is inflamed in enteritis?
   A. internal organs
   B. peritoneum
   C. intestines
   D. esophagus

7. What is the name of the valve that regulates movement of intestinal contents from the small intestine into the large intestine?
   A. jejunocecal valve
   B. ileocecal valve
   C. pyloric valve
   D. cecorectal valve

8. Cheilostomatoplasty is plastic surgery of which structures?
   A. tongue and mouth
   B. mouth and stomach
   C. gums and mouth
   D. lips and mouth

9. What is stagnation of the normal movement of food in the intestinal tract called?
   A. duodenitis
   B. enterostasis
   C. peristalsis
   D. peptic ulcer

10. Which of the following is an instrument designed for passage into the stomach to permit examination of its interior?
    A. gastrotome
    B. gastroscope
    C. gastric lavage
    D. gastrometer

11. Which of the following is a condition characterized by splitting of the lips and angles of the mouth?
    A. cheilosis
    B. stomatomycosis
    C. gingivostomatitis
    D. glossopharyngitis

12. Which surgical procedure might be used in cases of carcinoma of the tongue?
    A. glossectomy
    B. glossoplegia
    C. linguoplacement
    D. periodontal surgery

13. What is the long tube that carries food to the stomach called?
    A. ascending colon
    B. descending colon
    C. jejunum
    D. esophagus

14. Which of the following means surgical formation of an opening into the common bile duct through the abdominal wall?
    A. choledochostomy
    B. cholecystostomy
    C. esophagoduodenostomy
    D. gastroenterostomy

15. Which of the following is the most significant sign of diabetes mellitus?
    A. hyperlipemia
    B. hyperinsulinism
    C. hyperamylosis
    D. hyperglycemia

16. Why are the accessory glands important components of the digestive system?
    A. They are responsible for the mechanical breakdown of nurients.
    B. They are the driving force of ingestion.
    C. They are the primary providers of movement of food along the digestive tube.
    D. They produce digestive enzymes that aid in digestion and absorption of nutrients.

17. Which term means irrigation of the colon?
    A. colectasia
    B. coloclysis
    C. enterostasis
    D. peristalsis

18. Which of the following is an organ that produces insulin?
    A. appendix
    B. liver
    C. pancreas
    D. pylorus

19. Which of the following is *not* an accessory gland of the digestive system?
    A. duodenum
    B. gallbladder
    C. pancreas
    D. salivary glands

20. Which of the following is a disorder that is characterized by episodes of binge eating that are terminated by abdominal pain, sleep, self-induced vomiting, or purging with laxatives?
    A. anorexia nervosa
    B. bulimia
    C. Crohn's disease
    D. malabsorption syndrome

CASE STUDY

VII. Select A, B, C, or D for questions 1 through 5 after reading this information from a hospital record.

B. A. Stone (female, age 42)
Sx   Sudden onset of fever, nausea, and hyperemesis
PE   Tenderness in RUQ; intense midline abdominal pain; BP 160/90; flatulence
        Nothing else of significance
Abdominal US revealed numerous gallstones.
Dx   Cholecystitis/cholelithiasis
Treatment: Cholecystectomy

---

1. Hyperemesis is excessive
    A. hunger
    B. nausea
    C. urination
    D. vomiting

2. Flatulence is excessive
    A. air or gas
    B. swelling
    C. sensitivity to pain
    D. thirst

3. Cholecystitis is
    A. a cystic infection
    B. dilation of the bile ducts
    C. inflammation of the common bile duct
    D. inflammation of the gallbladder

4. The diagnosis was
    A. biliary abscess
    B. biliary dyskinesia
    C. cholecystitis resulting from gallstones
    D. tumors of the gallbladder and common bile duct

5. The treatment was
    A. anastomosis of the gallbladder and the stomach
    B. lithotripsy
    C. removal of cancerous tumors
    D. removal of the gallbladder

FILL IN THE BLANKS

VIII. Choose from the following terms to complete the paragraph:

absorption   large intestine
bolus   pyloric sphincter
cardiac sphincter   rugae
chyme   teeth
esophagus   villi

Imagine that you are eating a piece of bread. The (1) _____ grind and chew the food. The mass of bread is called a

(2) _____. A long tube, the (3) _____, carries the food to the stomach. The (4) _____

_____ guards the opening into the stomach. The inner mucosal layer of the stomach is arranged in temporary folds called

(5) _____. Food is churned and broken down in the stomach. The mixture of partly digested food and digestive secretions

is now called (6) _____. A muscle, the (7) _____ _____, regulates the outflow of churned

food from the stomach. This liquid mass is then passed to the small intestine, where digestion continues and (8) _____ of

nutrients occurs. Microscopic fingerlike structures called (9) _____ increase surface area of the small intestine. Later, in the

(10) _____ _____, much of the water is reabsorbed.

WRITING TERMS

IX. Write a term for each of the following meanings.

1. any disease of the liver   _____
2. any fungal disease of the mouth   _____
3. enzyme that breaks down milk   _____
4. excessive hunger   _____
5. incision of the vagus nerve   _____
6. increased lipids in the blood   _____
7. inflammation of a salivary gland _____
8. inflammation of the large intestine _____

9. inspection of the pylorus   _____
10. paralysis of the small intestine _____
11. pertaining to the common
    bile duct   _____
12. pertaining to the gums   _____
13. prolapse of the esophagus   _____
14. surgical fixation of the colon   _____
15. surgical repair of the tongue   _____

▶ **GREATER COMPREHENSION**

SPELLING

X. Circle all incorrectly spelled terms and write their correct spelling.

cholangiography   fluoroscopy   malocclusion   denchure   gastrick   periodontal
enteroclysis   lipopinia   retrocecal

INTERPRETING ABBREVIATIONS

XI. Write the meaning of these abbreviations:

1. GB _____
2. GI _____
3. IVC _____

4. NPO _____
5. TPN _____

PRONUNCIATION

XII. The pronunciation is shown for several medical words. Indicate which syllable has the primary accent by marking it with an ′.

1. cholecystogastric (**ko le sis to gas trik**)
2. choledochal (**ko led ə kəl**)
3. cholelithiasis (**ko le lǐ thi ə sis**)
4. colectasia (**ko lek ta zhə**)
5. fistula (**fis tu lə**)

6. hepatomegaly (**hep ə to meg ə le**)
7. jejunoileostomy (**jə joo no il e os tə me**)
8. proctoscopy (**prok tos kə pe**)
9. sigmoidoscope (**sig moi do skōp**)
10. sublingual (**səb ling gwəl**)

CATEGORIZING TERMS

XIII. Categorize terms as anatomical, diagnostic, surgical, radiological, or therapeutic by writing A, D, S, R, or T after each term:

1. anorexia _____
2. antiflatulents _____
3. approximation _____
4. cheilostomatoplasty _____
5. cholangiopancreatography _____
6. cholecystostomy _____
7. dyspepsia _____
8. esophagram _____
9. gastromalacia _____
10. lingual _____

DRUG CLASSES

XIV. Match the drug classes in the left column with their uses in the right column.

_____ 1. anorexiants
_____ 2. antidiabetics
_____ 3. antiemetics
_____ 4. antiflatulents

A. treat hyperglycemia
B. prevent formation of gas pockets
C. prevent motion sickness or vomiting
D. treat obesity

(Check your answers with the solutions in Appendix V.)

Listing of Medical Terms

absorption	caries	colic	duodenal ulcer
adipsia	cecoileostomy	colitis	duodenitis
alimentary tract	cecum	coloclysis	duodenography
alimentation	cheilitis	colon	duodenoscope
amylase	cheiloplasty	colonic stasis	duodenoscopy
amylolysis	cheilorrhaphy	colonoscopy	duodenostomy
anal	cheilosis	colopexy	duodenotomy
anastomose	cheilostomatoplasty	coloproctitis	duodenum
anastomosis	cholangiography	coloptosis	dysentery
anodontia	cholangiopancreatography	colorectal	dyspepsia
anorexia nervosa	cholangitis	coloscopy	dysphagia
anorexiant	cholecystectomy	colostomy	elimination
antacid	cholecystitis	cuspid	emaciation
antiemetic	cholecystogastric	defecation	emesis
antiflatulent	cholecystography	dental caries	emetic
antiodontalgic	cholecystogram	dental hygienist	enamel
antispasmodics	cholecystostomy	dentalgia	endodontitis
anus	choledochal	dentifrice	endodontium
aphagia	choledochitis	dentilingual	endogastric
appendectomy	choledochoduodenostomy	denture	endogenous
appendicitis	choledocholithiasis	descending colon	endoscope
approximation	choledochoplasty	diabetes mellitus	endoscopy
ascending colon	choledochostomy	diarrhea	enteral
bacteriophage	cholelith	digestion	enteritis
bicuspid	cholelithiasis	diverticulectomy	enteroclysis
biliary	cholestasis	diverticulitis	enterocolitis
bolus	chyme	diverticulosis	enterodynia
bradypepsia	cirrhosis	diverticulum	enteroplegia
bulimia	colectasia	duodenal	enterostasis
canker sores	colectomy	duodenal carcinoma	esophageal

Listing of Medical Terms—cont'd

esophagectasia
esophagitis
esophagoduodenostomy
esophagodynia
esophagogastroduodenoscopy
esophagogastroplasty
esophagogastroscopy
esophagogastrostomy
esophagogram
esophagojejunostomy
esophagomalacia
esophagoptosis
esophagoscopy
esophagram
esophagus
eupepsia
exogenous
extrahepatic
fissure
fistula
flatulence
fluoroscopy
fructase
fructose
fundus
fungal
gastralgia
gastrectasia
gastrectasis
gastrectomy
gastric carcinoma
gastric hypertrophy
gastric lavage
gastritis
gastrocele
gastroduodenal anastomosis
gastroduodenitis
gastroduodenostomy
gastrodynia
gastroenteritis
gastroenterocolitis
gastroenterology
gastroenterostomy
gastroesophageal reflux
    disease
gastrointestinal
gastrojejunostomy
gastromalacia
gastromegaly
gastropathy
gastropexy
gastroplasty
gastroptosis
gastropulmonary

gastrorrhaphy
gastroscope
gastroscopy
gastrostomy
gingiva
gingival
gingivalgia
gingivectomy
gingivitis
gingivoglossitis
gingivostomatitis
glossal
glossectomy
glossitis
glossopathy
glossopharyngeal
glossoplasty
glossoplegia
glossopyrosis
glossorrhaphy
glucose
glycolysis
hematemesis
hemorrhoidectomy
hemorrhoids
hepatectomy
hepatic
hepatitis
hepatocyte
hepatolith
hepatolytic
hepatoma
hepatomegaly
hepatopathy
hepatorrhagia
hepatosplenomegaly
hepatotomy
hepatotoxic
hernia
hiatal hernia
hiatus
hyperacidity
hyperalimentation
hyperemesis
hyperglycemia
hyperlipemia
hyperlipidemia
hypoglossal
hypoglycemia
ileitis
ileocecal valve
ileostomy
ileum
impaction

incisor
ingestion
inguinal
insulin
interdental
intestinal
jaundice
jejunoileostomy
jejunotomy
jejunum
lactase
lactose
laparocholecystotomy
laparocolostomy
laparocolotomy
laparocystectomy
laparocystotomy
laparogastrotomy
laparohepatotomy
lavage
lingual
lipase
lipoid
lipopenia
lithiasis
lithotripsy
macrodontia
malabsorption syndrome
malaise
malnutrition
malocclusion
mandibular
maxillary
metabolism
molar
mucoid
mucosa
mucous
mucus
mycosis
nasogastric
neoplasia
neoplasm
neoplastic
nutrition
obesity
oropharyngeal
orthodontics
pancreatectomy
pancreatic
pancreatitis
pancreatography
pancreatolith
pancreatolithectomy

pancreatolysis
pancreatopathy
pancreatotomy
paraappendicitis
paracolitis
parasplenic
parenteral
parietal peritoneum
parotid
parotitis
peptic ulcer
periappendicitis
pericolic
pericolitis
perihepatitis
periodontal
periodontics
periodontist
periodontitis
periodontium
peripancreatitis
peristalsis
peritoneum
peritonitis
peritonsillar
phagocyte
phagocytic
phagocytize
phagocytosis
photofluorogram
phrenogastric
polydipsia
polyphagia
postesophageal
precancerous
premolar
proctalgia
proctoclysis
proctodynia
proctologist
proctopexy
proctoplasty
proctoplegia
proctoptosis
proctorrhagia
proctorrhaphy
proctoscope
proctoscopy
protease
proteinase
proteinuria
proteolysis
proteuria
pyloric sphincter

Continued

Listing of Medical Terms—cont'd

pyloric stenosis	retrocecal	sphincter	temporomandibular joint
pyloromyotomy	retrocolic	stasis	topical
pyloroplasty	retroperitoneal	stomatitis	tracheoesophageal
pyloroscopy	rugae	stomatodynia	transhepatic
pylorostenosis	saliva	stomatomycosis	transverse colon
pylorotomy	salivary gland	stomatopathy	ulcer
pylorus	serosa	stomatoplasty	ulcerative colitis
pyorrhea	sialadenitis	stomatorrhagia	umbilical
rectocele	sialitis	subglossal	vagotomy
rectoplasty	sialography	sublingual	vagus
rectorrhaphy	sialolith	submaxillary	vermiform appendix
rectoscope	sigmoid colon	sucrase	villi
rectoscopy	sigmoidoscope	sucrose	viral
rectum	sigmoidoscopy	suprahepatic	visceral peritoneum

Español Enhancing Spanish Communication

English	Spanish (pronunciation)	English	Spanish (pronunciation)
appendix	apéndice (ah-PEN-de-say)	intestine	intestino (in-tes-TEE-no)
appetite	apetito (ah-pay-TEE-to)	laxative	purgante (poor-GAHN-tay)
belch	eructo (ay-ROOK-to)	lips	labios (LAH-be-os)
chew, to	masticar (mas-te-CAR)	liver	hígado (EE-ga-do)
constipation	estreñimiento (es-tray-nye-me-EN-to)	mouth	boca (BO-ka)
defecate	evacuar (ay-vah-coo-AR)	movement	movimiento (mo-ve-me-EN-to)
diabetes	diabetes (de-ah-BAY-tes)	milk	leche (LAY-chay)
digestion	digestión (de-hes-te-ON)	mucus	moco (MO-co)
enzyme	enzima (en-SEE-mah)	nutrition	nutrición (noo-tre-se-ON)
esophagus	esófago (ay-SO-fah-go)	pancreas	páncreas (PAHN-cray-as)
excretion	excreción (ex-cray-se-ON)	rectum	recto (REK-to)
feces	excremento (ex-cray-MEN-to)	saliva	saliva (sah-LEE-vah)
gallbladder	vesícula biliar (vay-SEE-coo-la be-le-AR)	starch	almidón (al-me-DON)
gallstone	cálculo biliar (CAHL-coo-lo be-le-AR)	stomach	estómago (es-TOH-mah-go)
glucose	glucosa (gloo-CO-sah)	swallow	tragar (trah-GAR)
gum, gingiva	encía (en-SEE-ah)	teeth	dientes (de-AYN-tays)
hernia	hernia (AYR-ne-ah), quebradura (kay-brah-DOO-rah)	thirst	sed (sayd)
		tongue	lengua (LEN-gwah)
hunger	hambre (AHM-bray)	vomiting	vómito (VOH-mee-toh)
insulin	insulina (in-soo-LEE-nah)		

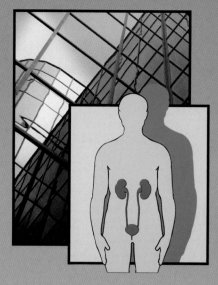

Urinary System

8

Outline

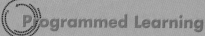
Principal Word Parts

COMBINING FORMS

albumin(o)	albumin
bacteri(o)	bacteria
cyst(o)	bladder, cyst, sac
dipl(o)	double
glomerul(o)	glomerulus
glyc(o), glycos(o)	sugar
gon(o)	genitals or reproduction
hydr(o)	water
ket(o), keton(o)	ketone bodies
lith(o)	stone, calculus
ne(o)	new
nephr(o), ren(o)	kidney
noct(i), nyct(o)	night
nos(o)	disease
olig(o)	few
py(o)	pus
pyel(o)	renal pelvis
staphyl(o)	grapelike cluster; uvula
strept(o)	twisted
tox(o)	poison
ur(o)	urine, urinary tract
ureter(o)	ureter
urethr(o)	urethra
urin(o)	urine

SUFFIXES

-cele	hernia
-rrhagia	hemorrhage
-rrhaphy	suture
-rrhea	flow or discharge
-rrhexis	rupture
-tripsy	surgical crushing

Learning Goals

▶ BASIC UNDERSTANDING

In this chapter, you will learn to do the following:

1. Identify the structures of the urinary tract and their functions.
2. Recognize the relationship between uremia and renal function.
3. Recognize that blood, glucose, ketones, and pus are not generally found in a catheterized urine specimen.
4. Distinguish the characteristics of the major shapes of bacteria and coccal arrangements.
5. Describe the significance of genitourinary infections and their association with some sexually transmitted diseases.
6. Write the meaning of the word parts associated with the urinary system and use them to build and analyze terms.

▶ GREATER COMPREHENSION

7. Identify the major structures of the nephron and their functions.
8. Categorize the terms as anatomical, diagnostic, radiological, surgical, or therapeutic.
9. Spell the terms accurately.
10. Pronounce the terms correctly.
11. Know the meanings of the abbreviations.
12. Identify the effects or uses of the drug classes presented in this chapter.

SECTION A

Urinary Tract

The urinary system plays an important part in excretion of waste products that are produced during cellular metabolism. It regulates the concentrations of various substances, including water, by controlling the amount that is excreted in the urine. There are several excretory routes through which the body eliminates wastes. You have studied how the lungs eliminate carbon dioxide and how the digestive system provides a means of expelling solid wastes. The skin also serves as an excretory organ by eliminating wastes in the form of perspiration. Another important mode of excretion is performed by the kidneys, which are part of the urinary system considered in this chapter. You will learn other vital functions of the kidneys, as well as several disorders of the urinary tract.

	8-1 The urinary system consists of paired kidneys, one on each side of the spinal column, a ureter for each kidney, a bladder, and a urethra. Figure 8-1 shows the location of these structures in the body.
	Read all of the information that accompanies Figure 8-1. Complete the blank lines 1 through 4 by reading the following information.
	Urine is formed in the kidneys. Label the left kidney (1). The ureters carry the urine to the urinary bladder. Label the left ureter (2). The bladder (3) is a temporary reservoir for the urine until it is excreted via the urethra (4).
urine	**8-2** The combining form ***urin(o)*** means urine. Urin/ary means pertaining to _____. The organs and ducts that are involved in the secretion and elimination of urine from the body are referred to as the urinary tract.
	You learned in Chapter 2 that ur(o) means urinary system or urine. In terms that use the combining form ur(o), you will need to decide which meaning is intended.
	8-3 Most of the work of the urinary system takes place in the kidneys. The average adult kidney is about 11 cm long by 6 cm wide (about 4 ½ by 2 ⅓ inches) and weighs about 145 grams (less than ½ lb.). Although the kidneys are best known for their life-maintaining function of regulating the volume and composition of blood plasma, they also have several other important functions that are summarized in Table 8-1.

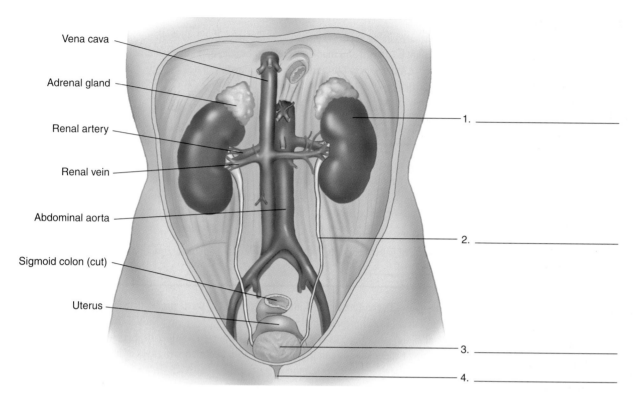

FIGURE 8-1

The urinary system. Adjacent vessels of the cardiovascular system are also shown. The right and left renal arteries branch off the abdominal aorta to transport blood to the kidneys. Urine, formed in the kidneys, leaves by way of the ureters and passes to the bladder, where it is stored. When voluntary control is removed, urine is expelled through the urethra. When blood is filtered, wastes are removed, but much of the water and other substances are reabsorbed. They enter the renal vein and are returned to the blood stream via the inferior vena cava.

TABLE 8-1   Major Functions of the Kidneys

Maintain plasma volume by varying the excretion of water
Maintain the chemical composition of the blood by selective excretion of solutes
Maintain blood pH, thus contributing to acid-base balance
Excretion of nitrogenous waste products of protein metabolism, mainly urea, uric acid, and creatinine
Production of renin (for regulation of blood pressure), erythropoietin (stimulates erythrocyte production), and prostaglandins (fatty acid derivatives that have effects on many organs)
Degrade insulin
Metabolize vitamin D to its active form

---

kidney
nephrectomy
(nə-frek′tə-me)

nephromegaly

8-4 Two combining forms, ***ren(o)*** and ***nephr(o),*** mean kidney. Renal (**re′nəl**) means pertaining to the _____. In a renal transplant the patient (recipient) receives a kidney from a suitable donor. The donated kidney is surgically removed from the donor. Build a word that means surgical excision of a kidney, using nephr(o) and the suffix for excision: _____.

When one kidney is removed, the opposite organ becomes enlarged. Enlargement of the kidney is _____.

renal	**8-5** If you debated using nephr(o) or ren(o) in the preceding frame, do not be concerned. Although renomegaly might be a word and many people might understand the meaning, nephromegaly is the commonly used term. Another way of stating the same thing might be _____ (pertaining to the kidney) enlargement.
kidneys	Renal clearance tests determine the efficiency with which the kidneys excrete a particular substance. Renal clearance tests are diagnostic evaluation of what organs? _____
urine blood	**8-6** Because the urinary system is responsible for removing harmful waste products from the blood, anything that interferes with excretion of wastes can be dangerous. Ur/emia (**u-re′me-ə**) is an accumulation of toxic products in the blood. This occurs when the kidneys fail to function properly. The meaning of ur/emia is implied. Write the meanings of its component parts: ur(o) means _____; -emia means _____.
uremia	An accumulation of waste products in the blood owing to inadequate functioning of the urinary system is called _____.
blood	**8-7** Kidney dialysis is required if the kidneys fail to remove waste products from the blood. This is also called hemo/dialysis, which means dialysis of the _____. Kidney dialysis or hemodialysis (**he″mo-di-al′ə-sis**) is the process of diffusing blood through a semipermeable membrane for the purpose of removing toxic materials and maintaining acid-base balance in cases of impaired kidney function. If uremia becomes severe, dialysis is required.
	Peritoneal dialysis is dialysis through the peritoneum, the dialyzing solution being introduced into and removed from the peritoneal cavity. Sometimes this type of dialysis is done as an alternative to hemodialysis.
making a record of the urinary system	**8-8** Remember that ur(o) also means the urinary system. Uro/graphy (**u-rog′rə-fe**) refers to the urinary system and means _____.
	Urography is making x-ray films of the entire urinary system or part of it after it has been rendered opaque by a radiopaque solution. Various structural abnormalities can be seen with urography.
ureter ureters	**8-9** Urine leaves the kidney by way of a ureter, which takes it to the bladder. The combining form *ureter(o)* means ureter. Ureter/al means pertaining to a _____. A ureteral dysfunction is a disturbance of the normal flow of urine through one or both _____.
bladder	**8-10** You learned earlier that cyst(o) means either cyst, bladder, or fluid-filled sac. Cystic (**sis′tik**) can have several meanings. It can mean pertaining to a cyst or pertaining to a fluid-filled sac such as the urinary _____.
urethra	**8-11** Urine leaves the bladder by way of the urethra and is expelled from the body. The combining form *urethr(o)* means urethra.
	Urethr/al means pertaining to the _____.

❏ SECTION A REVIEW 𝒰rinary Tract

This section review covers frames 8–1 through 8–11. Write combining forms or meanings for each of the following:

Combining Form	Meaning	Combining Form	Meaning
1. nephr(o)	_____	4. _____	urethra
2. ren(o)	_____	5. _____	urine
3. _____	ureter		

(Use Appendix V to check your answers.)

Kidneys and Ureters

Normal kidney function requires constant filtering of the blood, selective reabsorption, and formation of urine. About one million nephrons serve as the functional units of each kidney. Renal diagnostic and surgical terms frequently refer to anatomic features of the kidney. Anatomic features and terms are presented in this section along with information about the tubes that convey urine from the kidney to the bladder, the ureters.

inflammation of the kidney **nephritis**	**8-12** Nephr/itis (nə-fri′tis) is _____. Nephritis is also called Bright's disease. The most usual form is glomerulo/nephritis (**glo-mer″u-lo-nə-fri′tis),** in which glomeruli within the kidney are inflamed. Glomeruli are clusters of capillaries that act as filters. In glomerulonephritis, there is impairment of the filtering process. Inflammation of the kidney may be caused by microorganisms or their toxins or even by toxic drugs or alcohol. Regardless of the cause or the particular type, a word that means inflammation of the kidney is _____.
kidney **nephrolysis** (nə-frol′ə-sis)	**8-13** A substance that is nephro/toxic (**nef″ro-tok′sik)** is toxic or destructive to _____ cells. Build a word that means destruction of the kidney by combining nephr(o) with the suffix for destruction: _____. Nephrolysis is destruction of kidney tissue. It also means freeing of a kidney from adhesions.
heart **nephromalacia** (nef″ro-mə-la′shə)	**8-14** Cardio/nephric (**kar″de-o-nef′rik)** means pertaining to the _____ and the kidneys. Use nephr(o) to a build a word that means abnormal softening of the kidney: _____.
enlargement of the kidney **one kidney** **two (both) kidneys**	**8-15** Nephro/megaly (**nef″ro-meg′ə-le)** is _____. Kidney enlargement may involve one or both kidneys. Uni/lateral nephromegaly is enlargement of _____ _____; bi/lateral nephromegaly involves _____ _____.
kidney **nephrotomography** (nef″ro-to-mog′rə-fe) **nephrotomogram** (nef″ro-to′mo-gram)	**8-16** Nephro/sono/graphy (**nef″ro-so-nog′rə-fe)** is ultrasonic scanning of the _____. Nephromegaly, very small kidneys, cysts, and kidney stones can be observed in nephrosonography. Using nephrosonography as a model, write a word that means computed tomography of the kidney: _____. The film produced by nephrotomography is a _____.
nephropexy (nef′ro-pek″se)	**8-17** Use nephr(o) and -pexy to write a word that means surgical fixation of the kidney: _____. This type of surgery is often used to correct nephroptosis (**nef″rop-to′sis),** also called floating kidney, which is explained in Table 8-2. Other disorders or diseases of the urinary system are included in the table.

TABLE 8-2 Additional Diseases or Disorders of the Urinary System

chronic renal failure (CRF): A condition in which the kidney gradually ceases to remove metabolic wastes and excessive water from the blood. Uremia is a major characteristic. Kidney impairment is not reversible once the disease progresses to the end stage.

nephroptosis (**nef″rop-to′sis**): Gradual downward displacement of the kidney. Also called floating, hypermobile, or wandering kidney. Can occur when the kidney supports are weakened by sudden strain or a blow, or it may be present at birth. Can be corrected by nephropexy

nephrosclerosis (**nef″ro-sklə-ro′sis**): Sclerosis or hardening of the kidney

nephrosis (**nə-fro′sis**): Any disease of the kidney characterized by degenerative changes, especially the renal tubules, without the occurrence of inflammation

nephrotic syndrome: A classification that includes all diseases of the kidney characterized by chronic loss of protein in the urine and subsequent depletion of body protein, especially albumin.

polycystic kidney disease (**pol″e-sis′tik**): A renal disorder in which the kidneys are enlarged and contain many cysts. Also called polycystic renal disease

pyelonephritis (**pi″ə-lo-nə-fri′tis**): Inflammation of the kidney and its renal pelvis, owing to infection

pyonephrosis (**pi″o-nə-fro′sis**): Destruction of the kidney characterized by production of pus, with total or almost complete loss of renal function

renal artery stenosis: Severe narrowing of the renal artery, thus reducing blood flow to the kidney

urolithiasis (**u″ro-lĭ-thi′ə-sis**): Formation of urinary calculi

nephrosclerosis	**8-18** You know a great deal of medical vocabulary now, and you probably recognize many of the terms in Table 8-2; for example, hardening of the kidney is _____.
chronic	A condition in which the kidney gradually ceases to function properly and uremia develops is not acute, but _____, renal failure. A large percentage of patients with chronic renal failure have hypertension, which may be the cause or the result of CRF.
nephrosis	Degenerative changes of the kidney without inflammation is _____.
pyelonephritis	**8-19** The renal pelvis is a funnel-shaped structure located in the center of each kidney. The combining form for renal pelvis is *pyel(o)*. Write a term that means inflammation of the kidney and its renal pelvis by combining pyel(o), nephr(o), and -itis: _____.
cysts	Poly/cyst/ic kidney disease (Figure 8-2) is a renal disorder in which the kidneys are enlarged and contain many _____.
pus	**8-20** The combining form *py(o)* means pus. Pyo/nephrosis is destruction of the kidney characterized by production of _____.
stenosis	Looking again at Table 8-2, severe narrowing of the renal artery is renal artery _____.
kidneys	Pathologic changes to the renal arteries may result in drastically reduced blood flow through the kidneys. Reno/vascular means pertaining to the blood vessels of the _____.
	Renovascular disease, such as thrombosis or stenosis, results in ischemia and damage to the kidneys.
urolithiasis	Knowing that lith(o) means stone, build the word that means formation of urinary calculi by using ur(o), lith(o), and -iasis: _____.
kidney	**8-21** Nephro/lith/iasis (**nef″ro-lĭ-thi′ə-sis**) is a condition marked by the presence of _____ stones.
nephrolith (**nef′ro-lith**)	Another name for a renal calculus or a kidney stone is _____.

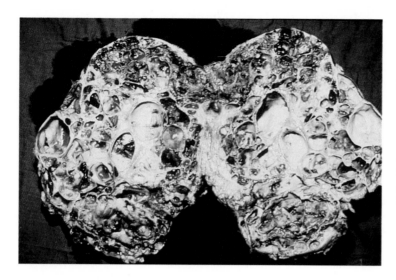

FIGURE 8-2
Polycystic kidney. There are many types, but this particular patient had an inherited type of polycystic kidney disease that accounts for about 10% of all patients with end-stage renal disease in the United States. Notice the replacement of normal tissue by numerous fluid-filled cysts. (From Zitelli BJ, Davis HW: *Atlas of pediatric physical diagnosis*, ed 3, 1997, St Louis, Mosby.)

	8-22 Urinary stones are often named according to their location: kidney, ureter, or bladder. They vary greatly in size, from small enough to pass through the ureter to large stones that occupy the entire renal pelvis, and have roughly the shape of a deer antler (staghorn calculi).
calculi (or stones)	Nephro/litho/tomy (**nef″ro-lĭ-thot′ə-me**) is removal of renal _____ by cutting through the body of the kidney. Notice that -tomy is used rather than -ectomy, because -tomy refers to incision of the kidney, and removal of the stone is only implied.
litholysis (li-thol′ĭ-sis)	Nephrolithotomy is necessary if the stone is too large to pass or break up, or if it will not dissolve. Increased water intake is often helpful in flushing out small stones from the kidney. Build a word by combining lith(o) and the suffix that means dissolving: _____.
	Litholysis is sometimes accomplished by drinking or injecting large amounts of fluid. Sometimes a stone is excreted, as in the case of many kidney stones.
stone **lithotripsy**	**8-23** Litho/tripsy (**lith′o-trip″se**) is surgical crushing of a _____. The suffix *-tripsy* means surgical crushing. Write the word that means surgical crushing of a stone: _____.
	Sometimes lithotripsy is successful with small stones and is accomplished by inserting a catheter through the urethra to the point where the stone is lodged. The stone is then crushed with an instrument called a lithotrite (**lith′o-trīt**).
outside the body	**8-24** Extracorporeal shock wave lithotripsy (ESWL) is a newer method of breaking up stones. You may remember that extracorporeal means _____.
	Extracorporeal shock wave lithotripsy uses ultrasonic energy from a source outside the body. This technique is used on stones that resist passage and is far less incapacitating than a full-scale surgery, such as nephrolithotomy.
nephroscope (nef′ro-skōp)	**8-25** Nephro/scopy (**nə-fros′kə-pe**) allows visualization of the kidney, using a fiberoptic instrument. Nephroscopy requires the use of an instrument that is inserted into a small incision in the renal pelvis (central cavity of the kidney) and allows the nephrologist to view inside the kidney. The instrument for nephroscopy is called a _____.

nephrostomy (nə-fros′tə-me) skin	**8-26** Using nephr(o), write another word that means creation of a new opening in the kidney (actually leading directly into the renal pelvis): _____. Percutaneous catheter nephrostomy provides for the diversion of renal output. Percutaneous tells us that the _____ is punctured to gain access to the kidney and then a catheter is placed into the renal pelvis. This procedure allows for drainage, drug instillation, and selected surgical procedures, including removal of calculi.
hydronephrosis (hi″dro-nə-fro′sis)	Write a word using nephrosis that literally means watery kidney condition: _____. This new term means distention of the renal pelvis with urine as a result of an obstructed ureter. Percutaneous catheter nephrostomy might be used as a temporary drain for renal output.
loss of kidney function chronic kidney stone	**8-27** Renal failure is _____. Acute means having severe symptoms and lasting for a short time. Chronic is the opposite of acute. Diseases of a chronic nature show little change or extremely slow progression over a long period. Acute renal failure shows symptoms that are more severe than _____ renal failure. Acute renal failure may be caused by nephritis or by anything that interferes with blood flow to the kidney or by those conditions that disrupt urinary output by the kidney. A nephrolith is an example of the latter; therefore, a nephrolith may be a cause of acute renal failure. A nephrolith is a _____ _____.
kidney **angiogram**	**8-28** Adequate blood circulation is essential for normal renal function. Anything that interferes with the normal circulation significantly reduces renal capabilities. Renal angio/graphy is radiographic study of the blood vessels of the _____. A renal _____ is the record of the renal blood vessels produced in renal angiography.
nephr(o)	**8-29** Anatomic features of the kidney are shown in Figure 8-3. Each kidney contains about one million microscopic nephrons, its functional units. The nephron (**nef′ron**) is named for the combining form _____, which means kidney. A nephron is shown in Figure 8-4. Its components are a glomerulus and tubules (**too′būlz**). Glomerulus comes from a word that means cluster. Each glomerulus is a cluster of capillaries.
glomerulus **glomerulopathy**	**8-30** The combining form *glomerul(o)* means glomerulus. Glomerulo/nephr/itis is a type of inflammation of the kidney in which the glomeruli (plural of glomerulus) are involved. Glomerul(o) is a combining form that means _____. Write a word that means any disease of the glomeruli (**glo-mer′u-li**): _____
proximal	**8-31** The glomerulus serves as a filter for the blood. It allows water, salts, wastes, and practically everything except blood cells and proteins to pass through its thin walls. Bowman's capsule collects the substances that filter through the glomerular walls and passes them to the long twisted tube, the tubule. The proxim/al tubule is that part of the tubule nearer the glomerulus. You learned that proxim(o) means near. That part of the renal tubule that is near the glomerulus and Bowman's capsule is the _____ tubule.

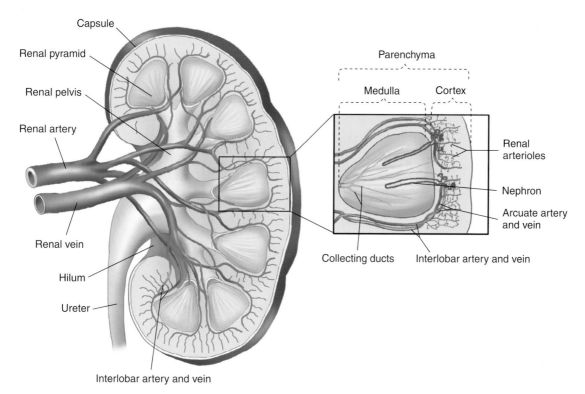

Capsule
Renal pyramid
Renal pelvis
Renal artery
Renal vein
Hilum
Ureter
Interlobar artery and vein

Parenchyma
Medulla   Cortex
Renal arterioles
Nephron
Arcuate artery and vein
Collecting ducts   Interlobar artery and vein

FIGURE 8-3

The kidney (sectioned). The kidney has a convex contour with the exception of the hilus (or hilum), a notch on the inner border. The hilus is the depression where the renal artery, renal vein, nerves, and lymphatics enter or leave the kidney. The kidney is encased in a fibrous capsule. A longitudinal section shows two distinct regions: the outer cortex and the inner medulla. The medulla has 10 to 15 triangular wedges called renal pyramids, made up of collecting ducts, lymphatics, and blood vessels. Cortical and medullary regions of each kidney contain approximately one million nephrons, the functioning units. A normal person can survive, although with difficulty, with less than 20,000 functioning nephrons. The kidneys are protected from direct trauma posteriorly by the ribs and muscle and anteriorly by the intestines.

---

glomerulus

tubule

8-32 Follow the long twisting tubule with a pencil. Notice that a tubule consists of a proximal tubule, a loop of Henle, and a distal tubule that opens into a collecting duct.

As fluid passes through the tubules, substances that the body conserves, such as sugar and much of the water, are reabsorbed into the blood vessels surrounding the tubules. The water and other substances remaining in the tubule become urine.

The function of a nephron is filtering of the blood and reabsorption of substances that the body conserves. Filtering occurs in what part of the nephron? _____

In what part of the nephron does reabsorption occur? _____

---

pyelitis (pi"ə-li′tis)

8-33 Waste products and some of the water remaining in the tubules after reabsorption become urine, which passes to the collecting duct. Thousands of collecting ducts deposit urine in the renal pelvis, the large central reservoir of the kidney.

Remembering that pyel(o) means renal pelvis, build a word that means inflammation of the renal pelvis: _____.

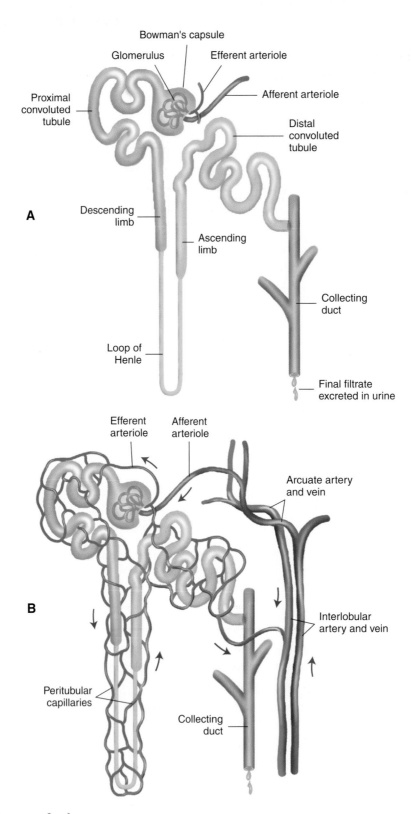

FIGURE 8-4

A, A nephron and surrounding capillaries. The renal arteries arise from the abdominal aorta. Each renal artery branches as it enters the hilus and after branching several times gives rise to the afferent arteriole. This terminates in capillary tufts called a glomerulus. Blood leaves the glomerulus through the efferent arteriole, which subdivides into peritubular capillaries. As the glomerular filtrate flows through the tubules, most of its water and varying amounts of solutes are reabsorbed into the peritubular capillaries. These capillaries join others and become the arcuate vein and eventually the renal vein, whereby blood leaves the kidney. **B,** As the filtrate passes through the tubular portion of the nephron, variable quantities of water, electrolytes, and other substances are reabsorbed into the body. Reabsorption occurs across the tubule walls into blood capillaries nearby (peritubular capillaries are shown).

pyelostomy (pi″ə-los′tə-me) **stone** **renal pelvis** **pyelolithotomy** **pyeloplasty** (pi′ə-lo-plas″te)	**8-34** Write a word that means formation of a new opening into the renal pelvis: _____ Pyelo/litho/tomy (**pi″ə-lo-lĭ-thot′ə-me**) is a surgical procedure to remove a _____ from the _____ _____. Literal translation of this term is incision of the renal pelvis for stones, and it is understood that the procedure is done for this purpose. Write the term: _____. Build another word that means plastic repair of the renal pelvis: _____.
renal pelvis **within**	**8-35** Sometimes dyes that are opaque to x-ray are used to make an internal organ visible. The film produced by radiography of the renal pelvis after injection of a contrast medium is a pyelo/gram (**pi′ə-lo-gram**). Pyelography (**pi″ə-log′rə-fe**) renders the _____ _____ visible, as well as other parts of the kidney and the ureters. In an intravenous (**in″trə-ve′nəs**) pyelogram (IVP), a contrast medium is injected into the vein at particular times and x-ray films are taken to observe kidney function. Remember that intra- means within. Intra/venous is _____ a vein.
ureter **ureterolith** (u-re′tər-o-lith″) **the presence** **(formation) of** **stones in a ureter**	**8-36** You learned that ureter(o) is the combining form for ureter (**u-re′tər**), the tube that carries urine from the kidney to the bladder. After urine collects in the renal pelvis, it drains to the bladder by passing through a tube called the _____. If a nephro/lith is a kidney stone, build a word that means stone in a ureter: _____. Uretero/lith/iasis (**u-re″tər-o-lĭ-thi′ə-sis**) is _____.
ureter **ureterectomy** (u″re-tər-ek′tə-me)	**8-37** Uretero/litho/tomy (**u-re″tər-o-lĭ-thot′ə-me**) is removal of a stone from the _____ by incision. Surgical removal of a ureter or part of it is _____.
ureteritis (u″re-tər-i′tis) **narrowing**	**8-38** Write another word that means inflammation of a ureter: _____. Uretero/stenosis (**u-re″tər-o-stə-no′sis**) is _____ of a ureter.
ureter **hydronephrosis** **hydroureter** **ureterostomy** (u″re-tər os′tə-me)	**8-39** Hydro/ureter (**hi″dro-u-re′tər**) is abnormal distention of a _____ with urine or watery fluid owing to obstruction. Compare the obstruction caused by a stone in the upper with obstruction in the lower part of the ureter in Figure 8-5. If the stone is in the upper part of the ureter, the condition may cause _____. If a stone or another obstruction occurs in the lower part of the ureter, the condition that results is called _____. This condition could require formation of a new opening through which the ureter could discharge its contents. Write a term that means formation of a new opening in a ureter: _____.
ureter **ureteroplasty** (u″re′tər-o-plast″te)	**8-40** Uretero/uretero/stomy (**u-re″tər-o-u-re″tər-os′tə-me**) is an interesting word. It uses the same combining form twice and has two meanings. It means formation of a connection from one _____ to another. It also means end-to-end anastomosis of two portions of a transected (cut) ureter. Write a word that means surgical repair of a ureter: _____.

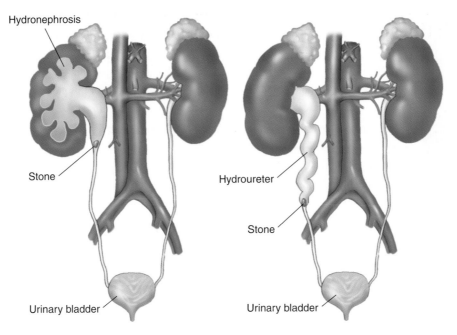

F I G U R E   8 - 5
Hydronephrosis and hydroureter. Hydronephrosis is caused by obstruction in the upper part of the ureter. Hydroureter is caused by obstruction in the lower part of the ureter.

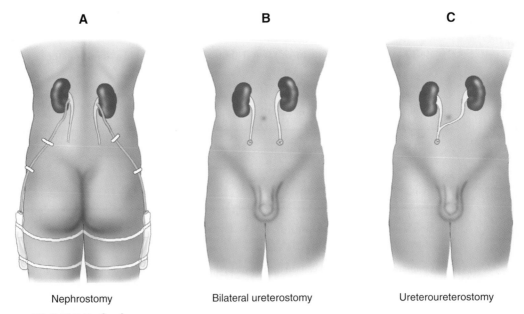

F I G U R E   8 - 6
Comparing nephrostomy and two ureterostomies. **A,** Nephrostomy. Percutaneous openings are made into the renal pelvis and urine is diverted to bags. **B,** Bilateral ureterostomy. Both ureters are brought out onto the skin for drainage of urine into bags. **C,** Ureteroureterostomy. One ureter is surgically attached to the other ureter which is brought out onto the skin for drainage of urine into a bag.

8-41 Various surgical procedures are performed for urinary diversion if the bladder is cancerous and must be removed. The type of surgical management depends on the type and stage of the cancer, as well as the patient's general health status. The ureters must be diverted into some type of collecting reservoir (pouch on the skin around the stoma or diversion of urine to the large intestine, so it is excreted with bowel movements). If the ureters are also removed, a nephrostomy is necessary. Nephro/stomy is a new opening into the kidney so that a catheter can be placed into the _____ _____ for the purpose of drainage. Compare nephrostomy and two types of ureterostomies in Figure 8-6.

renal pelvis

8-42 Build a word that means surgical excision of a kidney with the ureter (or part of it): _____.

nephroureterec-tomy
(nef″ro-u″rə-tər-ek′tə-me)

ureter
renal pelvis

Uretero/pyel/itis (**u-re″tər-o-pi-ə-li′tis**) is inflammation of a _____ and the _____ _____.

ureteropathy
(u-re″tər-op′ə-the)

Write a word that means any disease of a ureter: _____.

ureter

8-43 Uretero/cele (**u-re′tər-o-sēl**) is a hernia of the _____. The suffix -*cele* means hernia.

A hernia is a protrusion of an organ or part of the organ through an opening.

a hernia of the kidney

A nephro/cele (**nef′ro-sēl**) is _____.

❑ SECTION B REVIEW *K*idneys and Ureters

This section review covers frames 8–12 through 8–43. Write the word part for each of the following:

Combining Form	Meaning	Suffix	Meaning
1. _____	glomerulus	4. _____	hernia
2. _____	pus	5. _____	surgical crushing
3. _____	renal pelvis		

(Use Appendix V to check your answers.)

SECTION C

*B*ladder and Urethra

The urinary bladder is a collapsible muscular bag that serves as a reservoir for urine until it is expelled. It has a storage capacity in health of about 500 ml (1 pint) or more. The tube that leads from the bladder to outside the body, the urethra, is about 3.8 cm (1½ inches) long in adult females and about 20.3 cm (8 inches) long in adult males.

8-44 Cysto/graphy (**sis-tog′rə-fe**) uses radiopaque dyes to make the bladder visible. You learned that cyst(o) means a bladder or sac.

cyst(o)

The word part for bladder is _____. (When the word bladder is not identified, it usually means the urinary bladder.) A cysto/gram (**sis′to-gram**) is the film produced by radiography of the urinary _____.

bladder

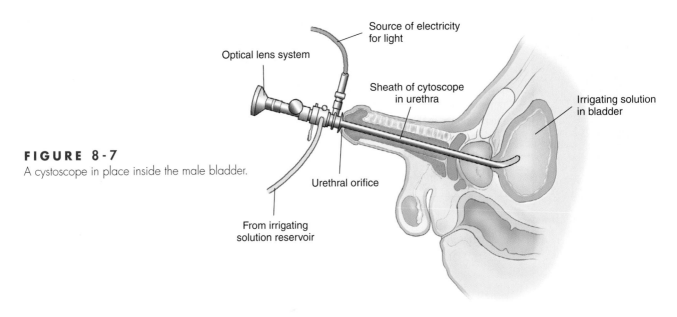

FIGURE 8-7
A cystoscope in place inside the male bladder.

(labels from figure:)
- Optical lens system
- Source of electricity for light
- Sheath of cytoscope in urethra
- Irrigating solution in bladder
- Urethral orifice
- From irrigating solution reservoir

abdomen **bladder** **cystoplegia** (sis″to-ple′-jə) **cystoplasty** (sis′to-plas″te)	**8-45** Abdomino/cystic (**ab-dom″ĭ-no-sis′tik**) pertains to the _____ and the _____. Using -plegia, write a word that means paralysis of the bladder: _____. Write another term that means surgical repair of the bladder: _____.
cystoscopy (sis-tos′kə-pe) **bladder**	**8-46** Write a term for visual examination of the bladder using special equipment: _____. In this type of examination, a hollow metal tube is passed through the urethra (**u-re′thrə**) and into the bladder. By means of a light, special lenses, and mirrors, the bladder mucosa is examined (Figure 8-7). The instrument used in cystoscopy is a cystoscope (**sis′to-skōp**). It allows one to see inside the _____.
ureters	**8-47** A bladder polyp is a growth protruding from the lining of the bladder. This abnormality is one of the things that might be seen by using a cystoscope. A polyp is any growth or mass protruding from a mucous membrane. Polyps may occur in the nose, ears, uterus, bladder, urethra, and anywhere there is mucous membrane. Cysto/uretero/scopy (**sis″to-u-re-tər-os′kə-pe**) is slightly more involved than a cystoscopy, because a cystoureteroscopy involves examination of the _____ and the bladder.
cystostomy (sis-tos′tə-me) **cystotomy** (sis-tot′ə-me)	**8-48** Write a word that means formation of a new opening into the bladder: _____. Using -tomy, build a word that means incision of the bladder: _____.
ureter, bladder	**8-49** Uretero/cysto/stomy (**u-re″tər-o-sis-tos′tə-me**) is formation of a new opening between a _____ and the _____. Ureterocystostomy involves surgical transplantation of the ureter to a different site in the bladder. This is also called uretero/neo/cysto/stomy (**u-re″tər-o-ne″o-sis-tos′tə-me**). The word part *ne(o)* means new.

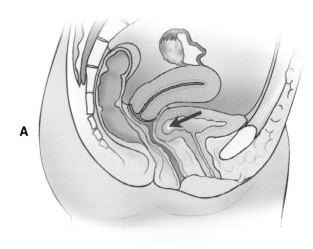
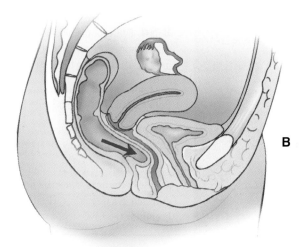

Cystocele   Rectocele

FIGURE 8-8
Comparison of a cystocele and a rectocele. **A,** Cystocele. The urinary bladder is displaced downward, causing bulging of the anterior vaginal wall. **B,** Rectocele. The rectum is displaced, causing bulging of the posterior vaginal wall.

cyst **bladder**	**8-50** Remembering the two meanings of cyst(o), write the two meanings of cyst/ectomy **(sis-tek′tə-me):** excision of a _____ or excision or resection (removal of a portion) of the urinary _____. Cyst(o) refers to any sac filled with fluid, including the urinary bladder. Written alone, a cyst is a pouch or sac that contains a fluid and develops abnormally in the body. A cyst may or may not be harmful. Poly/cystic **(pol″e-sis′tik)** means containing many cysts.
cystolith **(sis′to-lith)**	**8-51** Write a word that means a calculus in the urinary bladder: _____. Cystolithotomy **(sis″to-lĭ-thot′ə-me)** and cysto/lith/ectomy **(sis″to-lĭ-thek′tə-me)** both mean removal of a calculus by incision of the urinary bladder.
cystitis (sis-ti′tis) **difficult** **urination** **frequent urination** **cystorrhea** **(sis″to-re′ə)**	**8-52** Write a word that means inflammation of the bladder: _____. Dys/uria and poly/uria are frequently symptoms of cystitis. Dys/uria is _____ _____. Polyuria **(pol′e-u′re-ə)** is _____ _____. The sufix **-rrhea** means flow or discharge. Using -rrhea, write a term that means discharge from the bladder: _____.
cystocele **(sis′to-sēl)**	**8-53** Using -cele, write a word that means herniation of the bladder: _____. In a cystocele, the bladder hernia protrudes into the vagina (Figure 8-8). The posterior wall herniation that occurs in a rectocele is shown for comparison.

urethr(o)	**8-54** Filling of the bladder with urine stimulates receptors, producing the desire to urinate. Voluntary control prevents urine from being released. When the control is removed, urine is expelled through the urethra. The opening to the outside from the urethra is called the urinary meatus. You know that urethr(o) means urethra. The urethra is short in females and serves only to transport urine from the bladder to the outside. The combining form for urethra is _____. The male urethra is longer than that of the female. It has a dual role of conveying urine to the outside and serving as a passageway for sperm. Urgency, frequency, and hesitancy are terms that are often used to describe urination patterns. Urgency is a sense of the need to urinate immediately. Increased frequency is a greater number of urinations than expected in a given time. Hesitancy is a decrease in the force of the urine stream, often with difficulty in beginning the flow.
urethrography (u′rə-throg′rə-fe) bladder urethra	**8-55** Write a word that means roentgenography of the urethra (after injection of a radiopaque substance into it): _____. Cysto/urethro/graphy (**sis″to-u″rə-throg′rə-fe**) is making x-ray film of the _____ and _____. In a voiding cysto/urethro/gram (**sis″to-u-re′thro-gram**) (CUG), radiographs are made before, during, and after voiding (urination). It allows observation of the bladder as it empties and checks for reflux of urine into the ureters.
urethritis (u″rə-thri′-tis) cystourethritis (sis″to-u″re-thri′tis)	**8-56** Inflammation of the urethra is _____. Add a combining form to urethritis to write a new term that means inflammation of the urethra and bladder: _____. This means the same as urethrocystitis (**u-re″thro-sis-ti′tis**).
rectum and urethra urethra	**8-57** Recto/urethr/al (**rek″to-u-re′thrəl**) pertains to the _____. Urethro/rect/al (**u-re″thro-rek′təl**) also means pertaining to the urethra and rectum; however, not all words can be reversed like this! Urethro/vaginal (**u-re″thro-vaj′ĭ-nəl**) means pertaining to the _____ and the vagina.
urethrotomy (u″rə-throt′ə-me) urethrocele (u-re′ thro-sēl) urethrospasm (u-re′thro-spaz-əm) urethra	**8-58** Write terms for the following: Surgical incision of the urethra is _____. Herniation of the urethra is _____. Spasm of the urethra (actually, the muscular tissue of the urethra) is _____. Polyps are usually benign, but they may lead to complications or become malignant. For this reason, polyps are usually removed. Urethr/al polyps occur in the _____.
urethra urethra closed	**8-59** Remembering that trans- means through or across, trans/urethral (**trans″u-re′thrəl**) means through the _____. Transurethral surgery is performed by inserting an instrument through or across the wall of the _____. Transurethral surgery makes it possible to perform surgery on certain organs that lie near the urethra without having an abdominal incision. Urinary surgical procedures are classified as open (exposed through an incision) or closed (performed through cystoscopy, or visualization of structures by means of a fiberoptic cystoscope inserted into the urethra and bladder). Is transurethral surgery open or closed surgery? _____ In transurethral resection (TUR), small pieces of tissue from a nearby structure are removed through the wall of the urethra.

8-60 One surgery of this type is a transurethral resection of the prostate (TURP). In a TURP, surgery is performed on the prostate gland in males by means of an instrument passed through the wall of the urethra.

transurethral

In a TUR, an abdominal incision is not involved, since the surgeon approaches the prostate through the urethra. Small pieces of the prostate are removed with a special instrument. Because this surgery is performed by passing the instrument through the urethra, it is called _____ resection of the prostate. (Prostate is a frequently misspelled term. Note the difference in spelling of *prostate* and *prostrate*, which means lying in a face down, horizontal position.)

discharge from the urethra

8-61 Since -rrhea means flow or discharge, urethro/rrhea (**u-re″thro-re′ə**) means

_____.

There are three other suffixes that begin with the same letters as -rrhea and can easily be confused. The remainder of this section deals with these three suffixes: -rrhagia, -rrhexis, and -rrhaphy.

urethrorrhagia
(u-re″thro-ra′je-ə)

8-62 The suffix *-rrhagia* means hemorrhage. Hemorrhage, when broken into its component parts, means a bursting forth of blood. Write a word that means urethral hemorrhage: _____.

rupture of the bladder

Use *-rrhexis* to mean rupture. Cysto/rrhexis (**sis″to-rek′sis**) is

_____.

kidney
ureterorrhaphy
(u-re″tər-or′ə-fe)
urethrorrhaphy
(u″rə-thor′ə-fe)

Nephro/rrhaphy (**nef-ror′ə-fe**) is suture (surgical sewing) of the _____. Notice that -rrhaphy means suture. Write a word that means suture of a ureter: _____.

Suture of the urethra is _____.

❑ SECTION C REVIEW *B*ladder and Urethra

This section review covers frames 8–44 through 8–62. Complete the table by writing the meaning of the word part in the blank.

Combining Form	Meaning	Suffix	Meaning
1. ne(o)	_____	2. -rrhagia	_____
		3. -rrhaphy	_____
		4. -rrhea	_____
		5. -rrhexis	_____

(Use Appendix V to check your answers.)

SECTION D

*G*enitourinary Infections

Urinary tract infections are one of the more common infections, particularly in females. The close proximity of the reproductive organs and the anus makes possible the spread of infections of these areas to organs of the urinary system.

8-63 Genito/urinary (**jen′ĭ-to-u′rĭ-nar-e**) or uro/genital pertains to the genitals, as well as to the urinary organs. Microbes that cause sexually transmitted diseases sometimes gain entrance through the urinary tract. Write these two terms that pertain to both the genitals and the urinary tract:

genitourinary
urogenital

_____ and _____.

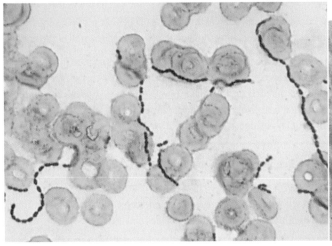
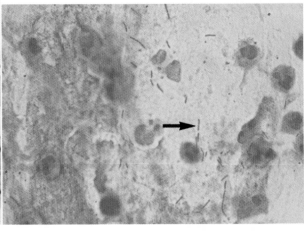

A   B

FIGURE 8-9
Gram stains of direct smears, body fluids collected, stained, and examined for the presence of leukocytes, bacteria, or other significant findings. **A,** Gram-positive cocci. The cocci are arranged in chains. Cells are also present on the smear. **B,** Gram-negative bacilli *(arrow)* are shown in the presence of numerous leukocytes. (**A,** From Murray PR, Rosenthal KS, Kobayashi GS, Pfaller MA: *Medical microbiology,* ed 3, St Louis, 1994, Mosby.) (**B,** From Forbes BA, Sahm DF, Weissfeld AS: *Bailey & Scott's diagnostic microbiology,* ed 10, St Louis, 1998, Mosby.)

	8-64 You learned that -rrhea means flow or discharge. You probably have heard of gono/rrhea, a sexually transmitted disease characterized by a heavy discharge from the vagina or from the urethra in either males or females. Sexually transmitted diseases were formerly called venereal (**və-nēr′e-əl**) diseases.
	Gonorrhea (**gon″o-re′ə**) is derived from *gon(o),* which means the genitals or reproduction. Many of the words in the medical dictionary that begin with gon(o) pertain to the gono/coccus, the type of bacteria that causes gonorrhea.
gonococcus (gon″o-kok′əs)	Write the name of the microorganism that causes gonorrhea: _____.
gonorrhea	**8-65** The gonococcus causes a sexually transmitted disease, _____. A sexually transmitted disease is one that may be acquired as a result of sexual contact with a person who has the disease.
inflammation of the urethra	Vaginitis (**vaj″ĭ-ni′tis**) or urethritis, or both, accompanied by a heavy discharge and dys/uria, are often symptoms of gonorrhea. Urethr/itis is _____.
difficult (or painful)	Dys/uria (**dis-u′re-ə**) is _____ urination.
	8-66 The gonococcus that causes gonorrhea is a bacterium, a single-celled microorganism that lacks a nucleus. Bacteria, combining form *bacteri(o),* are classified according to their shape as cocci, bacilli, or spirilla. Spherical bacteria are cocci, rod-shaped bacteria are bacilli, and spiral-shaped bacteria are called spirilla.
	The Gram's stain is a special staining technique that serves as a primary means of identifying and classifying bacteria. Gram-positive bacteria appear violet (purple) by this method and gram-negative bacteria appear pink or red. Observe the cocci and bacilli in Figuri 8-9, and then write answers in these blanks.
spherical **violet or purple**	The bacteria in Figure 8-9, *A,* are gram-positive cocci. This is noted by their shape, which is _____, and their color, which is _____.
elongated (rod-shaped) **pink or red**	The bacteria in Figure 8-9, *B,* are gram-negative bacilli. This is noted by their shape, which is _____, and their color, which is _____.

cocci (kok′si)	**8-67** Summarizing information in the previous frame, spherical-shaped bacteria are called _____.
bacilli (bə-sil′i) negative positive	Rod-shaped bacteria are called _____. Bacteria that stain pink or red after undergoing Gram's stain are called gram- _____, whereas bacteria that stain violet or purple are gram-_____.
	8-68 Cocci are often seen in particular arrangements when viewed with the microscope. For this reason, cocci are further classified according to their arrangement. Although there are others, three commonly seen arrangements are shown in Figure 8-10. Learning these arrangements will give more meaning when you hear words such as streptococcal (**strep″to-kok′əl**) (often shortened to strep) infections, staphylococcal (**staf″ə-lo-kok′əl**) (often shortened to staph) infections, or gonococcal infections.
twisted	The combining form **strept(o)** means twisted. Strepto/cocci (**strep″to-kok′si**) grow in _____ chains.
streptococci spherical bacteria in twisted chains	**8-69** Strept throat is a common way of saying strepto/coccal pharyngitis. In strep throat, inflammation of the throat is caused by what type of bacteria? _____ Not all streptococci cause pharyngitis. There are many types of streptococci. If streptococci were seen through a microscope, what would be their appearance? _____
streptococci	**8-70** Streptococc/emia (**strep″to kok se′me-ə**) is a serious condition. Streptococc/emia is the presence of _____ in the blood. The blood is normally free of all microorganisms. The presence of microbial toxins in the blood is tox/emia, a serious condition.
staphylococci (staf″ə-lo-kok′si)	**8-71** The combining form **staphyl(o)** means a grapelike cluster. Cocci that are arranged like a cluster of grapes are called _____. The combining form *staphyl(o)* is also used to mean uvula (**u′vu-lə**), a structure that hangs like a bunch of grapes from the soft palate in the back of the mouth. When staphyl(o) is joined to cocci, it refers to a type of bacteria. When it is not joined to cocci, you will have to decide which meaning is intended. Staphyl/itis (**staf″ə-li′tis**), for example, is inflammation of the
uvula	_____.
uvula staphylococci in the blood skin condition caused by staphylococcus	**8-72** Practice using staphyl(o) in the following. Staphyl/ectomy (**staf″ə-lek′to me**) is surgical removal of the _____. Staphylo/cocc/emia (**staf″ə-lo-kok-se′me-ə**) is _____. Staphylo/derma (**staf″ə-lo-dər′mə**) is a _____.
diplococci	**8-73** The combining form **dipl(o)** means double. When cocci occur in pairs, they are called diplococci (**dip″lo-kok′si**). The reason they remain in pairs is incomplete separation after cell division. Cocci in pairs (double cocci) are called _____.

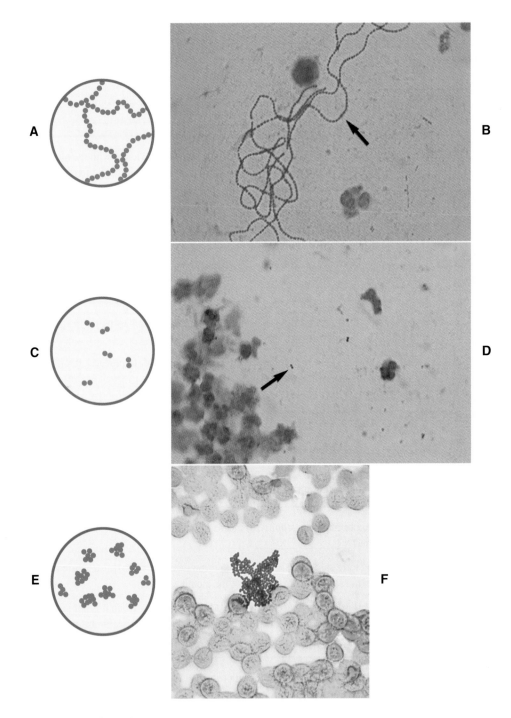

FIGURE 8-10

Three coccal arrangements. **A,** Schematic drawing of streptococci, cocci in chains. **B,** Streptococci in a direct smear. **C,** Schematic drawing of diplococci, cocci in pairs. **D,** Diplococci in a direct smear. **E,** Schematic drawing of staphylococci, cocci arranged in grapelike clusters. **F,** Staphylococci in a direct smear. (**C** and **D,** from Forbes BA, Sahm DF, Weissfeld AS: *Bailey & Scott's diagnostic microbiology,* ed 10, St Louis, 1998, Mosby. **F,** From Murray PR, Rosenthal KS, Kobayashi GS, Pfaller MA: *Medical microbiology,* ed 3, St Louis, 1994, Mosby.)

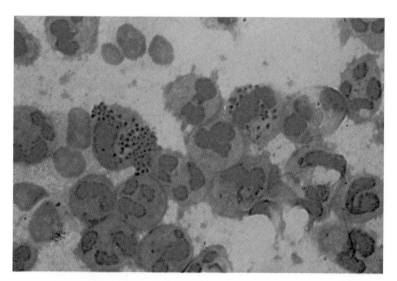

FIGURE 8-11
Gram-negative intracellular diplococci. The presence of gram-negative intracellular diplococci in a urethral smear is usually indicative of gonorrhea in males. The same finding in females is considered presumptive and is generally followed by culture to confirm the diagnosis. Note also the presence of many extracellular diplococci. (From Forbes BA, Sahm DF, Weissfeld AS: *Bailey & Scott's diagnostic microbiology*, ed 10, St Louis, 1998, Mosby.)

8-74 Most bacteria are helpful rather than harmful. They are responsible for decay and are used extensively in food production, as in vinegar, sour cream, and cheese. Bacteria are also beneficial in the intestinal tract, where they are responsible for production of vitamin K. Normal bacterial flora of the skin help prevent the establishment of pathogenic bacteria. Only a fraction of the total number of species of bacteria are pathogenic.

A special type of infection warrants consideration. It is called noso/comial (**nos″o-ko′me-əl**) infection. The combining form **nos(o)** means disease and "comial" comes from a word that means to care for. Nosocomial means pertaining to or originating in a hospital. Infections that are acquired in a hospital are called _____ infections.

nosocomial

8-75 You have seen that some types of bacteria can cause diseases of the urinary system. Other microorganisms, such as fungi and viruses, also cause urinary infections.

The gonococcus causes gonorrhea, a sexually transmitted disease that may spread to the urinary system. Gonococci (plural of gonococcus) are gram-negative intracellular diplococci. You learned earlier that intra- means within; intra/cellular means _____.

Intracellular diplo/cocci are cocci in _____ that are found within white blood cells (Figure 8-11).

within the cell

pairs

8-76 The presence of gram-negative intracellular diplococci is generally followed by a bacterial culture to confirm that the organisms are gonococci. Culturing is a technique for growing colonies of microorganisms. This technique of growing microorganisms, done for the purpose of identifying the pathogen, is called _____.

culturing

8-77 Bacterial cultures are commonly used to diagnose many types of infections, including streptococcal pharyngitis, urinary tract infections, as well as gonococcal infections. Spreptococcal pharyngitis is inflammation of the pharynx caused by _____.

streptococci

If a urinary tract infection (UTI) is suspected, urine is collected and cultured to identify the pathogen. Further testing of the colonies that grow in the culture determines the pathogen's sensitivity to various antibiotics. This is called an antibiotic sensitivity test. The two tests are commonly requested together and are called a culture and sensitivity (C & S).

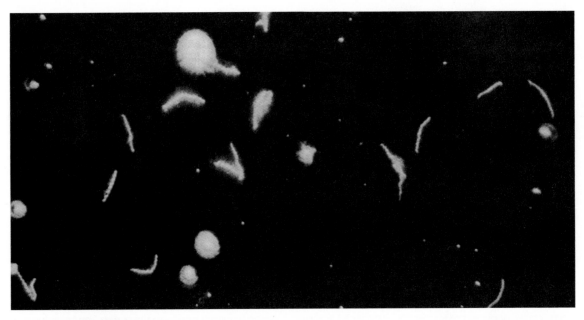

FIGURE 8-12
Dark-field preparation demonstrating the spirochete of syphilis. The organism, *Treponema pallidum*, can be observed in material from a chancre using a special dark-field preparation in the early stages of syphilis. The organisms are long, evenly tightly coiled spirals that are motile. (From Forbes BA, Sahm DF, Weissfeld AS: *Bailey & Scott's diagnostic microbiology*, ed 10, St Louis, 1998, Mosby.)

bladder	**8-78** Urinary tract infections are more common in women than in men and may be asymptomatic. UTI is usually characterized by urinary frequency, burning, pain with voiding, and if the infection is severe, visible blood and pus in the urine. Most urinary tract infections are cystitis or urethritis. Cyst/itis is inflammation of the _____. Treatment of urinary tract infections include antibiotics, analgesics, and increased intake of water.
	8-79 Micro/bio/logy (**mi″kro-bi-ol′ə-je**) is a special branch of biology. Micro/bio/logists study bacteria, fungi, viruses, and other small organisms. Very small or microscopic organisms are called micro/organisms. Viruses and some bacteria do not grow in commonly used culture media. They require living cells and in some cases are difficult or impossible to grow outside a host. One such organism is the spirochete that causes syphilis. Observe the spiral shape of the spirochete in Figure 8-12. The special technique called dark-field preparation is used to search for spirochetes that cause syphilis. The slide is examined microscopically using high-power magnification (HPF) or 400×.
high, low	**8-80** Laboratory reports often cite the number of organisms per microscopic high-power field, not just in reporting bacteria but also in other areas such as the study of the urine or in hematology. Sometimes, the number of organisms or cells per low-power field (LPF) is reported. HPF and LPF are abbreviations for microscopic _____ and _____ power fields.

❑ SECTION D REVIEW 𝒢enitourinary Infections

This section review covers frames 8–63 through 8–80. Write the meaning of each of the following:

Combining Form	Meaning	Combining Form	Meaning
1. dipl(o)	_____	4. staphyl(o)	_____
2. gon(o)	_____	5. strept(o)	_____
3. nos(o)	_____		

(Use Appendix V to check your answers.)

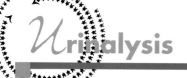

Urinalysis

A number of urine tests are available to evaluate the status of the urinary system. A urinalysis is a usual component of a physical examination but is particularly useful for patients with suspected urologic disorders.

8-81 The urinalysis is a test performed on urine. The complete urinalysis generally includes a physical, chemical, and microscopic examination performed in the clinical laboratory.

8-82 The urinalysis (u″rĭ-nal′ĭ-sis) often gives helpful information when the physician suspects a urinary tract infection. It is also helpful in assessing other aspects of health.

Urin/alysis was originally called urine analysis. It is often abbreviated UA or U/A. Examination of the urine is called _____.

urinalysis

8-83 Because the urine leaves the body by way of the urethra, in urethrorrhagia one would see blood in the urine. Join hemat(o) and -uria to form a word that means blood in the urine: _____.

Blood should not be present in the urine, so hematuria is considered an abnormal condition.

hematuria
(hem″ə-tu′re-ə)

8-84 Ammonia, creatinine, and salts are important waste products in urine, but another major waste is urea. Urea is a nitrogen compound that is the final product of protein metabolism. Its excess is one of the causes of uremia.

Several substances should not be present in normal urine, and their presence indicates various pathological states to the physician. Some abnormal components of urine are sugar, albumin, ketones, blood, pus, and microorganisms.

8-85 Protein/uria (pro″te-nu′re-ə) is _____.

The protein found in urine is usually albumin. The combining form *albumin(o)* means albumin. Albumin/uria (al″bu-mĭ-nu′re-ə) is _____.

Py/uria is also abnormal. Py/uria (pi-u′re-ə) is pus in the _____.

protein in the urine

albumin in the urine

urine

8-86 Sugar should not be present in the urine. When present, this is glycos/uria. The combining forms *glyc(o)* and *glycos(o)* means sweet or sugar. Many times glycosuria (gli″ko-su′re-ə) indicates diabetes. Glycosuria means _____.

It is not easy to remember which combining form is used to write a particular word. Notice that in the term *glycosuria*, glycos(o) is used instead of glyc(o).

sugar in the urine

8-87 Glucose is generally reabsorbed in the renal tubules. When the blood glucose rises above a certain level, the renal threshold for reabsorption is exceeded, and glucose is excreted in the urine. Write this term that means sugar in the urine: _____.

glycosuria

8-88 *ket(o)* and *keton(o)* mean ketone bodies. Keton/uria is ketones in the _____.
Ketone bodies are normal end products of lipid (fat) metabolism in the body. Excessive production of ketone bodies, however, leads to urinary excretion of ketones. Under normal conditions, ketones are not present in urine. Excretion of ketones in the urine is called _____.

urine

ketonuria
(ke″to-nu′re-ə)

ketoacidosis	**8-89** Ketone bodies are acids, and ketones are found in the urine when the body's fat stores are metabolized for energy, thus providing an excess of metabolic end products. This can occur in uncontrolled diabetes because of a deficiency of insulin. Use ket(o), acid(o), and -osis to write a term that means acidosis accompanied by an accumulation of ketones in the body: _____.
high power	**8-90** A microscopic study is generally part of a complete urinalysis. Body cells, crystals, and bacteria are some of the particles present in a microscopic study. These are generally reported as number/HPF. HPF means a microscopic _____ _____ field.
voids (or urinates) **catheter**	**8-91** Urine specimens are collected according to the laboratory or physician's instructions. A voided specimen is one in which the patient _____ into a container supplied by the laboratory or physician's office. A catheterized urine specimen is obtained by placing a _____ into the bladder via the urethra and withdrawing urine. This may be necessary to obtain an uncontaminated urine specimen or to measure the volume of urine retained in the bladder after urination. A 24-hour urine collection is collection of all of the urine voided in a 24-hour period.
retention (re-ten′shən)	**8-92** Retention means holding back or keeping in a position, as persistence in the body of material that is normally excreted. Accumulation of urine within the bladder because of inability to urinate is _____ of urine. Indwelling catheters are designed so that they are held in place in the urethra for the purpose of draining urine from the bladder. Continence* (kon′tĭ-nens) is the ability to control bladder or bowel function. Urinary incontinence (in-kon′ti-nens) is inability to control urination. This is loss of control of the passage of urine from the bladder. There are many causes of incontinence, such as loss of muscle tone, obesity, or unconsciousness. For the latter reason, indwelling catheters are used when one is anesthetized. Enuresis† (en″u-re′sis) also means the inability to control urination, and the term is applied especially to nocturnal bed-wetting. Nocturnal means pertaining to or occurring at night. Nocturia (nok-tu′re-ə), also called nycturia (nik-tu′re-ə), is excessive urination at night. Both *noct(i)* and *nyct(o)* mean night. Although it may be a symptom of disease, it also can occur in people who drink excessive amounts of fluids before bedtime or in people with prostatic disease.
diuretic (di″u-ret′ik) **absence of urination** **oliguria**	**8-93** Poly/uria is excretion of an abnormally large quantity of urine. Another name for increased or excessive urination is diuresis (di″u-re′sis). Sometimes diuretics are prescribed to increase urination. An agent that causes the body to eliminate more water in the form of urine is called a _____. Diuretics cause polyuria. The opposite of polyuria is an/uria (an-u′re-ə), which means _____. The full meaning of anuria is cessation of urine production or a urinary output of less than 100 ml (or a little more than 3 oz) per day. The patient who has less than 100 ml of urine output per day is described as anur/ic (an-u′rik). Compare the meaning of anuria and olig/uria (ol″ĭ-gu′re-ə), which means diminished capacity to form and pass urine of less than 500 ml per day. The combining form *olig(o)* means few. Write this term that means diminished urine production of less than 500 ml per day: _____.

*(Latin: *continere,* to contain.)
†(Greek: *enourein,* to urinate.)

8-94 Chemical analysis of urine is performed for the identification and quantification of any of a large number of substances. As a major way to rid the body of byproducts of metabolism, urine is examined to determine many aspects of the patient's health and the status of the urinary tract.

urinary tract

A uro/pathy (**u-rop′ə-the**) is any disease of the _____ _____.

❏ SECTION E REVIEW   𝒰rinalysis

This section review covers frames 8-81 through 8-94. Complete the table by writing the meaning of each combining form in the blank.

Combining Form	Meaning	Combining Form	Meaning
1. albumin(o)	_____	4. olig(o)	_____
2. glyc(o), glycos(o)	_____	5. noct(i)	_____
3. ket(o), keton(o)	_____	6. nyct(o)	_____

(Use Appendix V to check your answers.)

𝒯erminology Challenge

This section challenges you to read, write, and understand new terms or concepts about the urinary system. At times, you will use less familiar word parts that are covered more extensively in other chapters. It is important to remember the new terms introduced in this section.

anaerobic	**8-95** Most bacteria are aerobic (**ār-o′bik**), meaning they live and function in the presence of oxygen. Using an-, write a word that means able to function and grow without air or oxygen: _____. Some bacteria grow only in anaerobic conditions.
nephropyosis (**nef″ro-pi′o′sis**)	**8-96** Purulence means producing or discharging pus. Use nephr(o), the combining form for pus, and -osis to build a word that means purulence of a kidney: _____. (This is also called pyonephrosis.)
above bladder	**8-97** You learned that a catheter is used to drain urine from the bladder. The most common type of urinary catheter is placed in the bladder via the urethra. A suprapubic (**soo″prə-pu′bik**) catheter is inserted through the skin above the symphysis pubis, the bony eminence under the pubic hair. The prefix *supra-* means above or beyond. A supra/pubic catheter is inserted through an incision _____ the symphysis pubis. Suprapubic cystotomy is surgical incision of the _____ via an incision just above the symphysis pubis.
supra/renal (**soo″prə-re′nəl**) inter/renal (**in″tə-re′nəl**) extracystic (**eks″trə-sis′tik**)	**8-98** Renal means pertaining to the kidneys. Use supra- to write a term that means above a kidney: _____. Write a word that means between the kidneys: _____. The term *cystic* pertains to a *cyst,* the gallbladder, or the urinary bladder. Write a word that means outside a cyst or outside the bladder: _____.
	8-99 A kidney, ureter, and bladder x-ray (KUB) is radiology of the kidneys, ureters, and bladder. You will practice using the less familiar word parts in other chapters. For now, be able to read and write the new terms. There is no review for this section.

Study the following list of selected abbreviations. Then read through the Chapter Pharmacology and be sure you understand the effects and uses of the drug classes. When you are finished, work the Chapter Review. After completing the exercises, check your answers with the solutions in Appendix V.

You will find these items presented after the Chapter Review:
- Listing of Medical Terms
- Enhancing Spanish Communication

Selected Abbreviations

ADH	antidiuretic hormone		I & O	intake & output
A/G	albumin/globulin ratio		IVP	intravenous pyelogram
AGN	acute glomerulonephritis		KUB	kidney, ureter, and bladder
BPH	benign prostatic hypertrophy		LPF	low power field
BUN	blood urea nitrogen		pH	potential of hydrogen
C & S	culture and sensitivity		PKU	phenylketonuria
CGN	chronic glomerulonephritis		RP	retrograde pyelogram
CRF	chronic renal failure		STD	sexually transmitted disease
CUG	cystourethrogram		TUR	transurethral resection
cysto	cystoscopic examination		TURP	transurethral resection of the prostate
ESWL	extracorporeal shock wave lithotripsy		U/A	urinalysis
GC	gonococcus		UTI	urinary tract infection
GFR	glomerular filtration rate		VCUG	voiding cystourethrogram
GU	genitourinary		VD	venereal disease
HPF	high power field			

Chapter Pharmacology

Class	Effect and Uses
Antihypertensives (See Chapter Pharmacology, Chapter 5)	**Reduce Blood Pressure, Thus Reducing Blood Pressure in the Kidneys**
Antiinfectives trimethoprim (Trimpex) trimethoprim/sulfamethoxazole methylene blue nalidixic acid (NegGram) nitrofurantoin (Macrobid) penicillin G (Also see the antiinfectives in Chapter Pharmacology, Chapter 3.)	**Used Against Microorganisms** Used for UTIs Used for UTIs Used for UTIs Used for UTIs Used for UTIs Used for treating gonorrhea
Diuretics thiazide diuretics chlorothiazide (Diuril) (See Chapter Pharmacology, Chapter 5.)	**Increase Urination** Prevent formation and recurrence of kidney stones Prevents excess calcium loads in the urine
Uricosuric Drugs allopurinol	**Treat Gout** Manages gout attacks and treats uric acid stones

CHAPTER REVIEW 8

▶ **BASIC UNDERSTANDING**

REVIEWING WORD PARTS
I. Write a word (prefix, suffix, or combining form) for each clue.

CROSSWORD PUZZLE 8

Across
1   urinary tract
3   twisted
10 calculus
11 flow
13 sugar
14 that which causes
15 water
17 pelvis
18 glomerulus
19 the result of an action
20 side
21 urine
22 surgical crushing
24 instrument used for viewing
27 two
28 kidney
30 tumor
31 tissue
33 painful
34 rupture
36 genitals
38 bladder
39 repair (combining form)
41 without
42 urethra
44 color
46 medicine
47 distant
48 double
49 many

Down
2   discharge
3   grapelike cluster
4   pus
5   few
6   disease
7   ketone bodies
8   urine
9   bacteria
12 hemorrhage
16 albumin
17 disease
20 destruction
22 poison
23 to cut
25 production
26 suture
29 renal pelvis
32 ureter
35 process of recording
36 female
37 new
40 poison
43 kidney
45 characterized by

MATCHING

II. Match structures on the left with their functions:

_____ 1. bladder   **A.** cavity in the kidney that collects urine from many collecting ducts
_____ 2. nephron   **B.** carries urine from the bladder
_____ 3. renal pelvis   **C.** carries urine to the bladder
_____ 4. ureter   **D.** functional unit of the kidney
_____ 5. urethra   **E.** reservoir for urine until it is excreted

LABELING

III. Label the numbered structures with their corresponding combining form. Number 1 has two answers.

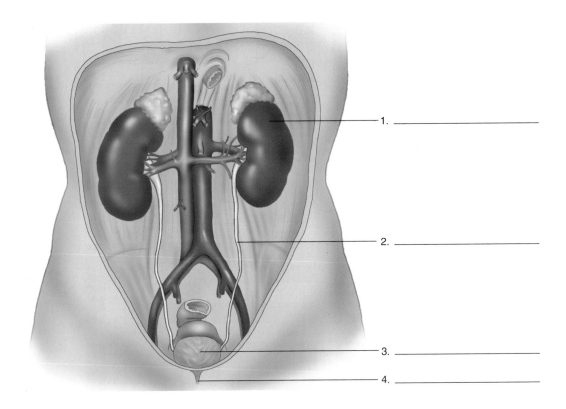

1. _____

2. _____

3. _____

4. _____

TRUE OR FALSE

IV. Read through this list. Write T for true if the characteristic is a function of the kidneys. Write F for false if the characteristic is not a kidney function.

_____ 1. degrade insulin
_____ 2. excrete waste products of metabolism
_____ 3. help maintain the chemical composition of the blood
_____ 4. maintain blood pH

_____ 5. manufacture vitamin K
_____ 6. produce erythropoietin
_____ 7. vary the excretion of water

MULTIPLE CHOICE

V. Select one answer (A–D) for each of the following multiple choice questions.

1. What does cystocele mean?
   A. resection of the bladder
   B. incision of the bladder
   C. inflammation of the bladder
   D. herniation of the bladder

2. Which of the following means excision of a renal calculus from the pelvis of the kidney?
   A. cystolithectomy
   B. pyelolithotomy
   C. lithotripsy
   D. pyelostomy

3. In which of the following is an instrument passed through the urethra in order to remove small pieces of the prostate gland?
   A. intravenous pyelogram
   B. retrograde pyelography
   C. transurethral resection
   D. urethrorrhaphy

4. What is glomerulonephritis?
   A. It is another name for floating kidney.
   B. It is surgical detachment of an inflamed kidney from nearby adhesions.
   C. It is inflammation of the kidney and bladder.
   D. It is inflammation of the kidney that involves primarily the tufts of capillaries that act as filters.

5. Which of the following means the same as nephromegaly?
   A. renal stone
   B. renal enlargement
   C. hypermobile kidney
   D. transplanted kidney

6. What is the diagnostic term for the condition that results whenever the tissue surrounding the kidney fails to anchor it to nearby structures and the kidney droops?
   A. renal failure
   B. renal colic
   C. nephroptosis
   D. nephropexy

7. What does glomerulopathy mean?
   A. any renal disease
   B. any disease of the filtering part of the kidney
   C. a disease of the renal tubules
   D. a disease of the renal pelvis

8. What is the term for examination of the interior of the bladder?
   A. cystoscopy
   B. pyeloscopy
   C. cystoscope
   D. pyeloscope

9. How does a proximal tubule compare to a distal tubule?
   A. The proximal tubule is nearer the renal pelvis.
   B. The proximal tubule is nearer the glomerulus.
   C. The proximal tubule is longer.
   D. The proximal tubule is thinner.

10. Which of the following is a rod-shaped bacterium?
    A. bacillus
    B. coccus
    C. enuresis
    D. spirochete

11. What does the term *urethrocele* mean?
    A. pertaining to the bladder and the urethra
    B. pertaining to the bladder and a ureter
    C. herniation of the urethra
    D. herniation of a ureter

12. Which of the following is the cause of gonorrhea?
    A. staphylococcus
    B. streptococcal bacilli
    C. gonococcus
    D. spirilla

13. What is the name of the instrument used to collect urine from the bladder?
    A. ureteral catheter
    B. urethral catheter
    C. intravenous cannula
    D. transurethral resector

14. Which of the following is a toxic condition of the body that occurs when the kidneys fail to function properly?
    A. uremia
    B. urography
    C. nephromalacia
    D. nephrolithiasis

15. What does glycosuria mean?
    A. increased blood sugar
    B. decreased blood sugar
    C. excretion of pus in the urine
    D. excretion of sugar in the urine

16. Which of the following means diffusing blood through a semipermeable membrane in order to remove toxic materials and maintain the acid-base balance?
    A. intravenous pyelography
    B. retrograde urography
    C. kidney clearance
    D. kidney dialysis

17. Which of the following is a normal substance in urine?
    A. blood
    B. glucose
    C. ketones
    D. urea

18. Which of the following terms refers to ultrasound of the kidney?
    A. nephrolithotomy
    B. nephroscopy
    C. nephrosonography
    D. nephrotomography

19. What is the meaning of urethrorrhagia?
    A. discharge from the urethra
    B. hemorrhage from the urethra
    C. rupture of the urethra
    D. suture of the urethra

20. What does urinary incontinence mean?
    A. excessive urination
    B. absence of urination
    C. inability to control urination
    D. none of the above

WRITING TERMS

VI. Write a term for each of the following:

1. abnormal softening of the kidney _____
2. any disease of the urinary system _____
3. between the kidneys _____
4. forming a new opening into the bladder _____
5. hemorrhage from the urethra _____
6. inflammation of the renal pelvis _____
7. ketones in the urine _____
8. pertaining to or originating in a hospital _____

9. pertaining to the kidney _____
10. presence of stones in a ureter _____
11. rupture of the bladder _____
12. sugar in the urine _____
13. surgical crushing of a stone _____
14. suture of the urethra _____
15. visual examination of the bladder _____

▶ **GREATER COMPREHENSION**

LABELING

VII. Choose from the following list to label parts of the nephron shown (1–5):

afferent arteriole   distal convoluted tubule   glomerulus   Bowman's capsule   efferent arteriole
proximal convoluted tubule   collecting duct

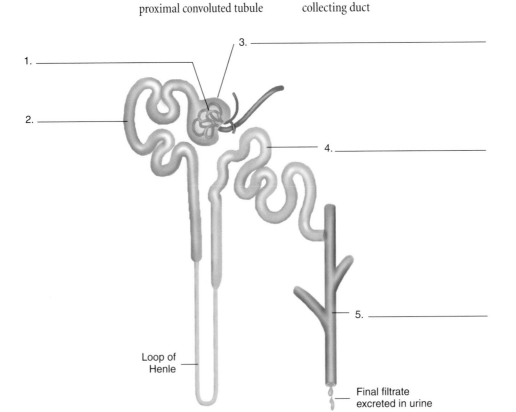

1. _____
2. _____
3. _____
4. _____
5. _____

Loop of
Henle

Final filtrate
excreted in urine

SPELLING

VIII. Circle all incorrectly spelled terms and write their correct spelling:

cardionefric   hematurea   reabsorption   glomerulopathy   hydroureter   staphylococcemia
gonococcus   polycystik   urethrarectal

FILL IN THE BLANKS

IX. Write words in the blanks to complete the following paragraph:

The renal arteries arise from the (1) _____ aorta. Each renal artery branches as it enters the hilus and, after branching

several times, it terminates in a group of capillary tufts called a (2) _____, which serves as a filter for the blood. The

structure that collects substances that filter through the glomerular walls is called (3) _____ _____.

(4) _____ of substances that the body conserves takes place in the tubules. Waste products and some of the water remain-

ing in the tubules become (5) _____, which passes to the collecting duct, where it is then deposited in the renal

(6) _____.

INTERPRETING ABBREVIATIONS

X. Write the meaning of these abbreviations:

1. BUN   _____
2. CGN   _____
3. CRF   _____
4. ESWL   _____
5. GFR   _____

6. GU   _____
7. I & O   _____
8. IVP   _____
9. LPF   _____
10. VCUG   _____

CASE STUDY

XI. Circle A, B, C, or D in questions 1 through 4 and write answers to 5 and 6 after reading this summary of an office visit:

Vinnie L. (23-year-old male)
Hx   Nothing significant reported, except patient expressed concern of "having GC."   No know allergies.
Sx   Purulent urethrorrhea and dysuria
PE   Normal
LAB   Urethral smear showed numerous WBCs and gram-negative intracellular diplococci. Urethral swab sent for culture.
Dx   gonorrhea

Rx   Probenecid, 1 g po 30 min before penicillin is given
              Procaine penicillin G, 4.8 million units IM (divided into 2 doses)
              1 month follow-up visit

1. GC is
   A. abbreviation for gonorrhea
   B. abbreviation for the bacteria that causes gonorrhea
   C. seldom transmitted to females
   D. very difficult to treat

2. Urethrorrhea is
   A. discharge from the urethra
   B. hemorrhage from the urethra
   C. inflammation of a ureter
   D. tenderness of a ureter

3. Dysuria means
   A. blood in the urine
   B. difficult or painful urination
   C. frequent urination
   D. red urine

4. The urethral smear showed
   A. many gonococcal erythrocytes
   B. many leukocytes containing possible gonococci
   C. normal numbers of cells and bacteria
   D. possible gonococci outside the cells

5. How is the oral prescription to be taken?

6. To which drug class does penicillin belong?

(Check your answers with the solutions in Appendix V.)

PRONUNCIATION

XII. The pronunciation is shown for several medical words. Indicate which syllable has the primary accent by marking it with an ′.

1. cysto/lith/ectomy (**sis to lĭ thek tǝ me**)
2. diuresis (**di u re sis**)
3. glomeruli (**glo mer u li**)
4. hemodialysis (**he mo di al ǝ sis**)
5. litho/tripsy (**lith o trip se**)

6. nephro/lith/iasis (**nef ro lĭ thi ǝ sis**)
7. nephro/sono/graphy (**nef ro so nog rǝ fe**)
8. pyelo/gram (**pi ǝ lo gram**)
9. pyonephrosis (**pi o nǝ fro sis**)
10. uro/graphy (**u rog rǝ fe**)

CATEGORIZING TERMS

XIII. Categorize each of the following terms by writing A, D, R, or T to indicate anatomical, diagnostic, radiological, surgical, or therapeutic. The first term is done as an example.

Category
(A, D, R, or T)

1. abdominocystic ___A___
2. cystectomy _____
3. cystostomy _____
4. hemodialysis _____
5. hydronephrosis _____

Category
(A, D, R, or T)

6. nephrosclerosis _____
7. proteinuria _____
8. renovascular _____
9. pyelogram _____
10. ureterolithotomy _____

Listing of Medical Terms

abdominocystic	cystocele	extracystic	loop of Henle
aerobic	cystogram	genitourinary	microbiology
albumin	cystography	glomeruli	microorganism
albuminuria	cystolith	glomerulonephritis	nephrectomy
anaerobic	cystolithectomy	glomerulopathy	nephritis
angiogram	cystolithotomy	glomerulus	nephrocele
anuria	cystoplasty	glycosuria	nephrolith
anuric	cystoplegia	gonococcus	nephrolithiasis
antihypertensive	cystorrhea	gonorrhea	nephrolithotomy
antiinfective	cystorrhexis	hematuria	nephrolysis
bacilli	cystoscope	hemodialysis	nephromalacia
bilateral nephromegaly	cystoscopy	hemorrhage	nephromegaly
bladder	cystostomy	hydronephrosis	nephron
bladder polyp	cystotomy	hydroureter	nephropexy
Bowman's capsule	cystoureteroscopy	incontinence	nephroptosis
Bright's disease	cystourethritis	interrenal	nephropyosis
cardionephric	cystourethrography	intracellular	nephrorrhaphy
catheter	diplococci	intravenous pyelogram	nephrosclerosis
catheterized specimen	distal tubule	ketoacidosis	nephroscope
chronic	diuresis	ketone	nephroscopy
cocci	diuretic	ketonuria	nephrosis
continence	dysuria	kidney dialysis	nephrosonography
cystectomy	enuresis	litholysis	nephrostomy
cystic	excretion	lithotripsy	nephrotomogram
cystitis	extracorporeal	lithotrite	nephrotomography

Listing of Medical Terms—cont'd

nephrotoxic	pyuria	urea	urethrography
nephroureterectomy	reabsorption	uremia	urethrorectal
nocturia	rectourethral	ureter	urethrorrhagia
nosocomial infection	renal calculus	ureteritis	urethrorrhaphy
nycturia	renal failure	ureterocele	urethrorrhea
oliguria	renal pelvis	ureterocystostomy	urethrospasm
peritoneal dialysis	renal transplant	ureterolith	urethrotomy
polycystic	renovascular	ureterolithiasis	urethrovaginal
polyuria	retention	ureterolithotomy	uricosuric
prostate	spirilla	ureteroneocystostomy	urinalysis
proteinuria	staphylococcemia	ureteropathy	urinary
proximal tubule	staphylococci	ureteroplasty	urogenital
purulence	stenosis	ureteropyelitis	urography
pyelitis	streptococcemia	ureterorrhaphy	urolithiasis
pyelogram	streptococci	ureterostenosis	uropathy
pyelography	suprapubic	ureterostomy	vaginitis
pyelolithotomy	suprapubic cystotomy	ureteroureterostomy	venereal disease
pyelonephritis	suprarenal	urethra	voided specimen
pyeloplasty	toxemia	urethritis	voiding cystourethrogram
pyelostomy	transurethral resection	urethrocele	
pyonephrosis	tubule	urethrocystitis	

Español

Enhancing Spanish Communication

English	Spanish (pronunciation)	English	Spanish (pronunciation)
acidity	acidez (ah-se-DES)	rupture	ruptura (roop-TOO-rah)
bladder	vejiga (vah-HEE-gah)	spiral	espiral (es-pe-RAHL)
calculus	cálculo (CAHL-coo-lo)	suture	sutura (soo-TOO-rah)
catheter	catéter (cah-TAY-ter)	urinalysis	urinálisis (oo-re-NAH-le-sis)
dialysis	diálisis (de-AH-le-sis)	urinary	urinario (oo-re-NAH-re-o)
excretion	excreción (ex-cray-se-ON)	urinate	orinar (o-re-NAR)
hemorrhage	hemorragia (ay-mor-RAH-he-ah)	urination	urinación (oo-re-nah-se-ON)
kidney	riñón (ree-NYOHN)	urology	urologia (oo-ro-lo-HEE-ah)
renal artery	arteria renal (ar-TAY-re-ah ray-NAHL)	voiding	urinar (oo-re-NAR)
renal calculus	cálculo renal (CAHL-coo-lo ray-NAHL)		

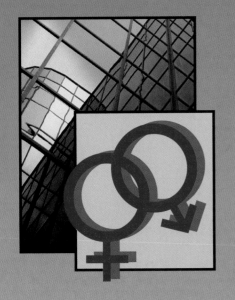

Reproductive System

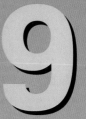

9

Outline

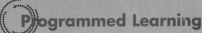
Principal Word Parts

COMBINING FORMS

amni(o)	amnion
cervic(o)	neck; cervix uteri
chori(o)	chorion
colp(o), vagin(o)	vagina
cry(o)	cold
crypt(o)	hidden
epididym(o)	epididymis
fet(o)	fetus
genit(o)	organs of reproduction
gynec(o)	female
hyster(o), uter(o)	uterus
lapar(o)	abdominal wall
men(o)	month
metr(o)	measure, uterine tissue
nat(o)	birth
o(o)	egg (ovum)
obstetr(o)	midwife
oophor(o), ovari(o)	ovary
orchi(o), orchid(o), test(o), testicul(o)	testicle
par(o)	bearing offspring
pen(o)	penis
perine(o)	perineum
prostat(o)	prostate
salping(o)	uterine tube
scrot(o)	scrotum
semin(o)	semen
sperm(o), spermat(o)	spermatozoa
sympt(o)	symptom
therm(o)	heat
vas(o)	vessel; ductus deferens
varic(o)	varicose vein
vulv(o)	vulva

PREFIXES

ante-, pre-	before
contra-	against
ecto-	situated on or outside
multi-	many
neo-	new
nulli-	none
post-	after; behind
primi-	first
pseudo-	false
quadri-	four

SUFFIXES

-an	pertaining to	-gravida	pregnant female
-blast	embryonic or early form	-para	woman who has given birth
-cidal	killing	-plasia	formation or development
-cyesis	pregnancy	-therapy	treatment
-genesis	origin or beginning		

Learning Goals

▶ BASIC UNDERSTANDING

1. Identify and know the functions of the major male and female reproductive structures.
2. Name the three types of uterine tissue.
3. Describe events that occur in the female reproductive cycle and how contraceptives prevent pregnancy.
4. Recognize the characteristics of several types of sexually transmitted diseases.
5. Write the meaning of the word parts and use them to build and analzye terms.

▶ GREATER COMPREHENSION

6. Recognize four types of uterine displacements.
7. Categorize terms as anatomical, diagnostic, radiological, surgical, or therapeutic.
8. Spell the terms accurately.
9. Pronounce the terms correctly.
10. Write the meanings of the abbreviations.
11. Identify the effects or uses of the drug classes presented in this chapter.

SECTION A

Structures of the Female Reproductive System

The male and female reproductive systems include the gonads, where sex cells and hormones are produced, and other organs, ducts, and glands that transport and sustain the egg or sperm cells. The female reproductive system includes the ovaries, uterine tubes, uterus, vagina, accessory glands, and external genital structures. Information about the breasts, often considered a part of this system, is found in Chapter 13, which covers hormones and the endocrine system.

genitalia	**9-1** The reproductive organs, whether male or female, are called the genitals or genitalia (jen″ĭ-tāl′e-ə). The combining form *genit(o)* refers to organs of reproduction. The genitalia include both external and internal organs. Another name for genitals is _____.
reproductive	Knowing that ur(o) means pertaining to urine or the urinary system, uro/genit/al means pertaining to the urinary and the _____ systems.
gynec(o) **gynecology** **females**	**9-2** The combining form that means woman or female is _____. The medical specialty that treats diseases of the female reproductive organs is _____. Gynecolog/ic (gi″nə-kə-loj′ik) means pertaining to gynecology or study of diseases that occur only in _____.

TABLE 9-1 The Female Genitalia

INTERNAL STRUCTURES	EXTERNAL STRUCTURES (VULVA)
Left ovary and associated left uterine tube	Mons pubis
Right ovary and associated right uterine tube	Labia majora
Uterus	Labia minora
Vagina	Clitoris
Special glands	Prepuce
	Openings for glands

internal

9-3 Examine Table 9-1. Note that the ovaries, the uterus, the vagina and several glands make up the _____ structures of the female genitalia.

Label these internal structures on Figure 9-1 as you read this frame. The right ovary (**o′və-re**) and left ovary are the primary reproductive structures because they produce ova (eggs) and hormones. The drawing in Figure 9-1 is a midsagittal view of the internal genitalia, so only one ovary is shown. Label line 1, the ovary. Ovaries are about the size and shape of an almond.

One uterine tube is associated with each ovary. Label line 2, the uterine tube. These tubes, also called fallopian tubes, are named uterine tubes because they extend laterally from the upper portion of the uterus to the region of the ovary. There is no direct connection between the ovary and the fingerlike projections of the uterine tube, the fimbriae. When an ovum (singular form of ova) is produced, the fimbriae create currents that sweep the ovum into the tube, and it is then carried along toward the uterus over the next 5 to 7 days. The uterine tube is the most common site of fertilization of the ovum by the male sex cell, the spermatozoa (often shortened to sperm), because the ovum is fertile only 24 to 48 hours.

The uterus (**u′tər-əs**) is a muscular organ that prepares to receive and nurture the fertilized ovum. Label line 3, the uterus. The uterus is hollow and pear shaped. The lower and narrower part that has the outlet from the uterus is the cervix uteri, commonly called the uterine cervix. When used alone, the term *cervix* (**sər′viks**) often means the cervix uteri. Label line 4 in the drawing, the cervix uteri.

The vagina (**və-ji′nə**) commonly called the birth canal, is muscular and capable of sufficient expansion for passage of the child during childbirth. It also serves as the repository for sperm during intercourse. The vagina is the connection between the internal genitalia and the outside through its opening called the vaginal orifice (opening). Label line 5, the vagina.

ovary

oophoropathy
(o-of″ə-rop′ə-the)

9-4 Two words parts mean ovary: *ovari(o)* and *oophor(o)*. The combining form *ovari(o)* is generally used to write terms that describe the structure of the ovary. The suffix *-an* means pertaining to. Ovari/an (o-var′e-ən) means pertaining to the _____. The combining form *oophor(o)* is used to write most diagnostic and surgical terms. Use oophor(o) to write a word that means any disease of the ovaries: _____.

salpingectomy
(sal″ping-jek′tə-me)

uterus

(your answer choice)

9-5 The combining form *salping(o)* means uterine tube. Write a term that means surgical removal of a uterine tube: _____.

Two combining forms that mean uterus are *uter(o)* and *hyster(o)*. You have already used the term *uterine* (**u′tər-in**), which means pertaining to the _____.

Write any word that you know that begins with hyster(o): _____.

Many students will think of words such as hysterics, hysterical, or hysterectomy. All of these words use the combining form hyster(o), which means uterus. According to Dunmore and Fleischer, the use of hyster(o) as a combining form originated with the ancient Greeks, who believed that women were especially susceptible to emotional disorders that arose from the womb. The Greeks used the word *hysterikos* to refer to suffering in the womb and the emotional upheaval caused by this suffering.

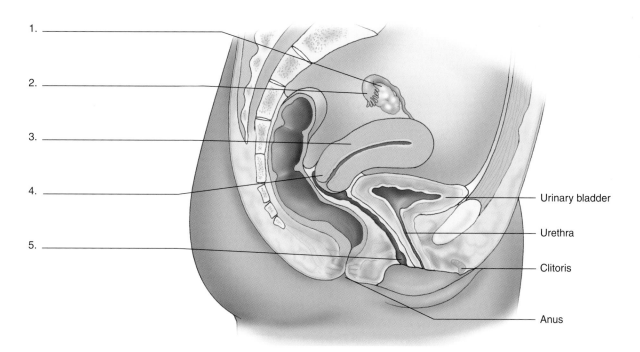

1. _____

2. _____

3. _____

4. _____

5. _____

— Urinary bladder

— Urethra

— Clitoris

— Anus

FIGURE 9-1

Female genitalia, midsagittal section. Identification of the genitalia is completed as you write the names of the structures in the blank lines. Structures other than the genitalia are shown with black labels and are included to show their close proximity to the reproductive structures. The urinary bladder and urethra are structures of the urinary apparatus; the anus is part of the digestive system.

vagina **vagina** **bladder**	**9-6** The vagina (və-ji′nə) is the birth canal, the receptacle for receiving sperm, and the passageway for menstrual flow. Both *vagin(o)* and *colp(o)* mean vagina. Vaginal (vaj′i-nəl) is an adjective and refers to the _____. Knowing that cyst(o) means bladder, colpo/cyst/itis is inflammation of the _____ and the urinary _____.
vulva	**9-7** Look again at the external structures that are listed in Table 9-1. The vulva refers to the external genitalia in the female, and the combining form is *vulv(o).* Vulv/ar (**vul′vər**) or vulv/al (**vul′vəl**) pertains to the _____.

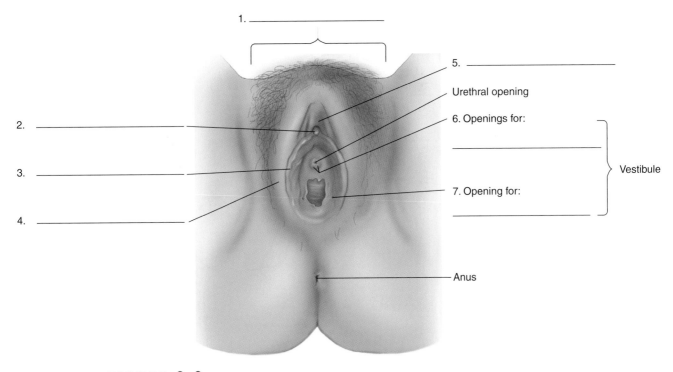

FIGURE 9-2
Female external genitalia. These structures are external to the vagina and are also called the vulva.

9-8 Look at Figure 9-2, noting the structures that compose the vulva. These structures are external to the vagina. Label the structures as you read the following material.

The mons* pubis **(monz pubis)** is a pad of fatty tissue and thick skin that overlies a bone called the symphysis pubis. The pubis is the anterior portion of the hip bones. After puberty, the mons pubis is covered with hair. Label line 1 in Figure 9-2, the mons pubis.

The clitoris **(klit′ə-ris)** is a small mass of erectile tissue and nerves that has similarities to the male penis. This small mass of erectile tissue becomes erect in response to sexual stimulation. Label line 2, the clitoris.

Two pairs of skin folds, the labia majora and the labia minora, protect the vaginal opening.

labia minora

The smaller pair of skin folds is called the _____ _____. Write the name of this structure on line 3 in the drawing.

majora

The larger pair of skin folds is called the labia **(la′be-ə)** _____. Write the name of this structure on line 4 in the drawing.

The labia minora merge and form a hood over the clitoris. This fold of skin that forms a retractable cover is called the prepuce **(pre′pūs).** Label line 5, the prepuce.

Label line 6, the paraurethral glands. The name of the para/urethral **(par″ə-u-re′thrəl)** glands tell us they

near

are located _____ the urethra.

Other glands, the vestibular glands, lie adjacent to the vaginal opening. Label line 7, the vestibular glands.

9-9 Vestibule **(ves′tĭ-bul)** is any space or cavity at the entrance to a canal. The vaginal vestibule is the space between the two labia minora into which the urethra and vagina open. The greater vestibular glands (Bartholin's glands) produce a mucuslike secretion for lubrication during sexual intercourse.

Another important locational term is perineum **(per″ĭ-ne′əm),** the area between the vaginal opening and the anus. The combining form *perine(o)* means perineum. Perine/al means pertaining to the

perineum

_____.

*(Latin: *mons*, mountain.)

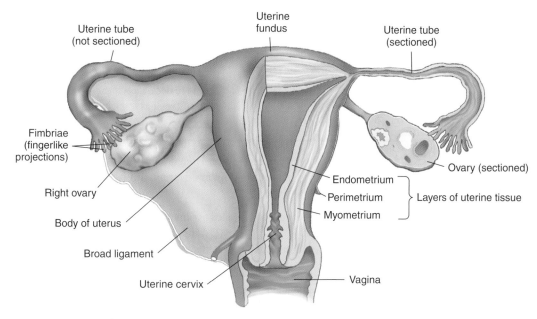

FIGURE 9-3
Organs of the female reproductive system, anterior view. The left ovary, left uterine tube, and left side of the uterus are sectioned to show their internal structure. Peritoneum and ligaments hold the reproductive structures in place.

	9-10 The uterus is the normal site where a fertilized ovum implants and develops. In the absence of a fertilized ovum, this is the organ from which menstruation (**men″stroo-a′shən**) flows. Examine the anterior view of the female genitalia in Figure 9-3.
fundus (fun′dəs) **body** **cervix**	The uterus consists of an upper portion, a large main portion, and a narrow region that connects with the vagina. The upper, bulging surface of the uterus, above the entrance of the uterine tubes, is called the uterine _____. The large, main portion is called the _____ of the uterus, and the narrow region is the uterine _____.
neck **cervix uteri**	**9-11** The word cervix refers to the neck itself or part of an organ that resembles a neck. The cervix uteri (**sər′viks u′tər-i**) specifically means the lower, necklike portion of the uterus, although it is common to see cervix written alone but meaning the cervix uteri. The word cervix means _____. The proper name of the uterine cervix is _____ _____.
neck **vagina and cervix uteri** **colpocervicitis** (kol-po-ser-vĭ-si′tis) **cervicocolpitis** (ser″vĭ-ko-kol-pi′tis) **cervicitis** (sər″vĭ-si′tis)	**9-12** The combining form *cervic(o)* means neck or cervix uteri. You can usually decide whether it refers to the neck itself or the cervix uteri by examining other parts of the word. For example, cervico/facial (**ser″vĭ-ko-fa′shəl**) refers to the _____ and face. Colpo/cervic/al (**kol-po-ser′vik-əl**) refers to the _____. Inflammation of the vagina and cervix is _____ or _____. Inflammation involving only the cervix is _____. Cervicitis refers specifically to inflammation of the cervix uteri.

measure
uterine tissue
uterine tissue

9-13 You have learned that uter(o) and hyster(o) mean uterus. A third combining form, **metr(o),** also means the uterus, and occasionally metr(o) means measure. The suffixes -*meter* and -*metry* are derived from the same root as metr(o), which means to measure.

Whenever you see metr(o) used in a word, you will need to decide if it means _____ or _____ _____. It is not as difficult as it might seem. For example, metr/itis (**mǝ-tri′tis**) could only refer to inflammation of _____ _____.

uterus

muscle
myometritis
(mi″o-mǝ-tri′tis)

endometrium

9-14 The uterus consists of three layers of tissue. From the outermost layer to the innermost layer, the layers are called perimetrium (**per″ĭ-me′tre-ǝm**), myometrium (**mi-o-me′tre-ǝm**), and endometrium (**en″do-me′tre-ǝm).**

The outer layer is visceral peritoneum and is called peri/metr/ium. Analyzing its word parts, peri- means around, metr(o) means _____, and -ium means membrane. In other words, perimetrium is a membrane that surrounds the uterus.

The myo/metr/ium is the thick muscular wall of the uterus. What does my(o) mean? _____ Write a term that means inflammation of the myometrium: _____.

The inner layer, the endo/metr/ium, is a mucous membrane. Write the name of this mucous membrane that lines the uterus: _____.

During much of a female's life, the endometrium goes through a monthly cycle of growth and discharge known as the menstrual cycle.

❏ SECTION A REVIEW   *S*tructures of the Female Reproductive System

This section review covers frames 9–1 through 9–14. Write a word part or its meaning as indicated in the following blanks.

Combining Form	Meaning	Combining Form	Meaning
1. _____	cervix uteri or neck	9. _____	uterine tube
2. colp(o)	_____	10. uter(o)	
3. genit(o)	_____	11. vagin(o)	
4. hyster(o)	_____	12. _____	vulva
5. metr(o)	_____	**Suffix**	**Meaning**
6. oophor(o)	_____	13. -an	_____
7. ovari(o)	_____		
8. _____	perineum		

(Use Appendix V to check your answers.)

Reproduction and the Female Reproductive Cycle

Sexual reproduction, the process by which a new individual is produced from male and female gametes, the sperm and ovum, is the way in which genetic material is passed from one generation to the next. The gonads produce ova and sperm, as well as hormones, that are necessary for proper functioning of the reproductive organs. Reproductive cycles normally occur in females from shortly after the onset of menstruation to menopause. These cycles reflect changes that are occurring in the ovaries (ovarian cycle) and the uterus (menstrual cycle).

9-15 The hypothalamus (part of the brain) and the pituitary gland, located just beneath the brain, secrete hormones that have significant roles in the control of reproductive functions. The hormones produced by these structures act on the ovaries to bring about two important functions: the production of additional hormones (estrogen and progesterone) and ova.

Female reproductive cycles begin at puberty (**pu´bər-tē**) and continue for about 40 years until menopause (**men´o-pawz**). Puberty is that stage of development when genitalia reach maturity and secondary sex characteristics appear. The onset normally occurs in females between 9 and 13 years of age with the development of breasts and menarche (**mə-nahr´ke**). Menopause, also called the climacteric, is the natural cessation of reproductive cycles and menstruation with the decline of reproductive hormones in later years. Menopause may occur earlier as a result of illness or surgical removal of the uterus or both ovaries.

Menarche is the first occurrence of menstruation (**men″stroo-a´shən**), the periodic bloody discharge caused by the shedding of the endometrium from the nonpregnant uterus. Write this term that means the first menstruation: _____.

menarche

Paying particular attention to its spelling, write the term that means the periodic (generally monthly) bloody discharge from the shedding of the endometrium: _____.

menstruation

9-16 The secretion of female reproductive hormones follows monthly cyclic patterns that affect the ovaries and uterus. Together, these cycles, called the ovarian cycle and the menstrual (uterine) cycle, make up the female reproductive cycle. The ovarian cycle reflects the changes that occur within the _____.

ovaries

The uterine (menstrual) cycle reflects the changes that take place in the _____.

uterus

See Figure 9-4 for the correlation of events in the ovarian and uterine cycles.

9-17 The ovarian and uterine cycles begin at puberty when certain unknown stimuli cause the hypothalamus to start secreting a hormone that acts on the pituitary gland. The pituitary gland then begins to secrete two hormones, follicle-stimulating hormone (FSH) and luteinizing hormone (LH). Looking at Figure 9-4, you see that FSH and LH act on follicles in the _____.

ovaries

The graafian follicle is a small ovarian recess or pit that contains fluid and surrounds an ovum (egg). Generally one ovum is released each month. The follicle produces hormones and grows in preparation for release of the ovum. These changes in the follicle are classified as the follicular phase, followed by the luteal phase. Find these two phases in the upper part of Figure 9-4. The follicular changes are represented by follicle development, _____, and _____ _____.

ovulation
corpus luteum

Ovulation (**ov″u-la´shən**) is the release of the ovum from the follicle. After the ovum is released, the ruptured follicle enlarges, takes on a yellow appearance, and is called the corpus luteum, meaning yellow body. The luteal phase is named after the yellowish structures called the _____ _____.

corpus
luteum

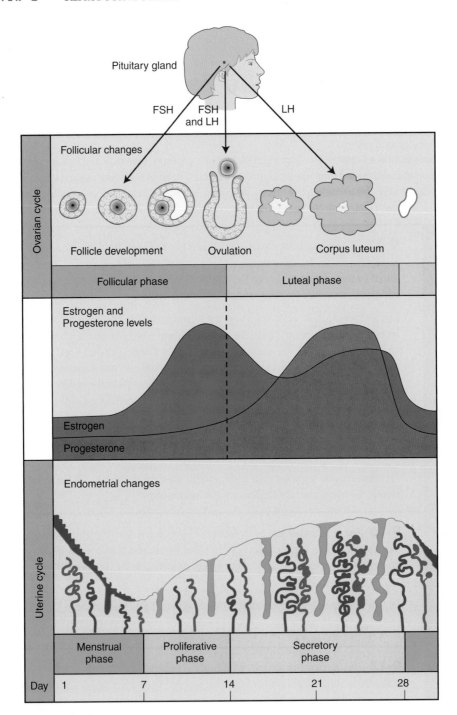

FIGURE 9-4

Correlation of events in the ovarian and uterine cycles. These two events make up the female reproductive cycle, with an average length of 28 days from the first day of bleeding of one cycle to the first day of bleeding of the next cycle.

TABLE 9-2 The Reproductive Cycle

DAYS	OVARIAN PHASE	UTERINE (MENSTRUAL) PHASE
1-5	*Follicular phase.* Growth of the follicle. Secretion of estrogen.	*Menses.* Blood is shed from the vagina.
6-12	Follicular phase continues.	*Proliferative phase.* Growth of the endometrium.
13-14	*Ovulation.* Ova is released by the follicle.	Proliferative phase continues.
15-28	*Luteal phase.* Follicle becomes corpus luteum. Secretes progesterone.	*Secretory phase.* Continued growth of endometrium, secretion of glycogen.

estrogen
(es′tro-jən)

progesterone
(pro-jes′tə-rōn)

9-18 Two important hormones that are secreted by the follicles influence the uterine cycle. During the follicular phase, increasing amounts of estrogen are secreted that stimulate repair of the endometrium. Estrogen reaches it peak near the middle of the cycle, then decreases until the next month. The corpus luteum secretes another important hormone, progesterone, which causes continued growth and thickening of the endometrium with additional preparatory activities to support a potential embryo. If fertilization (union of the ovum and sperm) does not occur, the corpus luteum begins to degenerate and the cycle starts again.

The initial hormone secreted by the ovarian follicle that causes the endometrium to thicken is

_____.

This is the same hormone that brings about female secondary sex characteristics, the external physical signs of sexual maturity, such as development of the breasts and pubic hair.

A second hormone is secreted by the corpus luteum. That hormone is called _____.

proliferative, secretory

9-19 The uterine cycle occurs simultaneously with the ovarian cycle and is the result of the estrogen and progesterone secretion by the ovaries. Looking again at Figure 9-4, write down the phases of the uterine cycle: the menstrual phase, the _____ phase, and the _____ phase.

The menstrual phase begins on day 1 of the cycle and continues for 3 to 5 days. The proliferative phase lasts for about 8 days. The name of this phase refers to the growth of the endometrium as it thickens and glands and blood vessels develop in the new tissue. The endometrium continues to grow and thicken in the secretory phase, and in addition, begins to secrete glycogen, which will nourish a developing embryo if fertilization occurs.

The term *menses* means the normal flow of blood during menstruation when fertilization has not occurred. Menses and menstruation are often used interchangeably. Several of the terms pertaining to the menstrual cycle use the combining form ***men(o),*** which means month. The events of the menstrual cycle are summarized in Table 9-2.

uterine tube

9-20 Estrogen and progesterone prepare the uterus for pregnancy. Fertilization, or conception, is the union of the sperm cell nucleus with an egg cell nucleus. This usually occurs in the _____ _____.

The fertilized ovum undergoes a series of cell divisions as it moves along the uterine tube, then enters into the uterine cavity. The embryo receives nourishment from the glycogen secreted by the endometrium. About the seventh day after ovulation, the fertilized ovum attaches to the endometrium. This is called implantation.

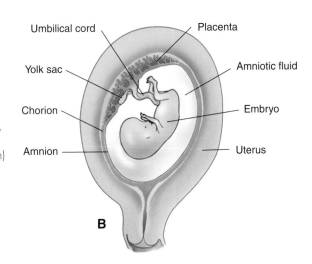

Four-cell stage
48 hours

Eight-cell stage
2 1/2 days

Morula
3 days

Blastocyst
5 days

Blastocyst begins
implantation
7 days

Two-cell stage
36 hours

A

Zygote

Ovulation

Fertilization

Umbilical cord

Placenta

Yolk sac

Amniotic fluid

Chorion

Embryo

Amnion

Uterus

B

FIGURE 9-5

Fertilization, implantation, and growth of the embryo. **A,** A mature ovum is released in ovulation. The ovum is fertilized by a sperm, and the product of fertilization, the zygote, undergoes rapid cell division known by these stages: 2-cell stage, 4-cell stage, 8-cell stage, morula, and blastocyst. The blastocyst implants in the endometrium. **B,** The placenta and extraembryonic membranes (the amnion and the chorion) form and surround the embryo, providing nourishment and protection. The human embryonic stage begins about 2 weeks after conception and lasts until about the end of the eighth week, after which time the fetal stage begins.

---

ovum, sperm

ovary

oogenesis
(o″o-jen′ə-sis)

9-21   A gamete (**gam′ēt**) is a reproductive cell (ovum or spermatozoon), and the union of the ovum and sperm is necessary in sexual reproduction to initiate the development of a new individual. The ovum, also called the egg, lives only a few days after ovulation, and the sperm have about the same time or less before they die after being discharged into the vagina. The gametes of reproduction are the _____ and the _____.

What organ is responsible for the production of ova? _____

Write a word that means formation of ova, using the combining form for ovum, **o(o),** and the suffix **-genesis,** which means origin or beginning: _____.

9-22 The product of fertilization is the zygote, which undergoes rapid cell divisions. The zygote is known by different names at various stages. Some of these stages between fertilization and implantation are shown in Figure 9-5, *A*. It is usually at the beginning of the third week that the developing offspring is called an embryo.* After the eighth week, it is called a fetus. Fetal means pertaining to the fetus.

It is during the embryonic stage that all of the organ systems form, making this the most critical time in development. This is also when the placenta and extraembryonic membranes form. Knowing that embryonic refers to the embryo, extra/embryonic means _____ the embryo.

Look at Figure 9-5, *B*, and locate two extraembryonic membranes, the amnion (**am′ne-on**) and the chorion (**kor′e-on**), that surround the embryo. These membranes provide protection by surrounding it with amniotic fluid. The amnion and the chorion, along with the placenta, are called the afterbirth and are shed shortly after birth.

The placenta is a highly vascular structure that nourishes the fetus. Oxygen, nutrients, and antibodies diffuse from the mother to fetal blood vessels, and fetal wastes diffuse from the fetal blood into the maternal blood. Maternal means from the mother. Membranes normally keep the fetal and maternal blood from actually mixing. Write the name of the structure that surrounds and nourishes the fetus: _____.

The placenta also secretes large amounts of progesterone, which is necessary for maintaining the uterus during pregnancy. The hormone that is responsible for maintaining the uterus throughout pregnancy is _____.

9-23 Within a few days after conception, the chorion starts producing a hormone, human chorionic gonadotropin (**gon″ə-do-tro′pin**) (HCG). It is present in body fluids (urine, blood) of pregnant females, and blood or urine is tested to determine if pregnancy exists. HCG can be detected long before other signs of pregnancy appear. The hormone that is tested for in pregnancy tests is HCG, or _____.

HCG can be demonstrated in the urine long before the fetal heart beat is heard.

9-24 The combining form *amni(o)* means amnion. Amniotic (**am″ne-ot′ik**) means pertaining to the _____. Amnionic also refers to the amnion, but amniotic is used more often.

Using amni(o) and the suffix -rrhea, which means flow, write a word that means discharge, or escape, of the amniotic fluid: _____.

Using -rrhexis, write a new word that means rupture of the amnion: _____.

Amniorrhexis occurs before the child is born and sometimes is the mother's first sign of impending labor. The "water breaks" or the "bag of water breaks" is a common saying that means amniorrhexis.

The word for deliberate rupture of the fetal membranes to induce labor is translated literally as "incision of the amnion." Write this new term: _____.

9-25 Use *chori(o)* to write words about the chorion. You have already used a word that means pertaining to the chorion, which is _____.

Amnio/chorionic (**am″ne-o-kor″e-on′ik**) pertains to two membranes, the _____ and the _____. Amnio/chorial (**am″ne-o-ko′re-əl**) is another word that means pertaining to the amnion and chorion.

9-26 The combining form o(o) means ovum (**o′vəm**). Oo/blast (**o′o-blast**) is an embryonic _____. (The suffix *-blast* means embryonic or early form.)

---

outside	
placenta (plə-sen′tə)	
progesterone (pro-jes′tə-rōn)	
human chorionic gonadotropin	
amnion	
amniorrhea (am″ne-o-re′ə)	
amniorrhexis (am″ne-o-rek′sis)	
amniotomy (am″ne-ot′ə-me)	
chorionic	
amnion chorion	
ovum	

*Embryo (Greek: *embryon,* to grow in).

TABLE 9-3 Selected Contraceptives*

METHOD	ACTION
Intrauterine device	Small plastic or metal device placed in the uterus that prevents fertilization or implantation; some release hormones
Oral contraceptives	Hormones, either progestin given alone or combined with estrogen, that prevent release of ova
Condom	Thin sheath (usually latex) worn over the penis to collect semen
Diaphragm	Soft rubber cup that covers the uterine cervix and prevents sperm from reaching the egg; holds spermicide
Cervical cap	Similar to diaphragm, but smaller, and covers cervix closely
Foams, creams, jellies, vaginal suppositories	Chemical spermicides inserted into the vagina before intercourse to prevent sperm from entering the uterus
Sponge	Acts as barrier to the sperm and releases spermicide
Implant (Norplant)	Capsules surgically implanted under the skin slowly release a hormone that blocks the release of ova
Injectable contraceptive	Hormonal injection on a specific schedule prevents ovulation
Calendar or rhythm method	Determine fertile period and practice abstinence (voluntarily avoiding sexual intercourse) during "unsafe" days
Basal body temperature (BBT)	Ovulation is determined by drop and subsequent rise in BBT; abstinence is practiced during fertile periods
Cervical mucus	Ovulation is determined by observing the changes in the cervical mucus; abstinence is practiced during fertile period
Symptothermal	A combination of observing symptoms and increase in body temperature (cervical mucus and BBT); abstinence is practiced on fertile days

*The order of the contraceptives is listed from lowest failure rates to the methods that have the highest failure rates. Hysterectomy, tubal ligation, and vasectomy are not included here because they are forms of sterilization, often permanent.

sperm sperm	**9-27** Use *spermat(o)* to mean spermatozoa (sper″mə-to-zo′ə) or sperm. A spermato/blast (sper′mə-to blast″) is an embryonic form of _____. A spermato/cyte (sper′mə-to-sīt″) is a cell that will become a mature, functioning _____.
	9-28 Write words for the following:
spermatopathy (sper″mə-top′ə-the)	any disease of sperm (or semen): _____
spermatoid (spər′mə-toid)	resembling a sperm: _____
spermatogenesis (sper″mə-to-jen′ə-sis)	formation (production) of sperm: _____
aspermatogenesis (a-spər″mə-to-jen′ə-sis)	absence of sperm production: _____
sperm condition	Sometimes spermat(o) is shortened to ***sperm(o)*** and used to form words about spermatozoa. A/sperm/ia means absence of sperm. Oligo/sperm/ia (ol″ĭ-go-sper′me-ə) means a deficiency in the number of sperm. Analyzing its parts, oligo- means few, sperm(o) means _____, and -ia means _____.
	In vitro fertilization (IVF) may be successful when failure to conceive is caused by insufficient numbers of sperm. In vitro fertilization is a method of fertilizing the ova outside the body by collecting mature ova and placing them in a dish with spermatozoa. Fertilized ova are then placed in the uterus for implantation.
sperm	**9-29** Spermato/cidal (sper″mə-to si′dəl) is the killing of _____ (-*cidal* means killing). Contraceptive foams and creams are spermatocides.
spermatolytic (sper′mə-to-lit′ik)	Build a word that means the same as spermatocidal by using the combining form for spermatozoa plus the suffix that means capable of destroying: _____.
conception (or pregnancy)	There are a variety of means of preventing pregnancy (Table 9-3). Prevention of conception is contraception (***contra-*** means against). A contraceptive is an agent that prevents _____.

uterus	**9-30** An intrauterine (**in″trə-u′tər-in**) device (IUD) is inserted into the _____ by the physician.
mouth	Oral contraceptives are what is meant when someone says she is on the pill. The word *oral* in the name tells us that the medication is taken by _____.
sympt(o), therm(o)	The sympto/thermal method of contraception introduces two new word parts: ***sympt(o)***, meaning symptom, and ***therm(o)***, meaning heat. The symptothermal method uses a combination of observing changes in the cervical mucus and body temperature. The word parts that refer to the change in cervical mucus and body temperature are _____ and _____, respectively.

9-31 Study Table 9-3 to learn additional means of preventing conception. Tubal ligation should be considered a permanent means of sterilization because it is not always reversible. Tubal ligation is constricting, severing, or crushing the uterine tubes.

Permanent sterilization in the male is a vas/ectomy (**və-sek′tə-me**). This is bilateral excision of the vas deferens (**vas def″ər-enz**), a duct that transports sperm.

❏ SECTION B REVIEW ℛeproduction and the Female Reproductive Cycle

This section review covers frames 9–15 through 9–31. Complete the tables by writing the meaning of each word part in the blanks.

Combining Form	Meaning		Prefix	Meaning
1. amni(o)	_____		9. contra-	_____
2. chori(o)	_____		**Suffix**	**Meaning**
3. men(o)	_____		10. -blast	_____
4. o(o)	_____		11. -cidal	_____
5. sperm(o)	_____		12. -genesis	_____
6. spermat(o)	_____			
7. sympt(o)	_____			
8. therm(o)	_____			

(Use Apendix V to check your answers.)

SECTION C

℘regnancy and Childbirth

Pregnancy is the process of growth and development of a new individual from conception through the embryonic and fetal periods to birth. Pregnancy lasts approximately 266 days from the day of fertilization. The birth of the baby is parturition.

before	**9-32** Gestation (**jes-ta′shən**) is another name for pregnancy. This is also called the prenatal period. The prefix ***pre-*** means before and ***nat(o)*** means birth. Pre/natal is that time _____ birth.

We saw in the previous section that the developing human individual is called an embryo at the beginning of the third week. By the end of the eighth week after fertilization, the developing individual is called a fetus, because by this time there are recognizable human features. Look at the timetable of prenatal development, Figure 9-6, and see the age when different features are present. Quickening, the first recognizable movements of the fetus in the uterus, occurs at about 18 to 20 weeks in a first pregnancy and slightly sooner in later pregnancies.

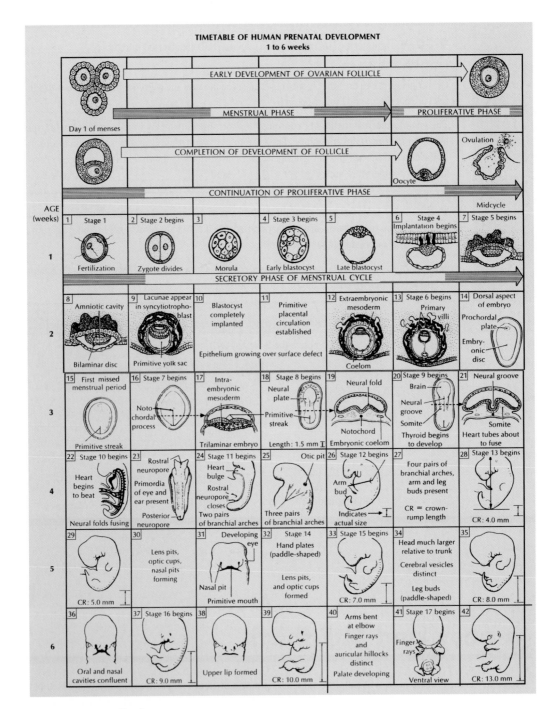

FIGURE 9-6

Timetable of prenatal development. Several significant events in the process of growth, maturation, differentiation, and development are shown in the timetable: development of the three germ layers; heart begins beating; fingers, eyelids, toes, and external genitalia are visible, and face has human appearance. (From Moore KL: *The developing human*, ed 3, Philadelphia, 1983, WB Saunders.)

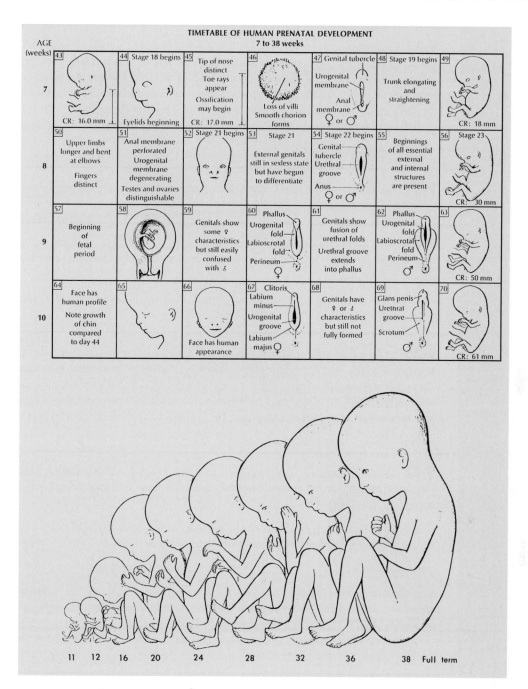

TIMETABLE OF HUMAN PRENATAL DEVELOPMENT
7 to 38 weeks

AGE (weeks)							
7	**43** CR: 16.0 mm	**44** Stage 18 begins Eyelids beginning	**45** Tip of nose distinct Toe rays appear Ossification may begin CR: 17.0 mm	**46** Loss of villi Smooth chorion forms	**47** Genital tubercle Urogenital membrane Anal membrane ♀ or ♂	**48** Stage 19 begins Trunk elongating and straightening	**49** CR: 18 mm
8	**50** Upper limbs longer and bent at elbows Fingers distinct	**51** Anal membrane perforated Urogenital membrane degenerating Testes and ovaries distinguishable	**52** Stage 21 begins	**53** Stage 21 External genitals still in sexless state but have begun to differentiate	**54** Stage 22 begins Genital tubercle Urethral groove Anus ♀ or ♂	**55** Beginnings of all essential external and internal structures are present	**56** Stage 23 CR: 30 mm
9	**57** Beginning of fetal period	**58**	**59** Genitals show some ♀ characteristics but still easily confused with ♂	**60** Phallus Urogenital fold Labioscrotal fold Perineum ♀	**61** Genitals show fusion of urethral folds Urethral groove extends into phallus	**62** Phallus Urogenital fold Labioscrotal fold Perineum ♂	**63** CR: 50 mm
10	**64** Face has human profile Note growth of chin compared to day 44	**65**	**66** Face has human appearance	**67** Clitoris Labium minus Urogenital groove Labium majus ♀	**68** Genitals have ♀ or ♂ characteristics but still not fully formed	**69** Glans penis Urethral groove Scrotum ♂	**70** CR: 61 mm

11 12 16 20 24 28 32 36 38 Full term

FIGURE 9-6, cont'd
For legend see opposite page.

9-33 The average period of gestation is about 266 days from the date of fertilization, but it is clinically considered to last 280 days from the first day of the last menstrual period (LMP). The expected date of delivery (EDD) is usually calculated on the latter basis. Termination of pregnancy before the fetus is capable of survival outside the uterus is an abortion. In lay language, a spontaneous or natural loss of the fetus is called a miscarriage, and abortion most often refers to a deliberate interruption of pregnancy. In the medical sense, both spontaneous loss and deliberate interruption of pregnancy are called abortion.

abortion

A miscarriage is a spontaneous _____.

fetography
(fe-tog′rə-fe)

9-34 The combining form *fet(o)* refers to fetus. Write a word that means radiology of the fetus in utero: _____.

fetoscope
(fe′to-skōp)

9-35 An endoscope for viewing the fetus in utero is a _____. A more common use of the term *fetoscope* is a special type of stethoscope used for monitoring the fetal heart beat through the mother's abdominal wall.

fetoscopy
(fe-tos′kə-pe)

The process of monitoring the fetal heart beat through the mother's abdominal wall is called

_____.

fetal monitor

9-36 Looking again at the information in Figure 9-6, see how early the heart begins to beat. Fetal heart beats are detectable early in pregnancy by auscultation, fetoscopy, or an electronic fetal monitor (EFM). The former is performed using the stethoscope. The latter is a device that provides information about the fetal heart rate (FHR). It may be used during prenatal visits to the doctor and during labor, when it also gives information about uterine contractions. The EFM may be applied either internally or externally. EFM means an electronic _____ _____.

9-37 Additional diagnostic techniques are used to assess the status of a developing fetus in utero.* Ultrasound imaging can be used to follow fetal growth and detect structural abnormalities (Figure 9-7). It often reveals the gender of the fetus.

Sometimes amnio/centesis (am″ne-o-sen-te′sis) is performed. Amniocentesis is surgical puncture of the amnion, the thin membrane that lies next to the fetus.

puncture

Amnio/centesis is surgical _____ of the amnion (am′ne-on).

Sometimes this is done to remove and study the amniotic fluid. The fluid may be cultured or studied chemically or cytologically to detect genetic disorders or fetal problems. One genetic disorder that can be detected by study of the amniotic fluid is Down syndrome. Patients with Down syndrome have an extra chromosome, usually number 21 or 22, and have moderate to severe mental retardation. This chromosomal aberration, also called trisomy 21 (tri- means three), is most often associated with late maternal age.

pregnancy

9-38 The suffix *-cyesis* means pregnancy. Pseudo/cyesis (soo″do-si-e′sis) is a term for false

_____.

The prefix *pseudo-* means false.

pseudocyesis

A condition in which the patient has signs and symptoms that suggest pregnancy, such as absence of menstruation, but is not pregnant is called _____. (This is also called pseudopregnancy.)

outside the usual place

9-39 Whenever a fertilized egg implants anywhere other than the uterus, this is an ectopic (ek-top′ik) pregnancy. The prefix *ecto-* means situated on or outside. The combining form top(o) refers to place. When ecto- and top(o) are combined, as in ectopic, it means outside the usual place. Where does the fertilized egg implant in an ectopic pregnancy? _____

ectopic

If the egg implants in a uterine tube, we call this a tubal pregnancy, or an _____ pregnancy.

*(Latin: *in utero,* within the uterus.)

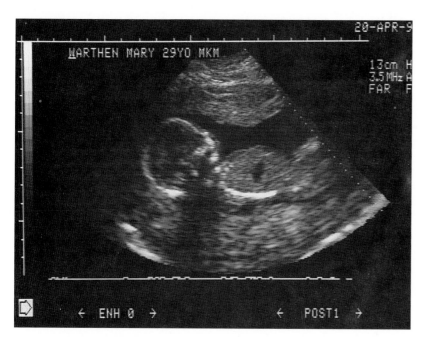

FIGURE 9-7
Ultrasound of fetus. Utilizing sound waves at high frequency, ultrasound imaging provides two-dimensional images of internal organs. (From Gerdin J: *Health careers today,* ed 2, St Louis, 1996, Mosby.)

TABLE 9-4   Complications of Pregnancy

TYPE OF COMPLICATION	MEANING
Abruptio placentae	Separation of the placenta from the uterine wall after 20 weeks or more or during labor, yet the fetus is implanted in a normal position.
Placenta previa	A condition in which the placenta is implanted abnormally in the uterus so that it impinges on or covers the internal os (opening at the upper end) of the uterine cervix.
Preeclampsia	A condition characterized by the onset of acute hypertension after the twenty-fourth week of gestation. The hypertension is often accompanied by proteinuria and edema. Preeclampsia may progress to the more severe form of pregnancy-induced hypertension, eclampsia, and can lead to convulsions and death if untreated.
Stillbirth	The birth of a fetus that died before or during delivery. A fetus that would usually have been expected to live but dies before or during delivery is also called a stillbirth.

---

outside

9-40 The prefix extra- also means outside. An ectopic pregnancy could also be called an extra/uterine pregnancy, meaning implantation of a fertilized egg outside the uterus.

Extrauterine means pertaining to _____ the uterus.

Ectopic pregnancy implantation sites include various places in the uterine tube, the ovary, the cervix, and the abdominal cavity. Ultrasound and radiography are important in diagnosing these abnormal pregnancies, and surgery is generally performed to remove the embryo or fetus, which seldom survives.

9-41 Four complications of pregnancy are summarized in Table 9-4.

placenta previa

Compare abruptio placentae (**ab-rup′she-o plə-sen′te**) and placenta previa (**pre′ve-ə**). In which condition is the fetus implanted too low in the uterus? _____ _____ (Figure 9-8)

eclampsia

Preeclampsia (**pre″e-klamp′se-ə**) is marked by acute hypertension. It may progress to a more severe form called _____, which can be life threatening.

FIGURE 9-8
Comparison of two complications of pregnancy.
A, Abruptio placentae. Separation of the placenta implanted in a normal position after 20 weeks or more before delivery of the fetus. This causes severe maternal hemorrhage that may be evident externally (as shown in this example), or the hemorrhage may be concealed within the uterus. **B,** Placenta previa. Abnormal implantation of the placenta too low in the uterus. Even slight dilation of the cervical opening can cause separation of an abnormally implanted placenta. This is the most common cause of painless bleeding in the third trimester.

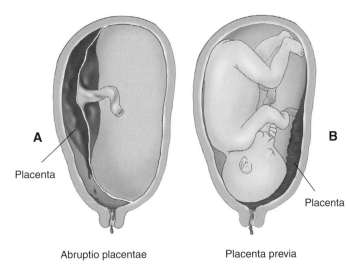

A   B

Placenta   Placenta

Abruptio placentae   Placenta previa

pregnant pregnant female second gravida III	**9-42** Gravid (**grav′id**) means pregnant, and gravida refers to a pregnant female. If a female is gravid, she is _____. Gravida (**grav′ĭ-də**) refers to a _____ _____. The female may be identified more specifically as gravida I, if pregnant for the first time, or gravida II, if pregnant for the _____ time. A designation for a female who has been pregnant three times is _____.
first pregnant	**9-43** The suffix *-gravida* refers to a pregnant female (with a specified number of pregnancies). The prefix *primi-* means first. A primi/gravida (**pri″mĭ-grav′ĭ-də**) is a female during her _____ pregnancy. This is the same as gravida I. The prefix *multi-* means many. Multi/gravida (**mul″tĭ-grav′ĭ-də**) means a female who has been _____ more than one time.
offspring	**9-44** A term that is used for a female who has produced viable offspring is *para*. A viable offspring is defined as one that has reached a stage of development that it can live outside the uterus and usually means a fetus that weighs at least 500 g (just over 1 lb) and has reached a gestational age of 20 weeks (22 weeks after fertilization). The term is used with numerals to indicate the number of pregnancies carried to more than 20 weeks' gestation, such as para III, indicating three pregnancies, regardless of the number of offspring produced in a single pregnancy or the number of stillbirths after 20 weeks. The combining form *par(o)* means producing or bearing viable offspring. Par/ous (**par′əs**) refers to producing viable _____.
para I para I para III	**9-45** The suffix *-para* refers to a female who has produced viable offspring. Determine the designation, para I, para II, or para III, for the following females. In each case, the pregnancies lasted more than 20 weeks. What is the para designation for a female who has one living child and has had no other pregnancies? _____ What is the para status of a female who has twins and has had no other pregnancies? _____ What is the para status of a female who has four children that resulted from three pregnancies and has had no additional pregnancies? _____

one	**9-46** A female who is designated as para I is also called a primi/para (**pri-mip′ə-rə**), which means that she has produced _____ viable offspring. (The number is implied from the prefix *primi-,* which means first.)
three	Since the number or prefix indicates how many pregnancies, a multiple birth counts as just one in the calculation. Secundipara* (**se″kən-dip′ə-rə**), or para II, designates that she has had two pregnancies that produced viable offspring. Additional successful pregnancies are designated as tripara (**trip′ə-rə**) for _____, and quadripara (**kwod-rip′ə-rə**) for four successful pregnancies. The prefix *quadri-* means four.
zero	The prefix *nulli-* refers to none. How many viable offspring have been produced by a nulli/para (**nə-lip′ə-rə**)? _____
many	This is the same as para 0. Translated literally, multi/para (**məl-tip′ə-rə**) has produced _____ (more than one).
parturition	**9-47** Parturition (**pahr″tu-ri′shən**) refers to childbirth, and labor is the process by which the child is expelled from the uterus. Labor is that time from the beginning of cervical dilation to the delivery of the placenta. Look closely at the term *dilation* and its three-syllable pronunciation: (**di-la′shən**). A synonym for dilation is dilatation (**dil″ə-ta′shən**). Both of the terms are derived from the same Latin root as the more familiar term *dilate.* Write the term that means childbirth: _____.
cervical	**9-48** Labor may be divided into three (or sometimes four) stages: cervical dilatation, expulsion, placental, and postpartum stages (Figure 9–9). Not everyone recognizes the postpartum stage as a stage of labor, since it occurs after childbirth. The first stage (cervical dilatation) begins with the onset of regular uterine contractions and ends when the _____ opening is completely dilated.
expulsion	The second stage (expulsion) extends from the end of the first stage until complete _____ of the infant. During this stage, the amniotic sac ruptures if that has not occurred already.
placenta	The third stage (placental) extends from the expulsion of the child until what structure and the membranes are expelled? _____ (The placenta is also called the afterbirth.)
	The fourth stage (postpartum) is the hour or two after delivery, when uterine tone is established. Post/partum means after childbirth because the prefix *post-* means after.
	Study Figure 9-9 and try to determine the stage of labor for each drawing. The fourth and final stage of labor is not shown. Notice how the fetal head turns in order to pass through the vaginal opening.
effacement	**9-49** Dilatation is the condition of being dilated or stretched beyond the normal dimensions. Cervical dilatation is the dilation or stretching of the cervical opening. The shortening and thinning of the cervix during labor is called effacement (**e-fās′mənt**). This term describes how the constrictive neck of the uterus is obliterated or effaced.
	Shortening and thinning of the cervix during labor is called _____. When this occurs, the mucus plug that fills the cervical canal dislodges.

*Secundipara (Latin: *secundus,* following, *parere,* to bring forth).

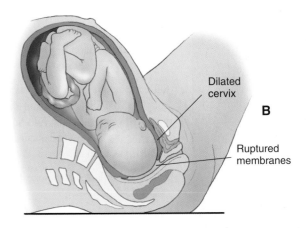

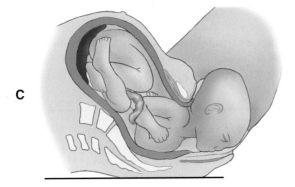
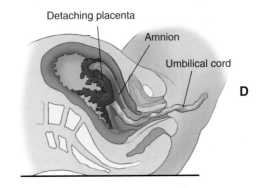

FIGURE 9-9
The fetus in utero before labor compared with three stages of labor. **A,** The normal position of the fetus shortly before labor begins. **B,** The first stage of labor (cervical dilatation) begins with the onset of regular uterine contractions and ends when the cervical opening is completely dilated. **C,** The second stage (expulsion) results in expulsion of the infant. **D,** The third stage (placental) ends when the placenta and membranes are expelled. A fourth stage (not shown) is sometimes identified as the hour or two after delivery, when uterine tone is established.

9-50 Fetal presentation describes the part of the fetus that is touched by the examining finger through the cervix or has entered the mother's pelvis during labor. The normal fetal presentation is cephalic, which means that the top of the head, the brow, the face, or the chin presents itself at the cervical opening during labor. To help you remember cephalic presentation, remember the meaning of cephalic, which is pertaining to the _____.

head

A breech presentation is one in which the buttocks or feet are presented. It occurs in approximately 3% of labors. Since the head is generally larger than the rest of the body, it may become trapped. If the buttocks or feet are felt by the examining finger during labor, it is called _____ presentation.

breech

Shoulder presentation is one in which the shoulder is presented at the cervical opening. This type of presentation, also called transverse presentation, almost always requires turning the fetus in utero or a cesarean section, a surgical procedure in which the abdomen and uterus are incised and the baby is removed. Compare the different types of presentations shown in Figure 9-10.

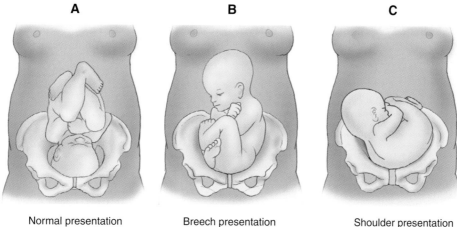

A   B   C

Normal presentation   Breech presentation   Shoulder presentation

FIGURE 9-10
Fetal presentation. **A,** Cephalic presentation, the normal presentation of the top of the head, the brow, the face, or the chin at the cervical opening. **B,** Breech presentation. **C,** Shoulder presentation.

abdominal wall **laparorrhaphy** (lap″ə-ror′ə-fe)	**9-51** A laparotomy (**lap″ə-rot′ə-me**) is necessary in cesarean sections and in all other abdominal surgeries that require opening of the abdominal cavity. Since ***lapar(o)*** means abdominal wall, laparo/tomy is incision of the _____ _____. If the abdominal wall is incised, it must be sutured (or stapled). Suturing of the abdominal wall is _____.
before **before birth** **parturition** **(childbirth)** **postpartum** **(or post partum)** **behind**	**9-52** You have learned that the prefix *pre-* means _____. Another prefix, ***ante-,*** also means before. Prenatal and ante/natal both refer to the time _____ _____. The prefix *ante-* is not always joined to the word, and sometimes there are two acceptable ways to write the same word. Either antepartum (**an″te-pahr′təm**) or ante partum is acceptable and means before _____. Write a term that means after childbirth: _____. Remember that post- also means behind, so postuterine means _____ the uterus.
birth **neonatologist** (ne″o-na′tol′ə-jist)	**9-53** Postnatal refers to the newborn and means the time after _____. Neo/natal (**ne-o-na′təl**) is a more specific term and refers to the period of time covering the first 28 days after birth. The prefix ***neo-*** means new. A neonate (**ne′o-nāt**) is a newborn child. Neonatology (**ne″o-na-tol′ə-je**) is the branch of medicine that specializes in the care of the newborn. Write the term for a physician who specializes in neonatology: _____.

❏ SECTION C REVIEW 𝒫regnancy and Childbirth

This section review covers frames 9–32 through 9–53. Complete the table by writing a word part or its meaning in each blank.

Combining Form	Meaning		Prefix	Meaning
1. _____	fetus		9. post-	_____
2. _____	birth		10. primi-	_____
3. _____	producing viable offspring		11. pseudo-	_____
			12. quadri-	_____
Prefix	**Meaning**		**Suffix**	**Meaning**
4. _____	situated on or outside		13. -cyesis	_____
5. _____	many		14. -gravida	_____
6. ante-, pre-	_____		15. -para	_____
7. neo-	_____			
8. nulli-	_____			

(Use Appendix V to check your answers.)

𝒢ynecologic Diagnosis, Pathology, and Treatment

SECTION D

Gynecologic and obstetric problems account for one fifth of all female visits to physicians. Annual gynecologic examinations are recommended for most adult females. Many diagnostic procedures and treatments are available to females with gynecologic disorders.

---

vaginal

speculum

9-54 The physical assessment of the female reproductive system includes examination of the breasts, the external genitalia, and the pelvis. A vaginal speculum (**spek′u-ləm**) is placed in the vagina and is used to view the cervix in a pelvic examination (Figure 9-11).

A speculum is an instrument for examining body orifices (openings) or cavities. A speculum that is used to examine the vagina is a _____ speculum.

A vaginal speculum is simply an instrument that can be pushed apart after it is inserted into the vagina to allow examination of the vagina and cervix. Write the word for this instrument: _____.

---

cells

9-55 Several specimens for cytology can be collected during the pelvic examination. Cyto/logy means the study of _____.

Cells of the cervix can be examined or cultured to detect vaginal infections with yeast, bacteria, or *Trichomonas,* a vaginal and urethral parasite. In addition, a Pap smear is performed to detect cancer of the cervix.

Pap smear

9-56 Pap smear is an abbreviated way of saying Papanicolaou smear or test. In a Pap smear, material is collected from areas of the body that shed cells. The cells are then studied microscopically. A shortened way of saying Papanicolaou smear is _____ _____.

The term *Pap smear* may refer to collection of material from other surfaces that shed cells, but it usually refers to collection and examination of cells from the vagina and cervix. Early diagnosis of cancer of the cervix is possible with the Pap test. When the Pap smear is examined, malignant cells have a characteristic appearance and indicate cancer, sometimes before symptoms appear.

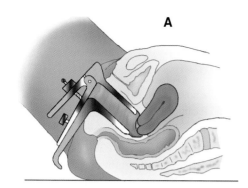

A

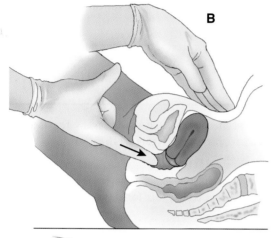

B

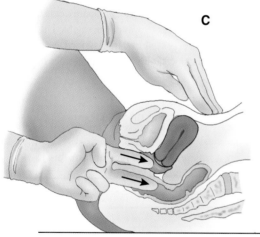

C

FIGURE 9-11

The gynecologic examination. **A,** Proper position of inserted speculum. **B,** The bimanual examination. The abdominal hand presses the pelvic organs toward the intravaginal hand. **C,** Rectovaginal examination. The examiner's index finger is placed in the vagina and the middle finger is inserted into the rectum. The gynecologic inspection consists of four parts: (1) Inspection of the external genitalia. (2) The speculum examination. The vaginal walls and cervix are inspected. Smears (Pap smear, for cytologic examination) are obtained. (3) Bimanual examination assesses the location, size, and mobility of the pelvic organs. (4) The rectovaginal examination is not always performed. In this examination, the posterior aspect of the genital organs and rectal tissue can be evaluated.

---

dysplasia

9-57 Cancer of the uterus may begin with a change in shape, growth, and number of cells, called dysplasia (**dis-pla′zhə**). The dysplasia is not cancer, but cells of this type tend to become malignant. This abnormality, which can be detected before cancer occurs, is called _____. The suffix *-plasia* means development or formation. Dysplasia means abnormal (bad) development. It is standard practice to grade Pap smears as class I, II, III, IV, or V. Class I is normal, and class V is definitely cancer. Most physicians recommend having Pap smears done on a routine basis.

If cancer of the cervix is detected in its early stage and treated, the prognosis* is quite good. Prognosis is prediction of the probable outcome of a disease. A word that means predicting the outcome of a disease is

prognosis

_____.

*Prognosis (Greek: foreknowledge).

colposcope (kol′po-skōp) cervix uterus	**9-58** Colposcopy (**kol-pos′kə-pe**) involves the use of a low-powered microscope to magnify the mucosa of the vagina and the cervix. The instrument used is a _____. Suspicious cervical or vaginal lesions may be seen during colposcopy. Some findings indicate the need for a cervical or endometrial biopsy. A cervical biopsy is removal of tissue from the _____. An endometrial biopsy requires collection of tissue from the lining of the _____.
	9-59 Regular Pap smears are an excellent method for early detection of cervical cancer, and it is possible that the lesion can be excised, thus preventing spread of cancer to nearby organs. Various treatments are used depending on the amount of dysplasia and may include cautery,* cryotherapy, and irradiation. Cautery (**kaw′tər-e**) is applying a caustic substance, a hot instrument, an electric current, or other agent to destroy tissue. Cryo/therapy (**kri″o-ther′ə-pe**) is a treatment that uses an extremely cold temperature to destroy tissue. The combining form **cry(o)** means cold, and **-therapy** is a suffix that means treatment. Irradiation uses radiant energy to destroy cancer cells.
removed	**9-60** Cancer can occur in any of the reproductive structures and spread to nearby organs. The stage of cancer is identified by the extent to which it has spread to other organs (Figure 9-12). Early removal of cancerous tissue is vital for preventing the spread of cancer. Removal of the uterus is also commonly performed for benign uterine tumors, sometimes called fibroids. Symptoms and treatment of fibroids vary widely. When a hyster/ectomy (**his″tər-ek′tə-me**) is performed, the uterus is _____.
vagina abdominal uterus, abdominal wall	**9-61** A hysterectomy is performed in one of three ways: abdominally, vaginally, or laparoscopically. A colpo/hyster/ectomy (**kol″po-his″tər-ek′tə-me**) is removal of the uterus by way of the vagina. This is also called a vaginal hysterectomy. Obstetrical and gynecological surgical procedures are classified as abdominal, vaginal, or laparoscopic. In a colpohysterectomy, an abdominal incision is not required, since the uterus is removed through the _____. An abdominal hysterectomy is removal of the uterus through an incision in the _____ wall. In a total abdominal hysterectomy (TAH), the uterus, the cervix, the uterine tubes, and the ovaries are removed through an abdominal incision. In a few cases, the uterus can be removed laparoscopically. A laparo/hyster/ectomy (**lap″ə-ro-his″tə-rek′tə-me**) is removal of the _____ through a small opening in the _____ _____.
ovaries, uterus	**9-62** Oophoro/hyster/ectomy is removal of the _____ and the _____. If the uterus and the ovaries are removed, the uterine tube is also removed. In an oophorohysterectomy, it is understood that the uterine tube is removed also; however, if one wanted to include all of these terms in one word, the word would be oophoro/salpingo/hyster/ectomy (**o-of″ə-ro-sal-ping″go-his″tər-ek′tə-me**).

*Cautery (Greek: *Kauterion*, branding iron).

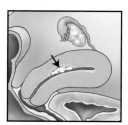

Stage I

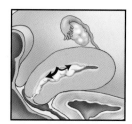

Stage II

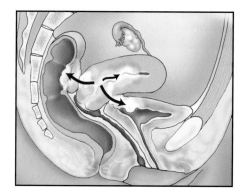

Stage III

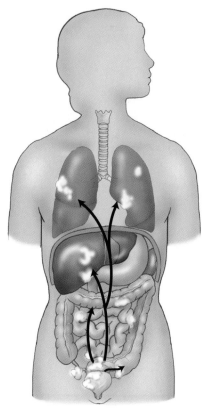

Stage IV

FIGURE 9-12
Staging uterine cancer. *Stage I:* Tumor is confined to the uterine corpus. *Stage II:* The cancer has invaded the cervix also. *Stage III:* The cancer has spread beyond the uterus but remains confined to the pelvis, such as in the bladder or rectum. *Stage IV:* The highest level of invasiveness; the cancer has spread beyond the pelvis, causing metastatic disease and large masses, such as in the liver or lungs. (From Polaski AL, Tatro SE: *Luckmann's core principles and practice of medical-surgical nursing,* Philadelphia, 1996, WB Saunders.)

---

oophorectomy
(o"of-ə-rek'tə-me)

without
oophorosalpingec-tomy
(o-of"ə-ro-sal"pin-jek'tə-me)
removal of a uterine tube and an ovary

9-63 Ovarian cancer is the leading cause of death from reproductive cancers because the disease has usually spread to other organs by the time it is discovered (Figure 9-13). Using oophor(o), write a term that means removal of the ovaries: _____.

Benign ovarian tumors may also be removed surgically, either using a laparoscope or open (abdominal) surgery. Ovarian cysts, globular sacs filled with fluid or semisolid material, are common and may be asymptomatic, or they may cause pelvic pain and menstrual irregularities. If a female is a/symptomatic, this means that she is _____ symptoms.

Build a word using oophor(o), the combining form for uterine tube, and the suffix for excision: _____. This is the same as salpingo-oophorectomy.

The word that you just wrote means _____.

Removal of an adult female's ovaries prohibits reproduction and prevents further production of ovarian hormones. Oophorectomy in a girl who has not reached puberty prevents development of secondary sex characteristics.

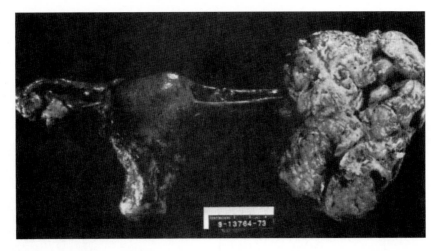

FIGURE 9-13
Carcinoma of the ovary. The specimen consists of the uterus with both uterine tubes and ovaries. The left ovary is enormously enlarged by a tumor; the right ovary shows a white area that also contains a tumor. Note the asymmetry of the body of the uterus (a congenital abnormality in this patient that is not related to ovarian carcinoma). (From Walter JB: *An introduction to the principles of disease,* ed 2, Philadelphia, 1982, WB Saunders.)

colpectomy (kol-pek′tə-me) **vaginectomy** (vaj″ĭ-nek′tə-me) **vulvectomy** (vəl-vek′tə-me)	**9-64** Vaginal and vulvar cancer are not common and occur mainly in women older than 50 years. Using colp(o) and vagin(o), write two terms, both meaning the removal of all or a part of the vagina: _____ and _____. (In vaginal cancer, this surgical procedure may be part of a radical hysterectomy—removal of ovaries, uterine tubes, lymph nodes, and lymph channels, as well as the uterus and cervix). Write a word that means removal of all or part of the vulva: _____.
laparoscope (lap′ə-ro-skōp″)	**9-65** Laparoscopy (**lap″ə-ros′kə-pe**) is abdominal examination using an endoscope. Build a word using lapar(o) for an instrument used in laparoscopy: _____. In addition to inspection of the ovaries and uterine tubes and identification of unexplained pelvic masses, this procedure is used for surgical procedures such as tubal ligation, ovarian biopsy, and in a few cases, removal of the uterus (Figure 9-14).
cervix **endometrium**	**9-66** A common surgical procedure that is performed for either diagnosis or treatment is dilation and curettage (**ku″rə-tahzh′**) (D & C). In this procedure, the cervix is dilated to allow the insertion of a curet into the uterus. The curet is a surgical instrument shaped like a spoon or scoop and is used for scraping and removal of material from the endometrium. In this procedure, called D & C, what structure is dilated? _____ What structure is scraped? _____ This surgical procedure is done to assess disease of the uterus, to correct heavy or prolonged vaginal bleeding, or to empty uterine contents of placental residue after childbirth.

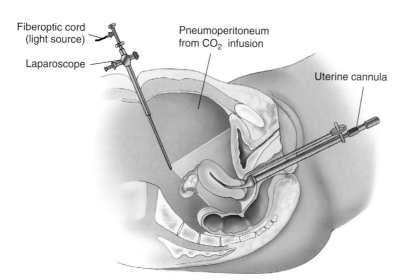

FIGURE 9-14

Laparoscopy. Using the laparoscope with fiberoptic light source, the surgeon can view the pelvic cavity and the reproductive organs. Further instrumentation, for example, for tubal sterilization, is possible through a second small incision. The purpose of the uterine cannula is to allow movement of the uterus during laparoscopy.

Fiberoptic cord (light source)

Laparoscope

Pneumoperitoneum from CO_2 infusion

Uterine cannula

---

menorrhea (men″o-re′ə)	**9-67** Menstrual disorders include painful menstruation, heavy or irregular flow, spotting, absence of or skipping periods, and premenstrual syndrome. Build a word by combining men(o) and -rrhea (flow or discharge): _____.
menstruation menses	Menorrhea means either normal menstruation or too profuse menstruation. Because of the double meaning of menorrhea, it would be clearer to use either of the following terms to mean the normal monthly flow of blood from the genital tract: _____ or _____.
menorrhagia (men″o-ra′jə)	The second meaning of menorrhea is profuse menstruation. Build a word that is a synonym for this meaning by using the combining form for month and the suffix for hemorrhage: _____.
	Menorrhagia is excessive bleeding at the time of a menstrual period, in the number of days, the amount of blood, or both.
hemorrhage of the uterus	**9-68** Metrorrhagia (me″tro-ra′je-ə) is uterine bleeding that occurs at completely irregular intervals, the period of flow sometimes being prolonged. The literal translation of metro/rrhagia is

_____.

Metrorrhagia may occur as spotting or outright bleeding, and is uterine bleeding other than that caused by menstruation. |
absence	**9-69** A/menorrhea is _____ of menstruation.
amenorrhea	Amenorrhea (ə-men″o-re′ə) is normal before puberty, after menopause, and during pregnancy. Underdevelopment of the reproductive organs or hormonal disturbances can cause absence of the onset of menstruation at puberty. This absence of menstruation is called _____.
	When menstruation has begun but then ceases, this is also called amenorrhea.
menstruation	Dys/menorrhea (dis-men″ə-re′ə) is painful or difficult _____.
premenstrual	**9-70** Premenstrual syndrome (PMS) is nervous tension, irritability, edema, headache, and painful breasts that can occur the last few days before the onset of menstruation. Various studies indicate that many females experience some degree of PMS but less than half experience symptoms that disrupt their lives. PMS means _____ syndrome.

9-71 In the next two frames, practice using oophor(o) to write several diagnostic and surgical terms pertaining to the ovaries.

pain in an ovary

Oophor/algia (o″of-ər-al′jə) is _____.

Oophoralgia is also called ovarian pain.

ovary

Oophoro/genous (o of″ə-roj′ə-nəs) means derived from or originating in the _____.

oophoritis
(o″of-ə-ri′tis)

Inflammation of an ovary is _____.

oophoropathy
(o-of″ə-rop′ə-the)

Any disease of an ovary is an _____.

9-72 Using oophor(o), write a word that means surgical fixation to correct an ovary that has lost its normal support: _____.

oophoropexy
(o-of′ə-ro-pek″se)

ovary

Oophoro/salping/itis (o-of″ə-ro-sal″pin-ji′tis) is inflammation of an _____ and a uterine tube.

9-73 Write words for the following:

salpingectomy
(sal″pin-jek′tə-me)

Excision of a uterine tube: _____

salpingopexy
(sal-ping′go-pek″se)

Surgical fixation of a uterine tube: _____

salpingorrhaphy
(sal″ping-gor′rə-fe)

Suture of a uterine tube: _____

9-74 A tubal ligation (lĭ-ga′shən) is one of several sterilization procedures in which both uterine tubes are constricted, severed, or crushed to prevent conception. The procedure originally involved the use of a ligature (a substance that tied or constricted), hence its name. This is now most often performed laparoscopically. Tubal ligation can be reversed in some cases by making a new opening to restore patency (condition of being open), but this is not always successful. Write a word that means making a new opening into a uterine tube: _____.

salpingo/stomy
(sal″ping-gos′tə-me)

Salpingostomy may be performed also for the purpose of drainage if a uterine tube is obstructed by infection or scar tissue.

9-75 Salpingo/cele (sal-ping′go-sēl) is hernial protrusion of a _____

uterine tube

_____.

Inflammation of a uterine tube is _____.

salpingitis
(sal″pin-ji′tis)

The uterine tubes are usually infected in pelvic inflammatory disease (PID). Without treatment, the uterine tubes can become obstructed and cause infertility. Pelvic inflammatory disease is any infection that involves the upper genital tract beyond the cervix. Untreated gonococcal or staphylococcal infections, for example, can spread along the endometrium to the uterine tubes and cause an acute salpingitis. If untreated or treated inadequately, the tubes can become obstructed. PID means _____ inflammatory disease.

pelvic

Septicemia and other severe complications rarely occur in PID as they do in toxic shock syndrome (TSS). A sudden high fever, headache, confusion, acute renal failure, and abnormal liver function are characteristic of TSS. This acute disease is caused by a type of staphylococcus and is most common in menstruating women who use tampons.

A

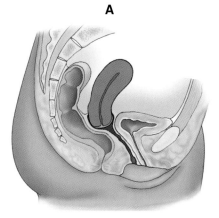

Grade I uterine prolapse

B

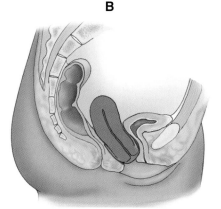

Grade II uterine prolapse

C

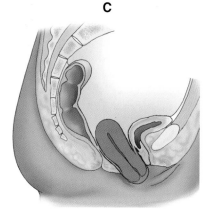

Grade III uterine prolapse

FIGURE 9-15

Three stages of uterine prolapse of increasing severity. Uterine prolapse may be congenital or may be caused by heavy physical exertion or other situations that weaken the pelvic supports. **A,** The uterus bulges into the vagina but does not protrude through the entrance. **B,** The uterus bulges farther into the vagina and the cervix protrudes through the entrance. **C,** The body of the uterus and the cervix protrude through the entrance to the vagina.

uterus, uterine **hysterosalpin-** **gogram** (his"tər-o-sal"ping′ go-gram)	**9-76** Hystero/salpingo/graphy (**his"tər-o-sal"pin-gog′rə-fe**) is radiological examination of the _____ and the _____ tubes after an injection of radiopaque material into those organs. Write the name of the record that is produced in hysterosalpingography: _____.
hysteropathy (his"tə-rop′ə-the) **hysteroscopy** (his"tər-os′kə-pe)	**9-77** Use hyster(o) in the next two frames to build words pertaining to the uterus. Write a word that means any disease of the uterus: _____. Write another word that means inspection of the uterus (using an endoscope): _____. Hysteroscopy is performed for several reasons, including the excision of cervical polyps, the collection of tissue for biospy, or removal of an intrauterine device. The hysteroscope is passed through the vagina and into the uterus.
hysteroptosis (his"tər-op-to′sis) **hysteropexy** (his′tər-o-pek-se)	**9-78** The uterus is normally held in its proper alignment with the vagina and the uterine tubes by ligaments that hold each structure in its proper place. Weakening of the ligaments causes a prolapsed uterus. Using -ptosis, write a word that means uterine prolapse: _____. A prolapsed uterus can be congenital or caused by heavy physical exertion. It is classified according to its severity (Figure 9-15). Build a word that means surgical fixation of a displaced uterus by adding -pexy to the combining form for uterus: _____. Laparo/hystero/pexy (**lap"ə-ro-his′tər-o-pek-se**) means fixation of the uterus to the abdominal wall. The uterus normally lies midline in the pelvis; however, some variations, called uterine displacements, occur (Figure 9-16). Mild degrees of these four types of displacements are common, may or may not cause symptoms, and may be determined by the position of the cervix when the pelvic examination is performed.

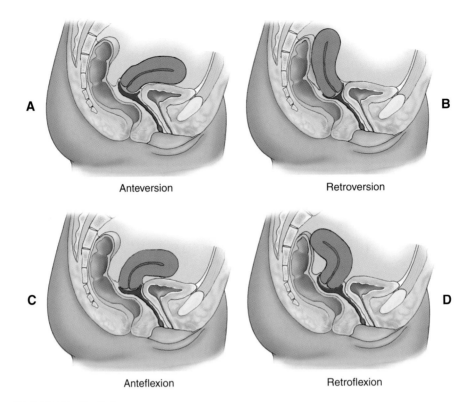

Anteversion

Retroversion

Anteflexion

Retroflexion

FIGURE 9-16
Normal versus abnormal (forward or backward) displacements of the uterus. **A,** anteversion, forward displacement of the body of the uterus toward the pubis, with the cervix tilted up; **B,** retroversion, tipped backward, the opposite of anteversion; **C,** anteflexion, bending forward; **D,** retroflexion, bending backward.

vagina, vaginal	**9-79** You learned that colp(o) means vagina. Colp/itis **(kol-pi′tis)** is inflammation of the _____. Colpitis means the same as _____ inflammation or irritation. This is more commonly called vaginitis.
vulva **vagina**	Vulvovaginitis **(vul″vo-vaj″ĭ-ni′tis)** is inflammation of the _____ and the _____.
vagina	**9-80** Colpo/dynia **(kol″po-din′e-ə)** is pain of the _____.
colporrhagia (kol″po-ra′jə)	Use colp(o) to write these words: Using -rrhagia, hemorrhage from the vagina is _____.
colporrhaphy (kol-por′ə-fe)	Using -rrhaphy, suture of the vagina is _____.
colpoplasty (kol′po-plas″te)	Surgical repair of the vagina is _____.

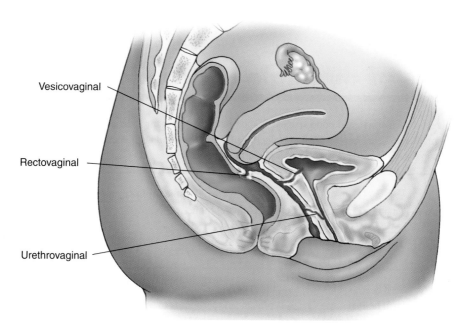

Vesicovaginal

Rectovaginal

Urethrovaginal

FIGURE 9-17
Sites of vaginal fistulas. Abnormal openings between the vagina and the bladder, rectum, and urethra are shown. These abnormal openings are called vesicovaginal fistula, rectovaginal fistula, and urethrovaginal fistula.

urethra	**9-81** Vaginal fistulas are abnormal openings between the vagina and the urethra, the bladder, or the rectum. Urethro/vaginal (**u-re″thro-vag′ĭ-nəl**) fistulas occur between the _____ and the vagina.
rectovaginal (rek′to-vag ĭ-nal)	Using urethrovaginal as a model, write a word to complete this blank: A _____ fistula is one that occurs between the rectum and the vagina.
bladder	Knowing that vesic(o) means bladder, a vesicovaginal (**ves- ĭ-ko-vaj′ĭ-nəl**) fistula occurs between the urinary _____ and the vagina.
	(See the locations of these types of fistulas in Figure 9-17.)

❑ SECTION D REVIEW 𝒢ynecologic Diagnosis, Pathology, and Treatment

This section review covers frames 9–54 through 9–81. Complete the table by writing the meaning of each word part listed.

Combining Form	Meaning	Suffix	Meaning
1. cry(o)	_____	2. -plasia	_____
		3. -therapy	_____

(Use Appendix V to check your answers.)

Structures of the Male Reproductive System

The male reproductive system produces, sustains, and transports sperm; introduces them into the female vagina; and produces hormones. The testes, the male gonads, are responsible for production of both sperm and hormones. All other organs, ducts, and glands in this system transport and sustain the sperm and are considered accessory reproductive organs.

testes	**9-82** The male gonads are the testes (**tes′tēz**), the primary organs of the male reproductive system. A gonad (**go′nad, gon′ad**) produces the reproductive cells. The ovaries are the female gonads. The _____ are the male gonads. Testes is the plural form of testis, which means the same as testicle.
copulation, coitus	**9-83** The penis (**pe′nis**), the male organ for copulation, transfers sperm to the vagina. The combining form *pen(o)* means penis. Pen/ile means pertaining to the penis. Copulation (**kop″u-la′shən**), also called coitus* (**ko′ĭ-tus**), is sexual union between male and female. Write these two terms that mean sexual union between male and female: _____ and _____.
	9-84 Study Figure 9-18 and write the names of the structures in the blank lines as you read the following information. Label the penis, line l. A loose fold of skin, the prepuce (line 2), covers the glans penis (line 3). Circumcision is surgical removal of the end of the prepuce and is commonly performed on the male infant at birth. Figure 9-18 is a midsagittal section, so only one testis is shown. Label the testis (line 4). Sperm leave the testes through ducts that enter the epididymis (**ep″ĭ-did′ə-mis**), a tightly coiled comma-shaped organ located along the superior and posterior margins of the testes. Label the epididymis (line 5). The testes and epididymis are contained in a pouch of skin that is posterior to the penis. This pouch of skin is called the scrotum (**skro′təm**). Label the scrotum (line 6). Each ductus deferens (line 7), also called the vas deferens, begins at the epididymis, continues upward, then enters the abdominopelvic cavity. Each ductus deferens joins a duct from the seminal vesicle (line 8) to form a short ejaculatory (**e-jak′u-lə-to″re**) duct. Label the ejaculatory duct (line 9), which passes through the prostate (**pros′tāt**) gland and then empties into the urethra. Label the prostate (line 10) and the urethra (line 11). Paired bulbourethral glands contribute an alkaline mucuslike fluid to the semen. Label the bulbourethral gland (line 12). Ejaculation (**e-jak″u-la′shən**) is the expulsion of semen (**se′men**) from the urethra.
scrotal (skro′təl) **testicle** **epididymis**	**9-85** In labeling Figure 9-18, you read that the scrotum is a pouch of loose skin that contains the two testes and their accessory organs. The combining form ***scrot(o)*** means scrotum. Use the suffix -al to write a term that means pertaining to the scrotum: _____. Four combining forms are used to write words about the testes: **orchi(o), orchid(o), test(o),** and **testicul(o).** Testicul/ar (**tes-tik′u-lər**) means pertaining to a _____, but most diagnostic and surgical terms will use either orchi(o) or orchid(o). Practice in later frames will help you remember which combining form to use. The combining form ***epididym(o)*** means epididymis. Epididymitis (**ep″ĭ-did-ə-mi′tis**) is inflammation of the _____.

*Coitus (Latin: *coitio,* a coming together, meeting).

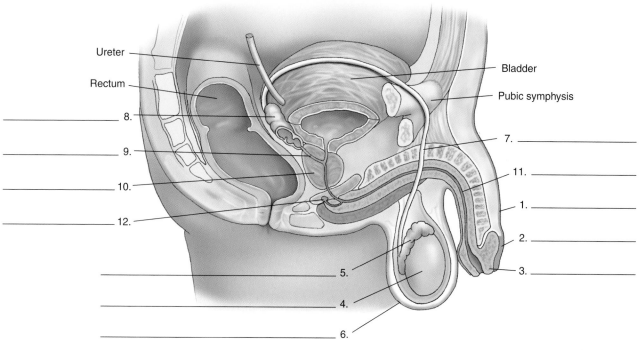

FIGURE 9-18
Structures of the male reproductive system, midsagittal section. The structures that are already labeled lie near, but are not part of, the male reproductive system.

9-86 The ductus deferens is a long duct that begins at the epididymis, enters the abdominal cavity, and connects with other structures of the internal reproductive tract. The combining form for ductus deferens is vas(o), which also means vessel. It will mean the ductus deferens most of the time in this chapter.

The combining form ***prostat(o)*** means the prostate. Using the suffix *-ic*, write a term that means pertaining to the prostate: _____.

The prostate, the seminal vessels, and the bulbourethral glands produce fluids that contribute to the semen and are necessary for the survival of the sperm. Semen is the secretion of the male reproductive organs that is discharged from the urethra during ejaculation.

prostatic
(pros-tat'ik)

☐ SECTION E REVIEW   *S*tructures of the Male Reproductive System

This section review covers from 9–82 through 9–86. Write the combining form or its meaning in each blank.

Combining Form	Meaning	Combining Form	Meaning
1. epididym(o)	_____	5. _____	scrotum
2. orchi(o), orchid(o)	_____	6. test(o), testicul(o)	_____
3. pen(o)	_____	7. vas(o)	_____
4. _____	prostate		

(Use Appendix V to check your answers.)

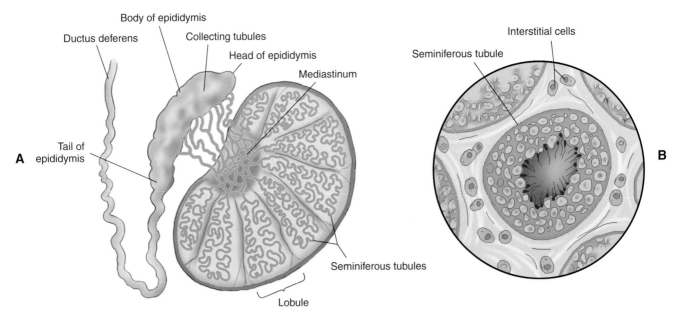

FIGURE 9-19
Sectional view of a testis. **A,** Each testis has about 250 lobules that contain as many as four seminiferous tubes where sperm are produced. **B,** Cross section of a seminiferous tube. The tubule is surrounded by interstitial cells, which are responsible for the production of testosterone.

Testes and Spermatogenesis

Each testis is capable of producing sperm and male hormones. Spermatogenesis is the formation of mature functional sperm capable of participating in conception.

9-87 The testes produce sperm and an important male hormone, testosterone. Sperm production requires a temperature slightly lower than normal body temperature. Because the scrotum is outside the body cavity, it provides the proper environment.

The testes are paired oval glands. Testis or testicle refers to one of these glands. In observing Figure 9-19, *A,* notice that a testis is divided into several compartments called lobules, and each lobule contains convoluted seminiferous tubules. Sperm are produced in these tubules. Lying just posterior to the testis is the epididymis, where sperm are stored until they are released. The duct leading from the epididymis is the

_____ _____.

A cross section of a seminiferous (**sem″ĭ-nif′ər-əs**) tubule (Figure 9-19, *B*) shows that seminiferous tubules are surrounded by cells called interstitial cells of Leydig. These cells produce a major male sex hormone, testosterone (**təs-tos′tə-rōn**).

ductus (vas) deferens

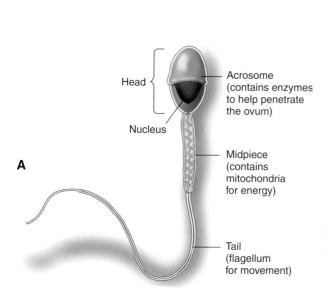

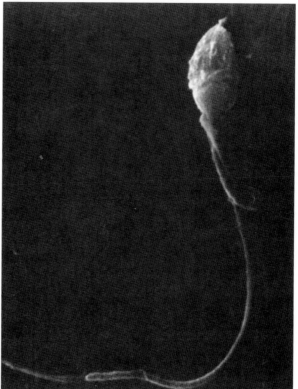

Head — Acrosome
(contains enzymes
to help penetrate
the ovum)

Nucleus

A

Midpiece
(contains
mitochondria
for energy)

Tail
(flagellum
for movement)

B

FIGURE 9-20

The human spermatozoon. **A,** A sperm in cross section. The nucleus contains the chromosomes and is located in the head. The tip of the head is covered by an acrosome, which contains enzymes that help the sperm penetrate the ovum, The midpiece contains mitochondria that provide energy, and the tail is a typical flagellum. **B,** Spermatozoon as seen using a scanning electron microscope. (Courtesy of Fisher Scientific Company.)

---

spermatozoon	**9-88** Sperm are produced within the seminiferous tubes. In the development of mature sperm, early spermatocytes (**sper′mə-to-sīts**) undergo a process called meiosis, which eventually results in mature, functional spermatozoa (Figure 9-20). The singular form of spermatozoa is spermatozoon. Write the singular form of spermatozoa: _____.
	Spermato/genesis (**sper′mə-to-jen′ə-sis**) is the formation of mature functional sperm. The hypothalamus, the pituitary gland, and the testes produce hormones that influence spermatogenesis (Figure 9-21).
testosterone	Follicle-stimulating hormone (FSH) and testosterone produced by the testes stimulate spermatogenesis. Luteinizing hormone (LH) acts on interstitial cells in the testes to produce testosterone. Testosterone also brings about male secondary sex characteristics, for example, enlarging of the sex organs, distribution of hair, deepening of the voice, and increased muscular development. Write the name of this hormone, which is often called the masculinizing hormone: _____.
seminal	**9-89** Spermatogenesis begins at puberty and normally continues throughout life, showing a decline in later years. Semen, also called seminal fluid, is a mixture of sperm cells and secretions from the accessory glands (prostate, seminal vesicles, and bulbourethral glands). The combining form **semin(o)** means semen. Write the other name for semen that uses this combining form: _____ fluid.
	There are usually millions of sperm each time semen is ejaculated, and although only one sperm fertilizes an ovum, it takes millions of sperm to ensure that fertilization will take place.

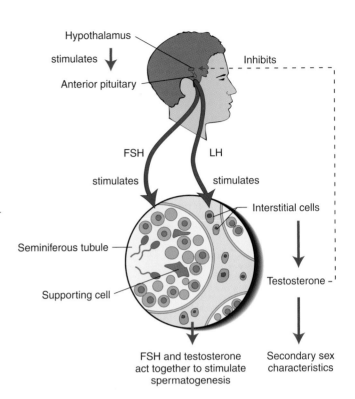

CHAPTER 9

FIGURE 9-21

Hormonal control of the testes. The hypothalamus produces hormones that stimulate the anterior pituitary to produce follicle-stimulating hormone (FSH) and luteinizing hormone (LH). Luteinizing hormone stimulates the interstitial cells of the testes to secrete testosterone. Acting together, FSH and testosterone stimulate spermatogenesis.

hidden
testes

cryptorchidism

9-90 The production of sperm outside the body cavity is necessary for the production of viable sperm. The testes develop in the abdominal cavity of the fetus and normally descend through the inguinal canal into the scrotum shortly before birth (sometimes shortly after birth). This provides a temperature about three degrees below normal body temperature. Cryptorchidism (**krip-tor′kĭ-diz″əm**) is a developmental defect characterized by the failure of one or both testes to descend into the scrotum. The combining form *crypt(o),* means hidden. The "o" in crypt(o) is usually omitted when joined to a combining form that begins with a vowel. Translated literally, crypt/orchid/ism means a condition of _____ _____.

Cryptorchidism is the same as undescended testicle. If the testes do not descend spontaneously or with hormonal injections, surgery is usually performed. Write the word that means the same as undescended testicle: _____.

Orchiopexy (**or″ke-o-pek′se**) is corrective surgery for cryptorchidism. Orchiopexy, sometimes called orchidopexy (**or′kĭ-do-pek″se),** is the attachment of the previously undescended testis to the wall of the scrotum.

❑ SECTION F REVIEW   *T*estes and Spermatogenesis

This section review covers frames 9–87 through 9–90. Write the combining form or its meaning in each blank.

Combining Form	Meaning		Combining Form	Meaning
1. crypt(o)	_____		5. scrot(o)	_____
2. epididym(o)	_____		6. semin(o)	_____
3. orchi(o), orchid(o)	_____		7. test(o), testicul(o)	_____
4. pen(o)	_____			

(Use Appendix V to check your answers.)

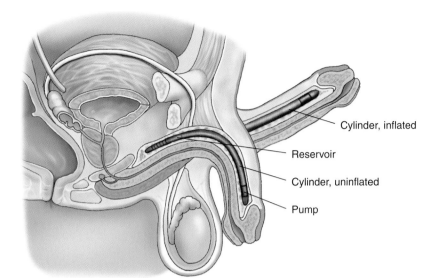

FIGURE 9-22

A penile prosthesis. One of several types of prostheses, this self-contained type consists of a pump, a cylinder filled with fluid, and a reservoir, all in one unit. The patient squeezes the pump just below the head of the penis to fill the cylinder and achieve erection. When an erection is no longer desired, the patient presses a release valve located behind the pump.

Cylinder, inflated

Reservoir

Cylinder, uninflated

Pump

Pathology, Diagnosis, and Treatment of Male Reproductive Structures

SECTION G

Urology is the branch of medicine that specializes in the male and female urinary tract and also includes male reproductive structures. The prostate is frequently affected by benign and malignant neoplasms, particularly in men over 50 years of age. A variety of disorders of the other male reproductive structures are also included.

absence	**9-91** A/spermia and oligo/spermia were discussed earlier in this chapter. Oligo/spermia means insufficient sperm in the semen. A/spermia is _____ of sperm. In addition to sufficient numbers, sperm must be actively motile and live long enough to reach the ovum. There are many causes of infertility besides insufficient sperm, and for this reason, it is best that the two partners are treated together.
penile	**9-92** Erection is the condition of swelling, rigidity, and elevation of the penis, and to a lesser degree in the clitoris of the female, caused by sexual arousal. It can also occur during sleep. Erection is necessary for the introduction of the penis into the vagina and for the emission of semen. The inability to achieve penile erection, alternating periods of normal function and dysfunction, or inability to ejaculate after achieving an erection is called erectile dysfunction, also known as male impotence. Vascular problems and various drugs cause sexual dysfunction. Treatment may include correction of the cause of the problem, such as interference of the flow of blood to the penis, or modifying medications that interfere with sexual activity. Surgical treatment includes injections and the use of penile prostheses **(pros-the′ses).** The term *prosthesis* means an artificial replacement for a body part (for example, an artificial arm or leg) or a device designed to improve function (for example, a hearing aid). The prosthesis that is designed to treat an erectile dysfunction is called a _____ prosthesis (Figure 9-22).

FIGURE 9-23

Vasectomy. This elective surgical procedure is performed as a permanent method of contraception (although it sometimes can be surgically reversed). It is usually performed under local anesthesia. A small incision is made in the scrotum, and a piece of the vas deferens is removed.

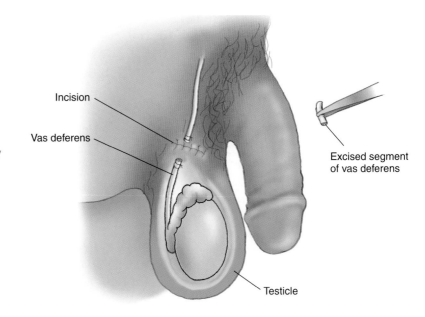

Incision

Vas deferens

Excised segment of vas deferens

Testicle

excision	**9-93** A vas/ectomy is _____ of the vas deferens or a portion of it (Figure 9-23).
	Bilateral vasectomy results in sterility.
	Unlike some combining forms with double meanings, it is not always obvious which meaning is implied by vas(o) in a word. For example, vas/ectomy refers only to excision of
vas deferens	the _____ _____.
incision	**9-94** Vaso/tomy (**va-zot′ə-me**) is _____ of the vas deferens.
vasostomy (va-zos′tə-me)	Write a word that means surgical formation of a new opening into the vas deferens: _____.
surgical anastomosis of the two cut ends of the vas deferens	Formulate a definition of vaso/vaso/stomy (**va″zo-va-zos′tə-me**): _____ _____.
vasovasostomy	Sometimes this surgical procedure is used to restore fertility in males who have had a vasectomy. Write this new word that means formation of new openings in the vas deferens: _____.
suture **scrotum**	**9-95** Vaso/rrhaphy (**vas-or′ə-fe**) is _____ of the vas deferens. In a vasectomy it is necessary to incise the pouch that contains the testes. This pouch is called the _____.
	9-96 It is unclear why the prostate is so frequently affected by benign and malignant neoplasms. Benign prostatic hyperplasia is a common disorder, particularly in men over 50 years of age. Hyperplasia is an increase in the size of an organ resulting from an increase in the number of cells. The condition is not malignant; however, it is usually progressive and may lead to obstruction of the urethra and to interference with urination (Figure 9-24). The increase in the number of cells (hyperplasia) results in prostatic enlargement (hypertrophy), so the condition is commonly known as benign prostatic hypertrophy (**hi-pər′tro-fe**) (BPH). The common name of the disorder that is nonmalignant and results in an enlarged prostate is
prostatic hyperplasia	benign _____ _____.
prostatitis (pros″tə-ti′tis)	Urinary frequency, pain, and urinary tract infections are characteristic of BPH. Inflammation of the prostate may also occur. Write a term that means inflammation of the prostate: _____.

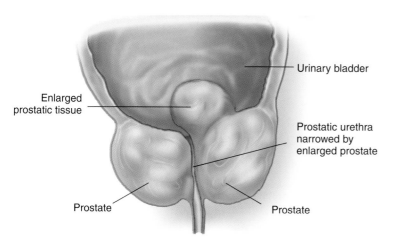

Urinary bladder

Enlarged
prostatic tissue

Prostatic urethra
narrowed by
enlarged prostate

Prostate

Prostate

FIGURE 9-24

Benign prostatic hyperplasia. This nonmalignant enlargement of the prostate is common among men over 50 years of age. As the prostate enlarges, it extends upward into the bladder, and inward, obstructing the outflow of urine from the bladder.

urethra	**9-97** A transurethral resection prostatectomy (TURP) may be necessary to correct the enlarged prostate of BPH. You learned in the last chapter that a transurethral resection is a surgical procedure that is performed through the _____. In a TURP, small pieces of the enlarged prostate are excised.
	9-98 Prostatic carcinoma, cancer of the prostate, also usually occurs after 50 years of age and is the most common cancer among men.
excision	There are several treatments for prostatic (**pros-tat′ik**) carcinoma, including radiation, hormonal therapy, and prostatectomy (**pros″tə-tek′tə-me**). A prostat/ectomy is _____ of all or part of the prostate gland.
testis	Prostatic cancer is more common after 50 years of age, but testicular (**tes-tik′u-lər**) cancer is more common in men between 15 and 35 years of age. Testicul/ar means pertaining to a _____.
excision	Orchiectomy is almost always performed when testicular cancer is suspected. Orchi/ectomy is _____ of the testis. Removal of both testes results in infertility.
	9-99 Several less severe problems occur within the scrotum, including hydrocele, spermatocele, and varicocele.
water	A hydro/cele is a mass, usually filled with a straw-colored fluid. For this reason, its name incorporates the combining form *hydr(o)*, which means _____. In this term, hydr(o) may help you remember that the swelling contains a straw-colored fluid.
sperm	A spermato/cele is a mass that contains _____. This develops on the epididymis. A spermatocele may be asymptomatic and may need no intervention.
orchialgia (or″ke-al′jə) orchidalgia (or″kĭ-dal′jə)	A varico/cele is a cluster of dilated veins that occur above the testis. The combining form **varic(o)** means a varicose vein. In many cases, varicoceles are asymptomatic but may contribute to infertility. Testalgia is testicular pain. Write two other words that mean testicular pain, using orchi(o) and orchid(o): _____ and _____.

orchiopathy (or″ke-op′ə-the)	**9-100** Write words using orchi(o) for the following:
	any disease of the testes: _____
orchiotomy (or″ke-ot′ə-me)	incision (and drainage) of a testis: _____
	Write words using orchid(o):
orchidorrhaphy (or″kĭ-dor′ə-fe)	suturing of a testicle: _____
anorchidism (an-or′kĭ-diz″əm)	absence of a testicle: _____
	Both anorchidism and an/orchism (**an-or′kiz-əm**) mean a congenital absence of the testis, which may occur unilaterally or bilaterally.
	Both orchiditis and orchitis (**or-ki′tis**) mean inflammation of a testis, marked by pain, swelling, and a feeling of weight.
epididymis	**9-101** Epididymitis (**ep″ĭ-did″ə-mi′tis**) is inflammation of the _____.
testis epididymis	Orchiepididymitis (**or″ke-ep″ĭ-did-ĭ-mi′tis**) is inflammation of a _____ and an _____.

❑ SECTION G REVIEW 𝒫athology, Diagnosis, and Treatment of Male Reproductive Structures

This section review covers frames 9–91 through 9–101. Complete the table by writing the meaning of the word part listed.

Combining Form   Meaning

1. varic(o)   _____

(Use Appendix V to check your answers.)

SECTION H

𝒮exually Transmitted Diseases

Sexually transmitted diseases are second only to the common cold and influenza as a leading cause of communicable disease in the United States. Without treatment, they can contribute to infertility, ectopic pregnancy, cancer, and death.

sexually transmitted	**9-102** Sexually transmitted diseases (STDs) are usually caused by infectious organisms that have been passed from one person to another through anal, oral, or vaginal intercourse. Some of the organisms that cause STDs are transmitted only through sexual intercourse, but others are transmitted also by infected blood or needles, by intrauterine transmission to the fetus, or by infection of the infant during birth. STDs were formerly called venereal (**və-nēr′e-əl**) diseases (VDs), named for Venus, goddess of love. These diseases are now called _____ _____ diseases.
discharge	**9-103** Different sexually transmitted diseases are caused by specific types of viruses, bacteria, protozoa, fungi, and parasites. One sexually transmitted disease, gonorrhea, was discussed in the previous chapter. Gonorrhea is caused by the gonococcus, a gram-negative intracellular diplococcus (see Figure 8-11). Gonorrhea causes a heavy urethral discharge in males, but females may be asymptomatic. The suffix, *-rrhea,* in gonorrhea means _____. Gonorrhea can usually be treated with penicillin or with another antibiotic in penicillin-sensitive persons.

9-104 The origin of syphilis is not clear, but an epidemic occurred in Europe in the late 15th century and the crew of Christopher Columbus was blamed for importing the disease from the New World. Write the name of this sexually transmitted disease, being careful of its spelling: _____.

syphilis

The first stage of syphilis is characterized by lymphadenopathy and by the appearance of a painless sore called a chancre **(shang′kər).** Do not confuse chancre with the word canker, which is an ulceration of the mouth or lips. The painless sore of syphilis that occurs usually on the genitals is called a

_____.

chancre

Material from a chancre may be examined for the spirochete that causes syphilis (see Figure 8-12).

lymph node

Lymphadenopathy means an enlarged or swollen _____ _____.

9-105 If not treated with penicillin or another antibiotic, the second stage of syphilis occurs 2 weeks to 6 months after the chancre disappears. The organisms spread throughout the body, and a generalized rash characterizes this stage. The second stage lasts 2 to 6 weeks and is followed by a fairly asymptomatic latent stage. Transmission of the disease can occur by blood donation to another person during the latent stage.

Only about one third of untreated individuals progress to the late stage, which has irreversible complications, including changes in the cardiovascular and nervous system and soft rubbery tumors, called gummas, on any part of the body.

syphilis

Congenital syphilis is acquired by the fetus in utero. The bacteria that cause syphilis can cross the placenta of an infected female and cause congenital _____. Infants who are born with congenital syphilis may have severe physical and mental defects and die within a few weeks after birth.

Several of the organisms that cause STDs can either cross the placenta and infect the fetus, sometimes causing physical and mental defects or stillbirth, or infect the infant during childbirth. A cesarean section is usually performed when the mother is known to be infected.

9-106 Fever therapy (such as intentional infection with malaria) was used to treat mental illness in past times. Some of the "psychotic" patients in mental hospitals were suffering from neuro/syphilis, a complication of late syphilis. Syphilitic patients who were infected with malaria developed high fever and improved. The organisms that cause syphilis, like many others, are adversely affected by high temperatures (sometimes a rise of as little as only one or two degrees). Fever can be an important body defense in many infectious diseases.

The stages of syphilis and information about additional STDs are summarized in Table 9-5.

9-107 Chlamydial **(klə-mid′e-əl)** infection, transmitted by intimate sexual contact, is the most common sexually transmitted disease in the United States. Read and answer questions about the characteristics of sexually transmitted diseases using the information in Table 9-5. Dys/uria means

difficult (painful) urination

_____ _____. Infected females may not have symptoms.

Undetected and untreated cases can progress to scarring and ulcerations of the epididymis in males or the uterine tubes in females, leading to subsequent infertility. Pelvic inflammatory disease (PID) is an inflammatory condition of the female pelvic organs that has spread from the genital tract.

ulceration

9-108 The major characteristic of chancroid **(shang′kroid)** is painful _____ of the genitals. Like other sexually transmitted diseases that are caused by bacteria, it can be treated with an antibiotic.

genital herpes

9-109 *Herpes genitalis* **(hər′pēz jen-ĭ-tal′is),** a viral infection, is also known as _____ _____. Genital blisters and ulceration are characteristic of this disease.

Active infection during pregnancy can lead to spontaneous abortion, stillbirth, or congenital birth defects. Delivery of the infant is often by cesarean section to prevent infection of the infant at the time of delivery.

TABLE 9-5 Sexually Transmitted Diseases and Their Causes

DISEASE OF THE GENITALS*	CAUSATIVE AGENT	CHARACTERISTICS
BACTERIAL		
Gonorrhea	*Neisseria gonorrhoeae*	Males: Urethral discharge, dysuria Females: Often asymptomatic
Syphilis	*Treponema pallidum* (a spirochete)	Primary stage: Painless chancre Secondary stage: Rash Late: Only about one third of untreated cases progress to syphilitic involvement of the viscera, the cardiovascular system, and the central nervous system
Chlamydial infection	*Chlamydia trachomatis*	Urethritis, dysuria, and frequent urination in males. In females, mild symptoms to none. One of the most common STDs in North America, often the cause of pelvic inflammatory disease and a frequent cause of sterility.
Chancroid (nonsyphilitic venereal ulcer)	*Haemophilus ducreyi*	Painful ulceration of the genitals, particularly on urination
Nonspecific genital infection	A variety of species, not all bacteria	Males: Nongonococcal urethritis Females: PID, cervicitis
VIRAL		
Herpes genitalis (genital herpes)	Herpes simplex virus (HSV 2)	Blisters and ulceration of the genitalia, fever, and dysuria
Condyloma acuminatum (genital warts)	Human papillomavirus (HPV)	Genital and anal warts
Acquired immunodeficiency syndrome (AIDS)	Human immunodeficiency virus (HIV)	A fatal late stage of infection with HIV that involves profound immunosuppression. To be diagnosed as having AIDS, one must be infected with HIV and have a clinical disease that indicates cellular immunodeficiency or have a specified level of CD4 and T-lymphocytes (T4). Characterized by opportunistic infections and malignant neoplasms that rarely afflict healthy individuals, especially Kaposi's sarcoma (Figure 9-25). Transmitted by infected body fluids (sexual contact, blood and blood products, breast milk).
Hepatitis B	Hepatitis B virus (HBV)	Symptoms vary from mild flulike symptoms to serious complications, cirrhosis, and hepatocellular carcinoma. Transmitted by contaminated blood or needles and sexual contact. (Hepatitis B vaccine is available for those at high risk. HBIG, hepatitis B immune globulin, provides postexposure passive immunity.)
Hepatitis C (non-A, non-B hepatitis)	Hepatitis C virus (HCV)	Symptoms are generally mild flulike symptoms. About 50% of the patients progress to chronic hepatitis. Transmitted mainly by blood products or sharing needles. Transmission to males is possible through contaminated menstrual blood or vaginal tears during intercourse.
Hepatitis D (delta hepatitis)	Hepatitis D virus (HDV)	Occurs only in patients infected with HBV. Usually develops into a chronic state. Transmitted through sexual contact and needle sharing. Prevention of hepatitis B with vaccine prevents hepatitis D.
PROTOZOA		
Trichomoniasis	*Trichomonas vaginalis*	Females: Frothy discharge of varying severity Males: Often asymptomatic
FUNGAL		
Candidiasis	*Candida albicans*	Vulvovaginitis: White patches, cheeselike discharge
ECTOPARASITIC		
Pubic lice	*Phthirus pubis*	Severe itching and erythema

*Although diseases of the genitals are given emphasis here, many of the organisms can infect other parts of the body as well. In addition, only the major STDs are included here.

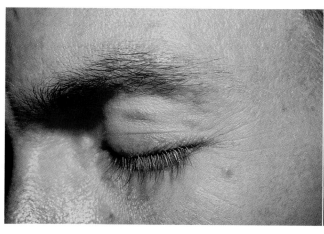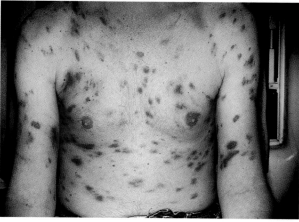

A   B

FIGURE 9-25
Kaposi's sarcoma. **A,** An early lesion of Kaposi's sarcoma. **B,** Advanced lesions of Kaposi's sarcoma. Note widespread hemorrhagic plaques and nodules. (From Noble J [editor]: *Textbook of primary care medicine,* St Louis, 1996, Mosby.)

genital warts	**9-110** *Condyloma acuminatum* (**kon″də-lo′mə ə-ku″mĭ-nāt′əm**) is commonly called _____ _____, which also describes its major characteristic. Persons who have had genital warts are at greater risk of genital malignancy, especially cervical cancer.
immunodeficiency (im″u-no-də-fish′ ən-se)	**9-111** The abbreviation *AIDS* means acquired _____ syndrome. As a result of the deficiency of antibodies, the immune response does not adequately protect the person from malignancies or opportunistic infections, infections that are caused by normally nonpathogenic organisms in someone whose resistance is decreased. HIV is spread by sexual intercourse or exposure to contaminated blood, semen, breast milk, or other body fluids of infected persons. The virus has a long incubation period (time between exposure and the onset of symptoms) and the disease we recognize as AIDS, which is the late fatal stage of infection.
liver	**9-112** Viral hepatitis is an inflammatory condition of the _____ caused by one of the hepatitis viruses, A, B, C, or D (delta). Hepatitis A is not considered a sexually transmitted disease, since transmission is generally through direct contact with fecally contaminated food or water. A vaccine is available. Hepatitis B is transmitted by sexual contact, blood products, and contaminated needles. Hepatitis B vaccine is available, required by various educational institutions, and recommended for healthcare workers and others at greater than usual risk. Hepatitis C is primarily transmitted by blood products and has a 50% chance of progressing to chronic hepatitis. Hepatitis D occurs only in patients who are infected with hepatitis B.
Trichomonas	**9-113** Trichomoniasis (**trik″o-mo-ni′ ə-sis**) is an infection caused by _____ *vaginalis,* a protozoon. Protozoa are single-celled, slightly more complex than bacteria, and the lowest (least complex) form of animal life. Symptoms of trichomoniasis are a frothy discharge in females and are minor or absent in males.
vulva vagina	**9-114** Candidiasis (**kan″dĭ-di′ə-sis**) is a fungal infection that is not limited to the genitals but can cause vulvovaginitis, which means inflammation of the _____ and the _____.

9-115 Pubic lice are sometimes included with STDs because they can be transmitted by sexual contact. They are also transmitted by close contact with contaminated objects, such as linens. They are commonly called crab lice and primarily infest the pubic region but are also found in armpits, beards, eyebrows, and eyelashes.

There is no review for this section.

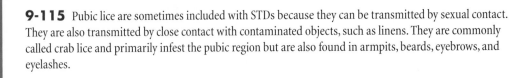

Terminology Challenge

Terms in this section are generally a greater challenge, since they require more than literal translation of word parts.

coitus	**9-116** Coitus* (**ko′ĭ-tus**) is sexual union in which the penis is inserted into the vagina. It is also called copulation. Write this word that means the same as sexual intercourse or copulation: _____.
white discharge	**9-117** Leukorrhea normally occurs in the adult female and is somewhat increased before and after the menstrual period. It may be abnormal if there is an increase in amount or changes in color or odor. Literal translation of leuko/rrhea (**loo″ko-re′ə**) is _____ _____. This new term specifically refers to a white, viscid discharge from the vagina and the uterine cavity.
	9-118 Mittelschmerz† (**mit′əl-shmertz**) means abdominal pain in the region of an ovary during ovulation. It is helpful in pinpointing the fertile period of the ovarian cycle.
endometriosis	**9-119** An abnormal gynecologic disorder, endometritis (**en″do-me-tri′tis**), is inflammation of the endometrium and is generally produced by bacterial invasion of the endometrium. Endometriosis (**en″do-me″tre-o′sis**), however, is an unusual condition in which tissue that contains typical endometrial elements is present outside the uterus, usually within the pelvic cavity. See the common sites of endometriosis in Figure 9-26. Endometrial tissue that is located outside the endometrium responds to hormonal changes and goes through cyclic changes of bleeding and proliferation. Scarring and adhesions result. Adhesions are abnormal adherence of structures that are not normally joined. A condition in which endometrium occurs in other places besides the uterus is called _____.
difficult episiotomy	**9-120** Dys/tocia‡ (**dis-to′shə**) means _____ labor. Abnormal or difficult labor is called dystocia. An episiotomy§ (**ə-piz″e-ot′-o-me**) facilitates delivery if the vaginal opening is too small. An episio/tomy is a surgical procedure in which an incision is made in the female perineum to enlarge her vaginal opening for delivery. The suffix -tomy will help you remember that an episiotomy§ involves an incision. Write this new term that means an incision that enlarges the vaginal opening to facilitate delivery: _____.

*Coitus (Latin: *coitio,* a coming together, meeting).
†Mittelschmerz (German: *mittel,* mid, middle + *schmerz,* pain, suffering).
‡Dystocia (dys- + Greek: *tokos,* birth).
§Episiotomy (Greek: *epision,* pubic region + -tomy).

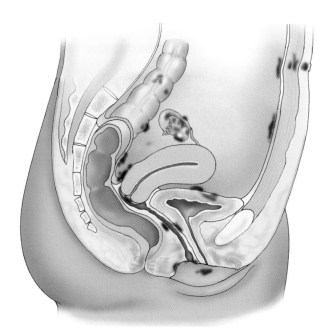

FIGURE 9-26
Common sites of endometriosis. The abnormal location of endometrial tissue is often the ovaries and less commonly other pelvic structures.

	9-121 Two disorders of the penis are phimosis* (**fi-mo′sis**) and balanitis (**bal″ə-ni′tis**). Phimosis occurs when the prepuce is constricted at the opening so that it cannot be retracted back over the glans penis. It is caused by inflammation or edema. It is sometimes accompanied by balanitis (balan[o], glans penis plus -itis, inflammation), inflammation of the glans penis.
phimosis	When the prepuce is constricted so that it cannot be retracted, the disorder is called _____.
balanitis	Inflammation of the glans penis is called _____.

*Phimosis (Greek: *phimgsis,* a muzzling or closure).

Study the following list of selected abbreviations. Then read through the Chapter Pharmacology section and be sure you understand the effects and uses of the drug classes that are presented. When you are finished, work the Chapter Review. After completing the exercises, check your answers with the solutions in Appendix V.

You will find these items presented after the Chapter Review:

• Listing of Medical Terms
• Enhancing Spanish Communication

Selected Abbreviations

AFP	alpha-fetoprotein (abnormal finding in certain liver diseases or embryonic cells)
AIDS	acquired immunodeficiency syndrome
BPH	benign prostatic hypertrophy
CPD	cephalopelvic disproportion
CS or C-section	cesarean section
Cx	cervix
D & C	dilation and curettage
DES	diethylstilbestrol (a synthetic estrogen; females who are exposed in utero are subject to increased risk of vaginal or cervical carcinomas)
EDD	expected delivery date
EFM	electronic fetal monitor
FHR	fetal heart rate
FSH	follicle-stimulating hormone
G	gravida (pregnant)
GC	gonococcus
GU	genitourinary
GYN	gynecology
HBV	hepatitis B virus
HCG	human chorionic gonadotropin
HCV	hepatitis C virus
HDV	hepatitis D virus
HIV	human immunodeficiency virus
HPV	human papillomavirus
HSV1	herpes simplex virus type 1 (oral herpes)
HSV2	herpes simplex virus type 2 (genital herpes)
IUD	intrauterine device
LH	luteinizing hormone
LMP	last menstrual period
NB	newborn
NGU	nongonococcal urethritis
OB	obstetrics
Pap	Papanicolaou smear, stain, or test
PID	pelvic inflammatory disease
PMS	premenstrual syndrome
STD	sexually transmitted disease
TAH	total abdominal hysterectomy
TUR, TURP	transurethral resection of the prostate
VD	venereal disease
VDRL	venereal disease research laboratory (also test for syphilis)

Chapter Pharmacology

Class	Effect and Uses
Anti-AIDS Drugs	**Used as Investigational Drugs to Treat AIDS**
didanosine (Videx)	An antiviral for advanced HIV infection
zidovudine (Retrovir)	
ribavirin (Virazole)	An antiviral for asymptomatic HIV-positive patients
aldesleukin (Proleukin)	A cytokine, involved in immune response
ganciclovir (Cytovene)	An antiviral
interferon β-1b (Betaseron)	A cytokine
Anti-Benign Prostatic Hyperplasia Drugs	**Used to Treat Benign Prostatic Hyperplasia**
finasteride (Proscar)	Inhibits androgen
terazosin (Hytrin)	Treats obstruction of urinary outflow
doxazosin (Cardura)	Treats obstruction of urinary outflow
tamsulosin (Flomax)	Treats obstruction of urinary outflow
Estrogen	**Used for Hormonal Replacement in Postmenopausal Females; Used in Combination Birth Control Products and Inoperable Prostatic Cancer**
conjugated estrogens (Premarin)	Used for hormonal replacement
estradiol (Estrace)	Used for hormonal replacement
(Climara)	A transdermal product
estropipate (Ogen)	A cream for intravaginal use

Chapter Pharmacology—cont'd

Class	Effect and Uses
Oral Contraceptives	**Used to Prevent Pregnancy**
Monophasic types	*Maintain a fixed dose of estrogen: progestin throughout the cycle*
mestranol/norethindrone (Ortho-Novum)	A fixed dose throughout the cycle
Biphasic types	*Progestin:estrogen varies throughout the cycle*
norethindrone/estradiol (Ortho-Novum 10/11)	Same ratio for first 21 days, then ratio changes for last 7 days of cycle
Triphasic types	*The estrogen remains the same or varies throughout the cycle; the progestin varies throughout the cycle*
levonorgestrel/ethinyl estradiol (Tri-Levlen)	Three colors of tablets for phases 1, 2, and 3
norethindrone/estradiol (Tri-Norinyl)	Three colors of tablets for phases 1, 2, and 3
Progestin only	*Uses the same dose at the same time every day*
norethindrone (Micronor)	Slightly higher failure rate than progestin:estrogen combinations
Ovulation Stimulants	**Used to Induce Ovulation in Selected Anovulatory Patients Who Desire Pregnancy**
chorionic gonadotropin (Profasi)	Used to induce ovulation
clomiphene (Clomid)	Used to treat ovulatory failure
danazol (Danocrine)	For treating endometriosis
dinoprostone (Prostin E$_2$)	Used to remove uterine contents after an intrauterine fetal death
ergonovine (Ergotrate Maleate)	Used to prevent and treat postpartum and postabortal hemorrhage
follitropin alfa (Gonal-F)	Used to treat ovulatory failure
oxytocin (Pitocin)	Used to induce labor
ritodrine (Yutopar)	Used to manage preterm labor
Progestins	**Used for Progesterone-like Effect to Prepare the Uterus for Implantation in Various Menstrual Disorders, Infertility, and Repeated Spontaneous Abortions**
medroxyprogesterone (Provera)	Used mainly for treatment of menopause in combination with estrogen
megestrol (Megace)	Used to relieve symptoms of advanced breast carcinoma
Testosterone	**Used for Testosterone Deficiency in Males; for Inoperable Breast Cancer in Females**
finasteride (Proscar)	Used for BPH and alopecia
fluoxymesterone (Halotestin)	For androgenetic alopecia and inoperable breast cancer

CHAPTER REVIEW 9

▶ BASIC UNDERSTANDING

REVIEWING WORD PARTS

I. Write a word (prefix, suffix, or combining form) for each clue.

CROSSWORD PUZZLE 9

Across

2 before
3 semen
5 varicose vein
12 heat
13 before
14 against
15 abdominal wall
16 vagina
17 many
18 testis
22 chorion
24 none
26 pregnancy
29 epididymis
30 penis
31 difficult
32 embryonic form
34 cell
36 ovary
37 poison
39 sperm
42 ovum
44 within
46 ductus deferens
48 new
49 body
50 inside
52 pregnant female
55 symptom
57 many
58 uterus
59 vagina
61 mucus

Down

1 first
2 after or behind
4 situated outside
6 uterine tissue
7 month
8 perineum
9 hidden
10 four
11 organs of reproduction
14 toward
16 killing
19 cold
20 midwife
21 uterine tube
22 cervix uteri
23 process of recording
24 birth
25 inflammation
27 prostate
28 uterus
31 distant
33 muscle
35 outside
38 amnion
40 false
41 treatment
43 ovary
44 between
45 testis
47 scrotum
49 viewing
51 tumor
53 vulva
54 fetus
56 resembling
60 pertaining to

MATCHING

II. Names of the three types of uterine tissue are in the left column. Match them with their locations in the uterus (A-C):

_____ 1. endometrium   **A.** Innermost
_____ 2. myometrium   **B.** Middle
_____ 3. perimetrium   **C.** Outermost

III. Match terms on the left with clues in the right column.

_____ 1. ovary   **A.** A gamete
_____ 2. ovum   **B.** A gonad
_____ 3. sperm   **C.** Normal site of implantation
_____ 4. testis   **D.** Product of fertilization
_____ 5. uterus   **E.** Receives the sperm during intercourse
_____ 6. uterine tube   **F.** Usual site of fertilization
_____ 7. vagina
_____ 8. zygote

IV. Match sexually transmitted diseases (STDs) in the left column with their characteristics in the right column. (More than one answer is possible.)

_____ 1. AIDS   **A.** A chancre occurs in the primary stage.
_____ 2. genital herpes **B.** Genital blisters, fever, and dysuria are characteristic of this disease.
_____ 3. gonorrhea   **C.** No immunization is available for this STD.
_____ 4. syphilis   **D.** Opportunistic infections and malignant disease are characteristic of this STD.
                             E. Penicillin is generally an effective treatment.
                             F. This STD is caused by bacteria.

LABELING

V. Label the diagram with the following combining forms that correspond to numbered lines 1 through 5 (the first one is done as an example): cervic(o), colp(o), hyster(o), oophor(o), salping(o).

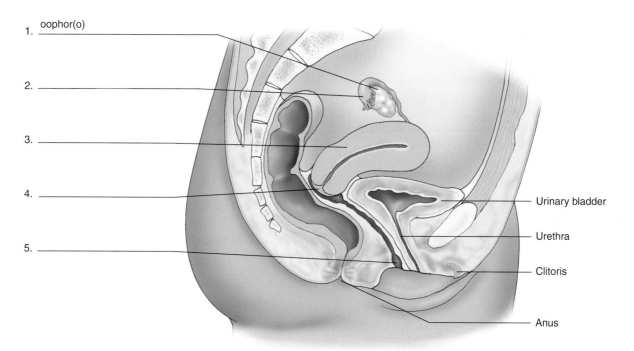

VI. Label the diagram with the following combining forms that correspond to numbered lines 1 through 12 (the first one is done as an example): epididym(o), orchi(o), pen(o), prostat(o), scrot(o), urethr(o), vas(o).

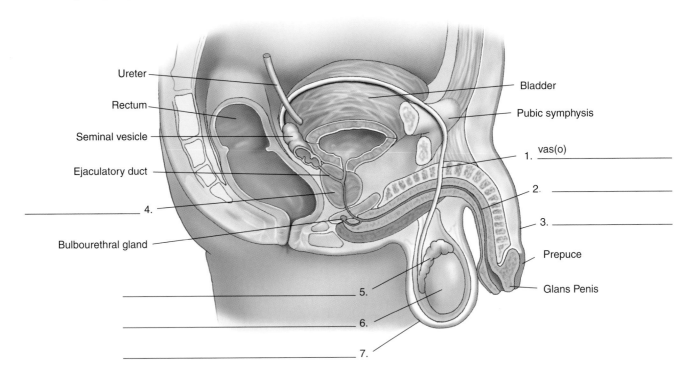

MULTIPLE CHOICE
VII. Select one answer (A–D) for each of the following multiple choice questions.

1. Which term means absence of a testis?
   A. anorchidism
   B. orchidectomy
   C. orchiectomy
   D. orchiorrhaphy

2. What does salpingostomy mean?
   A. any disease of an ovary and its uterine tube
   B. formation of an opening into a uterine tube
   C. hernia of a fallopian tube
   D. surgical fixation of a fallopian tube

3. Which term means the first occurrence of menstruation?
   A. amenorrhea
   B. dysmenorrhea
   C. menarche
   D. metrorrhagia

4. What is radiography of the uterus and uterine tubes after injection of opaque material called?
   A. hysterosalpingography
   B. oophorohysterectomy
   C. uteroplasty
   D. ureteroureterostomy

5. What does hysteropexy mean?
   A. ovarian tumor
   B. surgical fixation of an ovary
   C. surgical fixation of the uterus
   D. uterine tumor

6. Which term means examination of the abdominal cavity through one or more small incisions in the abdominal wall?
   A. hysteroscopy
   B. laparocystotomy
   C. laparoscopy
   D. phimosis

7. Which of these contraceptives acts as a physical barrier by covering the cervix during coitus?
   A. diaphragm
   B. symptothermal
   C. oral contraceptive
   D. vaginal suppository

8. What structures are inflamed in colpocervicitis?
   A. inner lining of the uterus
   B. uterine tissue itself
   C. uterus and an ovary
   D. vagina and cervix

9. How many viable offspring has a nullipara produced?
   A. many
   B. none
   C. one
   D. two

10. Which term means a condition in which the placenta is implanted abnormally in the uterus so that it impinges on or covers the uterine cervix?
    A. abruptio placentae
    B. eclampsia
    C. placenta previa
    D. stillbirth

11. What does dysmenorrhea mean?
    A. absence of menstruation
    B. painful menstruation
    C. profuse menstruation
    D. the monthly flow of blood from the female genital tract

12. What is another word for pregnant?
    A. gravid
    B. gravida
    C. primigravida
    D. tripara

13. Which of the following means a condition in which the patient has nearly all of the usual signs of pregnancy but is not pregnant?
    A. ectopic pregnancy
    B. multiparous
    C. pseudocyesis
    D. salpingocyesis

14. What is a word that means the time after birth?
    A. extrauterine
    B. intrauterine
    C. prenatal
    D. postnatal

15. What does the term *neonatologist* mean?
    A. a newborn child
    B. a physician who specializes in the treatment of neonates
    C. a physician who specializes in treating tumors
    D. a specialist who deals with pregnancy, labor, and delivery

16. What is the hormone that is present in body fluids of pregnant females and forms the basis of most pregnancy tests?
    A. amnion
    B. chorionic gonadotropin
    C. estrogen
    D. progesterone

17. What is the term for termination of pregnancy before the fetus is capable of survival outside the uterus?
    A. abortion
    B. auscultation
    C. gestation
    D. parturition

18. Which of the following is a contraceptive?
    A. dilation and curettage
    B. intrauterine device
    C. transurethral resection
    D. ultrasonography

19. Which of the following means removal of the cervix, uterus, uterine tubes, and ovaries through an incision in the abdominal wall?
    A. colpohysterectomy
    B. laparohysterectomy
    C. oophorosalpingectomy
    D. total hysterectomy

20. What is dilation and curettage?
    A. childbirth in the natural way
    B. collection of a Pap smear after insertion of a vaginal speculum
    C. dilatation of the cervical opening and scraping of the uterine wall
    D. irrigation of the dilated vagina

21. What is a term for undescended testicle?
    A. cryptorchidism
    B. orchidism
    C. orchidorrhaphy
    D. testalgia

22. Which statement is true of a bilateral vasectomy?
    A. It arrests sexual development in the female.
    B. It is excision of both uterine tubes.
    C. It generally results in male sterility.
    D. It is performed as an emergency procedure.

23. What is surgically removed in a circumcision?
    A. glans penis
    B. prepuce
    C. prostate
    D. testes

24. What is the proper term for a three-month-old developing human organism?
    A. a fetus
    B. a neonate
    C. a neoplasm
    D. an embryo

25. What is the ductus deferens?
    A. another name for a uterine tube
    B. another name for the vas deferens
    C. the female gonad
    D. the male gonad

FILL IN THE BLANKS
VIII. Write a word in each blank to complete this paragraph.

The female reproductive cycle is composed of two cycles that occur simultaneously. The (1) _____ cycle reflects the changes that occur in the ovaries. The changes in the ovarian follicle are called follicle development, (2) _____, and the corpus luteal stage. Two important hormones secreted by the follicles are (3) _____ and progesterone. The (4) _____ cycle is also called the menstrual cycle. In this cycle, the endometrium thickens and prepares for a developing embryo. If fertilization does not occur, the endometrial lining is shed, a process that is called (5) _____.

FILL IN THE BLANKS

IX. Write the missing word in these case summaries.

1. Bilateral _____, for sterility purposes, was performed on J. Smith, a 35-year-old male.

2. C. Well was found to have cervical erosion, as seen with a _____, a low-powered instrument that magnifies the vaginal and cervical mucosa.

3. Iva Flow had a _____ and _____, a surgical procedure in which the cervix was dilated and placental residual was removed from the uterus.

4. M. Karst underwent _____, surgical removal of the prostate.

5. Ima Parent delivered triplets with her first pregnancy. She is now classified as gravida _____.

WRITING TERMS

X. Write a term for each of the following:

1. childbirth	_____	7. removal of the ovaries	_____
2. female external genitalia	_____	8. rupture of the amnion	_____
3. inflammation of a uterine tube	_____	9. suture of the ductus deferens	_____
4. inflammation of the epididymis	_____	10. white, viscid vaginal discharge	_____
5. painful menstruation	_____		
6. release of an ovum from the ovarian follicle	_____		

▶ **GREATER COMPREHENSION**

LABELING

XI. The following diagrams represent displacements of the uterus. Label them as anteflexion, anteversion, retroflexion, or retroversion.

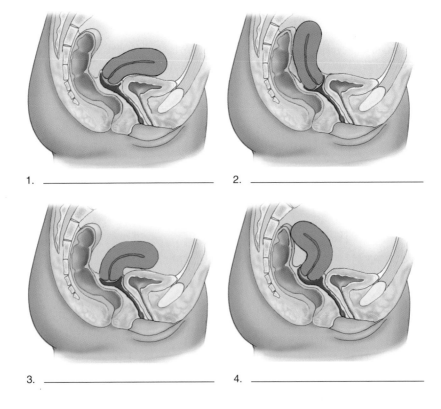

1. _____   2. _____

3. _____   4. _____

SPELLING

XII. Circles all incorrectly spelled terms and write their correct spelling.

displasia   ektopic   laparotomy   salpingosele   testosterone

INTERPRETING ABBREVIATIONS

XIII. Write the meaning of these abbreviations:

1. BPH _____
2. Cx _____
3. EDD _____
4. EFM _____
5. FHR _____

6. FSH _____
7. HBV _____
8. LH _____
9. NB _____
10. TURP _____

PRONUNCIATION

XIV. The pronunciation is shown for several medical words. Indicate which syllable has the primary accent by marking it with an ′.

1. amnio/chorial (**am ne o kor e əl**)
2. clitoris (**klit ə ris**)
3. colpo/cervic/al (**kol po sər vĭ kəl**)
4. colpoplasty (**kol po plas te**)
5. cryptorchidism (**krip tor kĭ diz əm**)

6. fetoscopy (**fe tos kə pe**)
7. myometritis (**mi o mə tri tis**)
8. neonate (**ne o nāt**)
9. phimosis (**fi mo sis**)
10. uni/para (**u nip ə rə**)

CATEGORIZING TERMS

XV. Categorize each of the following words as anatomical, diagnostic, radiological, surgical, or therapeutic by writing A, D, R, S, or T after each term:

A, D, R, S, or T

1. amenorrhea _____
2. amniotomy _____
3. bulbourethral glands _____
4. cryotherapy _____
5. fetography _____

A, D, R, S, or T

6. orchioplasty _____
7. prepuce _____
8. prostatitis _____
9. spermatocele _____
10. vasovasostomy _____

DRUG CLASSES

XVI. Match the drug classes in the left column with a use or effect in the right column. Use all choices only one time.

_____ 1. anti-benign prostatic hyperplasia drugs
_____ 2. estrogen
_____ 3. oral contraceptives
_____ 4. ovulation stimulants
_____ 5. progestins
_____ 6. testosterone

A. For progesterone-like effect
B. For testosterone deficiency in males
C. Hormonal replacement in postmenopausal women
D. To induce ovulation
E. To prevent pregnancy
F. To treat BPH

(Check your answers with the solutions in Appendix V.)

Listing of Medical Terms

abdominal hysterectomy
abruptio placentae
acquired immunodeficiency
    syndrome
amenorrhea
amniocentesis
amniochorial
amniochorionic
amnion
amniorrhexis
amniotic
amniotomy
anastomosis
anorchidism
anorchism
antenatal
antepartum
aspermatogenesis
aspermia
auscultation
balanitis
Bartholin's gland
bipara
bulbourethral glands
candidiasis
cautery
cervicitis
cervicocolpitis
cervix uteri
cesarean section
chancre
chancroid
chlamydial
chorion
circumcision
climacteric
clitoris
coitus
colpectomy
colpitis
colpocervical
colpocervicitis
colpocystitis
colpodynia
colpohysterectomy
colposcope
colposcopy
conception
condom
condyloma acuminatum
contraception
contraceptive
copulation
corpus albicans

corpus luteum
cryotherapy
cryptorchidism
cyesis
diaphragm
dilatation
dilation and curettage
ductus deferens
dysmenorrhea
dysplasia
dystocia
dysuria
eclampsia
ectopic pregnancy
effacement
ejaculation
ejaculatory
endometriosis
endometritis
endometrium
epididymis
epididymitis
episiotomy
estrogen
extraembryonic
extrauterine
fallopian tube
fetal
fetography
fetoscope
fetoscopy
fetus
fibroids
fimbria
fistula
follicle-stimulating hormone
follicular
gamete
genital herpes
genitalia
genitourinary
gestation
gonad
gonadotropin
gonorrhea
graafian follicles
gravid
gravida
gynecologic
gynecology
herpes genitalis
human chorionic
    gonadotropin
hydrocele

hydrocelectomy
hypothalamus
hysterectomy
hysteropathy
hysteropexy
hysteroptosis
hysterosalpingogram
hysterosalpingography
hysteroscopy
interstitial cells of Leydig
intrauterine device
Kaposi's sarcoma
labia majora
labia minora
laparohysterectomy
laparorrhaphy
laparoscope
laparoscopic hysterectomy
laparoscopy
laparotomy
leukorrhea
luteinizing hormone
lymphadenopathy
menarche
menopause
menorrhagia
menorrhea
menses
menstruation
metritis
metrorrhagia
mittelschmerz
mons pubis
multigravida
multipara
myometritis
myometrium
natal
neonatal
neonate
neonatologist
neonatology
nullipara
oligospermia
ooblast
oogenesis
oophoralgia
oophorectomy
oophoritis
oophorogenous
oophorohysterectomy
oophoropathy
oophoropexy
oophorosalpingectomy

oophorosalpingitis
oophorosalpingohysterectomy
orchialgia
orchidalgia
orchidorrhaphy
orchiopexy
orchiotomy
ovarian
ovary
ovulation
ovum
Pap smear
paraurethral gland
parous
parturition
pelvic inflammatory disease
penile
penis
perimetrium
perineal
perineum
phimosis
placenta
placenta previa
postnatal
postpartum
postuterine
preeclampsia
premenstrual syndrome
prenatal
prepuce
primigravida
primipara
progesterone
progestin
prognosis
prostate
prostatectomy
prostatic carcinoma
prostatic hyperplasia
prostatitis
pseudocyesis
puberty
quadripara
salpingectomy
salpingitis
salpingocele
salpingopexy
salpingorrhaphy
salpingostomy
scrotum
secundipara
semen
seminal vesicles

Listing of Medical Terms—cont'd

seminiferous
serosa
speculum
spermatoblast
spermatocidal
spermatocyte
spermatogenesis
spermatoid
spermatolytic
spermatopathy
spermatozoa
spermatozoon

symphysis pubis
symptothermal
syphilis
testalgia
testicular
testis
testosterone
toxic shock syndrome
trichomoniasis
tripara
tubal ligation
ultrasonography

unipara
urethrovaginal
urogenital
uterine tubes
uterus
vagina
vaginal
vaginal hysterectomy
vaginal speculum
vaginectomy
vaginitis
vas deferens

vasectomy
vasostomy
vasovasostomy
vestibular
vulva
vulval
vulvar
vulvectomy
vulvitis
vulvovaginitis
zygote

Español Enhancing Spanish Communication

English	Spanish (pronunciation)	English	Spanish (pronunciation)
birth	nacimiento (nah-se-me-EN-to)	ovarian	ovárico (o-VAH-re-co)
childbirth	parto (PAR-to)	ovary	ovario (o-VAH-re-o)
circumcision	circuncisión (ser-coon-se-se-ON)	parturition	parto (PAR-to)
conception	concepción (con-sep-se-ON)	penis	pene (PAY-nay)
condom	condón (con-DON)	pregnancy	embarazo (em-bah-RAH-so)
contraception	contracepción (con-trah-cep-se-ON)	pregnant	embarazada (em-bah-rah-SAH-dah)
cream	crema (CRAY-mah)	prostate	próstata (PROS-ta-tah)
diaphragm	diafragma (de-ah-FRAHG-mah)	prostatic	prostático (pros-TAH-te-co)
erection	erección (ay-rec-se-ON)	prostatitis	prostatitis (pros-ta-TEE-tis)
feminine	femenina (fay-may-NEE-na)	reproduction	reproducción (ray-pro-dooc-se-ON)
foam	espuma (es-POO-mah)	rhythm method	método de ritmo
heat	calor (cah-LOR)		(MAY-to-do day REET-mo)
hormone	hormona (or-MOH-nah)	sexual	sexual (sex-soo-AHL)
impotency	impotencia (im-po-TEN-se-ah)	symptom	síntoma (SEEN-to-mah)
intercourse, sexual	cópula (CO-poo-lah)	temperature	temperatura (tem-pay-rah-TOO-rah)
masculine	masculine (mas-coo-LEE-no)	testicle	testículo (tes-TEE-coo-lo)
menopause	menopausia (may-no-PAH-oo-se-ah)	uterus	útero (OO-tay-ro)
menstruation	menstruación (mens-troo-ah-se-ON)	vagina	vagina (vah-HEE-nah)
newborn	recién nacida (ray-se-EN nah-SEE-dah)		

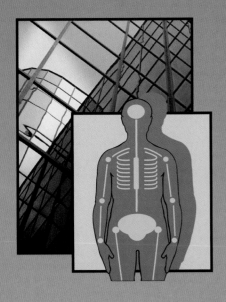

Muscular and Skeletal Systems

10

Outline

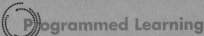
Principal Word Parts

COMBINING FORMS

ankyl(o)	stiff	carp(o)	wrist
arthr(o), articul(o)	joint; articulation	chondr(o)	cartilage
aut(o)	self	clavicul(o)	clavicle
blast(o)	embryonic form	coccyg(o)	coccyx
burs(o)	bursa	cost(o)	ribs
calc(i)	calcium	crani(o)	cranium
calcane(o)	heel bone	fasci(o)	fascia
		femor(o)	femur
		fibul(o)	fibula
		humer(o)	humerus
		ili(o)	ilium
		ischi(o)	ischium
		lumb(o)	lower back
		muscul(o)	muscle
		myel(o)	bone marrow or spinal cord
		orth(o)	straight
		oste(o)	bone
		patell(o)	patella
		pelv(i)	pelvis
		phalang(o)	phalanges
		pub(o)	pubis
		rach(i), rachi(o), spin(o)	spine
		radi(o)	radius (sometimes, radiant energy)
		sacr(o)	sacrum
		scapul(o)	scapula
		spondyl(o), vertebr(o)	vertebrae
		stern(o)	sternum
		synov(o), synovi(o)	synovial membrane
		tars(o)	tarsus (sometimes, edge of eyelid)
		ten(o), tend(o), tendin(o)	tendon
		tibi(o)	tibia
		troph(o)	nutrition
		uln(o)	ulna
		viscer(o)	viscera

PREFIXES

ab-	away from
ad-	toward
infra-	situated below
meta-	change or next
retro-	backward or behind
super-	above or excess
supra-	above
syn-	joined; together

SUFFIXES

-asthenia	weakness
-blast	embryonic form
-clasia	break
-desis	binding; fusion
-malacia	abnormal softening
-sarcoma	malignant tumor from connective tissue
-schisis	split
-trophy	nutrition

Learning Goals

▶ BASIC UNDERSTANDING

In this chapter, you will learn to do the following:
1. Recognize the major bones of the body.
2. Demonstrate an understanding of the functions of bones, muscles, and supporting structures.
3. Recognize the meaning of different types of body movements.
4. Differentiate between different types of fractures.
5. Write the meaning of the word parts and use them to build and analyze terms.

▶ GREATER COMPREHENSION

6. Demonstrate an understanding of the two divisions of the skeletal system and the major characteristics of a long bone.
7. Distinguish between the three different types of muscle tissue.
8. Spell the terms accurately.
9. Pronounce the terms correctly.
10. Know the meaning of the abbreviations.
11. Categorize the terms as anatomical, diagnostic, surgical, or radiological.
12. Identify the effects or uses of the drug classes presented in this chapter.

SECTION A

Structure and Function of the Skeletal System

The skeletal system consists of the bones and the cartilages, ligaments, and tendons that are associated with the bones. In addition to their primary function of support, the bones perform several other important functions.

skeleton	**10-1** The human skeleton* is the bony framework of the body. Skeletal means pertaining to the _____. The skeletal system consists not only of the bones, but also of the associated cartilages, ligaments, and tendons.

*Skeleton (Greek: a dried body or a mummy).

10-2 The most widely known function of the skeletal system is that of support, providing form and shape for the body. Four other functions are protection of soft body parts, movement, blood cell formation, and storage.

The delicate tissues of the brain are enclosed in the skull. This is an example of which function? _____

protection

Bones and muscles work together to enable us to bend our arms and legs, and turn our heads and perform other voluntary movements. This is an example of which function? _____

movement

Bone marrow is the soft tissue that fills the cavities of the bones. Red bone marrow functions in the formation of red blood cells, white blood cells, and platelets. In addition, bones store and release minerals, especially calcium, and are an essential part of mineral balance in the body. Fat is stored in the yellow bone marrow.

10-3 Bones may be classified as long, short, flat, or irregular. Examples of long bones are those in the arm, leg, and thigh. Bones of the wrist are examples of short bones. Most of the bones of the skull are flat bones, and bones of the spine are classified as irregular bones. The general features of a long bone are shown in Figure 10-1.

The intercellular substance of bone contains an abundance of mineral salts, primarily calcium phosphate and calcium carbonate, which gives bone its unique hardness.

Looking at the drawing, one sees that some parts of bone are hard and compact, whereas other parts are spongy. Which type of bony tissue do you suspect serves as protection and support, compact or spongy? _____

compact

The chief characteristic of bone is its rigid nature, but it is important to remember that bone contains living cells and is richly supplied with blood vessels and nerves.

10-4 Answer these questions as you look at Figure 10-1. The long shaft of the long bone is called the _____. This long shaft is thick compact bone that surrounds yellow marrow in adults.

diaphysis (di-af′ə-sis)

At each end of the diaphysis, there is an expanded portion called the _____. The epiphysis is spongy bone that is covered by a thin layer of compact bone. The two ends are covered by articular cartilage to provide smooth surfaces for movement of the joints. Except in the areas where there is articular cartilage, the bone is covered with a tough membrane called periosteum (per″e-os′te-əm). The combining form *oste(o)* means bone. Analyzing the word parts of peri/ost/eum will help you remember its meaning. The prefix *peri-* means _____, oste(o) means _____, and -ium means _____. (In writing periosteum, an "i" is omitted to facilitate pronunciation.)

epiphysis (ə-pif′ə-sis)

around, bone membrane

Note that bone is richly supplied with blood vessels. Similar to other body tissues, bone requires oxygen and nutrients and produces wastes, the end products of metabolism.

10-5 Add suffixes to oste(o) in the following to build new words concerning bone. Don't worry if you have forgotten a few of the suffixes. Looking them up in the word parts index will help you to remember them.

inflammation of a bone: _____

osteitis (os″te-i′tis)

resembling bone: _____

osteoid (os′te-oid)

surgical repair of bone: _____

osteoplasty (os′te-o-plas″te)

an instrument used to cut bone: _____

osteotome (os′te-o-tōm″)

measurement of bones: _____

osteometry (os″te-om′ə-tre)

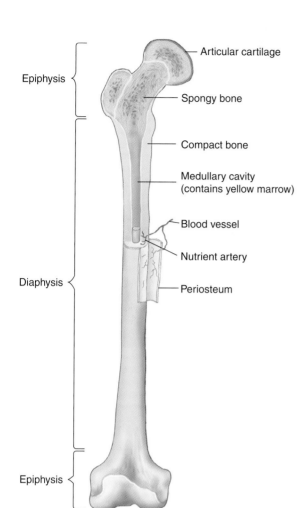

Epiphysis

Articular cartilage

Spongy bone

Compact bone

Medullary cavity
(contains yellow marrow)

Blood vessel

Nutrient artery

Periosteum

Diaphysis

Epiphysis

FIGURE 10-1

A typical long bone, partially sectioned. The outer part is compact, dense bone. The inner part is spongy and contains large spaces filled with bone marrow. Diaphysis is the long, main portion of a bone. Epiphyses are the knoblike ends of the bone.

---

osteectomy
(os″te-ek′tə-me)

osteocyte
(os′te-o-sīt″)

bone

10-6 Write a word that means excision of a bone (or a portion of it): _____.

(One "e" is often dropped, and this is written ostectomy.)

Write a word that means a bone cell: _____.

Osteocytes are embedded in the calcified intercellular substance of bone.

An osteo/blast (**os′te-o-blast″**) is an embryonic form of _____ cell, or osteocyte.

---

x-rays

10-7 Calcium in bone is radiopaque (**ra″de-o-pāk′**); hence bones can block x-rays so that they do not reach photographic plates. Bones are represented by white areas on an x-ray film (Figure 10-2). Unimpeded x-rays expose the x-ray film and cause it to blacken.

Metals, such as steel in a knife blade or metal of coins, are also radiopaque. This characteristic often enables the physician to know where a foreign object has lodged or if internal fixation devices are correctly positioned to align a bone.

Radiopaque means impenetrable to what type of rays? _____

(One "o" is omitted when radi[o] is joined with opaque, thus the spelling radiopaque.)

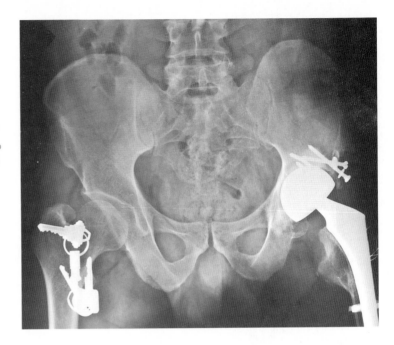

FIGURE 10-2
X-ray film of the pelvis. Keys were left in the pocket of a lightweight hospital robe during the examination, so radiography had to be repeated. Note also the metal fixation devices in the hip. Metal objects are radiopaque to x-rays. Bones appear white, and soft tissue appears gray. (Ballinger PW, Frank ED: *Mer atlas of radiographic positions and radiologic procedures*, vol 1, ed 9, St Louis, 1999, Mosby.)

calcium	**10-8** The combining form *calc(i)* means calcium. Calci/fication (**kal″sĭ-fĭ-ka′shən**) is the process by which organic tissue becomes hardened by deposit of what substance in tissue? _____
	Normally calcium is deposited in bone in large amounts to give bone its hardness. Calcification in soft tissue is abnormal.
calcium	Calci/uria means _____ in the urine. Although calcium may be present in normal urine in minute amounts, it is not readily detectable. (Urinary excretion of calcium is affected by several things, including diet.) Hyper/calciuria (**hi″pər-kal″se-u′re-ə**) is often seen in metastatic bone disease, in which there is rapid bone destruction.
osteosclerosis (**os″te-o-sklə-ro′sis**)	**10-9** There is a continuous remodeling of bone, with minerals being removed as bone is broken down and bone tissue is rebuilt. This remodeling is important in the regulation of the blood calcium level. Thus there is a delicate balance between bone destruction and bone formation. Excessive formation can lead to abnormal hardness and unusual heaviness of bone. Write a word that literally means hardening of bone: _____.
	Despite its density, osteosclerotic bone is brittle and subject to fracture.
calcium	**10-10** Vitamin D aids in the absorption of calcium from the intestinal tract. A deficiency of vitamin D results in insufficient calcium absorption and calci/penia (**kal″sĭ-pe′ne-ə**), a deficiency of _____ in the body.
calcium	Remember that de- means down or from. De/calci/fication (**de″kal-sĭ-fĭ-ka′shən**) is loss of _____ from bone or teeth.
ostealgia (**os″te-al′jə**) **osteodynia** (**os″te-o-din′e-ə**) **destruction of bone**	**10-11** Write two words, both of which mean pain in a bone, by adding appropriate suffixes to oste(o): _____ and _____. Softening and destruction of bone is called osteo/lysis (**os″te-ol′ĭ sis**). Paget's disease (named for Sir James Paget, an English surgeon) is a skeletal disease in which osteolysis is usually evident. Osteo/lysis is _____.

bone	**10-12** Osteo/genesis (**os″te-o-jen′ə-sis**) or ossification (**os″ĭ-fi-ka′shən**) is the formation of bone substance. Human embryos contain no bone but do contain cartilage, a more flexible tissue that is shaped like bone. Osteo/genesis is the process whereby cartilage is used as a model to form what kind of tissue? _____ Osteo/genesis is also called ossification. The Latin term for bone, *os* (plural, *ossa*), is often used in the naming of bones. For example, os coccygis is the formal name for the coccyx, or the tailbone. *Os* and *ossa* are not word parts but instead are Latin terms that mean bone and are commonly used in naming them.
bone osteotrophy	**10-13** Osteo/trophy (**os″te-ot′rə-fe**) is _____ nutrition. The combining form ***troph(o)*** means nutrition. The suffix is ***-trophy.*** Write the word that means bone nutrition: _____.
bone marrow spinal cord	**10-14** The compact tissue of bone is tunneled by a central canal that contains bone marrow. The combining form for bone marrow is ***myel(o).*** This combining form also means the spinal cord. Sometimes it is difficult to know if myel(o) in a word refers to bone marrow or the spinal cord, and in some words it can refer to either. For example, myel/itis (**mi″ə-li′tis**) means inflammation of either the _____ _____ or the _____ _____.
spinal cord bone marrow	**10-15** Myelo/encephal/itis (**mi″ə-lo-en-sef′ə-li′tis**), however, means inflammation of the brain and _____ _____. Think of the term *myelo/suppression* (**mi″ə-lo-sə-presh′ən**). Because it is unlikely that one would intentionally suppress the spinal cord, the meaning of myelo/suppression is inhibition of the _____ _____.
myelosuppressive (mi″ə-lo-sə-pres′iv) blood aspiration	**10-16** Cancer treatment often induces myelosuppression. Write a word that is an adjective that means inhibiting bone marrow activity: _____. (Drugs that inhibit bone marrow are called myelosuppressive agents or simply myelosuppressives.) A treatment that may be used in myelosuppression is hemo/therapy (**he″mo-ther′ə-pe),** or _____ treatment (transfusion). This is often necessary to sustain life if myelosuppression is severe. Sometimes the physician wants to know the extent of myelosuppression or has other reasons that indicate the need to study the bone marrow cells. In such cases, marrow is aspirated from the bone, using a needle. This is called bone marrow _____.
myeloblast (mi′ə-lo-blast) myelocyte (mi′ə-lo-sīt)	**10-17** The cells of red marrow are responsible for producing new blood cells. An embryonic bone marrow cell is called a _____. The myeloblast matures into another cell that, translated literally, means "bone marrow cell": _____. Myelocytes mature into leukocytes that are normally found in blood.

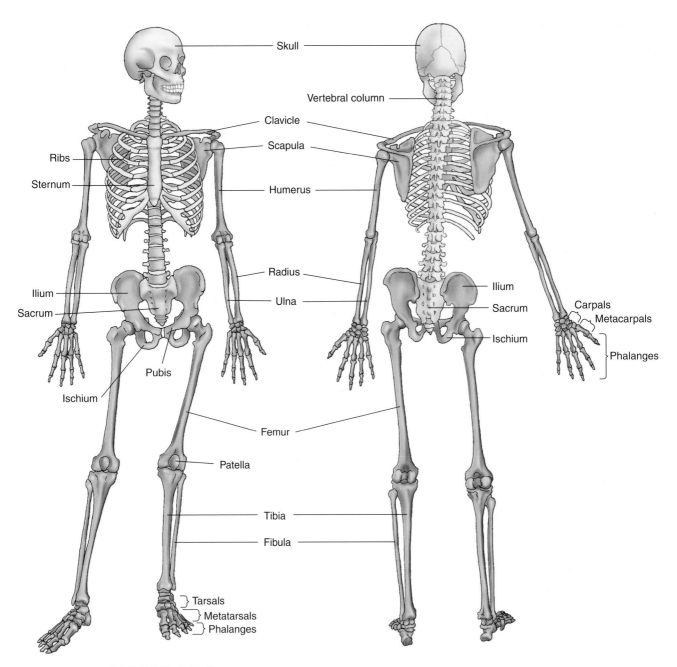

Skull

Vertebral column

Clavicle

Scapula

Ribs

Sternum

Humerus

Radius

Ilium

Ulna

Ilium

Sacrum

Sacrum

Ischium

Pubis

Carpals

Metacarpals

Ischium

Phalanges

Femur

Patella

Tibia

Fibula

Tarsals

Metatarsals

Phalanges

FIGURE 10-3

Anterior and posterior views of the human skeleton with major bones identified. The bones are grouped in two divisions: The axial skeleton forms the vertical axis of the body and is shown here as bone colored. The appendicular skeleton includes the free appendages and their attachments and is shown in blue.

10-18 The adult human skeleton usually consists of 206 named bones. There are also a few others that vary in number from one individual to another, so they are not counted with the other 206 bones. The major bones are identified in Figure 10-3. Study the names of the bones.

The skull serves as protection for the brain and forms the framework of the face. The vertebral column is attached at the base of the skull and is composed of 26 vertebrae, which protect the spinal cord.

sternum
(stər′nəm)

Locate the elongated, flattened breastbone, which is called the _____. Attached to the sternum are the ribs, which support the chest wall and protect the lungs and heart.

The bones just named comprise the axial skeleton. This part of the skeleton forms the vertical axis of the body.

10-19 The other division of the skeleton is called the appendicular skeleton, which includes the free appendages and their attachments to the axial skeleton. Locate the clavicle (**klav′ĭ-kəl**), also known as the collarbone. The two collarbones attach medially to the sternum.

The scapula (**skap′u-ləh**) is a large triangular bone that is commonly called the shoulder blade. It is joined to the longest bone of the arm, the humerus (**hu′mər-əs**), by muscles and tendons. The bones of the forearm are the ulna (**ul′nə**) and the radius (**ra′de-əs**). The wrist is composed of eight carpal bones,

carpals
(kahr′pəlz)

also called _____. Bones of the hand are metacarpals, and bones of the fingers are phalanges (**fə- lan′ jez**).

Three types of pelvic bones are shown: the ilium (**il′e-əm**), the ischium (**is′ke-əm**), and the

pubis (pu′bis)

_____.

femur (fe′mur)

The thigh bone, the longest bone of the leg, is called the _____. The patella is the kneecap, and the two bones of the lower leg are the tibia (**tib′e-ə**) and the fibula (**fib′u-lə**). The ankle is com-

tarsals (tahr′səlz)

posed of seven tarsal bones, also called the _____. Bones of the feet are metatarsals. Like bones of the fingers, those of the toes are called phalanges.

❏ **SECTION A REVIEW**   𝒮**tructure and Function of the Skeletal System**

This section review covers frames 10–1 through 10–19. Complete the table by writing a meaning in each blank.

Combining Form	Meaning		Suffix	Meaning
1. calc(i)	_____		5. -trophy	_____
2. oste(o)	_____			
3. myel(o)	_____			
4. troph(o)	_____			

(Use Appendix V to check your answers.)

TABLE 10-1 Named Bones of the Skull

CRANIAL BONES	FACIAL BONES	AUDITORY OSSICLES
Parietal (2)	Maxilla (2)	Malleus (2)
Temporal (2)	Zygomatic (2)	Incus (2)
Frontal (1)	Mandible (1)	Stapes (2)
Occipital (1)	Nasal (2)	
Ethmoid (1)	Palatine (2)	
Sphenoid (1)	Inferior nasal concha (2)	
	Lacrimal (2)	
	Vomer (1)	

Axial Skeleton

The axial skeleton is divided into the skull, the vertebral column and the thoracic cage. These bones form the vertical axis to which the appendicular skeleton attaches.

---

cranial (kra′ne-əl)	**10-20** The skull, the thoracic cage, and the vertebral column constitute the axial skeletal, which is made up of 80 bones. Only the major bones are considered here. The skull is composed of three types of bones: cranial bones, facial* bones, and the auditory ossicles, six tiny bones in the middle ear cavity (Figure 10-4). The bones that make up the skull are listed in Table 10-1. You learned that crani(o) means cranium or skull. The cranium is that portion of the skull that encloses and protects the brain. Write a word that means pertaining to the skull: _____. The opening at the base of the skull through which the spinal cord passes is called the foramen magnum.
skull **craniectomy** (kra″ne-ek′tə-me)	**10-21** Cranio/plasty (**kra′ne-o-plas″te**) is plastic surgery, or surgical repair, of the _____. Write a word using crani(o) that means excision of a segment of the skull: _____ (crani[o] and the suffix for excision).
craniotomy (kra″ne-ot′ə-me) **craniotome** (kra′ne-o-tōm″)	**10-22** Incision through the cranium is _____. Write the name of the instrument used in performing craniotomy: _____.
measuring **craniopathy** (kra″ne-op′ə-the)	**10-23** A cranio/meter (**kra″ne-om′ə-tər**) is an instrument for _____ the skull. Any disease of the skull is a _____.
thorax (or chest) **sternum** **intrasternal** (in″trə-stər′ nəl)	**10-24** Thoracic means pertaining to the _____. The bones of the thoracic cage are the thoracic vertebrae, the ribs, and the sternum. The scientific name of the breastbone is sternum. The combining form that means sternum is ***stern(o).*** Stern/al (**ster′nəl**) pertains to the _____. Write a word that means within the sternum: _____.

*Facial (Latin: *facialis,* from *facies,* face).

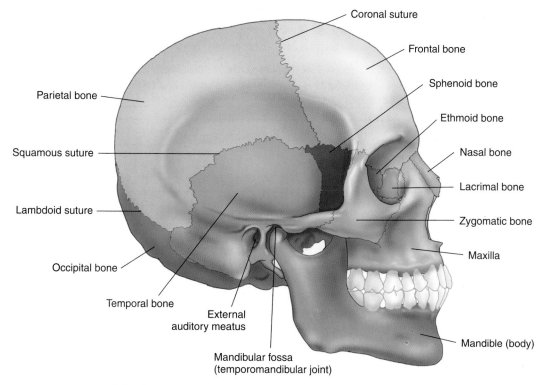

FIGURE 10-4
Major bones of the skull, lateral view. The cranium, that portion of the skull that encloses the brain, is composed of eight cranial bones. (The six types are parietal, temporal, frontal, occipital, ethmoid, and sphenoid.) Sutures are immovable fibrous joints between many of the cranial bones. The 14 facial bones form the basic framework and shape of the face. The auditory ossicles (not shown) are three tiny bones in each middle ear cavity. The external auditory meatus is the external opening of the ear.

sternotomy (stər-not′ə-me) **sternum**	**10-25** Incision of the sternum is _____. This is a common incision of open heart surgery. Stern/algia (**stər-nal′jə**) is pain in the _____.
substernal (səb-stər′nəl) **suprasternal** (soo″prə-ster′nəl) **sternum** **pericardium**	**10-26** Using the prefix *sub-*, write the word that means below the sternum: _____. Using *supra-*, which means above or beyond, write a term that means above the sternum: _____. Sterno/pericardi/al (**stər″no per″ĭ-kahr′de əl**) pertains to the _____ and the _____. Sometimes sternal punctures are done for the purpose of obtaining a sample of bone marrow, the soft material in the cavities of bones. Bone marrow samplings are examined for the presence of abnormal cells.
split	**10-27** The suffix *-schisis* means split.* The origin of -schisis is the same as part of a term you may know, schizophrenia, which was once believed to be a split personality. Sterno/schisis means _____ sternum. In sternoschisis (**stər-nos′kĭ-sis**), there is congenital fissure (split) of the sternum.

*(Greek: *schizein*, split.)

pertaining to the ribs	**10-28** The sternum is one of the bones that make up the thoracic cage, which protects the heart, lungs, and great vessels, and also plays a role in breathing (Figure 10-5). The 12 pairs of ribs (costae) are named according to their anterior attachments to the sternum. The combining form **cost(o)** means ribs (costae). Cost/al (**kos′təl**) means _____.
ribs **below a rib(s)**	**10-29** Inter/costal (**in″tər-kos′təl**) means between the _____. Intercostal muscles lie between the ribs and draw adjacent ribs together to increase the volume of the thorax in breathing. What is the location of sub/cost/al (**səb-kos′təl**)? _____
sternum **ribs** **pain in the ribs** **costectomy** **(kos-tek′tə-me)**	**10-30** Sterno/cost/al (**ster″no-kos′təl**) pertains to the _____ and the _____. Cost/algia (**kos-tal′jə**) is _____. Write a word that means excision of a rib: _____.
spine **rachialgia** **(ra″ke-al′jə)**	**10-31** The spine encloses and protects the spinal cord, supports the head, and serves as a place of attachment for the ribs and muscles of the back. The combining form **rach(i), rachi(o),** and **spin(o)** mean spine. Spinal means pertaining to the spine. Study these terms using rach(i) and rachi(o) to learn how they are used. Rachi(o) is more commonly used than rach(i). Rachio/dynia (**ra″ke-o-din′e-ə**) is a painful condition of the _____. Write another term using -algia that means a painful spine: _____.
neck **cervicodorsal** **(sər″vĭ-ko-dor′səl)**	**10-32** The spine extends from the base of the skull to the pelvis. It is also called the vertebral column because it is composed of vertebrae, which are named and numbered from above downward. Vertebrae is the plural form of vertebra (Figure 10-6). You previously learned that cervic(o) means neck. There are seven cervical (**sər′vĭ-kəl**) vertebrae located in the region near the _____. Write a word that means pertaining to the neck and back: _____.
chest **lower back** **thoracic, lumbar**	**10-33** Thorac/ic refers to the _____. The thoracic vertebrae are part of the posterior wall of the chest. The combining form **lumb(o)** means the lower back. The lumb/ar (**lum′bahr**) vertebrae are just below the thoracic vertebrae. In what part of the body are lumbar vertebrae located? _____ _____ Thoraco/lumbar (**thor″ə-ko-lum′bər**) means pertaining to two particular types of vertebrae. To what types of vertebrae does thoracolumbar refer? _____ and _____
sacrum **sacral (sa′krəl)**	**10-34** Use **sacr(o)** to write words about the sacrum, the triangular bone below the lumbar vertebrae. Sacro/dynia (**sa″kro-din′e-ə**) is pain of the _____. In adults, five vertebrae fuse to form the sacrum. Which vertebrae are fused into one bone, the sacrum? _____ vertebrae
coccygeal **(kok-sij′e-əl)** **coccygectomy** **(kok″sĭ-jek′tə-me)**	**10-35** The combining form **coccyg(o)** means coccyx, or the tailbone. In adults, the coccyx (**kok′ siks**) is the bone at the base of the vertebral column. It is formed by four fused vertebrae. Which vertebrae fuse to form the coccyx? _____ vertebrae Write a word that means excision of the coccyx: _____.

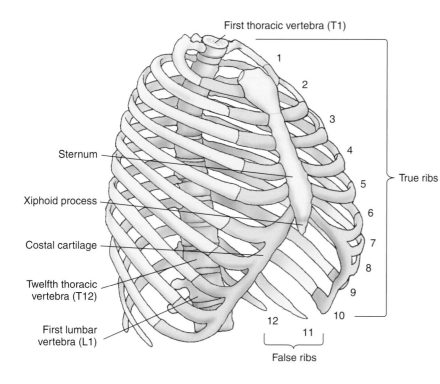

First thoracic vertebra (T1)

1
2
3
4
5
6
7
8
9
10
12
11

True ribs

False ribs

Sternum

Xiphoid process

Costal cartilage

Twelfth thoracic vertebra (T12)

First lumbar vertebra (L1)

FIGURE 10-5

The thoracic cage. The ribs exist in pairs, one on each side of the chest, and are numbered from the top rib, beginning with *one*. The upper seven pairs join directly with the sternum by a strip of cartilage and are called *true ribs*. The remaining five pairs are referred to as *false ribs* because they do not attach directly to the sternum. The last two pairs of false ribs, called *floating ribs,* are attached only on the posterior aspect.

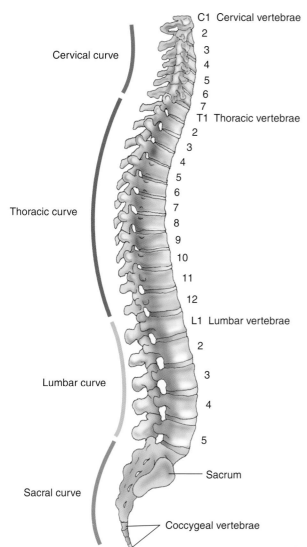

C1 Cervical vertebrae
2
3
4
5
6
7
T1 Thoracic vertebrae
2
3
4
5
6
7
8
9
10
11
12
L1 Lumbar vertebrae
2
3
4
5
Sacrum
Coccygeal vertebrae

Cervical curve

Thoracic curve

Lumbar curve

Sacral curve

FIGURE 10-6

The vertebral column with normal curvatures noted. The vertebrae are numbered from above downward. There are seven cervical vertebrae in the neck region, 12 thoracic vertebrae behind the chest cavity, five lumbar vertebrae supporting the lower back, five sacral vertebrae fused into one bone called the sacrum, and four coccygeal vertebrae fused into one bone called the coccyx.

vertebrectomy (ver″tə-brek′tə-me)	**10-36** Both *vertebr(o)* and *spondyl(o)* are combining forms that mean vertebrae. Write a word using vertebr(o) that means excision of a vertebra: _____.
vertebra, rib **vertebrosternal** (vər″tə-bro-stər′nəl) **sternovertebral** (stər″no-vər′tə-brəl)	**10-37** Vertebro/costal (**vər″tə-bro-kos′təl**) and costo/vertebral (**kos″to-vər′tə-brəl**) both mean pertaining to a _____ and a _____. Two other words that can be reversed in this way mean pertaining to the vertebrae and the sternum. Write these two words: _____ and _____.
pain in a vertebra **spondylitis** (spon″də-li′tis) **spondylomalacia** (spon″də-lo-mə-la′shə)	**10-38** Remembering that spondyl(o) also means vertebrae, write the meaning of spondyl/algia (**spon″dĭ-lal′jə**): _____. Using spondyl(o), form words that mean inflammation of vertebrae: _____. softening of vertebrae: _____.
vertebrae **vertebroplasty**	**10-39** Inter/vertebral (**in″tər-ver′tə-brəl**) means between two adjoining _____. Cushions of cartilage between adjoining vertebrae are called intervertebral disks. These layers of cartilage absorb shock. If they become diseased, sometimes they rupture, resulting in a herniated disk, popularly called a slipped disk. Vertebral fractures can sometimes be repaired by vertebro/plasty (**ver-te′bro-plas″te**). In this procedure, a plastic-like substance is injected on each side of the fractured vertebra to hold it in position while the bone heals. The name of the procedure used to assist the healing of a fractured vertebra is called _____.

❑ SECTION B REVIEW   *A*xial Skeleton

This section review covers frames 10–20 through 10–39. Complete the table by writing a word part or its meaning in each blank.

Combining Form	Meaning	Combining Form	Meaning
1. coccyg(o)	_____	7. _____	sternum
2. _____	ribs (costae)	8. vertebr(o)	_____
3. lumb(o)	_____	**Suffix**	**Meaning**
4. rach(i), rachi(o)	_____	9. -schisis	_____
5. _____	sacrum		
6. spondyl(o)	_____		

(Use Appendix V to check your answers.)

Appendicular Skeleton

Bones of the extremities and shoulder and pelvic girdles compose the appendicular skeleton. Many of the 126 bones that make up this group are small and are found in the hands and feet, but several of the remaining appendicular bones are the longest bones in the body. Bones of the appendicular skeleton are designed for movement.

---

ilium (il′e-əm) ischium (is′ke-əm) pubis (pu′bis)	**10-40** The pelvic girdle consists of two hip bones. Each of these bones consists of three separate bones in the newborn, but eventually the three fuse to form one bone. Names of the three bones are the ilium, the ischium, and the pubis: *ili(o)* means the ilium, the largest of the three bones; *ischi(o)* means the ischium, the posterior part of the pelvic girdle; and *pub(o)* means the pubis, the anterior and inferior part of the pelvic girdle. Ili/ac (**il′e-ak**) pertains to the _____. Ischi/al (**is′ke-əl**) pertains to the _____. Pub/ic (**pu′bik**) pertains to the _____.
ilium pubis pertaining to the ischium and pubis	**10-41** Examine Figure 10-7 and locate these three bones, which are fused to form each of the hip bones. Also compare the male pelvis with the female pelvis. Ilio/pubic (**il″e-o-pu′bik**) pertains to the _____ and the _____. Ischio/pubic (**is″ke-o-pu′bik**) means _____.
ischium coccyx ischium ischialgia (is″ke-al′jə)	**10-42** Ischio/coccyg/eal (**is″ke-o-kok-sij′e-əl**) pertains to the _____ and the _____. Ischio/dynia (**is″ke-o-din′e-ə**) is pain in the _____. Using a different suffix, write another word that means pain in the ischium: _____.
beneath the pubis pubes between	**10-43** Where is sub/pubic (**səb-pu′bik**) situated? _____ The hairs growing over the pubic region are called pubes (**pu′bēz**). This term is also used to denote the pubic region. The pubic region or the hairs that grow in this region are called the _____. The pubic symphysis is the inter/pubic (**in″tər-pu′bik**) joint _____ the two pubic bones.
head, pelvis cephalopelvic (sef″ə-lo-pəl′vik)	**10-44** The lower vertebrae make up part of the pelvis, the basinlike structure formed by the sacrum, coccyx, and pelvic girdle (hip bones). You learned in Chapter 3 that pelv(i) means pelvis. Cephalo/pelvic pertains to the fetal _____ and the maternal _____. If the head of the fetus is too large for the pelvis of the mother, this is called _____ disproportion. Birth by the usual means will be difficult or impossible in such cases.
shoulder blade scapula interscapular (in″tər-skap′u-lər)	**10-45** The combining form *scapul(o)* means scapula (shoulder blade). The scapula is a large, flat, triangular bone that joins on one end with the clavicle and on the other end with the upper arm bone. The common name of the scapula is the _____ _____. Scapul/ar (**skap′u-lər**) means pertaining to the _____. Write a term that means between the two shoulder blades: _____.

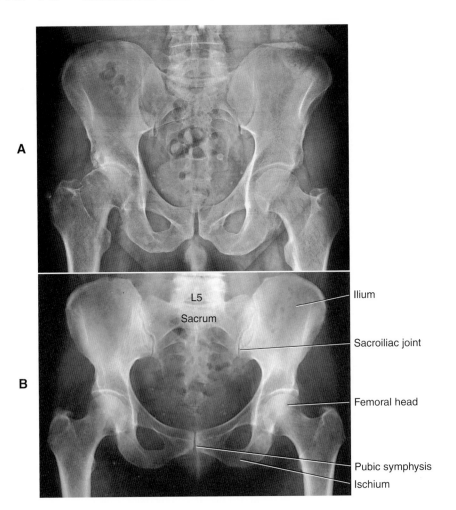

A

B

L5
Sacrum

Ilium

Sacroiliac joint

Femoral head

Pubic symphysis

Ischium

FIGURE 10-7
Radiographs comparing the male pelvis with that of the female, anterior views. **A,** Male pelvis. Bones of the male are generally larger and heavier. The pelvic outlet, the space surrounded by the lower pelvic bones, is heart shaped. **B,** Female pelvis. The pelvic outlet is larger and more oval than that of the male. The size and shape of the female pelvis varies and is important in childbirth. L5 is the fifth lumbar vertebra. The pubic symphysis is the joint where the two pubic bones are joined. (From Ballinger PW, Frank ED: *Merrill's atlas of radiographic positions and radiologic procedures*, vol 1, ed 9, St Louis, 1999, Mosby.)

sternum, clavicle **pertaining to the ribs and clavicle** **scapuloclavicular (skap"u-lo-klə-vik′ u-lər)**	**10-46** The clavicle is the collarbone. The combining form ***clavicul(o)*** means the clavicle. Sterno/clavicul/ar (**stər″no-klə-vik′u-lər**) pertains to the _____ and the _____. Costo/clavicular (**kos″to-klə-vik′u-lər**) means _____. Using costoclavicular as a model, write a word that means pertaining to the scapula and the collarbone: _____.
humerus **humeroscapular (hu″mər-o-skap′ u-lər)**	**10-47** The clavicle and the two scapulae form the connection between the arms and the axial skeleton. The major bones of the arm are the humerus, the ulna, and the radius. The humerus is the upper arm bone and has the combining form ***humer(o)***. Humer/al (**hu′mər-əl**) pertains to the _____. Use this new combining form and scapular to write a word that means pertaining to the humerus and scapula: _____.

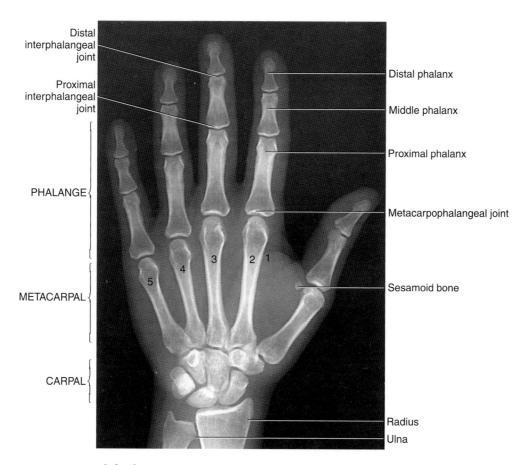

Distal interphalangeal joint
Proximal interphalangeal joint
PHALANGE
METACARPAL
CARPAL

5 4 3 2 1

Distal phalanx
Middle phalanx
Proximal phalanx
Metacarpophalangeal joint
Sesamoid bone
Radius
Ulna

FIGURE 10-8

Radiograph of the human hand, posteroanterior view. The ulna and radius, as well as the bones of the hand, are identified. Eight small carpal bones make up the wrist. The palm of the hand contains five metacarpal bones, which are numbered 1 to 5 starting on the thumb side. There are three phalanges in each finger (a proximal, middle, and distal phalanx) except the thumb, which has two. The sesamoid bone is a small round bone embedded in the tendon that provides added strength for the thumb. (Ballinger PW, Frank ED: *Merrill's atlas of radiographic positions and radiologic procedures*, vol 1, ed 9, St Louis, 1999, Mosby.)

ulnoradial (ul″no-ra′de-əl)	**10-48** The ulna and the radius are bones of the forearm, the portion of the arm between the elbow and the wrist. Use the combining forms ***uln(o)*** for ulna and *radi(o)* for radius. Also remember that radi(o) will sometimes refer to radiant energy, as you learned in Chapter 2. Use a combining form with radial to write a word that means pertaining to both the ulna and the radius: _____.
humeroradial (hu″mər-o-ra′de-əl)	**10-49** Write a word that means pertaining to the humerus and the radius: _____.
humeroulnar (hu″mər-o-ul′nər)	Use a combining form and ulnar to write a word that means pertaining to the humerus and ulna: _____.
	10-50 The combining form ***carp(o)*** means the carpus, or wrist. Observe in Figure 10-8 that the wrist consists of eight small bones, arranged in two transverse rows.
carpus	Carp/al (**kahr′pəl**) pertains to the _____.
carpals	Bones of the wrist are called carpals. Therefore a word that means the same as carp/al bones is _____.

carpals carpus	**10-51** Carp/ectomy (**kahr-pek′tə-me**) is excision of one or more of the _____. Carpo/ped/al (**kahr″po-ped′əl**) pertains to the _____ and the foot. A carpopedal spasm, for example, is involuntary contraction of the muscles of the hands and feet.
next carpal	**10-52** The metacarpals (**met″ə-kahr′pəlz**) connect the wrist bones (carpals) to the phalanges. You learned that *meta-* is a prefix that means a change or next, as in a series. The meta/carpals lie _____ to the carpals. The five metacarpals constitute the palm. The proximal ends of the metacarpals join with the distal row of what type of bones? _____
fingers phalangitis (**fal″ən-ji′tis**)	**10-53** The distal ends of the metacarpals join with the phalanges (**fə-lan′jēz**). The combining form *phalang(o)* means phalanges (Figure 10-8). The phalanges are bones of the _____ as well as bones of the toes. There are three phalanges in each finger (a proximal, middle, and distal phalanx) but not in the thumb. DIP means distal interphalangeal, and DIPJ means distal interphalangeal joint. Build a word that means inflammation of bones of the fingers or toes: _____.
carpus, phalanges phalangectomy (**fal″ən-jek′tə-me**)	**10-54** Carpo/phalang/eal (**kahr″po-fə-lan′je-əl**) pertains to the _____ and _____. Write a word that means excision of a bone of a finger or toe: _____.
femur iliofemoral (**il″e-o-fem′or-əl**)	**10-55** The lower extremities, like the two upper extremities, are composed of sixty bones. The femur, or thigh bone, is the longest and heaviest bone in the body (Figure 10-9). The combining form *femor(o)* means femur. Femor/al pertains to the _____. Using femoral, write a word that means pertaining to the ilium and the femur: _____.
pertaining to the pubis and the femur ischiofemoral (**is″ke-o-fem′o-rəl**)	**10-56** Using what you have learned in this chapter, determine the meaning of pubo/femor/al (**pu″bo-fem′ə-rəl**): _____. Write a word that means pertaining to the ischium and the femur: _____.
patella (**pə-tel′ə**) femur patellectomy (**pat″ə-lek′tə-me**)	**10-57** The patella, or kneecap, is anterior to the knee joint. The combining form *patell(o)* means patella. Patello/femoral (**pə-tel″o-fem′ə-rəl**) pertains to the _____ and the _____. Write a word that means removal of the patella: _____.
pain of the tibia pertaining to the fibula	**10-58** The lower leg is composed of two bones, the tibia and the fibula. The tibia, or shinbone, is the larger of the two bones. The combining form *tibi(o)* means tibia; the combining form *fibul(o)* means fibula. Tibi/algia (**tib″e-al′jə**) is _____. Fibul/ar (**fib′u-lər**) means _____.

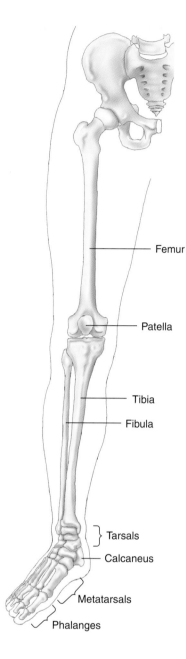

Femur

Patella

Tibia

Fibula

Tarsals

Calcaneus

Metatarsals

Phalanges

FIGURE 10-9

Right lower extremity, anterior view. The lower extremity consists of the bones of the thigh, leg, foot, and patella (kneecap). The lower leg has two bones, the tibia and the fibula. The foot is composed of the ankle, instep, and five toes. The ankle has seven bones, the calcaneus (heel bone) being the largest. The instep has five metatarsals, numbered 1 through 5 starting on the medial side. There are three phalanges in each of the toes, except in the great (or big) toe, which has only two.

10-59 The foot is composed of the ankle, the instep, and toes. The ankle, or tarsus, consists of a group of seven short bones that resemble the bones of the wrist but are larger. The combining form **tars(o)** means the tarsus. In addition, tars(o) means the edge of the eyelid. This is because a second meaning of tarsus is a curved plate of dense white fibrous tissue forming the supporting structure of the eyelid.

It is not always obvious, when looking at a word containing tars(o), which meaning is intended. Words used in the following frames refer to the ankle, but one should be aware that a second meaning of tarsus is the edge of the eyelid.

ankle

In these frames, tars(o) refers to the _____.

tarsus

10-60 Tars/optosis (**tahr″sop-to′sis**) is prolapse of the _____. This is commonly called flatfoot.

pertaining to the ankle (or tarsus)

Tars/al (**tahr″səl**) means _____.

One of the tarsal bones is the calcaneus, or heel bone.

calcaneus pain in the heel	**10-61** The combining form *calcane(o)* refers to the calcaneus. Calcane/al (**kal-ka′ne-əl**) pertains to the _____. Calcaneo/dynia (**kal-ka″ne-o-din′e-ə**) is _____.
calcaneus pertaining to the calcaneus and tibia	**10-62** Calcaneo/plantar (**kal-ka″ne-o-plan′tər**) pertains to the _____ and the sole. Plantar is a word that means concerning the sole. Calcaneo/tibial (**kal-ka″ne-o-tib′e-əl**) means _____.
calcaneofibular (kal-ka″ne-o-fib′u-lər) calcaneitis (kal-ka″ne-i′tis)	**10-63** Change the last part of calcaneotibial to write a word that means pertaining to the calcaneus and the fibula: _____. Write a word that means inflammation of the heel bone: _____
distal phalang(o)	**10-64** The bones between the tarsus and the toes are the metatarsals (**met″ə-tahr′səlz**). Which end of the metatarsals joins with the toes? _____ Bones of the toes are phalanges. Finger bones are also called phalanges. What is the combining form for phalanges? _____
phalanges many	**10-65** As shown in Figure 10-9, there are two bones in the great toe and three in each of the lesser toes. Bones of the toes are called _____. Each foot normally has five digits. Poly/dactyl/ism (**pol″e-dak′təl-iz-əm**) or poly/dactyly (**pol″e-dak′tə-le**) is the presence of _____ digits on the hands or feet. In either of these terms, it is understood that the number of digits is greater than the expected number of five.

❏ SECTION C REVIEW 𝒜ppendicular Skeleton

This section review covers frames 10–40 through 10–65. Complete the table by writing the combining form for each meaning.

Combining Form	Meaning	Combining Form	Meaning
1. _____	calcaneus	9. _____	patella
2. _____	wrist	10. _____	phalanges
3. _____	clavicle	11. _____	pubis
4. _____	femur	12. _____	radius
5. _____	fibula	13. _____	scapula
6. _____	humerus	14. _____	tarsus
7. _____	ilium	15. _____	tibia
8. _____	ischium	16. _____	ulna

(Use Appendix V to check your answers.)

TABLE 10-2 Types of Movement in Joints

TYPE OF MOVEMENT	EXAMPLES
Immovable: bones come in close contact and are separated only by a thin layer of fibrous connective tissue	Sutures in the skull
Slightly movable: Bones are connected by cartilage and joint allows slight movement only.	The symphysis pubis; joints that connect the ribs to the sternum
Freely movable: Ends of the opposing bones are covered with articular cartilage and separated by a space called the joint cavity. These joints are sometimes called synovial joints.	Shoulder, wrist, knee, elbow

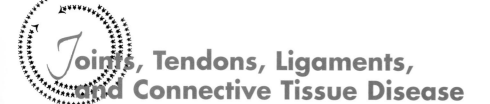

Joints, Tendons, Ligaments, and Connective Tissue Disease

SECTION D

Connective tissues include joints, tendons, and ligaments. Connective tissue diseases are discussed separately from other musculoskeletal conditions because most are classified as autoimmune diseases.

10-66 Connective tissues, characterized by an abundance of intercellular material with relatively few cells, support and bind other body tissue and parts. Bone is the most rigid of all of the connective tissues. The joints, tendons, and ligaments are also connective tissues.

10-67 A joint, or articulation (**ahr-tik″u-la′shən**), is a place of union between two or more bones. You are familiar with many joints: for example, the ankle, wrist, and knee. Joints are classified according to their structure and the amount of movement they allow. Joints are immovable, slightly movable, and freely moveable. Table 10-2 shows examples of the three types.

Two combining forms that mean joint are **articul(o)** and **arthr(o).** Most terms use arthr(o), but articul/ar (**ahr-tik′u-lər**) means pertaining to a _____.

joint

10-68 Most joints in the adult body are freely movable joints, also called synovial (**sĭ-no′ve-əl**) joints. Articular cartilage covers the ends of the opposing bones in a synovial joint, and they are separated by a space called the joint cavity that is filled with synovial fluid for lubrication (Figure 10-10).

The articular cartilage provides protection and support for the joint. Some joints also have pads and cushions that help stabilize the joint and act as shock absorbers. Bursae are fluid-filled sacs that help reduce friction. The combining form *burs(o)* means a bursa. Inflammation of a bursa is called _____.

bursitis
(bər-si′tis)

10-69 Note the location of the bursa in Figure 10-10. Bursae are commonly located between the skin and underlying bone or between tendons and ligaments.

Tendons are bands of strong, fibrous tissue that attach the muscles to the bones. Ligaments connect bones or cartilages and serve to support and strengthen joints. What type of connective tissue attaches the muscles to the bones? _____

tendons

What type of connective tissue connects bones or cartilages? _____

ligaments

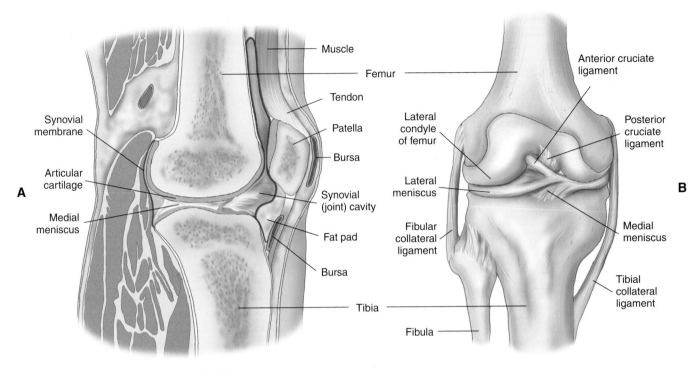

FIGURE 10-10
The knee joint. **A,** Lateral view, sagittal section. The hinged joint at the knee is a synovial joint. The ends of the opposing bones are covered by articular cartilage. The synovial membrane secretes synovial fluid into the joint cavity for lubrication. Menisci and bursae are special structures that act as protective cushions. **B,** Anterior view. Twelve ligaments, flexible bands of fibrous tissue, bind the structures of the knee to provide strength. Note how the anterior and posterior cruciate ligaments cross each other, a characteristic from which their name is derived (Latin: *crux*, cross and *ligare*, to bind).

10-70 Progressive deterioration and loss of articular cartilage is the major characteristic of degenerative joint disease (DJD), the most common type of connective tissue disease. Hips, knees, the vertebral column, and the hands are primarily affected because they are used most often and bear the stress of body weight. This disease is characterized by progressive deterioration and loss of articular

cartilage

_____.

inflammation

DJD is also called osteo/arthr/itis, but DJD is more accurate, since the inflammation of arthritis is secondary to loss of the cartilage. Arthr/itis is _____ of a joint or several joints. It is characterized by pain, swelling, heat, redness, and limitation of movement.

10-71 Possible causes of DJD include the wear and tear effects of aging, genetics, mechanical stress (abuse or overuse of certain joints), and certain metabolic diseases such as diabetes mellitus. Routine x-rays are often, but not always, helpful in confirming the diagnosis. CT and MRI may be used to determine vertebral involvement.

inflammation

Antiinflammatories are generally used to reduce inflammation and pain, especially drugs classified as nonsteroidal antiinflammatory drugs (NSAIDs). These drugs primarily reduce _____ that leads to pain.

joint

When other measures are inadequate to provide pain control for DJD, surgery may be indicated, often total joint replacement (TJR). Total joint replacement is the major arthroplasty that is performed. Arthro/plasty is surgical repair of a _____.

Replacement of hips, knees, elbows, wrists, shoulders, and joints of the fingers and toes are common. Replacement of ankles is less common.

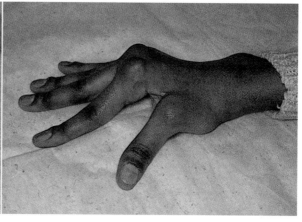

A

B

FIGURE 10-11
Hand deformities characteristic of chronic rheumatoid arthritis. **A,** Marked deformity of the metacarpophalangeal joints, causing deviation of the fingers to the ulnar side of the hand. **B,** Swan neck deformity, another abnormal condition of the fingers seen often in rheumatoid arthritis. (From Swartz MH: *Textbook of physical diagnosis: history and examination,* ed 2, Philadelphia, 1994, WB Saunders.)

synovitis
(sin-o-vi'tis)

10-72 Rheumatoid arthritis (RA) is the second most commonly occurring connective tissue disease. It is also the most destructive to joints. It is a chronic, progressive, systemic inflammatory process that affects primarily synovial joints. A systemic disease affects other areas of the body as well.

The combining forms ***synov(o)*** and ***synovi(o)*** mean synovial joint. The onset of RA is characterized by inflammation of the synovial joints. Using synov(o), write a word that means inflammation of the synovial joints: _____.

autoimmune

10-73 RA affects females more often than males and people with a family history of RA two or three times more often than the rest of the population. It is believed to be an autoimmune disease; that is, one that is characterized by an alteration of the immune system, resulting in the production of antibodies against the body's own cells. The combining form ***aut(o)*** means self. An alteration in the immune system, resulting in the production of antibodies against the body's own cells, is called an _____ disease.

Fever and fatigue are frequent findings in rheumatoid arthritis. As the disease worsens, the joints become progressively inflamed and painful. Joint deformity is common (Figure 10-11).

Many drugs are available to treat RA, in addition to those used to treat degenerative joint disease. Respiratory, heart, and other complications are common. Several laboratory tests help to support the diagnosis and progress of the disease, including the rheumatoid factor (RF), the antinuclear antibody (ANA) titer, and the erythrocyte sedimentation rate (ESR).

lupus

10-74 Lupus erythematosus is a third autoimmune disease, named for the characteristic butterfly rash that appears across the bridge of the nose in some cases (Figure 10-12).

There are two classifications of lupus: discoid* lupus erythematosus (DLE) and systemic lupus erythematosus (SLE). The discoid type affects only the skin. The systemic type can cause major body organs and systems to fail and is potentially fatal. Prolonged exposure to sunlight and other forms of ultraviolet lighting aggravates the skin rash. The name of this autoimmune disease is _____ erythematosus.

*Discoid (Greek: *diskos,* flat plate).

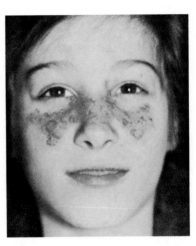

FIGURE 10-12
The characteristic "butterfly" rash of systemic lupus erythematosus. The word *lupus* is the Latin term for wolf. The rash is usually red, and thus the term *erythematosus*, a Latin word meaning reddened, was added in naming this disease. (From Nelson WE: *Textbook of pediatrics*, ed 15, Philadelphia, 1996, WB Saunders.)

skin	**10-75** Systemic scleroderma is another connective tissue disease. Translated literally, sclero/derma means hardening of the _____. Associated with a high mortality rate, systemic sclerosis is characterized by inflammation, fibrosis, and sclerosis of the skin and vital organs. The cause is unknown, but autoimmunity is suspected.
gout (gout)	**10-76** Gout, or gouty arthritis, is a systemic disease in which urate crystals deposit in the joints, myocardium, kidneys, and ears, causing inflammation. The disease can cause painful swelling of a joint, accompanied by chills and fever. Because the crystals are deposited in connective tissue, gout is classified as a form of arthritis. Males are affected more often than females, and diet is critical in the management of this disease called _____.
many **vessel** **pain of many muscles** **spine** **false**	**10-77** Several additional connective tissue diseases are included in Table 10-3. Polymyositis* (**pol″e-mi″o-si′tis**) is inflammation of _____ muscles, leading to atrophy (**at′rə-fe**) of the muscle. Atrophy is a wasting and decrease in the size of a organ, tissue, or part. In this case, atrophy leads to wasting and deformity of the muscle. Translated literally, vasculitis (**vas″ku-li′tis**) is inflammation of a _____. In systemic necrotizing vasculitis, arteritis leads to localized tissue death (necrosis). Remembering that my(o) means muscle, poly/my/algia (**pol″e-mi-al′jə**) means _____. The combining form **ankyl(o)** means stiff. Ankylosing spondylitis causes inflammation and stiffening of the _____. Ankylosis (**ang″kə-lo′sis**) is stiffening of a joint. You learned earlier that pseudo- means _____. Pseudogout (**soo′do-gout**) has goutlike symptoms but is not gout. Fibro/my/algia is characterized by pain of the torso, extremities, and the face. It may be attributable to deep sleep deprivation.
bursa **inflammation** **of a tendon**	**10-78** Two of the more common inflammatory conditions of connective tissue are bursitis and tendinitis. Both of these conditions involve specific connective tissues. You learned that bursitis is inflammation of a _____. Three combining forms—***ten(o), tendin(o)*** and ***tend(o)***—mean tendon. Tendin/itis (**ten″dĭ-ni′tis**) is _____. Both problems are related to overuse, repetitive motion, or irritation, and symptoms usually disappear with rest. Other diseases can lead to bursitis or tendinitis (also spelled tendonitis, not using the combining form).

*Myositis (Greek: *myos*, of muscle).

TABLE 10-3 Selected Connective Tissue Diseases

NAME OF THE DISEASE	MAJOR CHARACTERISTICS
Degenerative joint disease	Deterioration and loss of articular cartilage in joints
Rheumatoid arthritis	Systemic inflammatory disease that primarily affects synovial joints, resulting in joint deformities, but affects many other organs
Lupus erythematosus	Two types: discoid (involves only the skin) and systemic. Systemic can cause major organs to fail
Progressive systemic sclerosis	Inflammation, fibrosis, and sclerosis of the skin and vital organs. High mortality rate
Polymyositis/dermatomyositis	Inflammatory disease of striated muscle that causes weakness and atrophy. When a rash accompanies polymyositis, the disease is called dermatomyositis
Systemic necrotizing vasculitis	Arteritis that causes ischemia in tissues usually supplied by the vessels that are involved
Polymyalgia rheumatica	Stiffness, weakness, and aching of the shoulder and pelvic girdles. Systemic manifestations
Ankylosing spondylitis	Vertebral involvement that leads to spinal deformities. Also called rheumatoid spondylitis
Sjögren's syndrome	Inflammation and immune complexes obstruct secretory glands, resulting in dry eyes, dry mouth, and dry vagina
Infectious arthritis	Infectious invasion of the joints caused by microorganisms
Lyme disease	Circular rash, ill feeling, fever, headache, and muscle and joint aches caused by the bite of an infected deer tick. Prompt antibiotic treatment is effective. Without treatment, complications of arthritis and neurologic and cardiac problems are possible
Gout	Inflammation of joints caused by urate crystals deposited in joints
Pseudogout	Goutlike symptoms, but the crystals deposited in joints are different than those of gout
Fibromyalgia	Pain and muscle spasms of the torso, extremities, and face. Sometimes the result of deep sleep deprivation

---

pain **tenalgia** (te-nal′jə)	**10-79** Tenodynia may be caused by tendonitis. Teno/dynia means _____ in a tendon. Using ten(o), write another word that means painful tendon: _____.
incision of a tendon	Teno/tomy (**tə-not′ə-me**) is _____.
surgical repair of a tendon	Tendons may be damaged when a person suffers a deep wound. Tendo/plasty (**ten′do-plas″te**) is _____.
tenorrhaphy (tə-nor′ə-fe)	Write a word using ten(o) and -rrhaphy that means union of a divided tendon by a suture (suture of a tendon): _____.
bursectomy (bər-sek′to-me) **bursolith** (bər′so-lith)	**10-80** Write words that mean excision of a bursa: _____. a calculus in a bursa: _____.
several **pain of a joint** **arthrodynia** (ahr″thro-din′e-ə) **arthropathy** (ahr-throp′ə-the) **bones**	**10-81** There are many diagnostic and surgical terms that pertain to the joints. Polyarthritis (**pol″e-ahr-thri′tis**) means inflammation of _____ joints. Arthr/algia (**ahr-thral′jə**) is _____. Write another word that means pain in a joint, using a different suffix: _____. Write a word that means any disease of the joints: _____. An osteo/arthro/pathy is a disease of the _____ and joints.
spine **spondyloar-** **thropathy** (spon″də-lo-ahr- throp′ə-the) **pain in the back**	**10-82** Spondyl/arthr/itis (**spon″dəl-ahr-thri′tis**) is inflammation of the joints of the _____. (The "o" is sometimes dropped when spondyl[o] is combined with arthr[o].) Using the previous frame as a model, write a word that means any disease of the joints of the spine: _____. Many forms of arthritis are accompanied by pain and stiffness in adjacent parts. Spondylarthritis is accompanied by dors/algia (**dor-sal′jə**), which means _____.

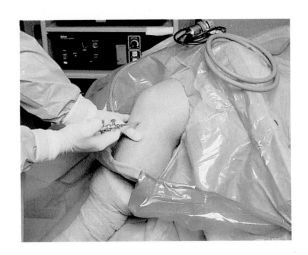

FIGURE 10-13
Arthroscopy of the knee. The examination of the interior of a joint is performed by inserting a specially designed endoscope through a small incision. This procedure also permits biopsy of cartilage or damaged synovial membrane, diagnosis of a torn meniscus, and in some instances, removal of loose bodies in the joint space. (From Mourad LA: *Orthopedic disorders*, St Louis, 1991, Mosby.)

hardening of the joints	**10-83** Arthro/scler/osis (**ahr″thro-sklə-ro′sis**) is _____.
	The tibio/femoral (**tib″e-o-fem′ə-rəl**) or knee joint is the largest joint of the body. The knee is a synovial joint. It is subject to many injuries, including dislocation, sprain, and fracture. The most common injury is tearing of the cartilage.
arthrotomy (ahr-throt′ə-me) **surgical repair of a joint**	Surgical removal of torn cartilage is sometimes necessary. Write a word that means incision of a joint using arthr(o) and the suffix that means incision: _____.
	Arthro/plasty (**ahr′thro-plas″te**) is _____.
arthroscopy (ahr-thros′kə-pe)	**10-84** An arthro/scope (**ahr′thro-skōp**) is a fiberoptic instrument used for direct visualization of the interior of a joint. The process is called _____.
	This procedure permits biopsy of cartilage or damaged synovial membrane, diagnosis of a torn meniscus, and in some instances, removal of loose bodies in the joint space (Figure 10-13).
arthrocentesis (ahr″thro-sen-te′sis)	Sometimes excessive fluid accumulates in a synovial joint after injury. It may be necessary to extract it with a needle. Write a word that means surgical puncture of a joint: _____.
x-ray of a joint	**10-85** Arthro/graphy (**ahr-throg′rə-fe**) is _____.
	This is usually done by an intraarticular injection of a radiopaque substance. Both intraarticular and
within	intra-articular mean _____ the joint.
arthrogram (ahr′thro-gram)	Write a word that means the roentgenographic record produced after introduction of opaque contrast material into a joint: _____.
excision of a joint	Arthr/ectomy (**ahr-threk′to-me**) is _____.
arthrodesis (ahr″thro-de′sis)	**10-86** The suffix *-desis* means binding or fusion. Use this suffix with arthr(o) to form a word that literally means fusion of a joint: _____.
	Arthrodesis is a surgical procedure that is used to immobilize a joint. It is artificial ankylosis. Fusing the bones together stabilizes painful joints that have become unable to bear weight. Thus a stiff but stable and painless joint results.

joint	**10-87** Arthro/clasia (**ahr″thro-kla′zhə**) is artificial breaking of an ankylosed _____ to provide movement. The suffix *-clasia* means break.
arthrolysis (ahr-throl′ə-sis)	Arthroclasia is a surgical procedure that is used to break adhesions of an ankylosed joint to provide movement. Another term that means operative loosening of adhesions in an ankylosed joint is formed by combining the word part for joint and the suffix that means dissolving or destruction. Use these word parts to write the new term: _____.
inflammation of cartilage pertaining to cartilage	**10-88** Embryos contain a great deal of translucent, elastic tissue that, for the most part, is transformed into bone as the embryo matures. This elastic tissue is cartilage. Not all cartilage becomes bone, as evidenced by cartilage found in several parts of the adult body, such as the nose and ear. The combining form *chondr(o)* means cartilage. Chondr/itis (**kon-dri′tis**) is _____. Chondr/al (**kon′drəl**) means _____.
vertebrae cartilage	**10-89** Vertebro/chondral (**vər″tə-bro-kon′drəl**) means pertaining to the _____ and the adjacent _____.
ribs	Chondro/costal (**kon″dro-kos′təl**) pertains to what structures and their associated cartilage? _____
chondrodynia (kon″dro-din′e-ə) chondralgia (kon-dral′jə) bone, cartilage	**10-90** Use two suffixes to write words that mean cartilage pain: _____ and _____. Osteo/chondr/itis (**os″te-o-kon-dri′tis**) is inflammation of what two structures? _____ and _____
cartilage	Chondritis means inflammation of cartilage. Arthro/chondr/itis (**ahr″thro-kon-dri′tis**) is inflammation of an articular _____.
resembling cartilage chondropathy (kon-drop′ə-the)	**10-91** Chondr/oid (**kon′droid**) means _____ _____. Write a word that means any disease of a cartilage: _____.
chondroma (kon-dro′mə)	**10-92** Using -oma, write a word that means a tumor (or tumorlike growth) of cartilage: _____.
cartilage	Adeno/chondr/oma (**ad″ə no-kon-dro′mə**) is a tumor containing elements of both a gland and _____. (This is also called chondroadenoma.)
destruction of cartilage	**10-93** Chondro/lysis (**kon-drol′ĭ-sis**) is _____.
chondroplasty (kon′dro-plas″te) chondrectomy (kon-drek′tə-me)	Surgical repair of cartilage is _____. This may be necessary if the cartilage becomes torn or displaced. A word that means surgical removal of cartilage is _____.
cartilage beneath the cartilage cartilages	**10-94** Perichondrium (**per″ĭ-kon′dre-əm**) is the membrane around the surface of cartilage. Peri/chondrial (**per″ĭ-kon′dre-əl**) means pertaining to or composed of perichondrium, the membrane around the _____, or concerning the perichondrium. What location is indicated by the word *sub/chondral* (**səb-kon′drəl**)? _____ Inter/chondral (**in″tər-kon′drəl**) means between two or more _____.

❑ SECTION D REVIEW *Joints, Tendons, Ligaments, and Connective Tissue Diseases*

This section review covers frames 10–66 through 10–94. Write the word part or its meaning in each blank to complete the table.

Combining Form	Meaning	Combining Form	Meaning
1. _____	stiff	6. synov(o), and synovi(o)	_____
2. arthr(o)	_____	7. ten(o), tend(o), tendin(o)	_____
3. articul(o)	_____	**Suffix**	**Meaning**
4. _____	bursa	8. _____	break
5. _____	cartilage	9. _____	binding or fusion

(Use Appendix V to check your answers.)

Muscles and Body Movement

Muscle functions in the movement of body parts and does so by contraction and relaxation of muscle fibers. Bones provide a place for muscles and supporting structures to attach. Because of the close association of the skeleton and muscles, the two systems are often referred to as one, as in musculoskeletal disorders. The muscular system is also closely associated with the nervous system, since a muscle fiber must first be stimulated by a nervous impulse before it can contract.

not	**10-95** There are three types of muscle tissue in the body: skeletal, visceral, and cardiac. Skeletal muscle, with the primary function of movement of the body and its parts, is voluntarily controlled by the nervous system. Visceral muscle, located in the walls of organs and blood vessels, is involuntary. In/voluntary means it is _____ voluntary, or not under our conscious control. (Visceral muscle is controlled by the autonomic nervous system.) The combining form ***viscer(o)*** means viscera, the internal organs enclosed within a body cavity, including the abdominal, thoracic, pelvic, and endocrine organs. Visceral means pertaining to the viscera.
heart	Cardiac muscle, myocardium, is also involuntary. Myo/cardium is _____ muscle. Characteristics of the three types of muscle tissue are shown in Figure 10-14.
chest	**10-96** Skeletal muscle makes up more than 600 muscles that are attached to and control the movement of the bones of the skeleton. The major muscles are shown in Figure 10-15. Most skeletal muscles have names that describe some feature of the muscle, sometimes with several features combined in one name. Muscle features such as size, shape, direction of fibers, location, number of attachments, origin, and action are often used in naming muscles. The name *pectoralis major* tells us it is a large muscle of the _____, and *major* indicates the large size of the muscle. The names of the muscles in the anterior view have been color-coded to indicate the origin of their names. For practice, color-code as many muscles shown in the posterior view as you can, using terms you have learned and a medical dictionary.
fascia	**10-97** A fibrous membrane called fascia (**fash′e-ə**) covers, supports, and separates muscles. The combining form for fascia is **fasci(o).** Fascial means pertaining to a _____. Most skeletal muscles are attached to bones by tendons that span joints. When the muscle contracts, one bone moves relative to the other bone, and muscles sometimes work in groups to perform a particular movement. Muscles are arranged in antagonistic pairs. This means that when one muscle of the pair is contracted, the other is relaxed. For example, the biceps brachii muscle on the anterior arm bends the forearm at the elbow. The triceps brachii muscle on the posterior arm straightens the forearm at the elbow. When the former
relaxed	muscle contracts, the other is _____.

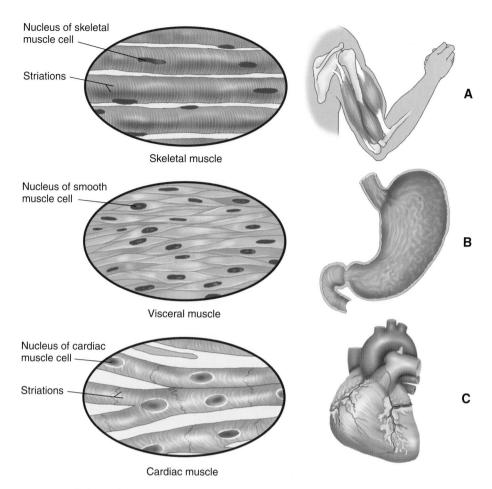

Nucleus of skeletal muscle cell

Striations

Skeletal muscle

A

Nucleus of smooth muscle cell

Visceral muscle

B

Nucleus of cardiac muscle cell

Striations

Cardiac muscle

C

FIGURE 10-14

Types of muscle. **A,** Skeletal muscle cells (fibers) are long and cylindrical with alternating light and dark bands that give the cell a striated appearance. Skeletal muscles are also known as voluntary muscles because we have conscious control over them. **B,** Visceral muscle cells are elongated, spindle-shaped, and involuntary. It is also called smooth muscle because it lacks striations. **C,** Cardiac muscle cells are cylindrical and are striated, but are shorter than skeletal muscle cells and are involuntary. These cells branch and interconnect.

flexion (flek′shən) **extension**	**10-98** Figure 10-16 gives information about some commonly used terms to describe particular movements. Use the information to write the answers in these blanks. The movement that means to bend a limb is _____. The movement that is the opposite, which straightens the limb, is called _____. The muscles responsible for these movements are called flexors and extensors.
abductors (ab-duk′tərz) **away from** **toward** **adductors** (ə-duk′tərz)	**10-99** Abduct/ion (**ab-duk′shən**) is the drawing away from the midline of the body, and the responsible muscles are called _____. The prefix **ab-** means away from, as in the word abduct. Abductors make movement possible _____ _____ the midline of the body. The prefix **ad-** means toward. If ab/duction is the drawing away from the midline of the body, ad/duction (**ə-duk′shən**) is drawing _____ the midline. The muscles responsible for adduction are called _____.

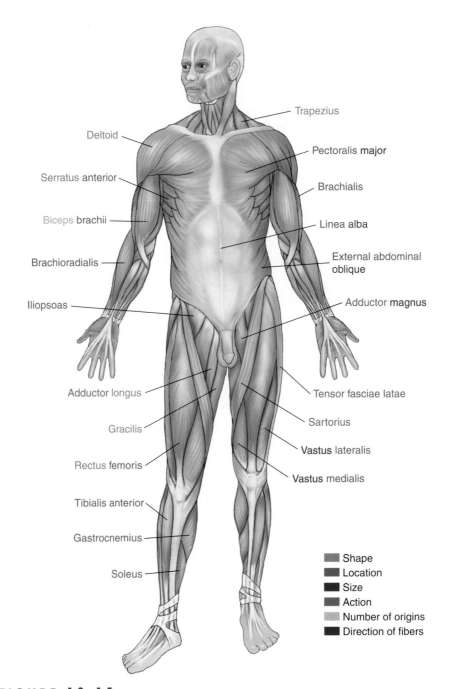

Deltoid

Serratus anterior

Biceps brachii

Brachioradialis

Iliopsoas

Adductor longus

Gracilis

Rectus femoris

Tibialis anterior

Gastrocnemius

Soleus

Trapezius

Pectoralis major

Brachialis

Linea alba

External abdominal oblique

Adductor magnus

Tensor fasciae latae

Sartorius

Vastus lateralis

Vastus medialis

Shape
Location
Size
Action
Number of origins
Direction of fibers

FIGURE 10-15

Major skeletal muscles of the body, anterior and posterior views. Muscle features such as size, shape, direction of fibers, location, number of attachments, origin, and action are often used in naming muscles. This is demonstrated by the use of color-coding of the names on the anterior view.

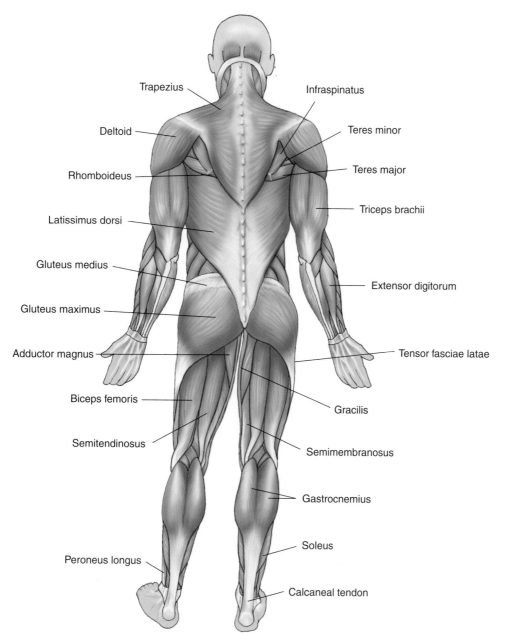

Trapezius
Deltoid
Rhomboideus
Latissimus dorsi
Gluteus medius
Gluteus maximus
Adductor magnus
Biceps femoris
Semitendinosus
Peroneus longus

Infraspinatus
Teres minor
Teres major
Triceps brachii
Extensor digitorum
Tensor fasciae latae
Gracilis
Semimembranosus
Gastrocnemius
Soleus
Calcaneal tendon

FIGURE 10-15, cont'd.
For legend, see opposite page.

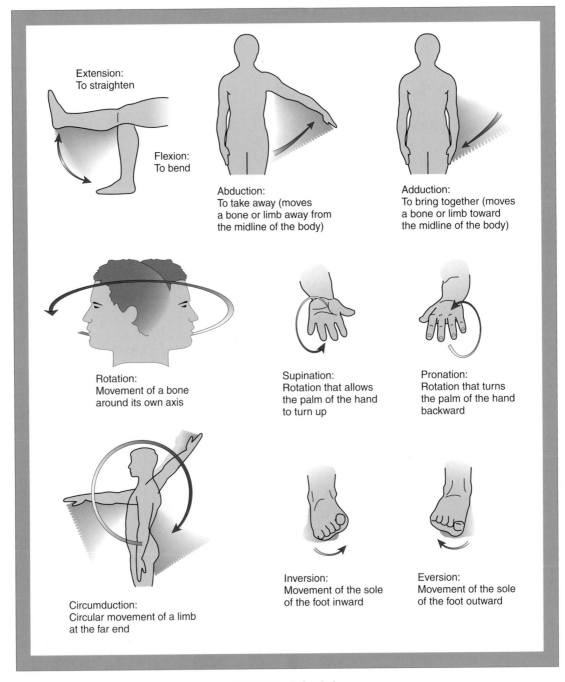

FIGURE 10-16
Types of body movements.

supination (soo″pǐ-na′shən) pronation (pro-na′shən) circumduction (ser″kəm-duk′shən) inversion (in-vər′zhən) eversion (e-ver′zhən)	**10-100** Rotation is the movement of a bone around its own axis. The rotation that allows the palm of the hand to turn up is called _____. The opposite movement is called _____. A circular movement of a limb at the far end is _____. Movement of the sole of the foot inward is _____, and the opposite movement is _____. Range of motion (ROM) is the maximum amount of movement that a healthy joint is capable of and is measured in degrees of a circle. Range-of-motion exercises are also used to increase muscle strength and joint mobility.
muscle electromyogram (e-lek″tro-mi′o- gram)	**10-101** You know that my(o) means muscle. Another combining form, _muscul(o),_ also means muscle. Muscul/ar means pertaining to _____. Before a skeletal muscle contracts, it receives an impulse from a nerve cell. The muscle exerts force on tendons, which in turn pull on bones, producing movement. Electro/myo/graphy (**e-lek″tro-mi-og′rə-fe**) is used to record the response of a muscle to electrical stimulation. This is particularly useful in studying nerve damage or other disorders. Electromyography is abbreviated EMG. The resulting record is called a _____.
	10-102 A muscle cramp is a painful, involuntary muscle spasm, often caused by inflammation of the muscle, but it can be a symptom of electrolyte imbalance. Muscle relaxants are prescribed to relieve muscle spasms. Tetany (**tet′ə-ne**) is a condition characterized by cramps, convulsions, twitching of the muscles, and sharp flexion of the wrists and ankle joints. It is caused by an imbalance in calcium metabolism.
atrophy hypertrophy	**10-103** A decrease in size of an organ or tissue is called atrophy. Muscle shrinks if a limb is immobilized. This type of atrophy is called disuse _____. Atrophy is noticeable in these cases, since the limb has decreased in size. Hyper/trophy (**hi-pər′tro-fe**) is an increase in the size of an organ, without an increase in the number of cells. An increase in the size of the heart resulting from an increase in the size of cardiac muscle cells is called cardiac _____.
size number	**10-104** Cardiomegaly or megalocardia means enlargement of the heart. It should be noted that although -megaly means enlarged, it gives no indication of the cause of the enlargement. Two suffixes that distinguish the cause of enlargement are -trophy and -plasia. In cardiac hypertrophy, is the enlargement of the heart caused by an increase in the _size_ of the existing cells or the _number_ of existing cells? _____ In contrast, an increase in the number of cells of a tissue or organ is called hyperplasia (**hi″pər-pla′zhə**). In hyperplastic bone marrow, for example, there is an increase in the _____ of bone marrow cells.
myasthenia (mi″əs-the′ne-ə)	**10-105** My/asthenia is a term specifically applied to muscle weakness. The suffix -_asthenia_ means weakness. Write this new word that means muscle weakness: _____. Myasthenia gravis is a disease of unknown cause, characterized by great muscle weakness. Death from this disease usually results from respiratory failure, but some cases of myasthenia are mild.

myolysis (mi'ol'ĭ-sis)	**10-106** Write a word that means destruction of muscle: _____.
softening	Myo/malacia (**mi″o-mə-la′shə**) is abnormal _____ of muscular tissue.
muscle pain	**10-107** My/algia (**mi-al′jə**) is _____ _____.
myodynia (mi″o-din′e-ə)	Another word that means the same as myalgia is a _____.
myopathy (mi-op′ə-the) myorrhaphy (mi-or′ə-fe) surgical repair of muscle surgical repair of muscle and tendon	**10-108** Any disease of muscle is called a _____. Write a word that means suture of a torn or cut muscle: _____. Myo/plasty (**mi′o-plas″te**) is _____. Teno/myo/plasty (**ten″o-mi′o-plas″te**) is _____.
muscle muscle muscular	**10-109** A myo/cele (**mi′o-sēl**) is herniation of a _____ through its ruptured sheath. Myo/fibr/osis (**mi″o-fi-bro′sis**) is a condition in which _____ tissue is replaced by fibrous tissue. A myo/fibr/oma (**mi″o-fi-bro′mə**) is a tumor composed of _____ and fibrous tissue.
muscles skeleton	**10-110** Musculo/skeletal (**mus″ku-lo-skel′ə-təl**) means pertaining to the _____ and _____. Because of the close association of the body's skeleton and muscles, the two systems are often referred to as one, as in musculoskeletal disorders. Additional diseases and disorders of these two systems are presented in the next section.
embryonic embryonic	**10-111** Cells of the musculo/skeletal system are derived from ancestral cells that mature and then begin to function as bone cells, muscle cells, etc. This is not unlike cells of other body systems. The combining form **blast(o)** means embryonic or early form. The suffix is -blast. A myo/blast (**mi′o-blast**) is an _____ cell that develops into muscle fiber. An osteo/blast (**os′te-o-blast″**) is an _____ bone cell.

❑ SECTION E REVIEW   *M*uscles and Body Movement

This section review covers frames 10–95 through 10–111. Complete the table by writing the word part or its meaning in each blank.

Combining Form	Meaning	Prefix	Meaning
1. _____	embryonic form	5. ab-	_____
2. _____	fascia	6. ad-	_____
3. muscul(o)	_____	**Suffix**	**Meaning**
4. _____	viscera	7. -asthenia	_____

(Use Appendix V to check your answers.)

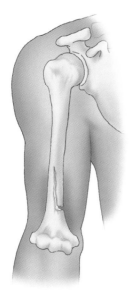
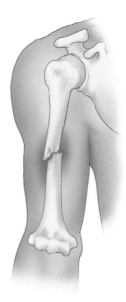
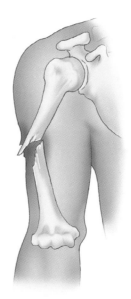

| Incomplete, simple (closed) | Complete, simple (closed) | Compound (open) |

FIGURE 10-17

Classification and description of the severity of fractures. Fractures are classified as either complete or incomplete and are described as either open or closed.

Musculoskeletal Injury and Diseases or Disorders

Injury to the musculoskeletal system, one of the primary causes of disability, ranges from simple muscle strains to severe bone fractures. Musculoskeletal disorders include bone tumors, metabolic bone diseases, and a variety of developmental bone abnormalities.

compound (or open)

10-112 Common musculoskeletal injuries include sprains, simple muscle strains, dislocations, and fractures.

A break in a bone is called a fracture. Fractures are classified as complete fractures, with the break across the entire width of the bone so it is divided into two sections, or incomplete fractures. They are also described by the extent of associated soft tissue damage as simple or compound.

The bone protrudes through the skin in a compound fracture, also called an open fracture. If a bone is fractured but does not protrude through the skin, it is called a simple or closed fracture (Figure 10-17). Which type of fracture is a broken bone that causes an external wound? _____.

An incomplete fracture in which the bone is bent and fractured on one side only as in Figure 10-17 is called a greenstick fracture and is seen principally in children.

spiral

across

10-113 Figure 10-18 illustrates four types of fractures. In an impacted fracture, one bone is firmly driven into the fractured end of another bone. Notice the many fragments of bone present in the comminuted (**kom′ĭ-noot″əd**) fracture. In which type of fracture is the bone twisted apart? _____

The bone is also displaced in the example. Displacement of a bone from a joint is also called a dislocation. The example of a transverse fracture, one in which the break is at right angles to the axis of the bone, also shows displacement. It will be helpful to remember that trans- in transverse means _____.

Dislocations and fractures are usually evident on x-ray films of the affected bones (Figure 10-19).

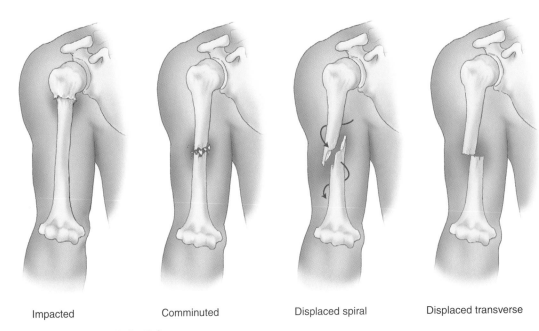

Impacted   Comminuted   Displaced spiral   Displaced transverse

FIGURE 10-18

Common types of fractures. The spiral and transverse fractures are also displaced. The ends of broken bones in displaced fractures often pierce the surrounding skin, resulting in open fractures; however, these two examples are closed fractures.

A   B   C

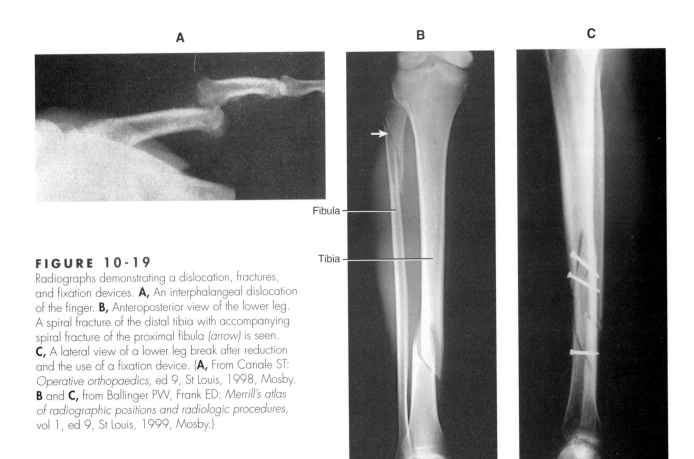

Fibula

Tibia

FIGURE 10-19

Radiographs demonstrating a dislocation, fractures, and fixation devices. **A,** An interphalangeal dislocation of the finger. **B,** Anteroposterior view of the lower leg. A spiral fracture of the distal tibia with accompanying spiral fracture of the proximal fibula *(arrow)* is seen. **C,** A lateral view of a lower leg break after reduction and the use of a fixation device. (**A,** From Canale ST: *Operative orthopaedics*, ed 9, St Louis, 1998, Mosby. **B** and **C,** from Ballinger PW, Frank ED: *Merrill's atlas of radiographic positions and radiologic procedures*, vol 1, ed 9, St Louis, 1999, Mosby.)

reduction	**10-114** Fractures are treated by reduction, pulling the broken ends into alignment. A cast immobilizes a broken bone until it heals. Correction of a fracture is called _____.
	A fracture is usually restored to its normal position by manipulation without surgery. This is called closed reduction. If the fracture must be exposed by surgery before the broken ends can be aligned, it is an open reduction. The fracture shown in Figure 10-19, *C,* was corrected by surgery that included internal fixation to stabilize the alignment.
	After a bone is broken, the body begins the healing process to repair the injury. Electrical bone stimulation, bone grafting, and ultrasound fracture treatment may be used when healing is slow or does not occur.
strain	**10-115** Although strains and sprains are not as serious as fractures, they are common traumatic injuries that cause much discomfort and can interfere with normal activities. A strain is damage, usually muscular, that results from excessive physical effort. Sprains are traumatic injury to the tendons, muscles, or ligaments around a joint, characterized by pain, swelling, and discoloration of the skin over the joint. Radiography is often needed to rule out fractures. If a muscle in the arm is very sore but shows no swelling or discoloration of the skin after many hours playing games at the computer, is this more likely to be a strain or a sprain? _____
spina bifida	**10-116** The skeletal system is affected by several developmental defects, including malformations of the spine. Some are congenital, and others can result from postural or nutritional defects or injury.
	Spina bifida (**spi′nə bif′ĭ-də**) is a congenital abnormality characterized by defective closure of the bones of the spine. It can be so extensive that it allows herniations of the spinal cord, or it might be evident only on radiologic examination. The name of this defect is _____ _____.
skull	A cranio/cele (**kra′ne-o-sēl**) is a hernial protrusion of the brain through a defect in the _____. This is the same as an encephalocele.
craniomalacia (kra″ne-o-mə-la′ she-ə)	Abnormal softness of the skull is _____.
split spine	Literal translation of rachi/schisis (**ra-kis′kĭ-sis**) is _____ _____. This is congenital fissure of one or more vertebrae.
scoliosis (sko″le-o′sis)	**10-117** Three important spinal deformities are scoliosis, lordosis, and kyphosis (Figure 10-20).
	Lateral curvature of the spine is present in which defect? _____
	Causes include congenital malformations of the spine, poliomyelitis, spastic paralysis, and unequal leg lengths.
	Lordosis (**lor-do′sis**) is abnormal concavity of the spine. Kyphosis (**ki-fo′sis**) is also an abnormal curvature of the spine, but the abnormality is increased convexity. These two abnormalities are most evident when viewed from the side.
osteopenia	**10-118** Musculoskeletal disorders include not only skeletal deformities, but also metabolic bone diseases, bone tumors, and a variety of syndromes.
	Osteo/penia (**os″te-o-pe′ne-ə**) is not a disease, but a condition that is common to metabolic bone disease. Osteopenia is a reduced bone mass, usually the result of synthesis not compensating for the rate of destruction of bone. Write this term that means a reduced bone mass: _____.
	Osteoporosis, osteomalacia, and osteitis deformans are three metabolic diseases that will be considered here.

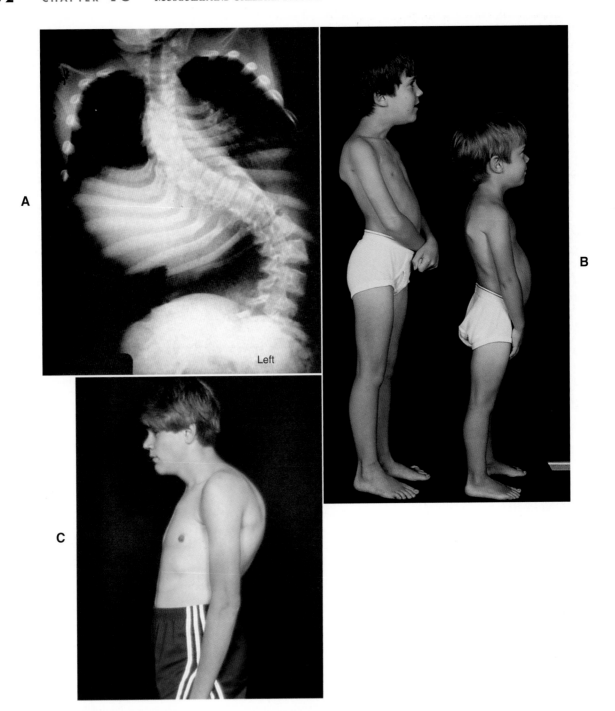

FIGURE 10-20
Three abnormal curvatures of the spine. **A,** Radiograph, posteroanterior view, showing extreme scoliosis of the spine of a 12-year-old boy with congenital spina bifida. **B,** Lordosis. **C,** Severe kyphosis of the thoracic spine. (**A,** From Laudicina PF: *Applied pathology for radiographers,* Philadelphia, 1989, WB Saunders. **B** and **C** from Zitelli BJ, Davis HW: *Atlas of pediatric physical diagnosis,* ed 3, St Louis, 1997, Mosby.)

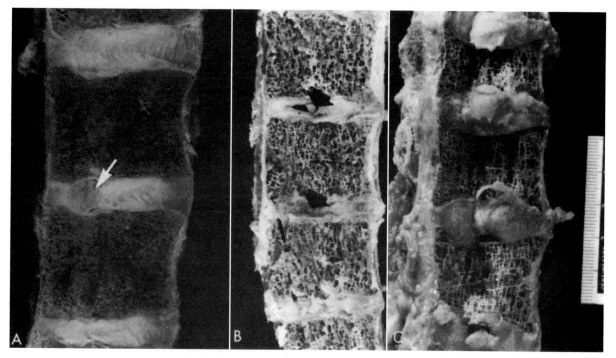

FIGURE 10-21

Normal versus osteoporotic vertebral bodies. **A,** Normal vertebral bodies. **B,** Vertebrae showing moderate osteoporosis. **C,** Vertebrae showing severe osteoporosis. The vertebral bodies are sectioned to show internal structure. *A* shows well-formed, normal vertebrae and disks. The white arrow points to a small focus of degeneration. In *B* the overall shape of the vertebrae is preserved, but osteoporosis is already well developed. The disks show severe degeneration (black arrows). Notice in *C,* severe osteoporosis, how the vertebrae have been compressed by the bulging disks. (From Walter JB: *An introduction to the principles of disease,* ed 2, Philadelphia, 1982, WB Saunders.)

---

osteoporosis

10-119 Osteo/porosis (**os"te-o-pə-ro'sis**) is a metabolic disease in which reduction in the amount of bone mass leads to subsequent fractures. It occurs most frequently in postmenopausal women, sedentary individuals, and patients on long-term steroid therapy. The bones appear thin and fragile, and fractures are common (Figure 10-21).

The metabolic bone disease in which there is a reduction in bone mass and increased porosity is called

_____.

It may cause pain, especially in the lower back, and loss of height, and spinal deformities are common. Figure 10-22 shows the effect of the disease on height and shape of the spine with advancing years. Estrogen therapy, begun soon after the start of menopause, has been found helpful in the prevention and maintenance of osteoporosis.

softening

10-120 Translated literally, osteo/malacia (**os"te-o-mə-la'shə**) means abnormal _____ of bone. It is a reversible metabolic disease in which there is a defect in the mineralization of bone, resulting from inadequate phosphorus and calcium.

The deficiency may be caused by a diet lacking phosphorus and calcium or vitamin D, which is necessary for bone formation. Other causes include malabsorption or a lack of exposure to sunlight, which is necessary for the body to synthesize vitamin D. Osteomalacia is the adult equivalent of rickets in children.

rickets
osteomalacia

Insufficient calcium for bone mineralization during the growing years causes rickets (**rik'əts**). Skeletal deformities of rickets are much more severe than those of osteomalacia in adults. In children, the disorder takes the form of _____.

In adults, the disorder is called _____.

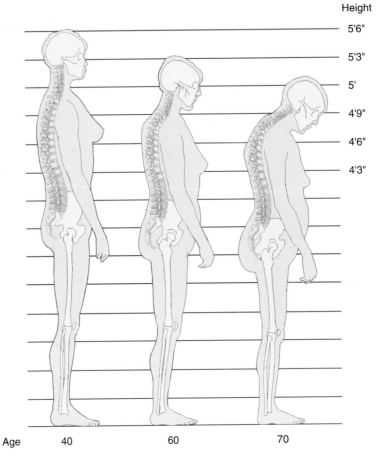

Height

5'6"

5'3"

5'

4'9"

4'6"

4'3"

Age   40   60   70

FIGURE 10-22
The effects of osteoporosis on height and shape of the spine. Compare the normal spine at age 40 with the changes that have occurred by ages 60 and 70. These changes can cause a loss of as much as 6 inches or more in height and can result in the so-called dowager's hump (far right) in the upper thoracic vertebrae.

Paget's

10-121 Osteitis deformans, also called Paget's disease, is a disorder characterized by excessive bone destruction and unorganized bone repair. First described by Dr. James Paget in 1876, the disease was thought to be an infectious inflammatory process and was named osteitis deformans. The other name for osteitis deformans is _____ disease.

marrow
inflammation

10-122 A term used to describe any infection of the bone is osteomyelitis. Analyze the word parts of the term: oste(o) means bone; myel(o) means _____, and -itis means _____.

It is caused by infectious microorganisms and is treated with antibiotics, although it often represents a difficult challenge.

bone

10-123 Benign bone tumors may be discovered on routine x-ray examination. Computed tomography, magnetic resonance imaging, biopsy, and bone scans are used to distinguish between benign and malignant tumors.

A bone scan is often useful in demonstrating malignant bone tumors, which appear as areas of increased uptake of radioactive material.

Malignant bone tumors may be primary (originating in the bone) or secondary (originating in other tissue and metastasizing to the bone). The latter greatly outnumber primary bone tumors. Osteosarcoma (os″te-o-sahr-ko′mə) is the most common type of primary _____ tumor. The suffix -sarcoma means a malignant tumor from connective tissue.

cartilage	**10-124** Three other types of primary bone tumors are chondrosarcoma, fibrosarcoma, and Ewing's sarcoma. A chondro/sarcoma (**kon″dro-sahr-ko′mə**) is derived from _____, spreads to the bone, and destroys it.
fibrous	A fibro/sarcoma (**fi″bro-sahr-ko′mə**) arises from _____ tissues. Ewing's sarcoma is an extremely malignant bone tumor.
herniated	**10-125** Acute back pain usually results from trauma. Pain resulting from pressure on spinal nerve roots is the most common symptom of a herniated disk, rupture of the disk surrounding a vertebra. This is also called a slipped disk, but a more appropriate name is a _____ disk. If bed rest does not alleviate the problem, a laminectomy may be indicated. This is surgical removal of the bony arch of a herniated disk.
wrist	**10-126** Three disorders of the hand that will be discussed are carpal tunnel syndrome (CTS), ganglion, and Dupuytren's contracture. Carp/al means pertaining to the _____. Carpal tunnel syndrome is a condition in which the median nerve in the wrist becomes compressed, causing pain and discomfort. Excessive hand exercise, a potential occupational hazard, can lead to a chronic condition of CTS. Surgery to relieve the pressure on the nerve may be necessary.
excision	**10-127** A ganglion is a round, cystlike lesion that often occurs over a wrist joint or a tendon. A ganglion is usually painless and can disappear, then recur. Fluid can often be removed with a needle (aspirated), but excision is more likely to resolve the problem. Dupuytren's contracture is a thickening and tightening of the palmar fascia, causing the fourth or fifth finger to bend into the palm and resist extension. When function becomes impaired, a partial fasciectomy is generally performed. A partial fasci/ectomy is _____ of fascia.
hallux valgus	**10-128** Four disorders of the foot that will be discussed are hallux valgus, hammertoe, Morton's neuroma, and tarsal tunnel syndrome. Hallux means the great toe. Hallux valgus is a deformity of the foot, sometimes called a bunion. The great toe deviates laterally at the metatarsophalangeal (MTP) joint. A bunionectomy involves removal of the bony overgrowth (Figure 10-23, *A*). The correct name for bunion is _____ _____.
osteotomy (os″te-ot′ə-me)	**10-129** A hammertoe is a toe that is permanently flexed at the midphalangeal joint, producing a clawlike appearance. This deformity often occurs simultaneously with hallux valgus (Figure 10-23, *B*). Hammertoe may be present in more than one digit, but the second toe is most often affected. Corns may develop on the dorsal side, and calluses may appear on the plantar surface. Surgery may be performed to correct the alignment of the toe. Write the name of this surgery by combining oste(o) and the suffix that means incision: _____.
tarsus (or ankle)	**10-130** In Morton's neuroma a small painful tumor grows in a digital nerve of the foot. Surgical removal of the neuroma is generally indicated if the pain persists and interferes with walking. Tarsal means pertaining to the _____. Tarsal tunnel syndrome is the ankle version of the carpal tunnel syndrome. Treatment is similar to that for carpal tunnel syndrome.

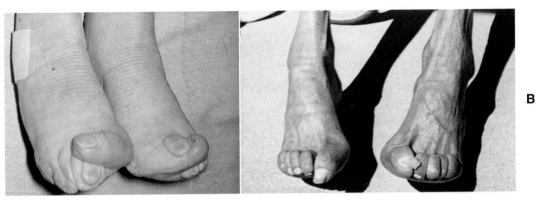

FIGURE 10-23
Deformities of the feet. **A,** Hallux valgus. The great toe rides over the second toe in this example.
B, Hammertoe. The toes are permanently flexed. Hallux valgus is also present. (From Kamal A,
Brockelhurst JC: *Color atlas of geriatric medicine,* ed 2. St Louis, 1991, Mosby.)

situated below	**10-131** Various prefixes denoting location are used to write words concerning bones of the body. The prefix *infra-* means situated below. You previously learned that sub- also means below. Sub- is used more often to form medical words, but you need to know that infra- also means _____ _____.
below the clavicle	Infra/clavicul/ar (**in″frə-klə-vik′u-lər**) means _____.
below the kneecap (patella)	Infra/patell/ar (**in″frə-pə-tel′ər**) means _____.
infrascapular (in″frə-skap′u-lər)	Use the previous example to write a word that means below the scapula: _____.
below infrasternal (in″frə-stər′nəl)	Infra/cost/al (**in″frə-kos′təl**) means _____ a rib. Using the previous example, write a word that means beneath the sternum: _____.
retrosternal (re″tro-ster′nəl)	**10-132** The prefix *retro-* is a prefix that means backward, or located behind. If infra/sternal means beneath the sternum, form a new word using retro- that means situated or occurring behind the breastbone: _____.
above	**10-133** You learned that super(o) means situated above or uppermost; *super-* is a prefix that has two meanings: above and excess; *supra-* is another prefix that means above. Super/ficial means situated on or near the surface. In this term, super- implies a location above other structures, since it means near the surface. Most medical words that refer to above a particular structure use supra- as the prefix. Supra/pubic (**soo″prə-pu′bik**) means _____ the pubis. Using supra-, write words that mean
suprapelvic (soo″prə-pel′vik)	above the pelvis: _____
suprasternal (soo″prə-stər′nəl)	above the sternum: _____
supracostal (soo″prə-kos′təl)	above a rib: _____ (Supracostal also means upon a rib.)

❑ SECTION F REVIEW 𝓜usculoskeletal Injury and Diseases or Disorders

This section review covers frames 10–112 through 10–133. Complete the table by writing a word part or meaning in each blank.

Prefix	Meaning	Suffix	Meaning
1. infra-	_____	5. -sarcoma	_____
2. _____	backward or located behind		
3. _____	above or excess		
4. _____	above		

(Use Appendix V to check your answers.)

𝓣erminology Challenge

Several terms in this chapter have been a challenge because they require more than literal translation of the word parts. Some additional challenges are included in this section.

---

syndactyly

10-134 An anomaly* (ə-**nom′**ə-**le**) is a deviation from what is regarded as normal, especially as a result of congenital defects.

Syndactyly (**sin-dak′tə-le**) is a congenital anomaly of the hand or foot, marked by persistence of the webbing between adjacent digits, so they are more or less completely attached. It can be so severe that there is complete union of the digits and fusion of the bones. Write this term that means a congenital anomaly marked by webbing between adjacent digits: _____. This is also called syndactylism (**sin-dak′tə-liz-əm**).

---

vertebra, joined (or together) binding or fusion

10-135 Analyze spondyl/syn/desis: spondyl(o) means _____;
syn- means _____;
-desis means _____.

Spondylosyndesis (**spon″də-lo-sin-de′sis**) is spinal fusion. It is fixation of an unstable segment of the spine, generally accomplished by surgical fusion with a bone graft or a synthetic device.

---

intrathecal

10-136 A lumbar puncture is performed for various therapeutic and diagnostic procedures. Diagnostic indications include obtaining cerebrospinal fluid, measuring its pressure, or injecting substances for radiographic studies of the nervous system. Therapeutic indications include removing blood or pus, injecting drugs, and introducing an anesthetic for spinal anesthesia (Figure 10-24).

An intraspinal injection is the introduction of drugs into the spine via a lumbar puncture. An intraspinal injection is the same as an intrathecal† (**in″trə-the′kəl**) injection.

An intraspinal injection is also called an _____ injection.

---

*Anomaly (Greek: *anomalos,* irregular).
†Intrathecal (intra- + Latin: *theca,* sheath).

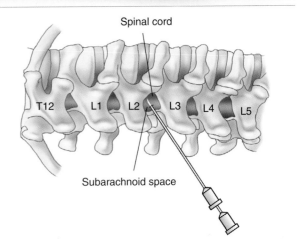

FIGURE 10-24
Lumbar puncture. The patient is generally positioned in the flexed lateral (fetal) position. The needle is inserted between the second and third or the third and the fourth lumbar vertebrae. Cerebrospinal fluid can be removed or its pressure can be measured, and drugs can be introduced as done for spinal anesthesia.

Spinal cord

T12   L1   L2   L3   L4   L5

Subarachnoid space

myocellulitis	**10-137** Cellul/itis (**sel″u-li′tis**) is an acute, spreading, swollen, pus-forming inflammation of the deep subcutaneous tissues. It may be associated with abscess formation. If the muscle is also involved, it is called myocellulitis (**mi″o-sel″u-li′tis).** You learned earlier that cellul(o) means small cell, but that may not be helpful in remembering this term. Write the term that means an acute, pus-forming inflammation of the tissues and muscle: _____.
muscular	**10-138** The suffix -trophy means nutrition. Dystrophy is any abnormal condition caused by defective nutrition. Muscular dystrophy is a group of inherited diseases that are characterized by weakness and atrophy of muscle without involvement of the nervous system. In all forms of muscular dystrophy, there is progressive loss of strength and disability. The name of this disease, the cause of which is unknown but appears to be an inborn error of metabolism, is _____ dystrophy.
muscle temporo-mandibular	**10-139** The temporomandibular (**tem″pə-ro-mən dib′u lər**) joint is one of a pair of joints connecting the mandible of the jaw to the temporal bone of the skull. It is abbreviated TMJ. An abnormal condition characterized by facial pain and by mandibular dysfunction, apparently caused by a defective or dislocated TMJ, is called TMJ pain dysfunction syndrome or is sometimes shortened to TMJ disorder. Some indications of this disorder are clicking of the joint when the jaw moves, limitation of jaw movement, and temporomandibular dislocation. It is sometimes associated with myofascial (**mi″o-fash′e-əl**) pain. Myofascial means pertaining to a _____ and its fascia. However, myofascial pain is jaw muscle distress associated with chewing or moving of the muscles associated with chewing. TMJ is an abbreviation for the _____ joint.

Study the following list of selected abbreviations. Then read through the Chapter Pharmacology section and be sure you understand the effects and uses of the drug classes that are presented. When you are finished, work the Chapter Review. After completing the exercises, check your answers with the solutions in Appendix V.

You will find these items presented after the Chapter Review:
• Listing of Medical Terms
• Enhancing Spanish Communication

Selected Abbreviations

ANA	antinuclear antibody	KJ	knee jerk
BK	below knee	lig	ligament
Ca	calcium	LS	lumbosacral
C-l, C-2, etc.	cervical vertebrae	L-l, L-2, etc.	lumbar vertebrae
CTS	carpal tunnel syndrome	NSAID	nonsteroidal antiinflammatory drug
CVA	costovertebral angle; cerebrovascular accident	RA	rheumatoid arthritis
DIP	distal interphalangeal	RF	rheumatoid factor
DIPJ	distal interphalangeal joint	ROM	range of motion
DJD	degenerative joint disease	SI	sacroiliac
DMARDs	disease-modifying antirheumatic drugs	SLE	systemic lupus erythematosus
DTR	deep tendon reflex	SLR	straight-leg raising
EMG	electromyography	T-l, T-2, etc.	thoracic vertebrae
ESR	erythrocyte sedimentation rate	TMJ	temporomandibular joint
fx	fracture	Tx	traction or treatment
jt	joint		

Chapter Pharmacology

Class	Effect and Uses	Class	Effect and Uses
Antiarthritics (NSAIDs)	**Relieve the Symptoms of Arthritis**	**Antigout (Uricosurics)—cont'd**	**Used to Treat Gout—cont'd**
celecoxib (Celebrex)	Selectively inhibits prostaglandin synthesis	probenecid (Benemid)	Increases the urinary excretion of uric acid
diclofenac (Voltaren)	Used in chronic arthritis and pain management	sulfinpyrazone (Anturane)	Increases the urinary excretion of uric acid
flurbiprofen (Ansaid)	Used in rheumatoid arthritis and osteoarthritis	**Antiinflammatories**	**Used to Relieve and Control Inflammation**
ibuprofen (Motrin)	Also used to treat pain	(See Pharmacology Section in Chapter 3.)	
ketoprofen (Orudis)	Also used to treat pain		
ketorolac (Toradol)	For relief of pain	**Neuromuscular Blocking Drugs**	
nabumetone (Relafen)	Used in treating acute arthritis	(See Pharmacology Section in Chapter 2.)	
naproxen (Naproxen)	Used in treating acute arthritis		
oxaprozin (Daypro)	Used in treating acute arthritis	**Radiopharmaceuticals**	**Used to Diagnose and Treat Metastatic Tumors**
sulindac (Clinoril)	For long-term management of both RA and DJD	Strontium-89 (Metastron)	Used both in bone scanning and in alleviating metastatic bone pain
Antigout (Uricosurics)	**Used to Treat Gout**		
allopurinol (Zyloprim)	Increases the urinary excretion of uric acid, thus decreasing uric acid in the serum		
colchicine (Colchicine)	Used to treat acute attacks of gout		

CHAPTER REVIEW 10

▶ BASIC UNDERSTANDING

REVIEWING WORD PARTS

I. Write a word (prefix, suffix, or combining form) for each clue.

CROSSWORD PUZZLE 10

Across

1 tarsus
4 split
6 bone marrow
8 fibula
9 around
11 bursa
12 new
14 cartilage
15 abnormal softening
17 process of measuring
19 spine
21 coccyx
23 large
25 nutrition (suffix)
26 stiff
29 backward or behind
30 clavicle
32 cell
34 fusion
36 skull
37 scapula
39 together
41 vertebrae
44 down, from, reversing
45 pelvis
46 vertebrae
48 wrist
49 bone
51 away from
52 humerus
53 situated below
55 straight
59 iodine (symbol)
60 ischium
62 swelling
64 formation of an
   artificial opening
65 self
66 sacrum
67 to cause an action

Down

1 nutrition (combining
   form)
2 tumor
3 break
5 sternum
7 femur
8 fascia
10 between
13 calcium
14 heel bone
16 weakness
17 softening
18 cutting instrument
20 articulation
22 phalanges
24 enzyme
27 pubis
28 muscle
31 toward
32 ribs
33 tendon
35 malignant tumor from
   connective tissue
38 above or excess
40 ulna
41 viscera
42 embryonic form
43 synovial membrane
47 patella
50 tibia
54 ilium
56 radius
57 many
58 change or next
59 membrane
61 equal
63 that which causes

MATCHING

II. Match the types of fractures in 1 through 5 with their meanings (A through E).

_____ 1. comminuted

A. A break in which there are many bone fragments

_____ 2. greenstick

B. Bone is bent and fractured on one side only

_____ 3. impacted

C. Bone is twisted apart

_____ 4. spiral

D. Break is at right angles to the axis of the bone

_____ 5. transverse

E. One bone is firmly driven into the other

III. Match the types of body movements in 1 through 10 with their meanings (A through J).

_____ 1. abduction

A. Circular movement of a limb at the far end

_____ 2. adduction

B. Movement of a bone around an axis

_____ 3. circumduction

C. Movement of the sole of the foot inward

_____ 4. eversion

D. Movement of the sole of the foot outward

_____ 5. extension

E. Rotation that allows the palm of the hand to turn up

_____ 6. flexion

F. Rotation that turns the palm of the hand backward (down)

_____ 7. inversion

G. To bend

_____ 8. pronation

H. To bring together

_____ 9. rotation

I. To straighten

_____ 10. suppination

J. To take away

LABELING

IV. Label the diagram with the combining form(s) for the bones that are indicated. For example, number 1 is clavicul(o).
(Number 5 has two combining forms.)

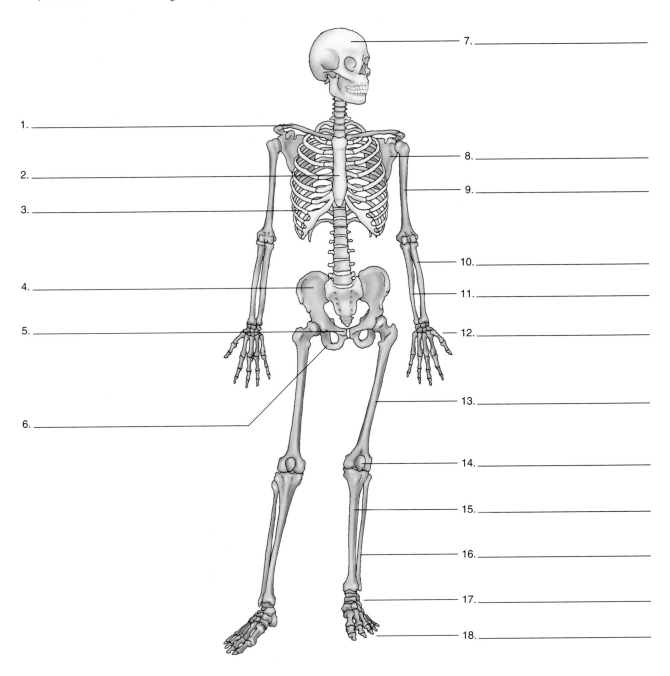

7. _____

1. _____

2. _____

3. _____

8. _____

9. _____

4. _____

10. _____

11. _____

5. _____

12. _____

6. _____

13. _____

14. _____

15. _____

16. _____

17. _____

18. _____

V. Match the bones in 1 through 10 with their common names (A through J):

_____ 1. carpal	**A.** Ankle bone	_____ 6. pelvis	**F.** Kneecap
_____ 2. clavicle	**B.** Bones of the fingers and toes	_____ 7. phalanges	**G.** Shoulder blade
_____ 3. coccyx	**C.** Breastbone	_____ 8. scapula	**H.** Tailbone
_____ 4. femur	**D.** Collarbone	_____ 9. sternum	**I.** Thigh bone
_____ 5. patella	**E.** Hip bone	_____ 10. tarsal	**J.** Wrist bone

SEQUENCING

VI. The five types of vertebrae are listed. Indicate their position by numbering them from uppermost (1) to the lowest (5):

cervical _____   sacral _____
coccygeal _____   thoracic _____
lumbar _____

MULTIPLE CHOICE

VII. Choose one answer (A–D) for each of the following multiple choice questions.

1. Which of the following is excision of the tail bone?
   A. coccygectomy
   B. phalangectomy
   C. sacrectomy
   D. vertebrectomy

2. What is sternoschisis?
   A. any morbid softening of the sternum
   B. congenital fissure of the breast bone
   C. excision of a rib from where it is attached to the breast bone
   D. sternal puncture for obtaining bone marrow samples

3. To what does iliac pertain to?
   A. a bone of the forearm
   B. a type of vertebra
   C. the ileum
   D. the ilium

4. Ulnoradial pertains to which two bones?
   A. forearm
   B. spine
   C. upper arm
   D. wrist

5. What is flexion?
   A. a specific type of muscle
   B. an internal organ enclosed within a cavity
   C. bending of a limb at a joint
   D. movement that brings a limb into a straight position

6. Dystrophy means any disorder arising from which of the following?
   A. difficult movement
   B. painful movement
   C. poor muscular coordination
   D. poor nutrition

7. Which term means any disease of the joints?
   A. arthropathy
   B. bursopathy
   C. chondropathy
   D. osteopathy

8. Which of the following procedures is used to record the response of a muscle to electrical stimulation?
   A. electromyography
   B. myelography
   C. sonography
   D. tomography

9. What does craniomalacia mean?
   A. abnormal softness of the skull
   B. an enlarged skull
   C. instrument for measuring the skull
   D. measurement of the skull

10. Which of the following is a break involving a fragmented bone that protrudes through the skin?
    A. compound comminuted fracture
    B. compound oblique fracture
    C. simple comminuted fracture
    D. simple oblique fracture

11. Which of the following means loss of calcium from bone?
    A. calcification
    B. calciuria
    C. decalcification
    D. osteogenesis

12. Where are intercostal muscles located?
    A. between the ribs
    B. between the vertebrae
    C. over the ribs
    D. over the vertebrae

13. What are metacarpals?
    A. bones of the ankle
    B. bones of the wrist
    C. bones that connect the ankle bones to the phalanges
    D. bones that connect the wrist bones to the phalanges

14. What is the presence of extra toes or fingers called?
    A. carpopedal disease
    B. Paget's disease
    C. phalangitis
    D. polydactyly

15. Where is the inflammation in myeloencephalitis?
    A. bone and bone marrow
    B. bone marrow and spinal cord
    C. brain and spinal cord
    D. spine and spinal cord

16. Which of the following is not a function of bones?
    A. blood cell formation
    B. protection of soft body parts
    C. providing energy
    D. storage of minerals

17. Which term means formation of bone?
    A. ossification
    B. osteocyte
    C. osteolysis
    D. osteoplasty

18. What is the name of the soft tissue that fills the cavity of a bone?
    A. diaphysis
    B. epiphysis
    C. marrow
    D. periosteum

19. Which of the following connects bones or cartilages and serves to support and strengthen a joint?
    A. bursa   C. ligament
    B. fascia   D. tendon

20. Which of the following is *not* a function of connective tissues?
    A. bind other structures together
    B. contain an abundance of intercellular material
    C. have a signficant role in body defense
    D. support other structures

FILL IN THE BLANKS

VIII. Write the missing word in each blank space.

1. Most of the bone is covered with a tough membrane called _____.

2. A deficiency of calcium in the body is called _____.

3. A term that means the same as "joint" is _____.

4. Bands of strong, fibrous tissue that attach the muscles to the bones are _____.

5. A chronic, systemic inflammatory process that affects primarily the synovial joints is _____ arthritis.

6. An autoimmune disease that is named for the characteristic butterfly rash that sometimes appears across the bridge of the nose is _____ _____.

7. Inflammation and stiffening of the spine is called _____ spondylitis.

8. A circular movement of a limb at the far end is called _____.

9. Lateral curvature of the spine is _____.

10. When a lumber puncture is performed and drugs are introduced into the spine, it is called an intraspinal injection, or an _____ injection.

WRITING TERMS

IX. Write a term for each of the following meanings:

1. an embryonic bone cell   _____
2. displacement of a bone from a joint   _____
3. excision of a cartilage   _____
4. incision of the breastbone   _____
5. inflammation of a bursa   _____
6. inflammation of the bone marrow   _____
7. morbid softening of muscle   _____
8. painful heel   _____
9. pertaining to the collarbone   _____
10. surgical repair of a joint   _____

▶ GREATER COMPREHENSION

SPELLING

X. Circle all incorrectly spelled terms and write their correct spelling.

karpectomy   myelosupression   osteitis   perichondrium   spondilitis

FILL IN THE BLANKS

XI. Use one of these terms to complete each blank in the following paragraphs:

appendicular   axial   cranial   diaphysis   epiphyseal   epiphyses   false   floating   red   sternum   true   yellow

The human skeleton is usually grouped into two major divisions. The (1) _____ skeleton consists of the skull, vertebral column and thoracic cage. Bones of the upper and lower extremities, as well as the shoulder and pelvic girdles, make up the

(2) _____ skeleton.

The long main portion of a long bone is called the (3) _____. The ends of the bone are called the (4) _____.

The skull is composed of three types of bones: (5) _____ bones, facial bones, and auditory ossicles. The ribs exist in pairs. The upper seven pairs are called (6) _____ ribs because they join directly with the (7)_____. The remaining five pairs are called (8) _____ ribs. The last two pairs are called (9) _____ ribs because they are attached only on the posterior side.

Bone marrow is of two types. (10) _____ marrow principally consists of fat cells and connective tissue. (11) _____ marrow is responsible for hematopoiesis.

XII. Write words in the blanks to complete the following:

There are three types of muscle tissue. That which is controlled by the conscious part of the brain is called (1) _____ muscle. Smooth muscle is located in the walls of hollow internal structures and is called (2) _____ muscle. Muscle tissue that forms the walls of the heart is called (3) _____.

Joints, tendons, and ligaments are types of (4) _____ tissues. The ends of the opposing bones in a synovial joint are covered with articular (5) _____, which provides protection and support for the joint. Fluid-filled sacs that are often near a joint and help reduce friction are called (6) _____. Degenerative joint disease is sometimes called (7) _____. A systemic disease in which urate crystals deposit in the joints and cause inflammation is called (8) _____.

INTERPRETING ABBREVIATIONS

XIII. Write the meaning of these abbreviations:

1. CTS _____
2. DIP _____
3. ESR _____

4. ROM _____
5. T-1 _____

PRONUNCIATION

XIV. The pronunciation is shown for several medical words. Indicate which syllable has the primary accent by marking it with a ′.

1. arthroclasia (**ahr thro kla zhə**)
2. arthroscopy (**ahr thros kə pe**)
3. chondrosarcoma (**kon dro sahr ko mə**)
4. fascia (**fash e ə**)
5. lumbar (**lum bahr**)

6. myalgia (**mi al jə**)
7. myasthenia (**mi əs the ne ə**)
8. osteoporosis (**os te o pə ro sis**)
9. sternocostal (**stər no kos təl**)
10. tibiofemoral (**tib e o fem ər əl**)

CATEGORIZING TERMS

XV. Categorize each of the following terms by writing A, D, R, or S to indicate if the term is anatomical, diagnostic, radiological, or surgical.

1. arthroclasia _____
2. arthrogram _____
3. carpophalangeal _____
4. craniotome _____
5. electromyography _____

6. hammertoe _____
7. laminectomy _____
8. rachischisis _____
9. spondylarthritis _____
10. tarsus _____

DRUG CLASSES

XVI. Match the drug classes in the left column with their uses in the right column.

_____ 1. antiarthritics   **A.** To diagnose and treat metastatic tumors
_____ 2. antigout   **B.** To increase the urinary excretion of uric acid
_____ 3. radiopharmaceuticals   **C.** To relieve the symptoms of pain and inflammation

(Check your answers with the solutions in Appendix V.)

Listing of Medical Terms

abduction	calcaneofibular	craniocele	humeroradial
abductor	calcaneoplantar	craniomalacia	humeroscapular
abduction	calcaneotibial	craniometer	humeroulnar
adductor	calcaneus	craniopathy	humerus
adenochondroma	calcification	cranioplasty	hypercalciuria
ankylosed	calcipenia	craniotome	hyperplasia
ankylosing spondylitis	calciuria	craniotomy	hypertrophy
ankylosis	carpal	cranium	iliac
anomaly	carpal tunnel syndrome	decalcification	iliofemoral
antarthritic	carpals	degenerative joint disease	iliopubic
antiarthritic	carpectomy	dermatomyositis	ilium
antiinflammatory	carpopedal	diaphysis	impacted fracture
appendicular	carpophalangeal	dislocation	infraclavicular
arthralgia	carpus	dorsalgia	infracostal
arthrectomy	cephalopelvic disproportion	Dupuytren's contracture	infrapatellar
arthritis	cervical	dystrophy	infrascapular
arthrocentesis	cervicodorsal	electromyogram	infrasternal
arthrochondritis	chondral	electromyography	interchondral
arthroclasia	chondralgia	epiphysis	intercostal
arthrodesis	chondrectomy	eversion	interpubic
arthrodynia	chondritis	Ewing's sarcoma	interscapular
arthrogram	chondrocostal	extension	intervertebral
arthrography	chondrodynia	extensor	intraarticular
arthrolysis	chondroid	fascia	intrasternal
arthropathy	chondrolysis	fasciectomy	intrathecal
arthroplasty	chondroma	femoral	inversion
arthrosclerosis	chondropathy	femur	ischial
arthroscope	chondroplasty	fibromyalgia	ischialgia
arthroscopy	chondrosarcoma	fibrosarcoma	ischiococcygeal
arthrotomy	circumduction	fibula	ischiodynia
articular	clavicle	fibular	ischiofemoral
articulation	coccygeal	flexion	ischiopubic
aspiration	coccygectomy	flexor	ischium
atrophy	coccyx	fracture	kyphosis
autoimmune	comminuted fracture	ganglion	lacrimal
axial	compound fracture	gout	laminectomy
bursa	costal	greenstick fracture	ligament
bursectomy	costalgia	hallux valgus	lordosis
bursitis	costectomy	hammertoe	lumbar
bursolith	costoclavicular	hematopoiesis	lupus erythematosis
calcaneal	costovertebral	hemotherapy	Lyme disease
calcaneitis	cranial	herniated disk	mandible
calcaneodynia	craniectomy	humeral	maxilla

Listing of Medical Terms—cont'd

metacarpal
metatarsal
metatarsophalangeal
Morton's neuroma
multiple sclerosis
muscular
muscular dystrophy
musculoskeletal
myalgia
myasthenia
myelitis
myeloblast
myelocyte
myeloencephalitis
myelography
myelosuppression
myelosuppressive
myoblast
myocele
myocellulitis
myodynia
myofascial
myofibrils
myofibroma
myofibrosis
myolysis
myomalacia
myopathy
myoplasty
myorrhaphy
nasal
oblique fracture
open fracture
ossification
ostealgia
osteectomy
osteitis
osteitis deformans
osteoarthritis
osteoarthropathy
osteoblast

osteochondritis
osteocyte
osteodynia
osteogenesis
osteoid
osteolysis
osteomalacia
osteometry
osteomyelitis
osteopenia
osteoplasty
osteoporosis
osteosarcoma
osteosclerosis
osteotome
osteotomy
osteotrophy
Paget's disease
patella
patellectomy
patellofemoral
pelvic
perichondrial
perichondrium
periosteum
phalanges
polyarthritis
polydactylism
polydactyly
polymyalgia rheumatica
polymyositis
pronation
pseudogout
pubes
pubic
pubis
pubofemoral
rachialgia
rachiodynia
rachischisis
radiopaque

radius
reduction
retrosternal
rheumatoid arthritis
rickets
sacral
sacrodynia
sacrum
scapula
scapular
scapuloclavicular
scleroderma
sclerosis
scoliosis
simple fracture
Sjögren's syndrome
sphenoid
spina bifida
spondylalgia
spondylarthritis
spondylarthropathy
spondylitis
spondylomalacia
spondylosyndesis
stapes
sternal
sternalgia
sternoclavicular
sternocostal
sternopericardial
sternoschisis
sternotomy
sternovertebral
sternum
subchondral
subcostal
subpubic
substernal
supination
supracostal
suprapelvic

suprapubic
suprasternal
syndactylism
syndactyly
synovial
synovitis
tarsal
tarsal tunnel syndrome
tarsoptosis
tarsus
temporal
temporomandibular
tenalgia
tendon
tendonitis
tendoplasty
tenodynia
tenomyoplasty
tenorrhaphy
tenotomy
tetany
thoracolumbar
tibia
tibialgia
tibiofemoral
transverse fracture
ulna
ulnoradial
vasculitis
vertebra
vertebrectomy
vertebrochondral
vertebrocostal
vertebroplasty
vertebrosternal
viscera
visceral
vomer
zygomatic

Español

Enhancing Spanish Communication

English	Spanish (pronunciation)
ankle	tobillo (to-BEEL-lyo)
arm	brazo (BRAH-so)
back	espalda (es-PAHL-dah)
bones	huesos (oo-AY-sos)
calcium	calcio (CAHL-se-o)
cartilage	cartílago (car-TEE-lah-go)
cheek	mejilla (may-HEEL-lyah)
chew (to)	masticar (mas-te-CAR)
collarbone	clavícula (clah-VEE-coo-lah)
cranium	cráneo (CRAH-nay-o)
elbow	codo (CO-do)
extremity	extremidad (ex-tray-me-DAHD)
face	cara (CAH-rah)
finger	dedo (DAY-do)
foot (pl. feet)	pie (PE-ay, PE-ays)
forearm	antebrazo (an-tay-BRAH-so)
fracture	fractura (frac-TOO-rah)
head	cabeza (cah-BAY-sah)
heel	talón (tah-LON)
hip	cadera (cah-DAY-rah)
jaw	mandíbula (man-DEE-boo-lah)
joint	articulacíon (ar-te-coo-lah-se-ON), coyuntura (co-yoon-TOO-rah)
knee	rodilla (ro-DEEL-lyah)
kneecap	rótula (RO-too-lah)
ligament	ligamento (le-gah-MEN-to)
movement	movimiento (mo-ve-me-EN-to)
neck	cuello (coo-EL-lyo)
nutrition	nutrición (noo-tre-se-ON)

English	Spanish (pronunciation)
phalanges	falanges (fah-LAHN-hays)
phosphorus	fósforo (FOS-fo-ro)
protection	protección (pro-tec-se-ON)
reduction	reducción (ray-dooc-se-ON)
rib	costilla (cos-TEEL-lyah)
sacrum	hueso sacro (oo-AY-so SAH-cro)
shoulder	hombro (OM-bro)
shoulder blade	espaldilla (es-pal-DEEL-lyah)
skeleton	esqueleto (es-kay-LAY-to)
skull	cráneo (CRAH-nay-o)
spinal column	columna vertebral (co-LOOM-nah ver-tay-BRAHL)
spine	espinazo (es-pe-NAH-so)
spiral	espiral (es-pe-RAHL)
sprain, to	torcer (tor-SERR)
sternum	esternón (es-ter-NON)
stiff	tieso (te-AY-so)
support	sustento (sus-TEN-to)
temple	sien (se-AYN)
tendon	tendón (ten-DON)
thigh	muslo (MOOS-lo)
thumb	pulgar (pool-GAR)
toe	dedo del pie (DAY-do del pe-AY)
vertebral column	columna vertebral (co-LOOM-nah ver-tay-BRAHL)
weakness	debilidad (day-be-le-DAHD)
wrist	muñeca (moo-NYAY-cah)
x-ray	radiografía (rah-de-o-grah-FEE-ah)

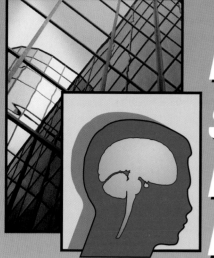

Nervous System and Psychological Disorders

11

Outline

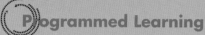
Principal Word Parts

COMBINING FORMS

algesi(o)	sensitivity to pain
arachn(o)	spider or arachnoid membrane
audi(o)	hearing
aut(o)	self
blephar(o)	eyelid
cerebell(o)	cerebellum
cerebr(o)	cerebrum
chem(o)	chemical
dacry(o), lacrim(o)	tear
dendr(o)	tree
esthesi(o)	feeling
gli(o)	neuroglia or a sticky substance
ir(o), irid(o)	iris
kerat(o)	cornea; hard, horny
kinesi(o)	movement
mening(o)	meninges
ment(o), psych(o)	mind
mon(o)	one or single
myel(o)	bone marrow or spinal cord
narc(o)	sleep
neur(o)	nerve
ocul(o), ophthalm(o)	eye
opt(o), optic(o)	vision
phren(o)	mind or diaphragm
pyr(o)	fire
schist(o), schiz(o)	split

PREFIXES

contra-	against
di-	twice
hemi-	half
idio-	individual
inter-	between
quadri-	four
semi-	half or partly

SUFFIXES

-esthesia	sensation, perception
-kinesia	movement
-lepsy	seizure
-mania	excessive preoccupation
-opia	vision
-phobia	abnormal fear
-tripsy	surgical crushing

Learning Goals

▶ **BASIC UNDERSTANDING**

In this chapter, you will learn to do the following:

1. Recognize descriptions of the major divisions and structures of the nervous system.
2. Identify the structural and functional characteristics of a neuron.
3. Describe the stimulus for the five types of receptors.
4. Use medical terminology to complete case studies.
5. Use the word parts to build and analyze terms concerning the nervous system.
6. Demonstrate understanding of several disorders of the nervous system.

▶ **GREATER COMPREHENSION**

7. Categorize terms as anatomical, diagnostic, or radiological.
8. Spell the terms accurately.
9. Pronounce the terms correctly.
10. Know the meanings of the abbreviations.
11. Identify the effects or uses of the drug classes presented in this chapter.

Divisions of the Nervous System and the Neuron

SECTION A

The nervous system is the control center and communications network. It stimulates movement and senses changes both within and outside the body. With the help of the hormonal system, the nervous system maintains homeostasis, a dynamic equilibrium of the internal environment of the body. The brain, a soft mass of tissue weighing approximately 1360 grams (3 pounds) in the average adult, receives thousands of bits of information and integrates all of the data to determine the appropriate response. The nervous system is the most complex of all body systems. Nerve cells called neurons are responsible for conducting impulses from one part of the body to another.

11-1 The nervous system, the body's most organized and complex system, affects both psychological and physiologic functions. In addition to being the center of thinking and judgment, the nervous system influences other body systems. For example, damage to the spinal nerves that supply nerve impulses to the diaphragm may result in respiratory arrest.

The various activities can be grouped as sensory, integrative, and motor functions. These functions keep us in touch with our environment, maintain homeostasis, and provide us with thought, learning, and memory.

11-2 Sensory receptors detect changes that occur inside and outside the body. For example, receptors monitor external changes such as light or room temperature. They also monitor changes within the body such as body temperature and blood pressure. The gathering of this type of information is the

sensory

_____ function of the nervous system.

Integrative functions create sensations, produce thoughts and memory, and make decisions based on sensory input.

The nervous system responds to sensory input and integration by sending signals to muscles or glands and causing an effect. Responding and causing an effect in muscles or glands is the motor function of the nervous system.

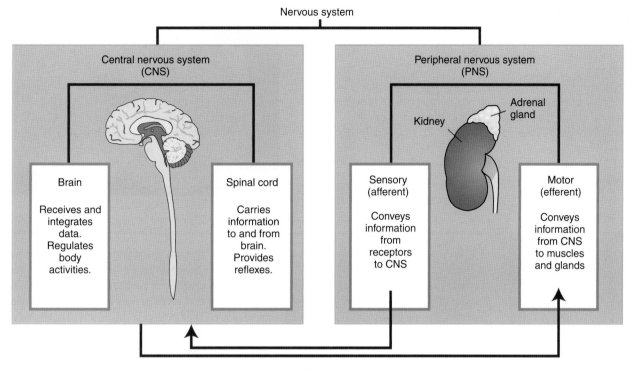

FIGURE 11-1
Major divisions of the nervous system.

central **peripheral** **brain, spinal cord**	**11-3** The two principal divisions of the nervous system are the central nervous system (CNS) and the peripheral (pə-rif′ə-rəl) nervous system (PNS). CNS is an abbreviation for _____ nervous system. PNS means _____ nervous system. Looking at Figure 11-1, you see that the CNS is composed of the brain and the spinal cord. This part of the system is the control center. It is composed of the _____ and the _____ _____.
efferent (ef′ər-ənt) **efferent** **afferent**	**11-4** The second division of the nervous system is the PNS, the various nerve processes that connect the brain and the spinal cord with receptors, muscles, and glands. Observing the diagram, you see that the PNS is divided into a sensory or afferent (af′ər-ənt) system and a motor or _____ system. Which system conveys information from the CNS to muscles and glands? _____ Which system conveys information from the receptors back to the CNS? _____
nerve **neurons, neuroglia**	**11-5** The nervous system is composed of two types or cells: neurons (noor′onz) and neuroglia (noo-rog′le-ə). You have learned that neur(o) means _____. Both types of cells that compose nervous tissue are named using neur(o). Write the names of the two types of cells: _____ and _____.

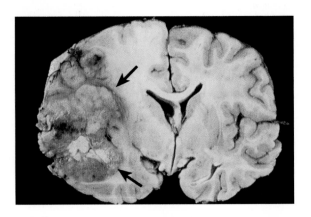

FIGURE 11-2
A primary brain tumor. This autopsy specimen of the brain shows a large tumor *(arrows)*. This patient had multiple distant metastases in the lung and spine. (From Osborn AG, Wintrhop S: *Diagnostic neuroradiology*, St Louis, 1994, Mosby.)

neuroglia

11-6 Neurons and neuroglia, or glial,* cells have different functions and appearances. Neurons conduct impulses either to or from the nervous system. Neuroglia provide special support and protection. If a neuron is destroyed, it cannot replace itself. On the other hand, neuroglia cells are far more numerous and, because they can reproduce, are the only source of primary malignant brain tumors, those originating in the brain. The tumors are called gliomas (gli-o′məz). The combining form *gli(o),* means neuroglia or a sticky substance. A gli/oma is a primary tumor of the brain and is composed of which type of nerve cell? _____

within

Tumors of the brain invade and compress brain tissue, which generally leads to increased intracranial pressure (ICP), headaches, and many neurologic problems. You know that crani(o) means the cranium, or skull, so intra/cranial means _____ the skull. Brain tumors can become quite large and occupy considerable intracranial space as shown in Figure 11-2.

tumor

Remembering that -oma means tumor, a neur/oma (noŏ-ro′mə) is a benign _____ composed chiefly of neurons and nerve fibers. Although they are benign, they can be painful (for example, a Morton's neuroma that occurs in the foot) or can compress brain tissue (an acoustic neuroma).

11-7 The neuron, or nerve cell, is the basic unit of the nervous system. Neurons carry out the function of the nervous system by conducting nerve impulses. Each neuron has a cell body, a single axon (ak′son), and one or more dendrites (den′drīts) (Figure 11-3).

The axon and dendrites are cytoplasmic projections, or processes, that project from the cell body. They are sometimes called nerve fibers. An axon carries impulses away from the cell body. Dendrites transmit impulses to the cell body. Which type of cytoplasmic projection carries a nervous impulse away from the cell body? _____

axon

dendrite

The combining form *dendr(o)* means tree. Which type of cytoplasmic projection has numerous branches? _____

gray

11-8 Many axons are surrounded by a white lipid covering called a myelin sheath. The myelinated axons appear whitish and are called white matter. Those that are not myelinated appear grayish, and are called _____ matter.

In a myelinated fiber, the nerve impulse "jumps" from one node of Ranvier (Figure 11-3) to the next and results in a faster rate of conduction than in an unmyelinated nerve fiber. If the myelin sheath becomes damaged, as it does in diseases like multiple sclerosis, conduction of the impulse is impaired.

nervous

An axon terminates in several short branches that together form a synaptic bulb. This is the region of communication between one neuron and another and is called the synapse (sin′aps). The synaptic bulb releases a neurotransmitter that either inhibits or enhances a nervous impulse. A neuro/transmitter is a chemical that transmits a _____ impulse that either inhibits or enhances a reaction.

*Glial (Greek: *glia,* glue + -al, pertaining to).

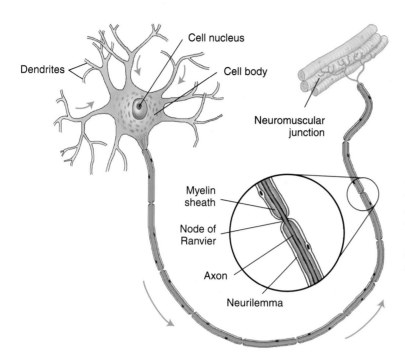

FIGURE 11-3
Structure of a typical neuron. The basic parts of a neuron are the cell body, a single axon, and several dendrites. Arrows indicate the direction that an impulse travels to or from the cell body. The axon is surrounded by a segmented myelin sheath with neurilemma that forms a tight covering over each segment. The unmyelinated regions between the myelin segments are called the nodes of Ranvier. A myelinated nerve fiber is capable of conducting an impulse many times faster than if it were not myelinated.

---

neurotransmitters

11-9 Some of the best known neurotransmitters are acetylcholine, epinephrine, dopamine, serotonin, and endorphins. To prevent prolonged reactions, a neurotransmitter is quickly inactivated by an enzyme. For example, acetylcholine is inactivated by acetylcholinesterase.

Disorders involving neurotransmitters have been implicated in the origin of various psychological disorders. The substances released at the synapse that either enhance or inhibit a nervous impulse are called _____.

---

nerves
muscles

11-10 Neuro/muscul/ar (**noor″o-mus′ku-lər**) means concerning both _____ and _____.

A neuro/muscular junction is the area of contact between a neuron and adjoining skeletal muscle.

When a nerve impulse reaches the neuromuscular junction, a substance called acetylcholine (**as″ə-təl-ko′lēn, as-ə-tēl-ko′ lēn**) is released, which leads to contraction of the muscle.

---

neuromuscular
acetylcholinesterase
(as″ə-təl-ko″lĭ-
nes′tə-rās, as″ə-tēl-
ko″lĭ-nes′tə-rās)

myospasm
(mi′o-spaz-əm)
neural (noor′əl)

11-11 Certain drugs can block transmission of impulses to the skeletal muscle. Blocking of the impulse is at the area of contact between a neuron and a skeletal muscle. This area is called the _____ junction.

Acetylcholine acts rapidly on muscle tissue, and most of it is then promptly inactivated. Write the name of the enzyme that is responsible for inactivating acetylcholine: _____.

There are also drugs that interfere with the action of acetylcholinesterase. If this occurs, acetylcholine accumulates and causes muscular spasm. A word you learned that means muscle spasm can be formed by using my(o). Write the word: _____.

Write a term that means pertaining to a nerve or nerves: _____.

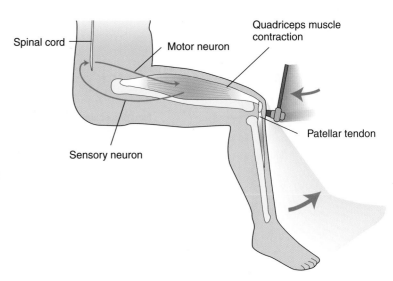

FIGURE 11-4

Conceptual drawing of the reflex arc. A receptor detects the stimulus, the tap on the patellar tendon with the reflex hammer. The sensory neuron transmits the nerve impulse to the spinal cord. The motor neuron conducts a nervous impulse that causes the quadriceps muscle to contract. Extension of the leg at the knee is the normal patellar response, also called knee jerk.

reflex

11-12 Conduction of nervous impulses is often described as a reflex arc. A reflex is an automatic, involuntary response to some change, either inside or outside the body. Reflexes help maintain homeostasis by making constant adjustments to our blood pressure, breathing rate, and pulse. A common reflex is that of quickly removing your hand from a hot object.

A deep tendon reflex (DTR) is one way of assessing the reflex arc. For example, a sharp tap on the tendon just below the kneecap normally causes extension of the leg at the knee. This is called the patellar response or knee jerk response. A normal response indicates an intact reflex arc between the nervous system and the muscles that are involved in the response. Other areas are also assessed for reflex activities. An automatic, involuntary response to some change, either inside or outside the body, is called a

_____.

11-13 The reflex arc involves two types of neurons: a sensory neuron and a motor neuron. Sensory neurons transmit nerve impulses toward the spinal cord and the brain. Motor neurons transmit nerve impulses from the brain and the spinal cord (Figure 11-4).

❑ SECTION A REVIEW 𝒟ivisions of the Nervous System and the Neuron

This section review covers frames 11–1 through 11–13. Complete the table by writing the meaning of each word part as shown.

Combining Form	Meaning	Combining Form	Meaning
1. dendr(o)	_____	2. gli(o)	_____

(Use Appendix V to check your answers.)

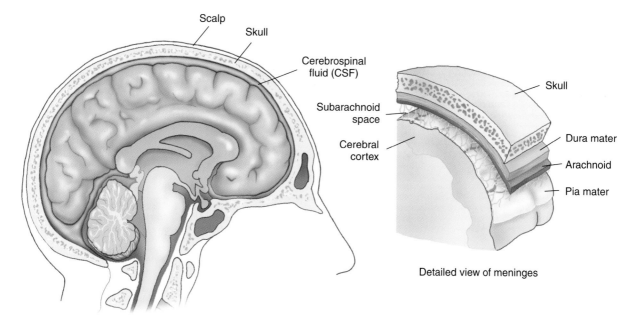

Detailed view of meninges

FIGURE 11-5

The brain and its protective coverings, the meninges. The tough outer membrane, the dura mater, lies just inside the skull. The threadlike strands of the middle layer, the arachnoid, resemble a cobweb. The pia mater is the innermost meningeal layer and is so tightly bound to the brain that it cannot be removed without damaging the surface.

Central Nervous System

The brain and spinal cord are protected by bone, the meninges, and circulating cerebrospinal fluid. Disturbances of the central nervous system vary from acute to chronic, short term to long term, and minor to life threatening.

11-14 The central nervous system consists of the brain and spinal cord. The brain is surrounded by the cranium (skull), and the spinal cord is protected by the vertebrae.

Three membranes collectively known as the meninges (singular, meninx) also provide protection (Figure 11-5). The tough outer layer, the dura mater* (**doo′rə ma′tər**) lies just inside the cranial bones and lines the vertebral canal. The middle layer is the arachnoid (**ə-rak′noid**), a thin layer with numerous threadlike strands that attach it to the innermost layer. The combining form *arachn(o)* means either the arachnoid membrane or spider. The innermost layer, the pia mater† (**pi′ə ma′tər, pe′ə mah′tər**), is thin and delicate and is tightly attached to the surface of the brain and spinal cord.

dura mater   The outer layer is the _____ _____.

arachnoid   The middle layer is the _____.

pia mater   The innermost layer is the _____ _____.

*Dura mater (Latin: *durus*, hard, *mater*, mother).
†Pia mater (Latin: *pia*, tender, *mater*, mother).

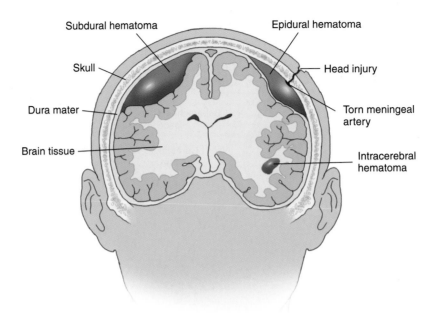

FIGURE 11-6
Three types of hematomas associated with head injuries: subdural hematoma, epidural hematoma, and intracerebral hematoma.

meninges (mə-nin′jēz) **brain, spinal cord** **meningeal** (mə-nin′ge-əl)	**11-15** The three membranes that cover the brain and the spinal cord are collectively called the _____. The combining form **mening(o)** refers to the meninges. The meninges are the membranes surrounding the _____ and the _____ _____. Use the suffix *-eal* to write a term that means pertaining to the meninges: _____.
below (or beneath) **subdural**	**11-16** Sub/dural (səb-doo′rəl) means _____ the dura mater, so it refers to the area between the dura mater and the arachnoid. The potential space between these two membranes is the _____ space. Accumulation of blood between the dura mater and the arachnoid is called a subdural hematoma. The acute form is often the result of a tear in the arachnoid associated with a head injury.
dura **mater** **epidural** (ep″ĭ-doo′rəl) **within** **cerebrum, brain**	**11-17** Three types of hematomas associated with head injuries are shown in Figure 11-6. Since epi-means above or on, epi/dural means situated on or outside of the _____ _____. Accumulation of blood in the epidural space is an _____ hematoma. This hematoma compresses the dura mater and thus compresses the brain. Notice that bleeding occurs _____ the brain in an intra/cerebral (in″trə-ser′ə-brəl) hematoma. Fortunately this type of hematoma is less common than a subdural or epidural hematoma. Intracerebral hematomas have a high mortality rate because of the damage they cause to brain tissue. The cerebrum is the largest and uppermost portion of the brain, and the combining form *cerebr(o)* means either the cerebrum or the brain in general. It is concerned with interpretation of impulses and all voluntary muscle activities. It is the center of higher mental faculties. The combining form *cerebr(o)* can mean either the _____ or the _____.

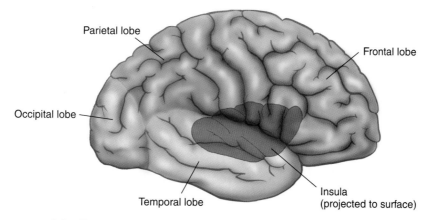

Parietal lobe

Frontal lobe

Occipital lobe

Insula
(projected to surface)

Temporal lobe

FIGURE 11-7

Lateral view of the cerebrum. The surface of the cerebrum is marked by convolutions. The pia mater closely follows the convolutions and goes deep into the grooves (sulci). Each cerebral hemisphere is divided into five lobes: the frontal lobe, the parietal lobe, the occipital lobe, the temporal lobe, and an insula that is covered by parts of the other lobes.

cerebrum	**11-18** Cerebr/al means pertaining to the _____.
cerebrotomy (ser″ə-brot′ə-me)	Write a word that means incision of the brain: _____.
craniocerebral (kra″ne-o-sər′e-brəl)	Write a word that means pertaining to the skull and the cerebrum: _____. (This is also called cerebrocranial [ser″ə-bro-kra′ne-əl].)
	11-19 The brain is that part of the CNS contained within the skull. A longitudinal fissure almost completely divides it into two cerebral hemispheres (**hemi-** means half). The surface of each hemisphere is covered with a convoluted layer of gray matter called the cerebral cortex. Division of the cortex into lobes provides useful reference points (Figure 11-7). The gray matter that covers the cerebrum is called the
cerebral cortex	_____ _____.
frontal	The lobe that is located near the front of the cerebrum is called the _____ lobe.
temporal (tem′pə-rəl)	**11-20** The region of the head in front of the ear is known as the temples. The part of the cerebrum that is located in the general area of the temples is called the _____ lobe.
occipital	Occipital (**ok-sip′ĭ-təl**) is an adjective that means concerning the back part of the head. The lobe that is located at the back part of the head, just behind the temporal lobe, is the _____ lobe.
parietal (pə-ri′ə-təl)	A remaining lobe, just above the occipital lobe, is the _____ lobe.
	It is interesting to note that different lobes are associated with different functions. The frontal lobe is associated with personality, behavior, emotion, and intellectual functions. The temporal lobe is associated with hearing and smell, the occipital lobe is associated with vision, and the parietal lobe is associated with language and the general function of sensation.
	11-21 The brain consists of several parts: the cerebrum, diencephalon, brain stem, and cerebellum (Figure 11-8).
diencephalon	The cerebellum lies just under the cerebrum, the largest portion of the brain. The thalamus and hypothalamus are parts of the _____.
stem	The midbrain, pons, and medulla are parts of the brain _____. The medulla is continuous with the spinal cord at an opening in the bone called the foramen* magnum.

*Foramen (Latin: hole).

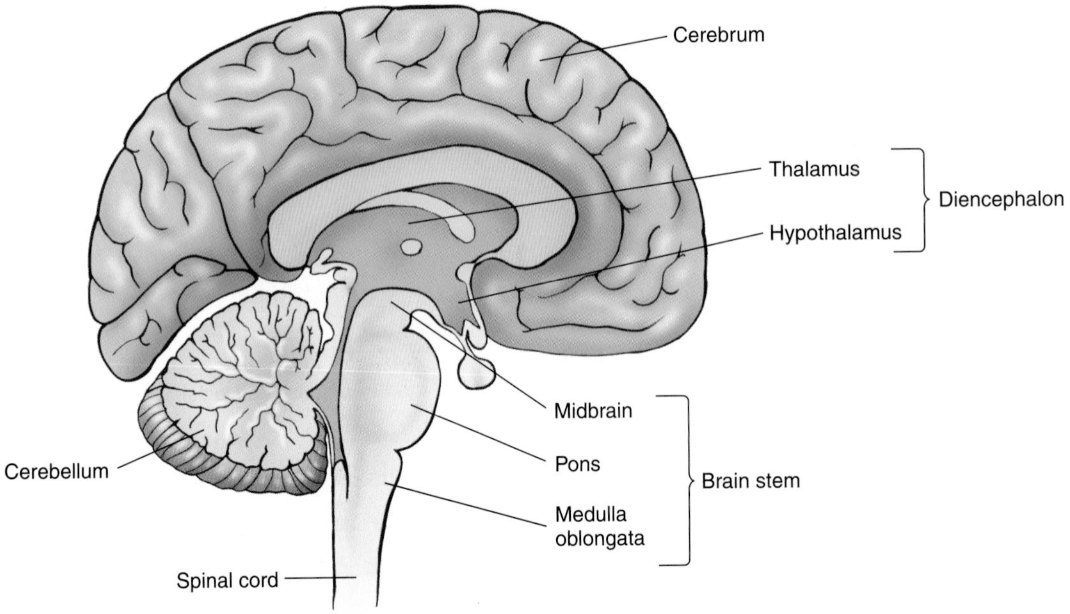

FIGURE 11-8

Principal structures of the brain. The brainstem consists of the midbrain, the pons, and the medulla. Its lower end is a continuation of the spinal cord. The diencephalon is above the brainstem and consists of the thalamus and the hypothalamus. The cerebrum is about seven eighths of the total weight of the brain and spreads over the diencephalon. The cerebellum is inferior to the cerebrum.

---

sciatic
(si-at′ik)

11-22 The spinal cord is a cylindrical structure located in the canal of the vertebral column. Thirty-one pairs of spinal nerves arise from the spinal cord and are named and numbered according to the region and level of the spinal cord from which they emerge (Figure 11-9).

The largest nerve in the body, arising from the sacral nerves on either side, is called the _____ nerve. Sciatica (si-at′ĭ-kə) is inflammation of the sciatic nerve, usually marked by pain and tenderness along the course of the nerve through the thigh and leg. This may arise from problems in the lower back as a result of a herniated vertebral disk or arthritis and is accompanied by lower back pain (LBP).

brain

11-23 In addition to the protection offered by the meninges, cerebrospinal fluid (CSF) surrounds and cushions the spinal cord and brain. Cerebro/spinal means pertaining to the _____ and the spinal cord.

water
head

Disorders, such as brain tumors, that interfere with the flow of CSF cause fluid accumulation in the skull, called hydrocephalus (hi-dro-sef′ə-ləs). Translated literally, hydro/cephalus means _____ in the _____. Hydrocephalus is a pathologic condition characterized by an abnormal accumulation of CSF within the skull and is usually accompanied by increased intracranial pressure. When this happens in an infant, before the cranial bones fuse, the cranium enlarges. In an older child or adult, the pressure damages the soft brain tissue. Diagnostic procedures include examination of the cerebrospinal fluid, computed tomography, encephalography, and angiography.

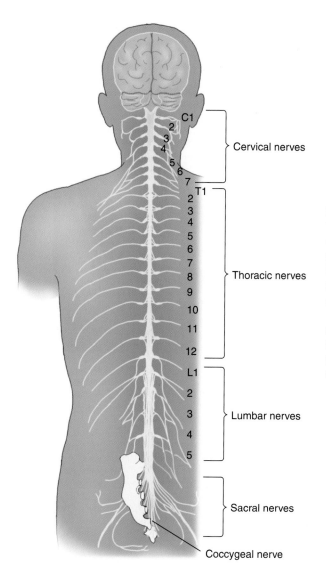

C1
2
3
4
5
6
7
⎫
⎬
⎭ Cervical nerves

T1
2
3
4
5
6
7
8
9
10
11
12
⎫
⎬
⎭ Thoracic nerves

L1
2
3
4
5
⎫
⎬
⎭ Lumbar nerves

⎫
⎬
⎭ Sacral nerves

Coccygeal nerve

FIGURE 11-9

The spinal cord and nerves emerging from it. The spinal cord, about 44 cm (16 to 18 inches) long, extends from the medulla to the second lumbar vertebra. It ends as the cauda equina (meaning horse's tail), a group of nerves that arise from the lower portion of the cord and hang like wisps of coarse hair. There are 31 pairs of spinal nerves: 8 cervical, 12 thoracic, 5 lumbar, 5 sacral, and 1 coccygeal. The sciatic nerve is the largest nerve in the body and supplies the entire musculature of the leg and foot. Irritation or injury to this nerve causes pain, often from the thigh down its branches into the toes. Neuralgia along the course of the sciatic nerve is called sciatica.

---

within
intrathecal
(in"trə-the'kəl)

11-24 The spinal puncture (usually a lumbar puncture) is performed for diagnostic purposes, as well as to introduce substances into the spinal canal. A word that means within the spinal canal is intra/thecal, which means _____ a sheath (or the spinal canal). Write the term that means within the spinal canal: _____.

The lumbar puncture is done in the lumbar area. It is performed not only for diagnostic purposes but also for the injection of an anesthetic solution for spinal anesthesia. Epidural anesthesia is injection of an anesthetic into the epidural space, which contains spinal fluid and spinal nerves. Epidurals, most commonly performed in the lumbar area, can be tailored to numb an area of the body from the lower extremities to the upper abdomen. They are often used in labor and childbirth.

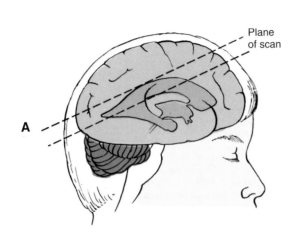

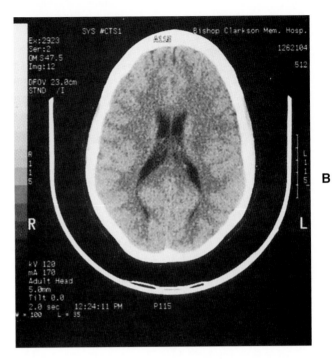

FIGURE 11-10
Computed tomography of the brain. **A,** Computed tomographic scans are taken at various cross sections of the brain. **B,** Tomogram of the plane shown in *A* provides a permanent record. The tomogram shows no gross abnormalities. (From Polaski AL, Tatro SE: *Luckmann's core principles and practice of medical-surgical nursing*, Philadelphia, 1996, WB Saunders.)

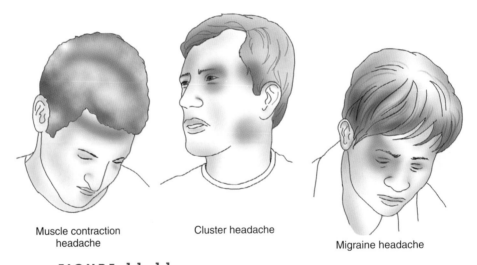

Muscle contraction
headache

Cluster headache

Migraine headache

FIGURE 11-11
Three types of headaches. Shaded areas show regions of most intense pain.

TABLE 11-1 Selected Diseases or Disorders of the Central Nervous System

Headaches	Tumors
Epilepsy	Meningoceles
Narcolepsy	Parkinson's disease
Infections (meningitis, encephalitis, myelitis, cerebellitis)	Alzheimer's disease
Strokes	Huntington's disease
Cerebral aneurysms	Multiple sclerosis
Head and spinal cord injuries	Amyotrophic lateral sclerosis

ventricles

ventricles

11-25 Cerebrospinal fluid is formed in the ventricles, four cavities in the brain. The fluid circulates through the ventricles, the subarachnoid space, and the central canal of the spinal cord. Cavities in the brain that produce CSF are called cerebral _____.

Ventriculo/graphy (**ven-trik″u-log′rə-fe**) is radiography of the cerebral _____ after introduction of air or a contrast medium. Ventriculography has been replaced by computed tomography (CT) in many cases.

ventriculogram
(ven-trik′u-lo-gram)

Write a word that means the record produced by ventriculography: _____.

Computed tomography and magnetic resonance imaging (MRI) are used in assessing the brain and spinal cord. CT is particularly helpful in detecting intracranial bleeding, lesions, cerebral edema, and changes in the brain structures (Figure 11-10).

radiography
of the brain

brain

11-26 Encephalo/graphy (**en-sef″ə-log′rə-fe**) is _____.

Pneumo/encephalo/graphy (**noo″mo-ən-sef″ə-log′rə-fe**) is radiographic visualization of the fluid-containing structures of the _____ after CSF is removed and replaced by air. This procedure has also largely been replaced by CT or MRI. It is a noninvasive technique for visualizing internal structures and creates images based on the magnetic properties of chemical elements within the body rather than using ionizing radiation such as x-rays.

Echo/encephalo/graphy uses ultrasonic waves beamed through the head to record structural aspects of the _____.

brain
echoencephalo-
gram
(ek″o-en-sef′ə-lo-
gram″)

The record produced by echoencephalography is an _____.

11-27 Dysfunctions of the nervous system range from a mild condition such as a headache to life-threatening situations. Table 11-1 lists several dysfunctions of the CNS.

A headache is pain in the head from any cause and is a symptom. Most headaches do not indicate serious disease. The most common types of headaches are pain related to the eyes, ears, teeth, and paranasal structures; tension (muscle contraction headaches); cluster; and migraine (Figure 11-11). Various drugs are used to treat headaches and their causes.

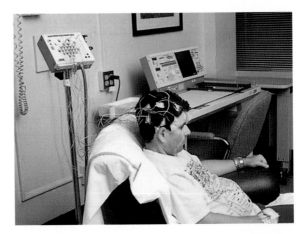

FIGURE 11-12
Electroencephalography. Electrodes are attached to various areas of the patient's head. The patient generally remains quiet with closed eyes during the procedure. In certain cases, prescribed activities may be requested. The test is used to diagnose epilepsy, brain stem disorders, lesions, and impaired consciousness. (From Chipps EM, Clanin NJ, Campbell VG: *Neurologic disorders,* St Louis, 1992, Mosby.)

tension	**11-28** Tension headaches result from the long-sustained contraction of skeletal muscles around the scalp, face, neck, and upper back. This is the primary source of many headaches associated with excessive emotional tension, anxiety, and depression. Also called muscle contraction headaches, _____ headaches result from long-sustained contraction of skeletal muscles of the head and upper back.
headache side	Cluster headaches, also referred to as histamine cephalgia, occur more frequently in men than in women and are unilateral. Ceph/algia means _____, and uni/lateral means occurring on one _____ only. Cephalalgia (**sef″ə-lal′jə**), formed by combining cephal(o) and -algia, meaning pain, is a synonym for cephalgia. They are very painful, occur in clusters, and fortunately, the headache does not last long. They were formerly believed to be caused by histamine and were so named.
fear light	A migraine headache is a vascular disorder characterized by recurrent throbbing headaches, often accompanied by loss of appetite, photophobia, and nausea with or without vomiting. Photophobia is sensitivity of the eyes to light. Translated literally, photo/phobia means an abnormal _____ of _____.
	Migraine headaches occur more often in females than in males and sometimes begin in childhood. The classic migraine begins with an aura of depression, irritability, restlessness, and perhaps loss of appetite. There may also be transient neurologic disturbances, including visual problems (flashes of lights, distorted or double vision, seeing spots), dizziness, and nausea. The headache increases in severity until it becomes intense and may last a few hours or up to several days if not treated.
seizures (or convulsions)	**11-29** Epilepsy (**ep′ĭ-lep″se**) is a group of chronic neurologic disorders characterized by recurrent episodes of convulsive seizures, sensory disturbances, loss of consciousness, or all of these. Seizures are also known as convulsions. Anti/convulsants are medications used to prevent or reduce the severity of _____.
electroencephalo-gram	The suffix *-lepsy* means seizure. A seizure is an abnormal, sudden, excessive discharge of electrical activity within the brain. This abnormal activity is assessed in electroencephalography, which is also used to diagnose brain stem disorders, lesions, and impaired consciousness. Electro/encephalo/graphy may be required to substantiate brain death, irreversible unconsciousness characterized by a complete loss of brain function. The record produced is called an _____ (Figure 11-12).
narcolepsy	**11-30** Narcolepsy (**nahr′ko-lep″se**) is uncontrollable, brief episodes of sleep and uses the combining form *narc(o),* which means sleep. In narcolepsy, the person cannot prevent a sudden attack of sleep while performing daytime activities. Its cause is unknown, and no pathologic lesions are found in the brain. The person may experience momentary loss of muscle tone. Visual or auditory hallucinations often occur at the onset of sleep. Stimulant drugs are often prescribed to prevent the sudden attacks of sleep at inappropriate times. The name of this disorder is _____.

meninges	**11-31** Infections of the CNS include encephalomyelitis, meningitis, and encephalitis. Encephalomyelitis (**en-sef″ə-lo-mi″ə-li′tis**) is inflammation of the brain and spinal cord. Mening/itis (**men″in-ji′tis**) is inflammation of the _____ of the brain and the spinal cord. Although other infectious organisms can invade the nervous system, bacterial and viral organisms are most often responsible for meningitis.
brain	**11-32** Encephal/itis is inflammation of the brain tissue. It is most often caused by a virus, usually having gained access to the blood stream from a viral infection elsewhere in the body. Encephalo/meningitis (**en-sef″ə-lo-men″in-ji′tis**) is inflammation of the _____ and its coverings.
slow	**11-33** Parkinson's disease is a slowly progressing, debilitating, neurologic disease that affects motor ability. It is characterized by muscle rigidity, bradykinesia, and tremor. The suffix -**_kinesia_** means movement. Brady/kinesia means _____ movement, or slowness of all voluntary movement or speech. Tremor is rhythmic, purposeless, quivering involuntary movements. A characteristic posture and masklike facial expression are often seen. Parkinson's disease occurs most often in people over 50 years of age and results from widespread degeneration of a part of the brain that produces dopamine. The cause is not known, but treatment usually includes the administration of dopaminergics, precursors to dopamine.
Alzheimer's	**11-34** Alzheimer's disease is chronic, progressive mental deterioration that is sometimes called dementia, Alzheimer's type. This accounts for more than half of the persons with dementia who are older than 65 years of age. It is less common in people in their 40s and 50s. Although the exact cause is not known, both chemical and structural changes occur in the brain. Alzheimer's disease is characterized by confusion, memory failure, disorientation, and inability to carry out purposeful activities. The patient becomes increasingly mentally impaired, severe physical deterioration takes place, and death occurs. The disease is called _____ disease.
Huntington's	**11-35** Huntington's disease, also called Huntington's chorea, is a hereditary disorder that affects both genders equally. Symptoms begin between 30 and 50 years of age. The two main symptoms are progressive mental status changes, leading to dementia, and rapid, jerky movements in the trunk, facial muscles, and extremities. Neurotransmitters have been implicated in the symptoms of this inherited disorder called _____ disease.
vessels	**11-36** In a cerebro/vascular (**ser″ə-bro-vas′ku-lər**) accident (CVA, stroke, or stroke syndrome), blood _____ in the brain have become diseased. Either the blood vessels have become narrowed, or one of the arteries may have ballooned out to form what is known as an aneurysm. The narrowed arteries then may become blocked, or the aneurysm may rupture to produce a cerebral hemorrhage. The types of stroke are shown in Figure 11-13.
brain	A cerebral embolus is a plug of matter (usually a blood clot) brought by the blood to the _____. A cerebral embolus is one cause of a CVA.
artery	Thrombotic strokes are caused by plaque deposits that build up on the interior of a cerebral _____.
hemorrhagic	Which type of stroke is caused by rupture of a cerebral artery? _____ Embolic or thrombotic strokes are frequently preceded by warning signs, such as a transient ischemic attack (TIA) that is caused by a brief interruption in cerebral blood flow. The term _ischemic_ pertains to deficient blood circulation (in this case, in the brain). TIA symptoms often include disturbance of normal vision, dizziness, weakness, and numbness. A transient ischemic attack is important because it may be a warning sign
stroke (CVA)	of an impending _____.

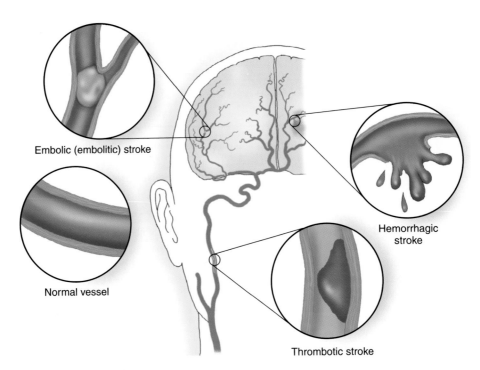

Embolic (embolitic) stroke

Normal vessel

Hemorrhagic stroke

Thrombotic stroke

FIGURE 11-13
Types of stroke. A cerebrovascular accident, commonly referred to as a stroke, is a disruption in the normal blood supply to the brain. An embolic stroke is caused by an embolus or a group of emboli that break off from one area of the body, often the heart, and travel to the cerebral arteries. Thrombotic strokes are caused by plaque deposits that build up on the interior of a cerebral artery, gradually occluding it. Hemorrhagic strokes are caused by rupture of a cerebral arterial wall.

cerebrum (or brain) excision	**11-37** An aneurysm is a ballooning out of the wall of a vessel, usually an artery, owing to congenital defect or weakness of the vessel wall. The potential danger is that the aneurysm will rupture. If a cerebral aneurysm ruptures, where does the hemorrhage occur? _____ An aneurysm/ectomy (**an″u-riz-mek′to-me**) is _____ of an aneurysm. Cerebral aneurysms are usually confirmed by cerebral angiography (Figure 11-14).
head	**11-38** Craniocerebral trauma is commonly called head trauma or head injury. It is a traumatic insult to the brain caused by an external physical force that may produce a diminished or altered state of consciousness. It may result in impairment of cognitive abilities (perception, reasoning, judgment, and memory) or physical functions and may be temporary or permanent. Cranio/cerebral trauma is commonly called _____ injury. Skull fractures, gunshot wounds, and knife injuries are examples of open head traumas. Blunt trauma as seen in motor vehicle accidents can lead to concussions (**kən-kush′ənz),** contusions (bruises), or tearing of the brain. Three types of hematomas that are associated with head injury were presented earlier in this section.

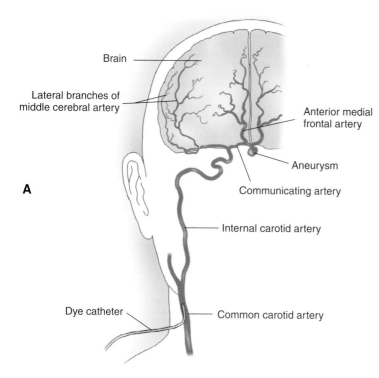

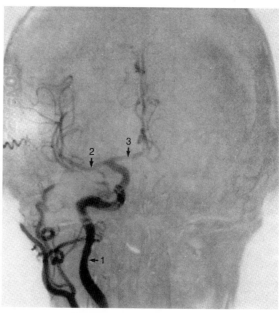

FIGURE 11-14

Cerebral aneurysm. **A,** Diagram of an aneurysm and the major cerebral arteries visible in cerebral angiography. **B,** A cerebral angiogram. Cerebral angiography is used to study intracranial circulation and is especially helpful in visualizing aneurysms and vascular occlusions. A contrast medium is used that outlines the vessels of the brain. (From Polaski AL, Tatro SE: *Luckmann's core principles and practice of medical-surgical nursing*, Philadelphia, 1996, WB Saunders.)

concussion	**11-39** Consciousness is responsiveness of the mind to the impressions made by the senses. A cerebral concussion usually causes loss of consciousness. A concussion is an injury resulting from impact with an object. A blow to the head can cause a cerebral _____.
semiconscious (sem"e-kon' shəs)	A person who is responsive to impressions made by the senses is said to be conscious. A person who is semi/conscious is only partially aware of his or her surroundings. A word that means only partially conscious is _____.
partly	**11-40** The prefix *semi-* means half, or partly. Semi/permeable means _____ permeable, or permitting passage of certain molecules but not all.
semicoma (sem"e-ko'mə)	A coma is a profound unconsciousness from which the patient cannot be aroused. Write a word that means a mild coma from which the patient can be aroused (partial coma): _____.
	11-41 Head injuries can also result in a spinal cord injury (SCI). Forceful injuries to the vertebral column can damage the spinal cord and lead to neurologic problems. Injuries to the vertebral column that can result in damage to the spinal cord include excessive rotation, hyperextension, hyperflexion, and vertical compression (Figure 11-15).

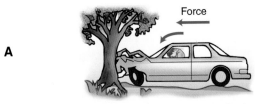

A

Hyperflexion injury of the cervical spine

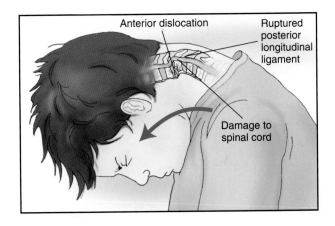

Anterior dislocation

Ruptured posterior longitudinal ligament

Damage to spinal cord

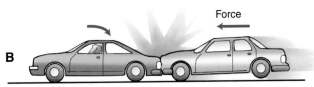

Force

B

Hyperextension injury of the cervical spine

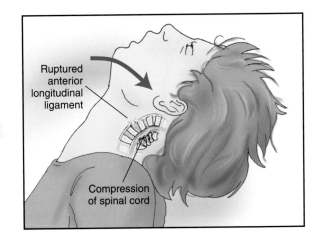

Ruptured anterior longitudinal ligament

Compression of spinal cord

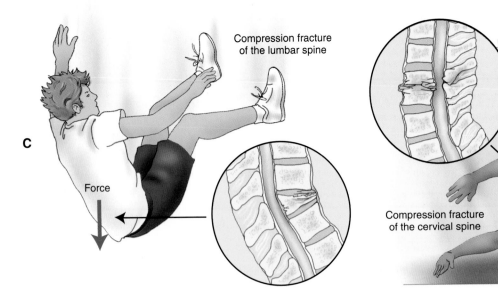

Compression fracture of the lumbar spine

C

Force

Compression fracture of the cervical spine

Force

FIGURE 11-15

Closed spinal cord injuries. Fractures and dislocations to the vertebral column can result in injury to the spinal cord. These types of vertebral injuries occur most often at points where a relatively mobile portion of the spine meets a relatively fixed segment. **A,** Hyperflexion of the cervical vertebrae. **B,** Hyperextension of the cervical vertebrae. **C,** Vertical compression of the cervical spine and the lumbar spine.

paralysis	**11-42** Paralysis is the loss of muscle function, loss of sensation, or both. It may be caused by trauma, disease, or poisoning. Injury to different areas of the spinal cord result in different types of paralysis. Remembering that -plegia means paralysis, in hemi/plegia (**hem″ĭ-ple′jə**), there is _____ of one half of the body (only one side).
one	The combining form ***mon(o)*** means one or single. Mono/plegia (**mon″o-ple′jə**) is paralysis of _____ limb.
both	Paralysis of both sides of the body is di/plegia (**di-ple′je-ə**). The prefix ***di-*** means twice or two. In diplegia, there is paralysis of similar parts on _____ sides of the body.
paralysis	**11-43** Quadri/plegia is _____ of all four extremities. The prefix ***quadri-*** means four.
quadriplegia (kwod″rĭ-ple′jə)	Paralysis of all four limbs is called _____.
paralysis	In para/plegia (**par″ə-ple′jə**), the upper limbs are not affected. Para/plegia is _____ of the lower portion of the body and both legs. The prefix *para-* means near, beside, or abnormal. Some interpretation is needed in the term *paraplegia*.
	Cerebral palsy (**pawl′ze**) is a motor function disorder caused by a permanent, nonprogressive brain defect present at birth or shortly thereafter. It may result in spastic paralysis in various forms, seizures, and varying degrees of impaired speech, vision, and hearing. It is often associated with asphyxia during birth.
neuralgia (nōō-ral′jə)	**11-44** Using -algia, write a word that means pain of a nerve: _____.
many	Poly/neur/algia (**pol″e-noo-ral′jə**) is pain of _____ nerves.
polyneuritis (pol″e-nōō-ri′tis)	Write a word that means inflammation of many nerves (simultaneously): _____.
a disease involving several nerves	A poly/neuro/pathy (**pol″e-nōō-rop′ə-the**) is _____.
joints	Neuro/arthro/pathy (**noor″o-ahr-throp′ə-the**) is any disease of the _____ associated with disease of the central or peripheral nervous system.
brain spinal cord	**11-45** An encephalo/myelo/pathy (**en-sef″ə-lo-mi″əl-op′ə-the**) is any disease involving the _____ and the _____ _____.
myelography (mi″ə-log′rə-fe)	Write a word that means making an x-ray film of the spinal cord (after injection of a contrast medium): _____.
myelogram (mi′ə-lo-gram)	The record produced in myelography is a _____.
pneumomyelography	Myelography can be useful in studying spinal lesions, spinal injuries, or disk disease. It is often supplemented by procedures such as tomography. Pneumo/myelography (**noo″mo-mi′ə-log′rə-fe**) is x-ray examination of the spinal cord after injection of air. Write this new word that means air myelography: _____.
myelomalacia (mi″ə-lo-mə-la′shə)	**11-46** Write a word that means morbid softening of the spinal cord: _____.
encephalomalacia (en-sef″ə lo-mə-la′shə)	Morbid softening of the brain is _____.
encephalosclerosis (en-sef″ə-lo-sklə-ro′sis)	Hardening of the brain is _____.

cerebellum cerebellitis (ser″ə-bel-li′tis)	**11-47** The combining form *cerebell(o)* means cerebellum. The cerebellum is located just below the cerebrum. Cerebell/ar (**ser″ə-bel′ər**) pertains to the _____. Inflammation of the cerebellum is _____.
meninges meninges spinal cord	**11-48** A meningo/cele (**mə-ning′go-sēl**) is hernial protrusion of _____ through a defect in the skull or vertebral column. Meningoceles are generally repaired by surgery. A meningo/myelo/cele (**mə-ning″go-mi′ə-lo-sēl**) is hernial protrusion of part of the _____ and _____ _____ through a defect in the vertebral column.
multiple sclerosis without, muscle nutrition	**11-49** Multiple sclerosis (MS) is a progressive degenerative disease that affects the myelin sheath and conduction pathway of the central nervous system. One of the earliest signs is paresthesia, abnormal sensations in the extremities or on one side of the face. The disease is characterized by periods of remission and exacerbation (flare). Disability increases as the disease progresses and the periods of exacerbation become more frequent. In multiple sclerosis, the myelin sheath deteriorates and is replaced by scar tissue that interferes with normal transmission of the nerve impulse. This disease that is named for the multiple areas of sclerotic tissue that replaces the myelin sheath is _____ _____. Amyotrophic lateral sclerosis (ALS) is another progressive degenerative disease of the nervous system. It is also called Lou Gehrig's disease. It is characterized by atrophy (wasting) of the hands, forearms, and legs. The disease results in paralysis and death. The cause of the disease is unknown. Analyzing the parts of a/myo/trophic, a- means _____, my(o) means _____, and -trophic means _____. Dyslexia is an impairment of the ability to read and results from a variety of pathologic conditions, some of which are associated with the nervous system. Dyslexic persons often reverse letters and words, cannot adequately distinguish the letter sequences in written words, and have difficulty determining right from left. Dyslexia is unrelated to intelligence, and the exact cause is not known.
tetanus botulism	**11-50** You learned that meningitis and myelitis are caused by infectious microorganisms. Three other diseases that have a devastating effect on the central nervous system are tetanus, botulism, and poliomyelitis. Tetanus (**tet′ə-nəs**), also known as lockjaw, is caused by a bacteria and is easily preventable through immunization. The infection is frequently transmitted through a wound contaminated with the bacteria. The bacterial toxin attacks the nervous system and results in muscle rigidity and spasms. Taking its name from the "locked jaw" rigidity that results, this disease is known as _____. Botulism (**boch′u-liz-əm**) is caused by a bacteria that is toxic to nervous tissue and causes paralysis of both voluntary and involuntary motor activity. Most cases are caused by eating improperly canned foods. Symptoms usually appear 12 to 36 hours after eating contaminated food in this neurotoxic disease, called _____. Poliomyelitis (**po″le-o-mi′ə-li′tis**) is an acute viral disease that attacks the gray matter of the spinal cord and parts of the brain. It can be asymptomatic, mild, or paralytic. This disease is rarely seen in North America, since it can be prevented by immunization. It is informally called polio.*

*Polio (Greek: *polios*, gray).

❏ SECTION B REVIEW 𝒞entral Nervous System

This section review covers frames 11–14 through 11–50. Complete the table by writing the word part or meaning as indicated.

Combining Form	Meaning	Prefix	Meaning
1. _____	arachnoid membrane or spider	7. di-	_____
2. _____	cerebellum	8. hemi-	_____
3. _____	cerebrum or brain	9. semi-	_____
4. _____	meninges		
5. mon(o)	_____	**Suffix**	**Meaning**
6. _____	sleep	10. _____	seizure
		11. _____	movement

(Use Appendix V to check your answers.)

Peripheral Nervous System and the Sense Organs

SECTION C

The peripheral nervous system (PNS) is that portion of the nervous system that is outside the central nervous system. The PNS consists of the nerves that branch out from the brain and spinal cord to form the communication network between the central nervous system and the rest of the body.

11-51 The peripheral nervous system (PNS) is composed of the network of nerves that link the central nervous system with all parts of the body. It is further divided into the sensory (afferent) and motor (efferent) systems.

Special sense organs have receptors that detect sensations, and then sensory neurons transmit the information to the CNS. Motor neurons carry impulses that initiate muscle contraction.

Peripheral means located away from the center. The PNS is located away from the nervous system control center, the CNS or the _____ nervous system.

central

11-52 Receptors are sensory nerve endings that respond to various kinds of stimulation. The awareness that results from the stimulation is what we know as sensation. The major senses are pain, sight, hearing, smell, taste, touch, and pressure. Receptors are _____ nerve endings.

sensory

The PNS consists of nerves that connect with skin and muscles that are involved in conscious activities (somatic tissues) and also nerves that link the CNS to the visceral organs, such as the stomach and heart, that function without conscious effort (autonomic tissues). These further divisions of the PNS are illustrated in Figure 11-16.

The autonomic (**aw″to-nom′ik**) system regulates and coordinates visceral activities without our conscious effort. This helps maintain a stable internal environment. It has two divisions, the sympathetic and parasympathetic nervous systems.

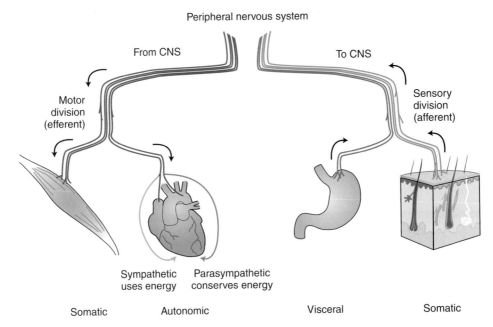

FIGURE 11-16
Schematic drawing of the divisions of the peripheral nervous system. The motor (efferent) division is further divided into the somatic and autonomic systems. The sensory (afferent) division is further subdivided into the visceral and somatic systems.

autonomic	**11-53** Sympathetic and parasympathetic systems are divisions of the _____ nervous system. In general, impulses transmitted by the nerve fibers of one division stimulate an organ, whereas impulses from the other division decrease or halt organ activity.
	Sympathectomy (**sim″pə-thek′tə-me**) is a surgical procedure in which a sympathetic nerve or nerves are severed. This surgery has special uses, including alleviation of pain.
parasympathetic (par″ə-sim″pə-thet′ik)	Activation of the sympathetic division causes a series of physiological responses called the fight-or-flight response. These responses increase the heart and breathing rates and prepare the body for fighting off danger. When danger is past, which system would counteract these responses? _____ system
cholinergic (ko″lin-ər′jik) **adrenergic** (ad″ren-ər′jik) **acetylcholine**	**11-54** Sympathetic and parasympathetic nerve fibers, like other axons of the nervous system, release neurotransmitters and are classified on the basis of the substance produced. Cholinergic fibers release acetylcholine. Adrenergic fibers release epinephrine. (Epinephrine is also called adrenaline, hence the term adren/ergic.) Write the names of these two types of nerve fibers: _____ and _____ . Cholinergic fibers release _____ .
epinephrine (ep″ĭ-nef′rin)	Adrenergic fibers release _____ .

11-55 Special sense organs, the eyes, the ears, the skin, the mouth, and the nose, have receptors that enable us to see, hear, feel, taste, and smell. The receptors that detect changes in our environment can be grouped into five types: chemoreceptors, mechanoreceptors, photoreceptors, thermoreceptors, and nociceptors.

The combining form ***chem(o)*** means chemicals. Chemo/receptors are nerve endings adapted for excitation by what type of substances? _____

Taste buds contain chemoreceptors (**ke″mo-re-sep′tərz**) for sweet, sour, bitter, and salty tastes. Receptors that are stimulated by chemical stimuli are called _____. The nose and tongue have chemo/receptors, which detect chemicals.

chemical

chemoreceptors

11-56 Mechano/receptors that are sensitive to changes in touch or pressure are widely distributed in the skin. Mechanoreceptors (**mek″ə-no-re-sep′torz**) for hearing are located within the ear.

The eyes have photoreceptors (**fo″to-re-sep′torz**) that detect _____.

Thermoreceptors are located immediately under the skin and are widely distributed throughout the body. Thermo/receptors detect changes in temperature. There are cold receptors and, as the name implies, _____ receptors.

The sense of pain is initiated by special receptors that are widely distributed throughout the skin and the internal organs.

light

heat

11-57 The eyes contain photoreceptors and are responsible for vision. Ophthalm/ic means pertaining to the _____. Ocular also means pertaining to the eye, because ***ocul(o)*** also means eye.

Intra/ocular (**in″trə-ok′u-lər**) means _____ the eye, and extra/ocular (**eks″trə-ok′u-lər**) means _____ the eye.

Write a word that means between the eyes: _____.

Using ophthalm(o) and the suffixes *-meter, -malacia, rrhagia,* and *-scopy,* write terms that mean the following:

an instrument for measuring the eye _____.

abnormal softening of the eye _____.

hemorrhage from the eye _____.

visual examination of the eye with an ophthalmoscope _____.

eye

within
outside

interocular

ophthalmometer

ophthalmomalacia

ophthalmorrhagia

ophthalmoscopy

11-58 The structures of the eye and nose are shown in Figure 11-17. Although it probably is not necessary to memorize the structures that make up these two sense organs, it is important to recognize names associated with them.

Eyelids open and close the eye and keep foreign objects from entering the eye. The eyelids, as well as the anterior portion of the sclera, are lined with a mucous membrane called conjunctiva (**kən-jənk′ti-və**). Conjunctivitis (**kən-junk″tĭ-vi′tis**) is inflammation of the conjunctiva and is caused by a bacterial or viral infection, allergy, or irritants. What is referred to as bloodshot eyes is probably inflammation of the conjunctiva, called _____.

conjunctivitis

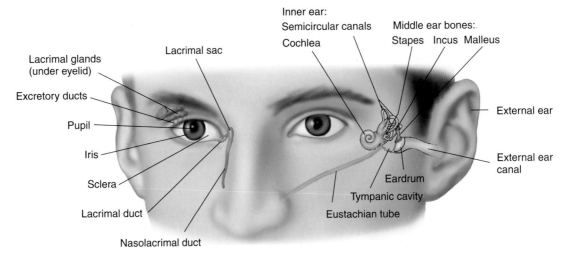

FIGURE 11-17
Structures of the ear and eye.

---

keratitis
(ker″ə-ti′tis)

11-59 The cornea is the convex, transparent structure at the front of the eyeball that helps focus light rays entering the eye. Corneal (**kor′ne-əl**) problems are the leading cause of visual problems in the United States. The cornea was one of the first organs transplanted, and rejection of the transplanted tissue is uncommon.

The combining form **kerat(o)** means the cornea, but it also means hard, like horn. Write a term that means inflammation of the cornea: _____.

The lens of the eye is located just beneath the pupil and is responsible for focusing the light rays so they form a perfect image on the retina. A cataract (**kat′ə-rakt**) is an abnormal progressive condition of the lens, characterized by loss of transparency. Cataracts are usually treated with removal of the cataract. To prevent the need for a special contact lens or glasses, an intraocular lens (IOL) is sometimes surgically implanted when the cataract is removed. The name of this disorder is _____.

cataract

---

iritis (i-ri′tis)

11-60 Both **ir(o)** and **irid(o)** mean the iris, the pigmented portion that accounts for blue, brown, gray, green, and combinations of these colors in eyes. Using ir(o), write a term that means inflammation of the iris: _____.

Glaucoma (**glaw-ko′mə**) is an abnormal condition of increased pressure within the eye. Prolonged pressure can damage the retina and optic nerve. Several drugs and laser surgery are used to relieve the increased pressure.

---

retina

11-61 The retina, located in the posterior part of the eye, contains photoreceptors (rods and cones). The retina is continuous with the optic nerve, which carries the nervous impulse to the cerebrum and enables vision. Examine the appearance of the optic nerve and retina in Figure 11-18.

Any disease of the retina is a retinopathy. A detached retina is separation of the retina from the back of the eye (Figure 11-19). Although it can be caused by severe trauma, most cases are associated with internal changes within the eye. Retinal detachment requires surgical treatment to avoid deterioration that can lead to blindness in the affected eye. This disorder is called detached _____.

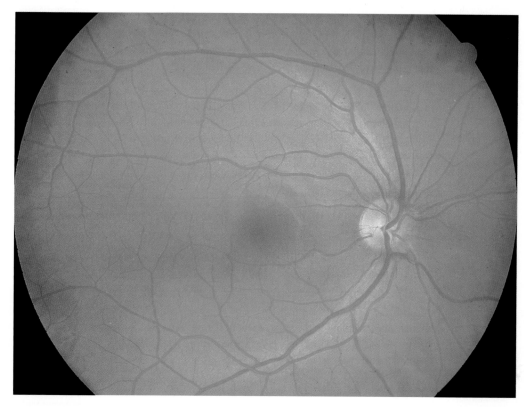

FIGURE 11-18
Ophthalmoscopic view of the interior of the eye. A normal retina and optic nerve are shown. The normal retina and blood vessel walls are mainly transparent. Note that the branching points of the blood vessels "point" toward the optic nerve. (From Palay DA, Krachmer JH, editors: *Ophthalmology for the primary care physician,* St Louis, 1997, Mosby.)

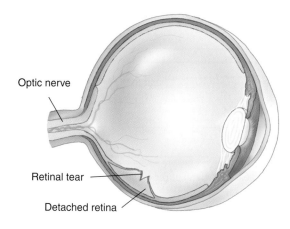

Optic nerve

Retinal tear

Detached retina

FIGURE 11-19
Retinal detachment. The onset of separation of the retina from the back of the eye is usually sudden and painless. The person may experience bright flashes of light or floating dark spots in the affected eye. Sometimes there is loss of visual field, as though a curtain is being pulled over part of the visual field. Retinal detachments are usually visible using ophthalmoscopy.

crying	**11-62** The combining forms *dacry(o)* and *lacrim(o)* mean tear, as in crying. The lacrim/al gland produces fluid (tears) that keeps the eye moist. (Refer again to Figure 11-17.) If more lacrimal (**lak″rĭ-məl**) fluid is produced than can be removed, we say that the person is _____. (This is also called tearing.)
tears eyelid	Lacrim/ation (**lak″rĭ-ma′shən**) refers to crying, or the production and discharge of _____. Lacrimation can cause blephar/edema (**blef″ar-ə-de′mə**), which is swelling of the _____. Blepharedema can also be caused by other things, such as infection.
pain in the eye calculus presence of lacrimal calculi	**11-63** Ophthalm/algia (**of″thəl-mal′jə**) may be due to an eye infection. This can lead to excessive lacrimation. Ophthalm/algia is _____. Concretions (calculi) can form in the lacrimal passages. A dacryo/lith (**dak′re-o-lith″**) is a lacrimal _____, or a tear stone. Dacryo/lith/iasis (**dak″re-o-lĭ-thi′ə-sis**) is the _____.
lacrimal nose inflammation of the lacrimal sac	**11-64** Tears produced by the _____ gland wash over the eyeball and are drained off through small openings in the inner corner of the eye. Tears pass through these openings into small ducts that lead to the lacrimal sac. From here they pass into the large nasolacrimal duct that ends in the nasal cavity. Naso/lacrimal pertains to the _____ and the lacrimal apparatus. Another name for the lacrimal sac is dacryo/cyst. Dacryo/cyst/itis (**dak″re-o-sis-ti′tis**) is _____.
dacryocystotomy (dak″re-o-sis-tot′ ə-me) lacrimal sac, nose	**11-65** Write a word that means incision of the lacrimal sac: _____. Dacryo/cysto/rhino/stomy (**dak″re-o-sis″to-ri-nos′tə-me**) is surgical creation of a passageway between the _____ _____ and the _____.
lacrimal sac radiography of the lacrimal sac	**11-66** Dacryo/sinus/itis (**dak″re-o-si″nəs-i′tis**) is inflammation of the _____ _____ and the sinus. Dacryo/cysto/graphy (**dak″re-o-sis-tog′rə-fe**) is _____.
eye nose tear stone	**11-67** Oculo/nasal (**ok″u-lo-na′səl**) refers to the _____ and the _____. A rhino/dacryo/lith (**ri″no-dak′re-o-lith″**) is a _____ _____ in the nasal duct.
blepharoplasty (blef′ə-ro-plas″te)	**11-68** A sty (also spelled stye) is an infection of a sebaceous gland of the eyelid. It usually affects only one eye at a time. Blepharoptosis (**blef′ə-rop-to′sis**), also simply called ptosis, is drooping of the upper eyelid (Figure 11-20). It can be congenital or can result from muscle dysfunction or other causes. If vision or appearance is adversely affected, blepharoptosis can be corrected by plastic surgery. Write the name of this surgery: _____.

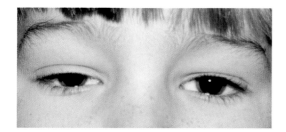

FIGURE 11-20
Blepharoptosis. Note the drooping of the right upper lid. (From Palay DA, Krachmer JH, editors: *Ophthalmology for the primary care physician*, St Louis, 1997, Mosby.)

---

myopia (mi-o′pe-ə)
hyperopia
(hi″pər-o′pe-ə)
astigmatism
(ə-stig′mə-tiz-əm)

11-69 Three common irregularities in vision are explained in Figure 11-21. These are refractive disorders, since light rays are not focused appropriately on the retina.

Another name for nearsightedness is _____. Farsightedness is the same as _____. Uneven focusing of the image, resulting from distortion of the curvature of the lens

cornea

or cornea, is _____.

Corrective glasses or contact lenses can often correct these types of defective vision. In some cases of myopia, radial keratotomy (**ker″ə-tot′ə-me**) may be performed to reduce or eliminate the need for further correction. Kerato/tomy is incision of the _____.

The excimer laser is used in this type of corneal surgery and creates minimal damage to adjacent cells.

11-70 The ears have receptors that detect touch, pain, heat, and cold, but the mechanoreceptors that enable us to hear usually come to mind when we think of the ear as a sense organ. We depend on our ears not only for hearing but also for the sense of equilibrium, both functions of mechanoreceptors.

outer

Anatomically, the ear is divided into the external ear, middle ear, and inner ear (refer again to Figure 11-17). The part of the ear that is visible is the _____ ear. With the function of collecting sound waves and directing them into the ear, the outer ear ends at the tympanic membrane (eardrum).

The middle ear is an air-filled cavity and has three tiny bones. When the eardrum vibrates, these bones transmit the vibrations to fluids in the inner ear. The cochlea (**kok′le-ə**) contains receptors that enable us to hear. The semicircular canals enable us to maintain a sense of balance.

---

otoscope
(o′to-skōp)

11-71 Otoscopy (**o-tos′kə-pe**) makes it possible to inspect the tympanic membrane (Figure 11-22). The instrument used in otoscopy is an _____.

The thin membrane that we call the eardrum can become ruptured or perforated by shock waves from an explosion, deep sea diving, trauma, or acute middle ear infections as seen in Figure 11-22, *D*.

---

otitis

pain in the ear

11-72 Write a word that means inflammation of the ear: _____.

Otitis may produce otalgia. Ot/algia (**o-tal′je-ə**) is _____.

This is called an earache.

---

inflammation

11-73 Otitis media (**o-ti′tis me′de-ə**) is _____ of the middle ear. The middle ear is separated from the external ear by the eardrum.

A discharge from the ear may accompany otitis. Write a word that means discharge from the ear: _____.

otorrhea
(o″to-re′ə)

Otorrhea may contain blood, pus, or even spinal fluid. Ear infections are just one cause of otorrhea.

Mastoid/itis (**mas″toid-i′tis**) is an infection of one of the mastoid bones, usually an extension of a middle ear infection. It is difficult to treat and hearing loss can result. Antibiotic therapy is aimed at treating middle-ear infections before they progress to mastoiditis.

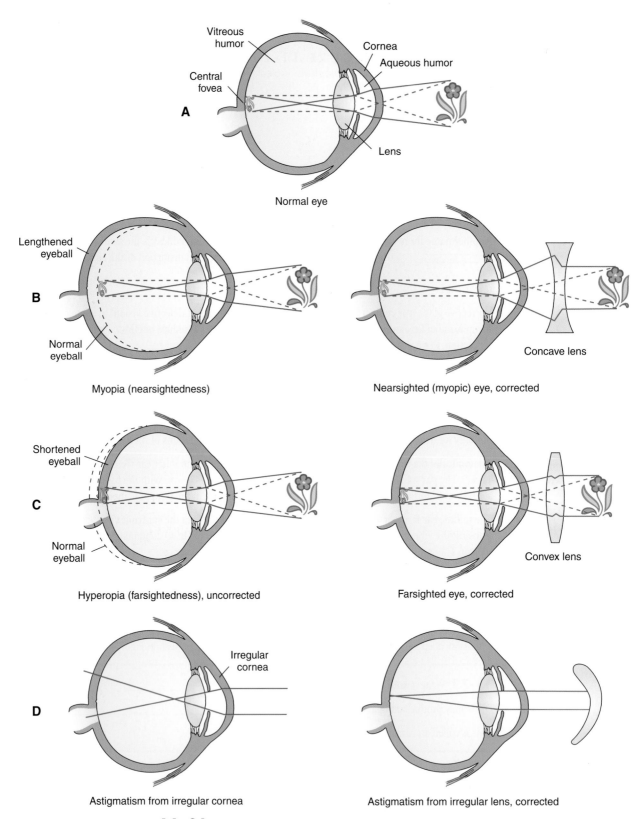

FIGURE 11-21

Normal and abnormal refraction in the eyeball. **A,** In the normal eye, a clear image is formed when light rays from an object are bent properly and converge on the center of the retina. **B,** In myopia (nearsightedness), the image is focused in front of the retina and is corrected by use of a concave lens. **C,** In hyperopia (farsightedness), the image is focused behind the retina and is corrected using a convex lens. **D,** In astigmatism, the curvature of the cornea or lens is uneven and results in the image being focused at two different points on the retina. A cylindrical lens is used to correct astigmatism.

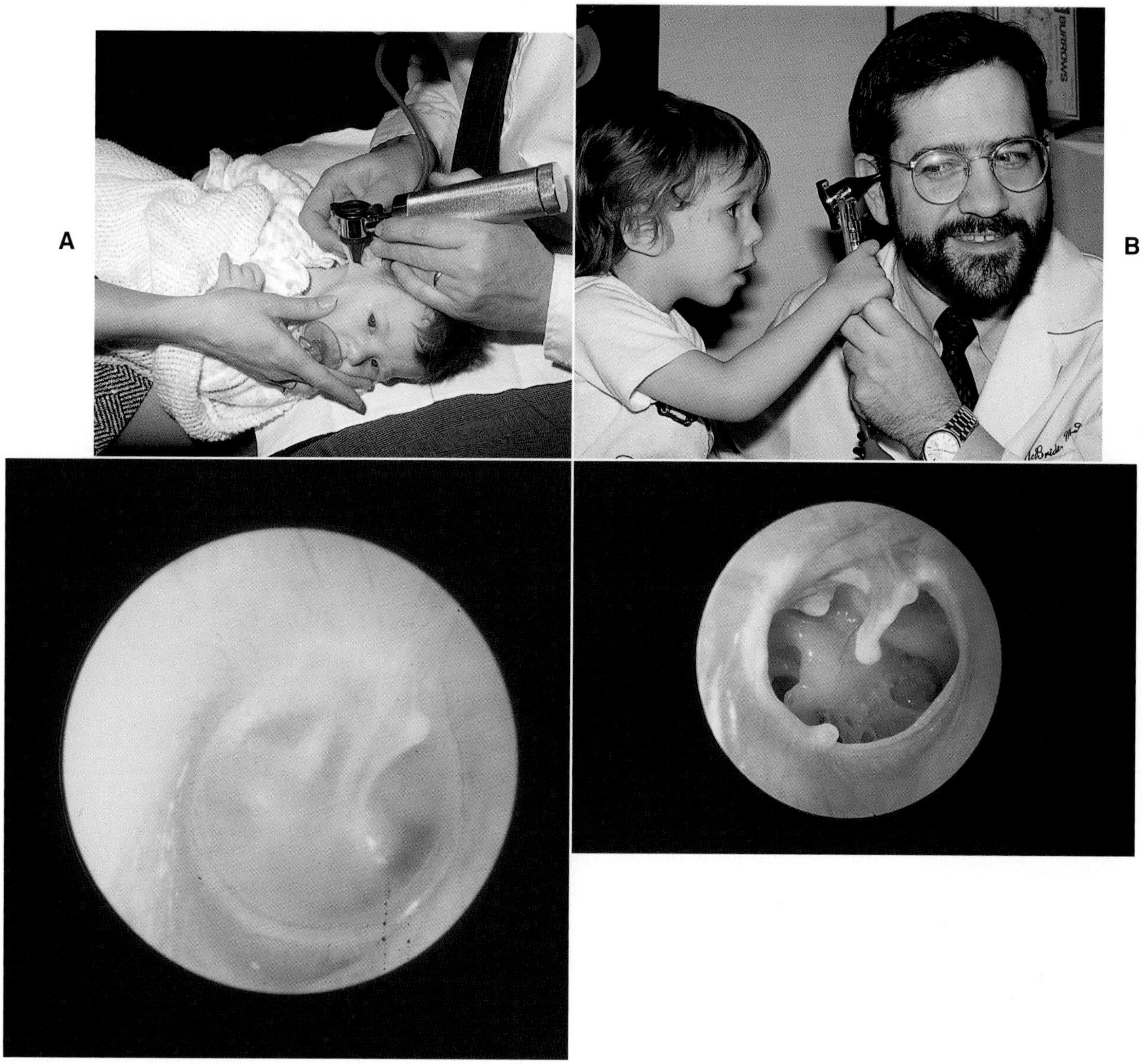

FIGURE 11-22

Otoscopy. **A,** An otoscope is used to examine the eardrum visually. **B,** Making a game of blowing out the otoscope light or allowing a young child first to check the examiner communicates that otoscopy does not hurt. **C,** Otoscopic view of a normal intact eardrum. **D,** Otoscopic view of a perforated eardrum. (**A** and **B,** from Zitelli BJ, Davis HW, Oski FA: *Pediatric physical diagnosis,* ed 2, London, 1992, Mosby–Wolfe. **C** and **D,** From Ignatavicius DD, Workman ML, Mishler MA: *Medical-surgical nursing across the health care continuum,* ed 3, Philadelphia, 1999, WB Saunders.)

otosclerosis (o"to-sklə-ro′sis)	**11-74** Write a word that means hardening of the ear: _____. This condition is caused by formation of spongy bone around structures of the middle and inner ear, and it leads to hearing impairment.
	11-75 Tinnitus* (**tin′ĭ-təs, tĭ-ni′təs**), noise in the ears, is one of the most common complaints of persons with ear or hearing disorders. The noise includes ringing, buzzing, roaring, or clicking. It may be a sign of something as simple as accumulation of ear wax or cerumen† (**sə-roo′mən**) or as serious as Meniere's (**men"e-ārz′**) disease. The latter is a chronic disease of the inner ear with recurrent episodes of hearing loss, tinnitus, and vertigo (**vər′tĭ-go**). Dizziness is also called vertigo.
tinnitus, vertigo	Ringing in the ears is called _____, and dizziness is _____.
hearing **hearing**	**11-76** The combining form **audi(o)** means hearing. Audi/ble pertains to _____. An audio/meter (**aw"de-om′ə-tər**) is a device for measuring _____. (The record produced is an audiogram.)
audiologist (aw"de-ol′ə-jist)	Audio/logy is the science of hearing, particularly the study of impaired hearing that cannot be improved by medication or surgery. A person skilled in audiology is an _____.
	11-77 The skin contains numerous sense receptors for heat, cold, pain, touch, and pressure. Hair has no receptors, but the movement of hair can be detected by receptors near the hair follicle. The skin and many tissues have pain receptors. Pain is the most common symptom for which patients seek medical advice. The combining form **algesi(o)** means sensitivity to pain. Algesia is a word that refers to
sensitivity to pain	_____.
increased	**11-78** Hyper/algesia (**hi"pər-al-je′ze-ə**) is _____ sensitivity to pain.
decreased sensitivity to pain	Hyp/algesia (**hi"pal-je′ze-ə**) or hypo/algesia is _____.
sensitive	An/algesic (**an"əl-je′zik**) means relieving pain or not _____ to pain. Agents that relieve pain without causing loss of consciousness are also called analgesics.
	Three well-known analgesics are aspirin, ibuprofen, and acetaminophen (Tylenol).
	11-79 Three terms that pertain to changes in the way our nervous system responds to sensory stimuli are hyp/esthesia (**hīp"əs-the′zhə**), hyperesthesia (**hi"pər-es-the′zə**), and pseudesthesia (**soo"dəs-the′zə**). The suffix -**esthesia** means sensation or perception. Hypesthesia is also called hypoesthesia and means lessened or below normal sensitivity to touch.
increased	Hyperesthesia is _____ sensitivity to sensory stimuli, such as pain or touch. Pseudesthesia is an imaginary or false sensation, as that felt in an arm that has been removed.
	11-80 My/asthenia gravis, meaning grave muscle weakness, is a chronic neuromuscular disease characterized by great muscular weakness and fatigue.
inflammation	Translated literally, poly/neur/itis (**pol"e-noo-ri′tis**) means _____ of several nerves. Because inflammation is not necessarily present in polyneuritis, the term poly/neuropathy (**pol"e-noo-rop′ə-the**) is often used. Damage to cranial or peripheral nerves can lead to various neuropathies that may be evidenced by tingling, burning, or decreased sensitivity in an extremity.
	11-81 Facial paralysis, or Bell's palsy, is a neuropathy that drastically affects the body image. The cause is unknown, the onset is acute and is characterized by a drawing sensation and paralysis of all facial muscles on the affected side. Bell's palsy is acute paralysis of a cranial nerve affecting one side of the face
facial	and is also called _____ paralysis.

*Tinnitus (Latin: *tinnire*, to tinkle).
†Cerumen (Latin: *cera*, wax).

carpoptosis (kahr″pop-to′sis)	**11-82** The peripheral nerves are subject to many types of trauma. Those of the extremities are commonly affected. An example is wristdrop, in which nerve damage results in the hand remaining in a flexed position at the wrist, and it cannot be extended. Write the term that means wristdrop by combining carp(o) and -ptosis: _____.
hardening **neurectomy** (noo-rek′to-me) **neurorrhaphy** (noo-ror′ə-fe)	**11-83** Neuro/scler/osis (noor″o-sklə-ro′sis) is _____ of nervous tissue. Using -ectomy and -rrhaphy, write words that mean the following: excision of (part of) a nerve _____. suturing of a nerve _____.
destruction of nerve(s) **nervous**	**11-84** Neuro/lysis (noo rol′ĭ-sis) is _____. Neurolysis has several meanings, but all of them have to do with nervous tissue. The word is used to mean release of a nerve sheath by cutting it longitudinally, loosening of adhesions surrounding a nerve, or disintegration of nerve tissue. Neuro/genic (noor″o-jen′ik) means originating in _____ tissue. It also means resulting from nervous impulses.
nerve **neurotripsy** **neuroplasty** (noor′o-plas″te)	**11-85** Neuro/tripsy (noor″o-trip′se) is surgical crushing of a _____. Write the new term that means surgical crushing of a nerve: _____. Write a word that means surgical repair of a nerve: _____.
against **side**	**11-86** The prefix *contra-* is used to mean against or opposed. You have also learned that anti- means against. Practice will help you remember which prefix to use. A contra/indication (kon″trə-in″dĭ-ka′shən) is any condition that renders a particular treatment improper or undesirable. Contra- means _____. Contra/lateral (kon″trə-lat′ər-əl) means associated with a particular part on an opposite _____.

❏ SECTION C REVIEW   𝒫eripheral Nervous System and the Sense Organs

This section review covers frames 11–51 through 11–86. Complete the table by writing a word part or its meaning in each blank.

Combining Form	Meaning	Combining Form	Meaning
1. algesi(o)	_____	8. lacrim(o)	_____
2. audi(o)	_____	9. ocul(o)	_____
3. _____	chemical	**Prefix**	**Meaning**
4. dacry(o)	_____	10. contra-	_____
5. ir(o)	_____	**Suffix**	**Meaning**
6. irid(o)	_____	11. -esthesia	_____
7. kerat(o)	_____		

(Use Appendix V to check your answers.)

Psychological Disorders

Psychological disorders are unlike most diseases or disorders that health professionals are confronted with because there often is no change in the body structure or chemistry, thus making the abnormalities difficult to demonstrate and treat in the usual sense.

psychiatry psych(o), phren(o)	**11-87** A psychologist is a nonmedical person who is trained in methods of psychological analysis, therapy, and research. The medical specialty that deals with the diagnosis, treatment, and prevention of mental illness is _____. In addition to **ment(o),** you have learned two combining forms that mean mind. They are _____ and _____.
mind **mind**	**11-88** Psycho/analysis (**si″ko-ə-nal′ĭ-sis**) is a method of diagnosing and treating disorders of the _____. This is accomplished by ascertaining and studying the facts of the patient's mental life. Psycho/therapy (**si″ko-ther′ə-pe**) is treatment of disorders of the _____. Therapy means treatment, and in psychotherapy, treatment is by mental rather than physical means.
mind	**11-89** Psycho/pharmacology (**si″ko-fahr″mə-kol′ə-je**) is the study of the action of drugs on functions of the _____. Anti/depressants are medications that prevent or relieve depression. Anti/psychotics are medications that are used to treat the symptoms of severe psychiatric disorders. Tranquilizers are prescribed to calm anxious or agitated persons, ideally without decreasing their consciousness. Narcotic drugs produce stupor or sleep.
mind **mind**	**11-90** Only a few psychological disorders have observable pathologic conditions of the brain. Some examples of observable pathologic conditions are mental retardation, dementia, and Alzheimer's disease. The combining form **ment(o)** means mind. You already use this word part when you write ment/al, which means pertaining to the _____. Mental retardation is a disorder characterized by subaverage general intelligence with deficits or impairments in the ability to learn and to adapt socially. Mental retardation is abnormally low intellectual functioning of the _____, or deficient intellectual development.
mind	**11-91** De/mentia (**də-men′shə**) is loss of function of the _____. This irreversible mental state, which is characterized by absence or reduction of intellectual faculties, is due to organic brain disease. Although it is considered incurable, conditions that cause the decline may be treatable or partially reversible.
autism **movement**	**11-92** Signs of psychological disorders can appear in a very young child. Such is the case with mental retardation, autism (**aw′tiz-əm**), and attention deficit disorder. Autism is characterized by extreme withdrawal and impaired development in social interaction and communication. Write the name of this disorder characterized by extreme withdrawal: _____. Attention-deficit hyperactivity disorder is abbreviated ADD or ADHD. It is characterized by short attention span, hyperactivity, and poor concentration. Hyperactivity is also called hyperkinesia. Translated literally, hyper/kinesia or hyper/kinesis is above normal _____.

mind	**11-93** Anxiety disorders are characterized by anticipation of impending danger and dread, the source of which is largely unknown or unrecognized. An anxiety attack is an acute, psychobiologic reaction that usually includes several of the following: restlessness, tension, tachycardia, and breathing difficulty. A psycho/biologic response involves both the _____ and the physical body.
	Phobias are obsessive, irrational, and intense fears of an object, an activity, or a physical situation. The suffix -*phobia* means abnormal fear. Phobias range from abnormal fear of public places, agoraphobia **(ag″o-rə-fo′be-ə),** to abnormal fear of animals, zoophobia **(zo″o-fo′be-ə),** and even include an abnormal fear of acquiring a phobia, phobophobia **(fo″bo-fo′be-ə).**
acrophobia (ak″ro-fo′be-ə)	Write a word that means an irrational fear of heights by using the combining form for extremity and -phobia: _____.
fear	Claustro/phobia **(klaws″tro-fo′be-ə)** is a morbid _____ of closed places. (A claustrum is a barrier.)
pyrophobia (pi″ro-fo′be-ə)	An abnormal fear of fire is _____.
after	**11-94** An obsession is a persistent thought or idea that occupies the mind and cannot be erased by logic or reasoning. A compulsion is an irresistible, repetitive impulse to act contrary to one's ordinary standards. An obsessive-compulsive disorder is a pattern of persistent behaviors that involve compulsion to act on an obsession.
	A posttraumatic stress disorder is characterized by an acute emotional response _____ a traumatic event or situation involving severe environmental stress, such as military combat.
	11-95 A panic disorder or panic attack is an episode of acute anxiety that occurs unpredictably with feelings of intense apprehension or terror, accompanied by dyspnea, dizziness, sweating, trembling, and chest pain.
	11-96 A manic episode is a distinct unstable period in which there is a persistently elevated, expansive, and irritable mood. A bipolar disorder is a major mental disorder characterized by the occurrence of manic episodes and major depressive episodes.
bipolar	In an extreme manic episode, a delusion of grandeur may occur. Megalo/mania **(meg″ə-lo-ma′ne-ə)** is an abnormal mental state in which one believes oneself to be a person of great importance, power, fame, or wealth. Megalomania may occur in an extreme manic episode of _____ disorder.
excessive preoccupation excessive preoccupation	**11-97** As a suffix, -*mania* means excessive preoccupation. Phago/mania **(fag″o-ma′ne-ə)** is _____ _____ with eating. A phago/maniac **(fag″o-ma′ne-ak)** has an insatiable craving for food.
	Pyro/mania **(pi″ro-ma′ne-ə)** is _____ _____ with fires. A pyro/maniac has an obsessive preoccupation with fires. The combining form *pyr(o)* means fire. Pyro/mania is a compulsion to set fires or watch fires.
false	**11-98** Klepto/mania* **(klep″to-ma′ne-ə)** is characterized by an abnormal, uncontrollable, and recurrent urge to steal.
	Pseudo/mania **(soo″do-ma′ne-ə)** is a _____ or pretended mental disorder.
false	Pseudo/plegia **(soo″do-ple′jə)** is hysterical paralysis. There is loss of muscle power without real paralysis. Pseudo in the name tells us that the paralysis is _____.
weakness	**11-99** The suffix -*asthenia* means weakness. Neur/asthenia **(noor″əs-the′ne-ə)** is a nervous disorder (neurosis) characterized by _____ and sometimes nervous exhaustion. It generally follows a depressed state and is believed by some to be psychosomatic.

*Kleptomania (Greek: *kleptein,* to steal; *mania,* madness).

11-100 Schizophrenia (**skiz″o-fre′ne-ə, skit″so-fre′ne-ə**) is any of a large group of psychotic disorders characterized by gross distortion of reality, hallucinations, disturbances of language and communication, and disorganized or catatonic behavior (psychologically induced immobility with muscular rigidity that is interrupted by agitation). Notice the two pronunciations of the term *schizophrenia.* The combining forms ***schiz(o)*** and ***schist(o)*** mean split. Either *skiz o,* or *skit so* is correct pronunciation in schizophrenia.

A psychotic disorder, or psychosis, is any major mental disorder characterized by a gross impairment in reality testing.

split mind

Translated literally, schizo/phrenia means _____ _____ , and relates to the splitting off of a part of the psyche, and the part that is expressed may be contrary to the original personality of the person.

against

11-101 A number of personality disorders exist with which you may already be familiar. These include antisocial behavior, paranoia, and others. Anti/social behavior acts _____ the rights of others. Paranoia (**par″ə-noi′ah**) is characterized by persistent delusions of persecution, mistrust, and combativeness. Additional information about psychological disorders can be found in the *Diagnostic and Statistical Manual of Mental Disorders* (DSM).

❑ SECTION D REVIEW   𝒫sychological Disorders

This section review covers frames 11–87 through 11–101. Complete the table by writing the meaning of each word part listed.

Combining Form	Meaning		Suffix	Meaning
1. ment(o)	_____		4. -mania	_____
2. pyr(o)	_____			
3. schist(o), schiz(o)	_____			

(Use Appendix V to check your answers.)

𝒯erminology Challenge

The nervous system and associated terminology is one of the most complicated body systems. Many functions are still not well understood, and great progress is expected in the treatment of these disorders. This section challenges you to read, write, and understand new terms or concepts about the nervous system and psychological disorders.

11-102 You learned in Chapter 5 that the combining form, ventricul(o), means ventricle. The word part can refer to a ventricle in either the brain or the heart.

inflammation of a ventricle

Ventricul/itis (**ven-trik″u-li′tis**) is

_____ .

Although it is not obvious, ventriculitis refers especially to inflammation of a ventricle of the brain.

electroencephalog- raphy (e-lek"tro-ən-sef" ə-log'rə-fe) electroencephalo- graph e-lek"tro-ən-sef' ə-lo-graf")	**11-103** You are probably familiar with the term *electrocardiography,* which means the process of recording the electrical activity of the heart. Use electro/cardio/graphy as a model to write a word that means the process of recording the electrical activity of the brain: _____. The instrument used in electroencephalography is an _____. Electrodes are attached to various areas of the patient's head using a special gel. During neurosurgery, the electrodes can be applied directly to the brain. Electroencephalography is used to diagnose several disorders, including seizures, lesions, and impaired consciousness.
electroencephalo- gram (e-lek"tro-en-sef' ə-lo-gram")	**11-104** Although the legal definition of brain death varies from state to state, it is generally defined as an irreversible form of unconsciousness characterized by a complete loss of brain function while the heart continues to beat. A diagnosis of brain death may require demonstrating that electrical activity of the brain is absent. The record produced by the electrical activity of the brain is an _____.
false pseudesthesia (soo"dəs-the'zhə)	**11-105** Pseudesthesia, like many situations that involve the nervous system, is not well understood. Pseud/esthesia is a sensation occurring in the absence of the appropriate stimulus. In other words, pseudesthesia is a _____ sensation. (Pseudesthesia is also called pseudoesthesia. It is notable that two spellings are accepted for many terms in which pseud[o] is joined to a combining form that begins with a vowel.) Pseudesthesia can occur in a lost arm or leg after amputation. This imaginary or false sensation is termed _____.
anotia (an-o'shə)	**11-106** A developmental anomaly is any congenital defect that results from interference with the normal growth and differentiation of the fetus. Because the nervous system functions as the major regulating and communicating system of the body, malfunction, paralysis, or other developmental defects are sometimes obvious at birth. They range from minor to life-threatening situations. One developmental defect that is not life threatening but life altering is absence of one or both ears. Write a word that means absence of the ear: _____. Anotia is absence of one or both external ears. It is generally accompanied by lack of an internal ear also. Cosmetic reconstructive surgery is generally performed while the child is still young, but this does not, of course, correct the deafness.
abnormal fear	**11-107** Rabies is an acute, often fatal, disease of the central nervous system transmitted to humans by infected animals. After introduction of the virus into the human body, often by an animal bite, the virus travels along nerve pathways to the brain and later to other organs. Without medical intervention and possibly the use of vaccine, coma and death are likely. A nontechnical term for rabies that is obsolete is hydrophobia **(hi"dro-fo'be-ə).** Literal translation of hydro/phobia is _____ _____ of water. The name hydrophobia was given after observation that rabid animals avoid water. Infected animals avoid water because paralysis prevents them from being able to swallow.

There is no review for this section.
Study the following list of selected abbreviations. Then read through the Chapter Pharmacology section and be sure that you understand the effects and uses of the drug classes that are presented. When you are finished, work the Chapter Review. After completing the exercises, check your answers with the solutions in Appendix V.
You will find these items presented after the Chapter Review:
• Listing of Medical Terms
• Enhancing Spanish Communication

Selected Abbreviations

ACh	acetylcholine	EEG	electroencephalogram
AD	right ear (Latin: *auris dextra*)	ENT	ear, nose, and throat
ADD	attention deficit disorder	EOM	extraocular movements
ADHD	attention-deficit hyperactivity disorder	ICP	intracranial pressure
ALS	amyotrophic lateral sclerosis	KJ	knee jerk
ANS	autonomic nervous system	MA	mental age
AS	left ear (Latin, *auris sinistra*)	MMPI	Minnesota Multiphasic Personality Inventory
ATS	anxiety tension state	MRI or RI	magnetic resonance imaging
CA	chronological age; cancer	MS	multiple sclerosis
CNS	central nervous system	OCD	obsessive-compulsive disorder
CSF	cerebrospinal fluid	PEG	pneumoencephalography
CSM	cerebrospinal meningitis	PET	positron emission tomography
CT	computed tomography	PNS	peripheral nervous system
CVA	cerebrovascular accident, costovertebral angle	REM	rapid eye movement
DSM	*Diagnostic and Statistical Manual of Mental Disorders*	SCI	spinal cord injury
		SNS	somatic nervous system
DT	delirium tremens	TIA	transient ischemic attack
DTR	deep tendon reflex		

Chapter Pharmacology

Class	Effect and Uses
Antialcoholic Drugs	**For Management of Chronic Alcoholics Who Want or Need Enforced Sobriety**
disulfiram (Antabuse)	Must be used with the patient's knowledge
Analgesics	**For Relief of Pain**
(See Chapter Pharmacology of Chapter 2.)	
Anesthetics	**For Loss of Sensation**
(See Chapter Pharmacology of Chapter 2.)	
Anti-Alzheimer Drugs	**Cholinesterase Inhibitors Relieve the Deficiency of Acetylcholine That Is Believed to Exist in Alzheimer's Disease**
donepezil (Aricept)	Used to treat mild to moderate dementia
tacrine (Cognex)	Used to treat mild to moderate dementia
Antianxiety Drugs	**Used to Relieve the Symptoms of Anxiety**
meprobamate (Equanil)	Used for short-term relief of symptoms
Benzodiapines	***Used to treat anxiety disorders and are processed by the kidneys***
alprazolam (Xanax)	Also used for panic disorders
chlordiazepoxide (Librium)	Also used in alcohol withdrawal
oxazepam (Serax)	Used for short-term relief
lorazepam (Ativan)	Used for short-term relief
diazepam (Valium)	Also used for the relief of tension before surgery
clorazepate (Tranxene)	Also used for acute alcohol withdrawal

Chapter Pharmacology—cont'd

Class	Effect and Uses
Miscellaneous	*Lack prominent sedative effects*
buspirone (BuSpar)	Used in anxiety disorders
doxepin (Sinequan)	Used in depression or anxiety
hydroxyzine (Atarax)	Also used for pruritis
Tricyclic drugs	
amitriptyline (Elavil)	Used in depression
amoxapine (Asendin)	Used in depression
clomipramine (Anafranil)	Used in obsessive-compulsive disorders
imipramine (Tofranil)	Used for enuresis in children
nortriptyline (Pamelor)	Used in depression
Tetracyclic drugs	*Used in depression*
bupropion (Wellbutrin)	Used to treat symptoms of depression
maprotiline (Ludiomil)	Used to treat symptoms of depression
mirtazapine (Remeron)	Used to treat symptoms of depression
trazodone (Desyrel)	Used to treat symptoms of depression
venlafaxine (Effexor)	Used to treat symptoms of depression
Selective serotonin reuptake inhibitors	*Used in depression*
fluoxetine (Prozac)	Used in depression, bulimia nervosa
fluvoxamine (Luvox)	Used in OCD
paroxetine (Paxil)	Used in panic disorders also
sertraline (Zoloft)	Multiple uses
Monoamine oxidase inhibitors (MAOIs)	*Used in depression that is not responsive to other antidepressive therapy*
phenelzine (Nardil)	Used in atypical depression
tranylcypromine (Parnate)	Used in depression
Anticonvulsants	**Prevent or Reduce the Severity of Epileptic or Other Convulsive Seizures**
Hydantoins	
mephenytoin (Mesantoin)	Inhibits seizure activity
phenytoin (Dilantin)	Used to control grand mal seizure
Succinimides	
ethosuximide (Zarontin)	Used in petit mal seizures
phensuximide (Milontin)	Used in petit mal seizures
Oxazolidinediones	
trimethadione (Tridione)	Used in petit mal seizures
Benzodiazepines	
clonazepam (Klonopin)	Used in petit mal seizures
clorazepate (Tranxene)	Used to manage partial seizures
diazepam (Valium)	Used with other drugs to prevent convulsions
Miscellaneous	
carbamazepine (Tegretol)	Also used to treat trigeminal neuralgia
gabapentin (Neurontin)	Used in partial seizures
lamotrigine (Lamictal)	Used in partial onset seizures
topiramate (Topamax)	Used to treat a broad spectrum of epileptic activity
valproic acid (Depakote)	Also used in manic episodes of bipolar disorder

Continued

Chapter Pharmacology—cont'd

Class	Effect and Uses
Antiemetic Drugs (See Chapter Pharmacology in Chapter 7.)	**Used to Relieve or Prevent Vomiting and Lightheadedness**
Antimigraine Drugs	**Used to Relieve Migraine Headaches**
rizatriptan (Maxalt)	Not intended for prevention of migraines
sumatriptan (Imitrex)	Used for treatment of acute migraine or cluster headache
zolmitriptan (Zomig)	Used for treatment of acute migraine with or without aura
Antiparkinson Drugs	**Used to Relieve the Symptoms of Parkinson's Disease**
amantadine (Symmetrel)	Is thought to release dopamine
benztropine (Cogentin)	Used as an adjunct treatment for all types of Parkinson's disease
levodopa (Dopar)	Used in combination with other drugs of this type
pramipexole (Mirapex)	Used for certain types of Parkinson's disease
procyclidine (Kemadrin)	Also used as antispasmodic
selegiline (Eldepryl)	Used in combination with other drugs of this type
tolcapone (Tasmar)	Used if patient doesn't respond to other drugs
trihexyphenidyl (Artane)	Used in all forms of Parkinson's disease
Antimanic Drug	
lithium	Used in manic episodes of manic depression
Antipsychotic Drugs	**Used to Relieve the Symptoms of Psychoses**
Phenothiazines	
chlorpromazine (Thorazine)	Also used for manic-depressive disorder
fluphenazine (Prolixin)	Used to manage psychotic symptoms
mesoridazine (Serentil)	Used in schizophrenia
prochlorperazine (Compazine)	Also used for nausea and vomiting
promazine (Sparine)	Used to manage psychotic symptoms
thioridazine (Mellaril)	Also used for severe combativeness in children
trifluoperazine (Stelazine)	Also used for short-term relief of anxiety
Phenylbutylpiperadines	
haloperidol (Haldol)	Also used in Tourette's syndrome
Dibenzapines	
clozapine (Clozaril)	Used for severe schizophrenia
loxapine (Loxitane)	Manages manifestations of psychoses
olanzapine (Zyprexa)	Manages manifestations of psychoses
benzisoxazole	
risperidone (Risperdal)	
Emetic	
ipecac	Used for drug overdoses and poisonings

CHAPTER REVIEW 11

▶ **BASIC UNDERSTANDING**

REVIEWING WORD PARTS

I. Write a word (prefix, suffix, or combining form) for each clue.

CROSSWORD PUZZLE 11

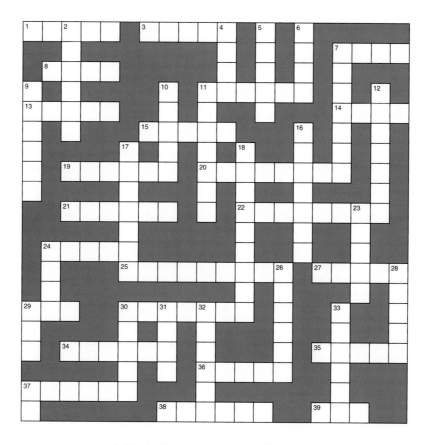

Across

1 seizure (suffix)
3 excessive preoccupation
7 one
8 fire
11 against
13 discharge
14 individual
15 nerve
19 cornea
20 eyelid
21 tear

22 feeling (suffix)
24 twitching
25 eye
27 chemical
29 resembling
30 sensitivity to pain
34 four
35 sleep
36 iris
37 tree
38 abnormal fear
39 muscle

Down

2 mind
4 self
5 mind
6 vision
7 meninges
9 surgical crushing
10 spinal cord
11 brain
12 movement
16 arachnoid membrane
17 tear

18 cerebellum
23 between
24 half
26 vision
28 eye
29 pertaining to
30 hearing
31 neuroglia
32 split
33 surgical repair
37 twice

MATCHING

II. Assign structures in the left column to the correct division of the nervous system by choosing either A or B.

_____ 1. brain   **A.** Central nervous system
_____ 2. chemoreceptors   **B.** Peripheral nervous system
_____ 3. pain receptors
_____ 4. sense organs
_____ 5. spinal cord

III. Match the types of receptors in the left column with the appropriate stimulus in the right column (A-E).

_____ 1. chemoreceptors   **A.** Change in chemical concentration of substances
_____ 2. mechanoreceptors   **B.** Changes in temperature
_____ 3. nociceptors   **C.** Light
_____ 4. photoreceptors   **D.** Movement in fluids or changes in pressure
_____ 5. thermoreceptors   **E.** Tissue damage

MULTIPLE CHOICE

IV. Choose one answer (A, B, C, or D) for each of the following:

1. Which of the following is the innermost meningeal membrane?
   A. arachnoid
   B. dura mater
   C. epidural
   D. pia mater

2. Which of the following is the correct name for a stroke?
   A. cerebrovascular accident
   B. craniocerebral trauma
   C. monoplegia
   D. polyneuropathy

3. Which term means an irrational fear of heights?
   A. acrophobia
   B. agoraphobia
   C. claustrophobia
   D. zoophobia

4. Which of the following means hernial protrusion of the spinal cord through a defect in the vertebral column?
   A. myeloblast
   B. myelocele
   C. rachischisis
   D. sternoschisis

5. Where is the mass of blood located in a subdural hematoma?
   A. between the spinal cord and its bony encasement
   B. between two of the meninges
   C. within the bone marrow
   D. within the spinal canal

6. What is cerebral meningitis?
   A. inflammation of the cerebellum
   B. inflammation of the medulla
   C. inflammation of the meninges of the brain
   D. inflammation of the meninges of the spinal cord

7. Which term means incision of the lacrimal sac?
   A. cholecystotomy
   B. cystolithectomy
   C. dacryocystotomy
   D. dacryolithiasis

8. Which of the following involves irreversible loss of memory, disorientation, and speech and gait disturbances and is a form of presenile dementia resulting from atrophy of frontal and occipital lobes?
   A. Alzheimer's disease
   B. Lou Gehrig's disease
   C. Meniere's syndrome
   D. Parkinson's disease

9. Which of the following terms means radiology of the spinal cord after injection of a contrast medium?
   A. myelography
   B. myelogram
   C. pneumo-encephalography
   D. tympanoplasty

10. Which term means paralysis of one side of the body?
    A. diplegia
    B. hemiplegia
    C. paraplegia
    D. quadriplegia

11. What is narcolepsy?
    A. a seizure characterized by convulsive attacks
    B. a seizure or sudden attack of sleep
    C. addiction to narcotics
    D. treatment of disease with narcotics

12. What is the term for any condition that renders a particular treatment improper or undesirable?
    A. a contraindication
    B. a contralateral situation
    C. an anticonvulsant
    D. an antipyretic

13. What does interocular mean?
    A. between the ears
    B. between the eyes
    C. within the ear
    D. within the eye

14. What does algesia mean?
    A. pain
    B. oversensitivity to pain
    C. sensitivity to pain
    D. undersensitivity to pain

15. What is the term for the occurrence of a sensation in the absence of the appropriate stimulus?
    A. hyperesthesia
    B. hypesthesia
    C. pseudesthesia
    D. pseudomania

16. What is the disease in which there is progressive deterioration of the myelin sheaths of neurons to form many scleroses?
    A. angiosclerosis
    B. arteriosclerosis
    C. idiopathic epilepsy
    D. multiple sclerosis

17. Which term means a pathologic condition of the ear in which there is formation of spongy bone and usually results in hearing loss?
    A. hyperalgesia
    B. ophthalmodynia
    C. otalgia
    D. otosclerosis

18. What does lacrimation mean?
    A. a cytoplasmic process on a neuron
    B. a nervous disorder with anxiety as its major symptom
    C. demyelination of nerve cells
    D. discharge of tears

19. What is a word that means resulting from nervous impulse?
    A. neurogenic
    B. neuroplasty
    C. neurosis
    D. neurotripsy

20. What is neurotripsy?
    A. loosening of adhesions surrounding a nerve
    B. plastic repair of a nerve
    C. spontaneous disintegration of nerve tissue
    D. surgical crushing of a nerve

CASE STUDIES

V. Write the appropriate term in these case studies.

1. B. Bocher, a 70-year-old female, was brought to the emergency room by her daughter. The patient complained of weakness, headache, nausea, and abdominal pain. When Dr. Fast asked about her diet, she said the only unusual food she had eaten was some home-cured sausage for dinner the previous evening. Dr. Fast requested blood tests, including a blood culture and abdominal x-rays. Within 30 minutes after entering the emergency room, Mrs. Bocher developed double vision and began vomiting. Suspecting a severe form of food poisoning called _____, Dr. Fast ordered that antitoxin be administered immediately.

2. Jimmy Schooler experienced loss of consciousness after what his mother described as a convulsion. His teacher had told her that Jimmy "blanks out at times" but responds after a few seconds. The electroencephalogram showed excessive electrical activity. The CT and MRI did not show a lesion, and all other tests were normal. On the basis of the abnormal EEG, the most likely diagnosis is _____.

3. E.Z. Speed was checking out his new sports car and lost control while rounding a curve. When the paramedics arrived on the accident scene, E.Z. was barely conscious, complained of his neck hurting, and said he had no feeling in his legs. Paralysis of the legs and lower portion of the body is called _____.

4. Madeline, a 4-year-old, has recurring otitis media. Sometimes this is accompanied by _____, which means a discharge from the ear.

5. A 20-year-old adult with a history of unrealistic interpretation of things that happen, standing for long periods in one place with a fixed gaze, hearing voices, and showing a great deal of anger and frustration at times probably has a psychotic disorder called _____.

FILL IN THE BLANKS

VI. Write the appropriate word in each blank.

Three membranes collectively known as (1) _____ cover the brain and spinal cord. The largest and uppermost portion of the brain is the (2) _____. A fluid called (3) _____ fluid surrounds and cushions the brain and spinal cord.

The nervous system is composed of two types of cells. The basic unit of the nervous system is called a (4) _____. The other type of cell that serves as support is a (5) _____ cell.

A cytoplasmic projection that carries impulses away from the cell body of the neuron is called a (6) _____. Another type of cytoplasmic process that carries an impulse to the cell body is a (7) _____.

A chemical that transmits a nervous impulse across a synapse is called a (8) _____.

The peripheral nervous system has two parts, the sensory system and the motor system. Which of these two systems carries a message from receptors to the central nervous system? (9) _____ The motor system is divided into the somatic nervous system and the autonomic nervous system. Which system, somatic or autonomic, is responsible for voluntary movement? (10) _____ Which system is subdivided into the sympathetic and parasympathetic nervous system? (11) _____

WRITING TERMS

VII. Write one term for each of the following meanings:

1. an abnormal fear of fire _____
2. between the two cerebral _____
   hemispheres
3. destruction of nerve tissue _____
4. excessive sensitivity to pain _____
5. inflammation of the cerebellum _____

6. measurement of hearing _____
7. pertaining to a nerve _____
8. pertaining to the tears _____
9. radiology of the spinal cord _____
10. within the skull _____

▶ **GREATER COMPREHENSION**

FILL IN THE BLANKS

VIII. Write the correct term to complete each of the blanks in the following sentences.

1. The white, lipid covering on axons that enhance the rate of conduction of a nervous impulse is called a _____ sheath.

2. The area of contact between a neuron and adjoining skeletal muscle is called a _____ junction.

3. When a nerve impulse reaches the junction between the neuron and the skeletal muscle, a substance called _____ is released, which leads to contraction of the muscle.

4. An area between two neurons is a _____.

5. The part of the brain that connects the cerebral hemispheres with the spinal cord is the brain _____, and it is composed of the medulla, the pons, and the midbrain.

6. The _____ consists of the thalamus and the hypothalamus.

7. The part of the brain that is responsible for interpretation of sensory impulses and all voluntary muscle activities is the _____.

8. Adrenergic fibers release the neurotransmitter _____.

9. Cholinergic fibers release the neurotransmitter _____.

10. The various activities of the nervous system can be grouped as sensory, integrative, and _____ functions.

INTERPRETING ABBREVIATIONS

IX. Write the meanings of the following abbreviations:

1. ADD _____
2. ALS _____
3. CNS _____
4. CSF _____
5. CVA _____

6. DSM _____
7. EEG _____
8. ICP _____
9. MS _____
10. TIA _____

PRONUNCIATION

X. Pronunciation is shown for several terms. Mark the primary accent in each term with an ´.

1. audiometer (aw de om ə ter)
2. cerebellar (ser ə bel ər)
3. cerebrospinal (ser ə bro spi nəl)
4. encephalocele (en sef ə lo sēl)
5. monoplegia (mon o ple jə)

6. neuroarthropathy (noor o ahr throp ə the)
7. neuroglia (noo rog le ə)
8. neurolysis (noo rol ĭ sis)
9. phagomania (fag o ma ne ə)
10. rhinodacryo/lith (ri no dak re o lith)

CATEGORIZING TERMS

XI. Categorize each of the following terms by writing A, D, R, or S for anatomical, diagnostic, radiological, or surgical:

1. arachnoid _____
2. cochlea _____
3. cornea _____
4. dacryocystography _____
5. dyslexia _____

6. keratotomy _____
7. mastoiditis _____
8. meningocele _____
9. ptosis _____
10. tinnitus _____

SPELLING

XII. Circle terms that are spelled incorrectly and write their correct spelling.

afferent   dimentia   mastoiditis   neurasthenia   pyrofobia

DRUG CLASSES

XIII. Write a term in each blank to complete these sentences.

1. A drug class called _____ is used for relief of pain.

2. Another drug class called _____ is used to provide loss of sensation.

3. Anti _____ drugs are used to relieve the symptoms of anxiety.

4. _____ prevent or reduce the severity of seizures.

5. Antiemetic/antivertigo drugs are used to relieve or prevent _____ and lightheadedness.

6. Anti _____ drugs are used to relieve the symptoms of psychoses.

7. _____ are used to induce vomiting in drug overdoses or poisonings.

(Check your answers with the solutions in Appendix V.)

 Listing of Medical Terms

acetylcholine	audiology	cerebral ventricle	dacryolithiasis
acetylcholinesterase	audiometer	cerebrocranial	dacryosinusitis
acrophobia	autism	cerebrospinal fluid	dementia
adrenaline	autonomic	cerebrotomy	dendrite
adrenergic	axon	cerebrovascular accident	diencephalon
afferent	blepharedema	cerebrum	diplegia
agoraphobia	blepharoplasty	cerumen	dopamine
algesia	blepharoptosis	chemoreceptor	dura mater
Alzheimer's disease	botulism	cholinergic	dyslexia
amyotrophic lateral sclerosis	bradykinesia	claustrophobia	echoencephalogram
analgesic	brain stem	cochlea	echoencephalograph
anesthetic	carpoptosis	concussion	echoencephalography
aneurysm	cataract	conjunctivitis	efferent
aneurysmectomy	central nervous system	contraindication	electroencephalogram
anotia	cephalalgia	contralateral	electroencephalograph
antianxiety	cerebellar	contusion	electroencephalography
anticonvulsant	cerebellitis	corneal	emetic
antidepressant	cerebellum	craniocerebral	encephalitis
antiemetic	cerebral angiography	dacryocystitis	encephalography
antipsychotic	cerebral concussion	dacryocystography	encephalomalacia
arachnoid	cerebral cortex	dacryocystorhinostomy	encephalomeningitis
astigmatism	cerebral hemisphere	dacryocystotomy	encephalomyelitis
audiologist	cerebral palsy	dacryolith	encephalomyelopathy

Continued

Listing of Medical Terms—cont'd

encephalosclerosis
endorphin
epidural hematoma
epilepsy
epinephrine
extraocular
glaucoma
glioma
hemiplegia
homeostasis
Huntington's disease
hydrocephalus
hydrophobia
hypalgesia
hyperalgesia
hyperesthesia
hyperkinesia
hyperkinesis
hyperopia
hypesthesia
hypoalgesia
hypothalamus
intercerebral
interocular
intracerebral
intracranial
intraocular
intrathecal
iritis
keratitis
kleptomania
lacrimal gland
lacrimation
mania
mastoiditis
mechanoreceptor
medulla
megalomania
Meniere's disease
meningeal

meninges
meningitis
meningocele
meningomyelocele
mental retardation
midbrain
monoplegia
multiple sclerosis
myasthenia gravis
myelogram
myelography
myelomalacia
myopia
myospasm
narcolepsy
nasolacrimal duct
neural
neuralgia
neurasthenia
neurectomy
neuroarthropathy
neurogenic
neuroglia
neurology
neurolysis
neuroma
neuromuscular
neuron
neuroplasty
neurorrhaphy
neurosclerosis
neurotransmitter
neurotripsy
nociceptor
occipital
oculonasal
ophthalmalgia
ophthalmic
ophthalmomalacia
ophthalmometer

ophthalmorrhagia
ophthalmoscopy
otalgia
otitis
otitis media
otorrhea
otosclerosis
otoscope
otoscopy
palsy
paranoia
paraplegia
parasympathetic
Parkinson's disease
peripheral nervous system
phagomania
phagomaniac
phobophobia
photophobia
photoreceptor
pia mater
pneumoencephalography
pneumomyelography
poliomyelitis
polyneuralgia
polyneuritis
polyneuropathy
pons
pseudesthesia
pseudoesthesia
pseudomania
pseudoplegia
psychiatric
psychiatry
psychoanalysis
psychobiologic
psychologist
psychopharmacology
psychosis
psychotherapy

ptosis
pyromania
pyromaniac
pyrophobia
quadriplegia
rabies
radial keratotomy
retinal detachment
retinopathy
rhinodacryolith
schizophrenia
sciatic
sciatica
semicoma
semiconscious
semipermeable
sensory
serotonin
somatic
stye
subdural hematoma
sympathectomy
sympathetic
synapse
temporal
tetanus
thalamus
thermoceptor
tinnitus
transient ischemic attack
tympanic membrane
unilateral
ventricle
ventriculitis
ventriculogram
ventriculography
vertigo
zoophobia

Español *Enhancing Spanish Communication*

English	Spanish (pronunciation)
adrenaline	adrenalina (ah-dray-nah-LEE-nah)
anxiety	ansiedad (an-se-ay-DAHD)
brain	cerebro (say-RAY-bro)
concussion	concusión (con-coo-se-ON)
conscious	consciente (cons-se-EN-tay)
consciousness	conciencia (con-se-EN-se-ah)
convulsion	convulsión (con-vool-se-ON)
cranium	cráneo (CRAH-nay-o)
dizziness	vértigo (VERR-te-go)
ear	oreja (o-RAY-hah)
epilepsy	epilepsia (ay-pe-LEP-se-ah)
eye	ojo (O-ho)
eyeball	globo del ojo (GLO-bo del O-ho)
eyebrow	ceja (SAY-hah)
eyelash	pestaña (pes-TAH-nyah)
fainting	languidez (lan-gee-DES), desmayo (des-MAH-yo)
fatigue	fatiga (fah-TEE-gah)
fear	miedo (me-AY-do)
fiber	(FEE-brah)
fire	fuego (foo-AY-go)
gray	gris (grees)
headache	dolor de cabeza (do-LOR day cah-BAY-sa)
heat	calor (cah-LOR)

English	Spanish (pronunciation)
light	luz (loos)
lobe	lóbulo (LO-boo-lo)
neck	cuello (coo-EL-lyo)
nerve	nervio (NERR-ve-o)
nervous	nervioso (ner-ve-O-so)
neurology	neurología (nay-oo-ro-o-HEE-ah)
optic	óptico (OP-te-co)
painful	doloroso (do-lo-RO-so)
paralysis	parálisis (pah-RAH-le-sis)
psychiatry	psiquiatría (se-ke-ah-TREE-ah)
psychology	psicología (se-co-lo-HEE-ah)
seizure	ataque (ah-TAH-kay)
sensation	sensación (sen-sah-se-ON)
sleep	sueño (soo-AY-nyo)
spasm	espasmo (es-PAHS-mo)
spinal column	columna vertebral (co-LOOM-nah ver-tay-BRAHL)
stroke	ataque de apoplejía (ah-TAH-kay de ah-po-play-HEE-ah)
tear	lágrima (LAH-gre-mah)
trauma	daño (DAH-nyo)
vision	visión (ve-se-ON)
white	blanco (BLAHN-co)

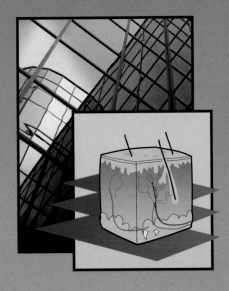

Integumentary System

12

Outline

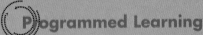

Principal Word Parts

COMBINING FORMS

adip(o), lip(o)	fat
alb(o), albin(o)	white
axill(o)	axilla (armpit)
bacter(i), bacteri(o)	bacteria
cry(o)	cold
cutane(o), derm(o), dermat(o)	skin
cyan(o)	blue
erythemat(o)	erythema or redness
follicul(o)	follicle
heli(o)	sun
hidr(o)	sweat
hydr(o)	water
ichthy(o)	fish
kerat(o)	horny or cornea
leuk(o)	white
melan(o)	black
myc(o)	fungus
necr(o)	dead or death
onych(o), ungu(o)	nail
pil(o), trich(o)	hair
rhytid(o)	wrinkle
seb(o)	sebum
seps(o)	infection
sept(o)	infection or septum
therm(o)	heat
xer(o)	dry

PREFIXES

dia-	through
in-	in, into, or not
ecto-	outside
meso-	middle
sub-	under

SUFFIXES

-cidal	killing
-derm	skin or germ layer
-phoresis	transmission

Learning Goals

▶ BASIC UNDERSTANDING

In this chapter, you will learn to do the following:

1. Demonstrate an understanding of the structure and functions of the skin.
2. Recognize the functions of accessory structures associated with the skin.
3. Write the meaning of word parts pertaining to the integumentary system, and use them to build and analyze medical terms.
4. Recognize descriptions of different types of skin lesions.
5. Describe several diseases or disorders of the skin.
6. Demonstrate an understanding of several methods for administering medications.

▶ GREATER COMPREHENSION

7. Categorize burns based on descriptions of the depths of the burns.
8. Classify skin diseases or eruptions as being caused by bacteria, fungi, viruses, or parasites.
9. Spell the terms accurately.
10. Pronounce the terms correctly.
11. Know the meaning of the abbreviations.
12. Categorize terms as diagnostic, anatomical, radiological, therapeutic, or surgical.
13. Identify the effects or uses of the drug classes presented in this chapter.

Structures and Functions of the Integumentary System

The skin is the integument or external covering of the body. Because it is on the outside of our bodies, we are more familiar with the skin than with any other organ. Its accessory structures are the hair, nails, and sebaceous and sweat glands.

above the dermis	**12-1** The integumentary (**in-teg-u-men′tar-e**) system is the skin and its glands, hair, nails and other structures that are derived from it. The skin consists of two main parts: the epidermis (**ep″ĭ-dər′mis**) and the dermis (**dər′mis**) (Figure 12-1). Remembering that epi- means above or on, where is the epi/dermis located? _____
hard	The epidermis consists of four to five layers. The palms and soles have the greatest number of layers. The outermost layer of epidermis consists of cells that are nonliving and are constantly being shed and replaced. These cells contain keratin (**ker′ə-tin**), a scleroprotein. Sclero/protein (**sklēr″o-pro′tēn**) identifies the protein as being _____, or horny.
horny	**12-2** The combining form *kerat(o)* means horny or the cornea—the convex, transparent structure at the front of the eye. When kerat(o) is used in discussions regarding the skin, it means hard or horny. Kerato/genesis (**ker″ə-to-jen′ə-sis**) is the formation of keratin, a _____ material. A kerat/oma (**ker″ə-to′mə**), also called a callus, is a flat, poorly defined mass on the sole over a bony prominence and is caused by pressure. A corn is also caused by pressure or friction but, unlike a callus, is round or conical and usually painful.

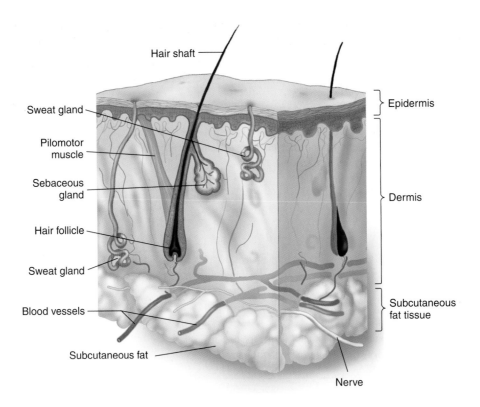

Hair shaft

Sweat gland

Pilomotor muscle

Sebaceous gland

Hair follicle

Sweat gland

Blood vessels

Subcutaneous fat

Epidermis

Dermis

Subcutaneous fat tissue

Nerve

FIGURE 12-1
The skin. The epidermis, the thin outer layer, is composed of four to five layers. Underneath the epidermis is the thicker dermis, composed of connective tissue containing lymphatics, nerves, blood vessels, hair follicles, sebaceous glands, and sweat glands. Beneath the dermis is a layer of subcutaneous adipose tissue.

---

keratosis
(ker″ə-to′sis)

sebum

12-3 A condition of the skin characterized by the formation of horny growths or excessive development of the horny growth is called a _____.

One type of keratosis, seborrheic keratosis, is a consequence of aging and another type, actinic keratosis, is a premalignant lesion that is common in people with chronically sun-damaged skin.

Sebo/rrhea (**seb″o-re′ə**) means overproduction of sebum (**se′bəm**), the oily secretion of the sebaceous glands of the skin. The combining form for sebum is **seb(o)**. Write the name of the oily secretion of the sebaceous glands: _____.

The lesion of seborrheic keratosis is a common benign lesion that may occur anywhere on the body of an older person, but is more commonly found on the face, neck, upper trunk, and arms (Figure 12-2). Lesions like this with well-defined edges and definite boundaries are described as circumscribed lesions because it would be possible to draw a circle around a lesion of this type.

Actinic* (**ak-tin′ik**) keratoses are premalignant lesions, and progression to skin cancer may occur if the lesions are not removed.

*Actinic (Greek: *aktis*, ray).

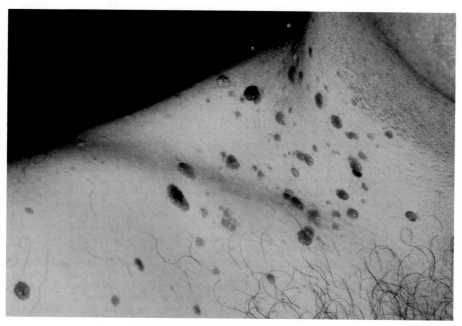

FIGURE 12-2
Seborrheic keratoses. This elderly man's back is covered by numerous seborrheic keratoses, some of which are deeply pigmented with melanin. The large lesions show the characteristic stuck-on appearance. Seborrheic keratoses are benign tumors that can be removed by curettage, cryosurgery, and application of caustic agents. (From Bork K, Bräuninger W: *Skin Diseases in Clinical Practice*, ed 2, Philadelphia, 1998, Saunders.)

dermis

12-4 The dermis, also called the corium (**ko′re-əm**), is the thicker layer of the skin. It is a noncellular connective tissue that is composed of collagen and elastic fibers that provide strength and flexibility.

Decreased blood flow that occurs with aging results in a decreased thickness of both the dermis and the subcutaneous fat layer. Decreased tone and elasticity lead to wrinkles, and thin, transparent skin is more susceptible to injury. A reconstructive technique in plastic surgery uses collagen injections to enhance the lips or "plump" sagging facial skin. The collagen injections are replacement of the lost collagen and elastic from which layer of the skin? _____

The dermis contains numerous blood vessels, nerves, and glands. Hair follicles are also embedded in this layer.

The upper region of the dermis has many fingerlike projections. The ridges marking the outermost layer of the skin are caused by the size and arrangement of these projections. The ridge patterns on the fingertips and thumbs (fingerprints) are different for each person.

below the skin

12-5 Locate the subcutaneous (**sub″ku-ta′ne-əs**) adipose (**ad′ĭ-pōs**) tissue in Figure 12-1. Sub/cutaneous means _____.

The subcutaneous adipose layer lies just under the dermis. It serves as a cushion against shock and insulates the body. The combining form *adip(o)* means fat.

fat

Adipose means pertaining to _____.

TABLE 12-1 Functions of the Skin

FUNCTION	EXPLANATION
Protective covering	Intact skin protects underlying tissue from microorganisms and damaging effects of ultraviolet light and mechanical, chemical, and thermal injury.
Water balance	The skin helps prevent fluid loss from the body. It also prevents too much water from entering the body during swimming or bathing.
Temperature regulation	The skin helps maintain the normal body temperature of 37° C (98.6° F) by dilation and constriciton of blood vessels in the skin and by perspiration.
Sensory reception	Receptors for heat, cold, pain, touch, and pressure relay information to the brain.
Vitamin D synthesis	Skin cells contain a precursor molecule that is converted to vitamin D when the precursor is exposed to ultraviolet rays in sunlight.
Psychosocial function	The appearance of the skin is an important part of body image.

skin	**12-6** Remembering that derm(a) and dermat(o) mean skin, a dermato/logist is a physician who specializes in treating the _____.
skin **below the skin**	Another combining form, ***cutane(o),*** also means skin. Cutane/ous pertains to the _____. Sub/cutaneous means _____.
	A sub/cutaneous wound is one in which there is no break in the skin or with only a small opening through the skin.
dermabrasion	**12-7** Derm/abrasion (dər″mə-bra′shən) is a treatment for removing superficial scars on the skin. This physical "sanding of the skin" to reduce facial scars is called _____. This procedure is also used to remove tattoos.
	12-8 Alternatives to dermabrasion are chemical peels or laser destruction of the outermost epidermal layers. Chemical peels use a strong chemical solution to reduce wrinkles, blemishes, and sun-damaged areas of the skin. The top layers peel away, and new, smoother skin layers replace the old ones.
wrinkles	**12-9** A combining form that means wrinkle or wrinkles is ***rhytid(o).*** Rhytidoplasty means face-lift. Literal translation of rhytido/plasty (rit′ĭ-do-plas″te) means surgical repair for _____.
rhytidoplasty	Skin of the face is tightened, wrinkles are removed, and the skin is made to appear firm and smooth. Write the name of this surgical procedure that means face-lift: _____.
	12-10 Increased expenditures on cosmetics, sunscreens, and treatments to improve our appearance attest to how we value the skin as the protective covering that is presented to our external environment. Read about other important functions of the skin that are listed in Table 12-1.
	12-11 The skin is derived from a tissue layer called ectoderm that forms during embryonic development. Soon after fertilization, the fertilized egg undergoes cell division, producing a ball of cells that eventually differentiates into three distinct layers: endoderm, mesoderm, and ectoderm. The suffix ***-derm*** means either skin or a germ layer. Here it is used to refer to a germ layer, a primary layer of cells of the developing embryo from which various organ systems develop.
ectoderm (ek″to-dərm)	Endo/derm (en′do-dərm) is the innermost germ layer. The outermost layer is the _____.
middle	Meso/derm (mez′o-dərm) is the middle germ layer. The prefix ***meso-*** means middle. Meso/derm is the _____ germ layer.
ectoderm	Skin is derived from which germ layer? _____

❏ SECTION A REVIEW   *S*tructures and Functions of the Integumentary System

This section review covers frames 12–1 through 12–11. Complete the table by writing a word part or its meaning in each blank.

Combining Form	Meaning	Prefix	Meaning
1. adip(o)	_____	6. _____	middle
2. cutane(o)	_____	**Suffix**	**Meaning**
3. kerat(o)	_____	7. -derm	
4. rhytid(o)	_____		_____
5. seb(o)	_____		

(Use Appendix V to check your answers.)

---

*A*ccessory Skin Structures

The accessory skin structures include hair, nails, sebaceous glands, and sweat glands. Sebaceous glands generally arise from the walls of hair follicles and produce sebum, the oily substance responsible for lubrication of the skin. Sweat glands are found in most parts of the skin, being most numerous in the palms and soles.

12-12 The nails, hair, sweat glands, and sebaceous glands are derived from the epidermis and are embedded in the dermis.

Hair protects the scalp from injury. Eyebrows and eyelashes protect the eyes, and hair in the nostrils and external ear canal protects these structures from dust and insects. The differing distribution of hair in the male and female is controlled by hormones. At puberty, hair develops in the armpit and pubic regions and, in the male, on the face and other parts of the body.

---

armpit

axillary

12-13 The combining form *axill(o)* means axilla (**ak-sil′ə**) or armpit. Hair develops in the axill/ary region at puberty. The axillary (**ak′sĭ-lar″e**) region is the area of the _____.

Write the word that means pertaining to the armpit: _____.

---

trichopathy
(**trĭ-kop′ə-the**)

trichoid (trik′oid)

trichophobia
(**trik″o-fo′be-ə**)

12-14 A combining form that means hair is *trich(o)*. Write words for the following:

any disease of the hair: _____.

resembling hair: _____.

abnormal dread (fear) of hair _____.

This is an abnormal dread of hair or of touching it.

---

condition

destruction
electrical

12-15 The literal translation of trich/osis (**tri-ko′sis**) is an abnormal _____ of the hair. Its extended meaning is abnormal growth or development of hair in an unusual place. Electro/lysis (**e-lek″trol′ə-sis**) is sometimes used to destroy the hair follicles when hair is growing in an undesirable place. By its word parts, you know that electro/lysis is _____ of a substance by passing _____ current through it. Most electrolysis is done for aesthetic reasons, for example, getting rid of facial hair.

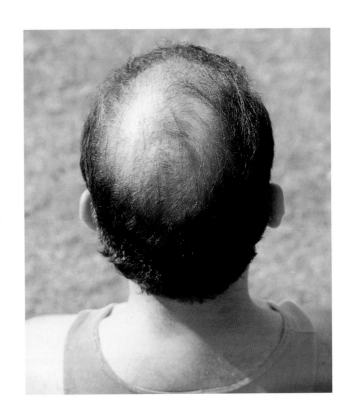

FIGURE 12-3

Alopecia prematura. This man is in his early thirties and is experiencing premature baldness. (From Ignatavicius DD, Workman ML, Mishler MA: *Medical-surgical nursing across the health care continuum*, ed 3, Philadelphia, 1999, WB Saunders.)

alopecia	**12-16** An equally important problem is loss of hair. Baldness is alopecia* **(al″o-pe′she-ə).** Write this new word for baldness: _____.
	Alopecia prematura is baldness that occurs early in life (Figure 12-3).
	The most popular aesthetic plastic surgery for males is hair transplantation. Grafts or plugs of skin containing hair follicles are transplanted from some part of the body to the head. An oral medication is effective in restoring hair in certain types of alopecia but must be taken the remainder of one's life to prevent hair loss.
epidermis	**12-17** Observe the structure of a hair in Figure 12-4. The hair root is embedded in the dermis and is the portion of the hair below the surface. The shaft protrudes above the surface of the skin, or above what layer? _____
	The combining form **pil(o)** also means hair.
sebaceous (sə-ba′shəs) **sweat**	The arrector pilli muscles contract under stresses of cold or fright, straighten the hair follicles, and raise the hairs, producing goose bumps or gooseflesh. Observing Figure 12-4, write the name of two glands that are directly connected with the hair follicle: _____ gland and the apocrine _____ gland. Most sebaceous glands are structurally associated with hair follicles, but those of the eyelids, the nipple, and genitalia are freestanding.

*Alopecia (Greek: *alopex*, fox mange).

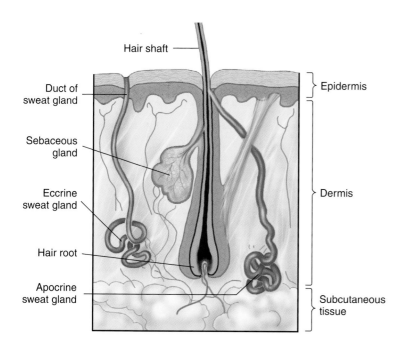

Hair shaft

Duct of
sweat gland

Sebaceous
gland

Eccrine
sweat gland

Hair root

Apocrine
sweat gland

Epidermis

Dermis

Subcutaneous
tissue

FIGURE 12-4
The structure of hair and associated glands. The hair shaft extends beyond the surface of the epidermis, and the root is the portion of the hair that is below the surface of the skin. Straight hair occurs when the hair shaft is round; wavy, if it is oval; curly or kinky, if it is flat. Hair can be cut without pain because it contains no nerves. The cuticle is the outermost covering and is the part that wears away at the tip of the shaft, resulting in split ends. Two types of glands (sebaceous glands and apocrine sweat glands) have ducts that open into hair follicles, and their secretions are transported to the skin surface. Stimulation of the eccrine sweat glands causes perspiration through ducts that open onto the surface of the skin. This is the single most important factor in the regulation of body temperature.

sebaceous

12-18 Sebaceous glands are found in all areas of the body that have hair. Sebum, the oily material secreted by the sebaceous gland, keeps hair and skin soft and pliable and also inhibits growth of bacteria on the skin. The increased activity of the sebaceous glands at puberty may block the hair follicle and cause blackheads. Bacteria can infect the blocked follicle and result in a pus-filled pimple. Acne occurs where sebaceous glands are most numerous. Acne results from bacterial infection of blocked _____ glands.

Treatment of acne includes the use of topical and oral antibiotics, topical and oral retinoids, and special skin washes. Topical* means pertaining to the surface of a part of the body. Retinoids are compounds that are structurally related to substances that exhibit Vitamin A activity, such as retinal and retinol. Retinoids increase the sloughing off of epithelial cells and cause extrusion of the blackheads.

skin

12-19 You learned that seb(o) means sebum, and seborrhea means excessive production of sebum. Seborrheic dermatitis is an inflammatory condition of the _____ that begins with the scalp but may involve other areas, particularly the eyebrows.

seborrheic
(seb"o-re'ik)

Seborrheic dermatitis is commonly called dandruff. The cause is not known, but the sebaceous glands become overactive and the hair and scalp are excessively oily. This skin condition is known as _____ dermatitis.

*Topical (Greek: *topos*, place).

sweat	**12-20** Another type of gland found in the skin is a sweat* gland or sudoriferous **(soo″do-rif′ər-əs)** gland. Another name for a sudoriferous gland is a _____ gland.
	Look again at Figure 12-4 and study the two types of sweat glands. Those that are associated with the hair follicles interact with bacteria on the skin to produce a characteristic body odor.
	Sweat glands that are not associated with hair follicles open to the surface of the skin through pores. When stimulated by temperature increases or emotional stress, these glands produce perspiration that evaporates on the skin surface and has a cooling effect.
sudoriferous	Perspiration, or sweat, is the substance produced by the sweat or _____ glands.
temperature	Sweat is a mixture of water, salt, and other waste products. Although elimination of waste is a function of the sweat glands, their principal function is to help regulate body temperature. As sweat evaporates on the skin surface, the skin is cooled and the body temperature is lowered. The principal function of sweat glands is to help regulate body _____.
water, sweat (or perspiration) sweat gland	**12-21** Use hidr(o) to write terms pertaining to sweat. Do not confuse hidr(o) and hydr(o). The combining form **hydr(o)** means _____, whereas hidr(o) means _____. Hidr/aden/itis **(hi″drad-ə-ni′tis)** is inflammation of a _____ _____. (Hidr[o] frequently loses the "o" when joined with aden[o].)
transmission excessive sweating (or perspiration) against	**12-22** Diaphoresis **(di″ə-fo-re′sis)** means excessive sweating. The suffix *-phoresis* means transmission. Translated literally, dia/phoresis means _____ through, so you will need to remember that diaphoresis means _____ _____. Antiperspirants act _____ perspiration or, in other words, inhibit perspiration.
heat coldness	**12-23** Remember that therm(o) means heat. In hypo/thermia **(hi″po-thər′me-ə),** the amount of _____ in the body is below normal. Exposure to very low temperatures can cause hypothermia. Acro/hypo/therm/y **(ak″ro-hi″po-thər′me)** is abnormal _____ of the hands and feet.
hyperthermia (hi″pər-ther′me-ə) heat	**12-24** Using hypothermia as a model, write a word that means a greatly increased body temperature: _____. In a healthy person, internal body temperature is maintained within a narrow range by thermo/regulatory centers in the hypothalamus. The thermoregulatory centers bring about a balance between generation and conservation of _____. Pyrexia **(pi-rek′se-ə),** or fever, is an elevated body temperature that is mediated by an increase in the heat regulatory set point. In contrast, hyperthermia overrides or bypasses normal heat regulation.
heat heat paralysis	**12-25** Heat stroke and sunstroke are examples of hyperthermia. In both there is a profound disturbance in the thermoregulatory system, or _____ -regulating system. They are caused by prolonged exposure to excessive heat or the sun and are life-threatening situations. Thermo/plegia **(thər″mo-ple′jə)** is another name for heatstroke or sunstroke. Translated literally, thermoplegia means _____ _____.

*Sweat (Latin: *sudor*).

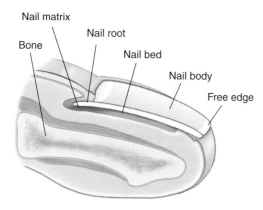

Nail matrix
Bone
Nail root
Nail bed
Nail body
Free edge

FIGURE 12-5

Structures of the nail. Each nail has a free edge, a nail body (the visible part), and a nail root, which is covered with skin. The nail bed is thickened to form the nail matrix, which is responsible for growth of the nail. The matrix is under the part of the nail body that appears as a whitish, crescent-shaped area called the lunula. Nails appear pinkish because of the rich supply of blood vessels in the underlying dermis.

12-26 Fingernails and toenails, modifications of the horny epidermal cells, are composed of keratin. (See the fingernail components in Figure 12-5.)

Nails are thin plates of dead epidermis that contain a very hard type of keratin. The cuticle is not shown in the illustration. The nail matrix is responsible for growth of the nail and appears as a whitish, crescent-shaped area called the lunula (**loo′nu-lə**). Nails appear pink because of the rich supply of blood vessels in the underlying dermis. The part that is responsible for growth of the nail is called the nail

matrix

_____.

The combining form _onych(o)_ means nail. An onycho/phag/ist (**on″ĭ-kof′ə-jist**) habitually bites the

nails

_____.

habit of nail-biting   What is onychophagia (**on″ĭ-ko-fa′jə**)? _____

---

tumor   **12-27** An onych/oma (**on″ĭ-ko′mə**) is a _____ of the nail or the nail bed.

onychectomy   Write a word that means removal (excision) of the nail: _____.
(**on″ĭ-kek′tə-me**)

(Declawing of an animal is also called onychectomy.)

---

fungal condition of   **12-28** Onycho/myc/osis (**on″ĭ-ko-mi-ko′sis**) is a _____.
the nails

Write words for the following:

onychomalacia   softening of the nails: _____.
(**on″ĭ-ko-mə-la′shə**)

onychopathy   any disease of the nails: _____.
(**on″ĭ-kop′ə-the**)

Another combining form, _ungu(o),_ also means nail. It is used to write an adjective, ungual (**ung′gwəl**),

nail   that means pertaining to the _____.

12-29 The nails, hair, sweat glands, and sebaceous glands are derived from the same germ layer as the skin. That particular germ layer is outermost in the developing embryo and is called the

ectoderm

_____.

Sense receptors of the skin, as well as other parts of the nervous system, are also derived from ectoderm.

❑ SECTION B REVIEW *Accessory* Skin Structures

This section review covers frames 12–12 through 12–29. Complete the table by writing the meaning of each word part:

Combining Form	Meaning	Combining Form	Meaning
1. axill(o)	_____	6. ungu(o)	_____
2. hidr(o)	_____	**Suffix**	**Meaning**
3. onych(o)	_____	7. -phoresis	_____
4. pil(o)	_____		
5. trich(o)	_____		

(Use Appendix V to check your answers.)

Skin Lesions

A skin lesion is any visible, local abnormality of the tissues of the skin, such as a sore, a rash, or a tumor. Most skin lesions are benign, but one type is among the most malignant of all kinds of cancer.

lesion	**12-30** Diagnosis of skin disorders includes identifying lesions or changes in the skin. A skin lesion is defined as any visible, local abnormality of the tissues of the skin. This not only includes spots that appear on the skin but also swellings and changes of shape, such as an underlying tumor. Any visible, local abnormality of the tissues of the skin is called a _____.
	The superficial appearance of most lesions gives a great deal of information; however, palpation* (**pal-pa′-shən**)—using the fingers to feel the texture, size, and consistency—often gives additional information. Observe the two types of lesions shown in Figure 12-6.
cyst **nodule** (**nod′ūl**)	Both a cyst and a nodule cause a raised area of the overlying skin, but the _____ is filled with fluid or a semi-solid material, whereas the _____ is solid.
	12-31 Examine the appearance of other types of lesions presented in Figure 12-7.
	The lesions are primary lesions because they are initial reactions to an underlying problem. A freckle is a nonraised small dark spot on the skin, so it is called a _____.
macule (**mak′ūl**)	
papule (**pap′ūl**)	Both papules and plaques are elevated and circumscribed, but which type is less than 1 cm in diameter? _____ A small mole is a papule. Dandruff represents a type of plaque.
	Vesicles (**ves′ĭ-kəlz**), bullae (**bul′e**), and pustules (**pus′tūlz**) are blisterlike and contain fluid. The lesions of acne are filled with pus, so they are called _____.
pustules	
bullae	Vesicles and bullae are differentiated by size. Which one is larger? _____
urticaria	**12-32** Urticaria (**ur″tĭ-kar′e-ə**) is an allergic skin eruption characterized by transient elevated, irregularly-shaped lesions that are called wheals (**hwēlz, wēlz**). Treatment includes antihistamines and removal of the stimulus or allergen. This allergic skin reaction, also called hives, is _____ (Figure 12-8).

*Palpation (Latin: *palpare,* to touch gently).

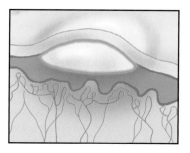

A cyst is a sac filled with
fluid or semi-solid material.

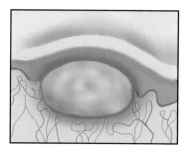

A nodule is a marble-like,
solid lesion more than 1cm
wide and deep.

FIGURE 12-6
Schematic drawing of two types of lesions in cross section. Palpation will usually distinguish
between a fluid-filled cyst and a solid nodule.

12-33 Secondary lesions are changes in the appearance of the primary lesion and can occur with normal progression of the disease. See Figure 12-9 and use the accompanying information to write words in the blanks in this frame.

fissure (fish′ər)

Athlete's foot produces linear cracks in the epidermis and is an example of a _____.

ulcers

Deep, irregular erosions that extend into the dermis are called _____.

Atrophy (at′rə-fe) of the skin is characterized by thinning with loss of skin markings. Stretch marks are an example of atrophy.

Dried serum, sebum, blood, or pus on the skin surface produces a crust. Crusts frequently result from broken vesicles, bullae, or pustules.

Scales are dried fragments of sloughed epidermis. They appear dry and irregular in size and shape and are usually whitish. They are frequently seen in psoriasis, a common chronic skin disease characterized by circumscribed red patches covered by thick, dry silvery scales (Figure 12-10, *A*).

12-34 A verruca (və-roo′kə) is a benign warty skin lesion with a rough surface, caused by a common contagious virus (Figure 12-10, *B*). Treatment includes salicylic acid and electrodessication. In electro/dessication, tissue is destroyed by _____. The term for a warty skin lesion is

electricity
verruca

_____.

Petechiae* (pə-te′ke-e) are tiny purple or red spots appearing on the skin as a result of tiny hemorrhages within the dermal or submucosal layers (Figure 12-10, *C*). They are flush with the skin and range in size from pinpoint to pinhead size. Write this term for the spots that result from tiny hemorrhages in the skin:

petechiae

_____.

An ecchymosis (ek″ĭ-mo′sis) is a hemorrhagic spot, larger than a petechia. It forms a nonelevated blue or purplish patch (Figure 12-10, *D*). Write the term for this large hemorrhagic spot: _____.

ecchymosis

---

*Petechiae (Italian: *petecchie,* flea bite).

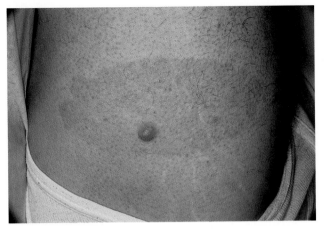

Macules
Nonraised, discolored spots less than 1 cm in diameter

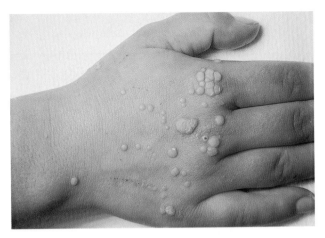

Papules
Elevated lesion less than 1 cm in diameter

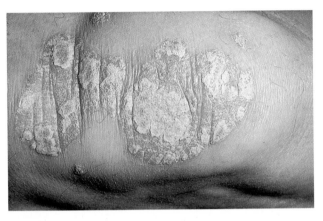

Plaques
Elevated and circumscribed patches more than 1 cm in diameter

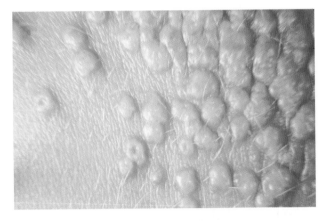

Vesicles
Blisters less than 1 cm and filled with clean fluid

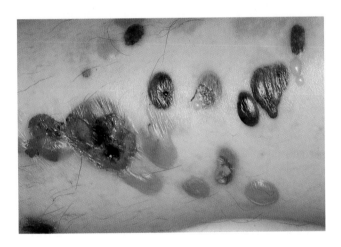

Bullae
Blisters greater than 1 cm and filled with clean fluid

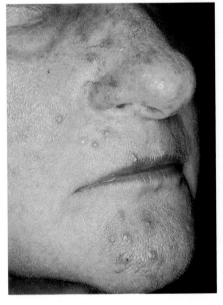

Pustules
Vesicles filled with cloudy fluid or pus

FIGURE 12-7
Primary lesions of the skin. These are initial reactions to an underlying problem that alters one of the structural components of the skin. (From Noble J, editor: *Textbook of primary care medicine*, St Louis, 1996, Mosby.)

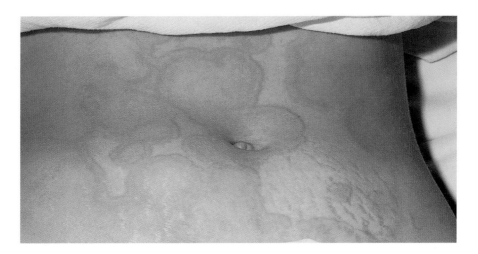

FIGURE 12-8
Wheals. This elevated, irregularly shaped lesion is seen in urticaria (hives), an allergic skin eruption. Notice the irregular shape, which is caused by edema. (From Noble J, editor: *Textbook of primary care medicine*, St Louis, 1996, Mosby.)

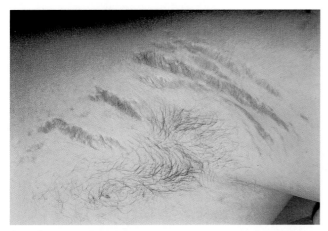

Atrophy
Wasting of the epidermis. Skin appears thin and transparent

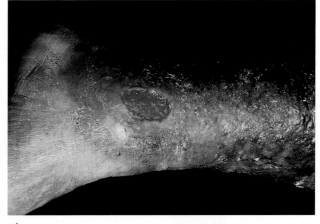

Ulcer
Irregularly shaped erosions that extend into the dermis

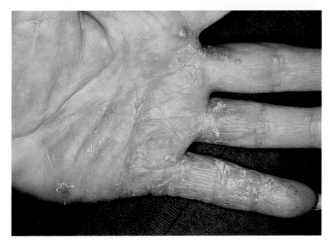

Fissures
Deep linear splits through the epidermidis into the dermis

FIGURE 12-9
Secondary lesions of the skin. The linear lines of atrophy, ulcerations, and fissures result from changes in the initial skin lesion. (From Noble J, editor: *Textbook of primary care medicine*, St Louis, 1996, Mosby.)

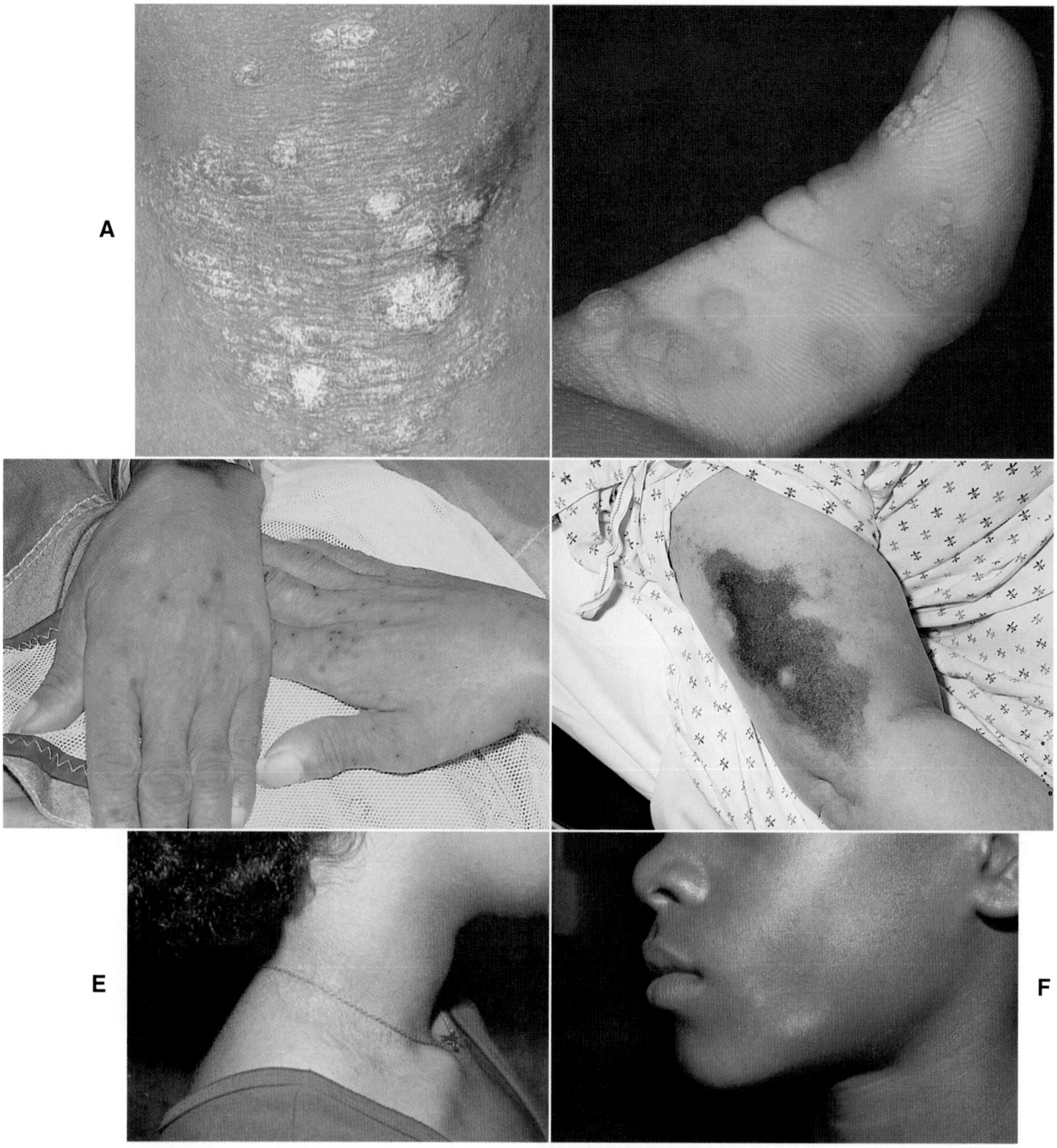

FIGURE 12-10

Common benign disorders of the skin. **A,** Psoriasis is characterized by circumscribed red patches covered by thick, dry silvery scales. **B,** A verruca, commonly called a wart, has a rough surface. **C,** Petechiae appear on the skin as a result of tiny hemorrhages beneath the surface. **D,** An ecchymosis is a hemorrhagic spot. **E,** Nickel dermatitis is a type of contact dermatitis. **F,** Hypopigmented lesions occur mainly in children. (**A** and **B,** From Habif TP: *Clinical dermatology: a color atlas guide to diagnosis and therapy,* ed 3, St Louis, 1990, Mosby. **C,** From Ignatavicius DD, Workman ML, Mischler MA: *Medical-surgical nursing across the health care continuum,* ed 3, Philadelphia, 1999, WB Saunders. **D,** From Noble J, editor: *Textbook of primary care medicine,* St Louis, 1996, Mosby. **E,** From Weston WI, Lane AT: *Color textbook of pediatric dermatology,* ed 2, St Louis, 1996, Mosby. **F,** From Behrman: *Nelson textbook of pediatrics,* ed 15, Philadelphia, 1996, WB Saunders.)

inflammation	**12-35** Dermatitis, also called eczema (ek′zə-mə), is _____ of the skin. There are several kinds of dermatitis, including seborrheic dermatitis and contact dermatitis. Contact dermatitis is a skin rash resulting from exposure to an irritant or antigen. Figure 12-10, *E,* shows the appearance of a person's skin who is allergic to a necklace that contains nickel.

A type of skin disorder that results in hypopigmented lesions usually occurs in children (Figure 12-10, *F*). The cause of these lesions is unknown, dryness seems to be a contributing factor, and they eventually disappear. |
dry condition	A term for dry skin is xerosis. The combining form *xer(o)* means dry. Literal translation of xer/osis is a _____ _____, but the term is used to refer to dry skin. The mucous membranes are often dry also. This is more common in older persons, particularly in the winter when there is less moisture in the air.
pressure	**12-36** A pressure ulcer is a special type of injury to the skin that occurs almost exclusively in people with limited mobility. Also called bedsores or decubitus ulcers, these sores occur as a result of mechanical trauma and lack of adequate blood circulation to the affected area. Once formed, they are slow to heal. Ulcerations that occur almost exclusively in persons with limited mobility are called _____ ulcers.
nevus	**12-37** A new growth of tissue characterized by a disordered growth of cells is a tumor, also called a neoplasm. Several benign tumors have already been discussed, for example, seborrheic keratoses, warts, and moles. Another term for a mole is a nevus (ne′vəs). The plural is nevi (ne′vi). Write this term that means a mole: _____.
black tumor	Because about half of malignant melanomas arise from moles, nevi with irregular edges or variegated colors are usually removed and examined to determine whether they are malignant melanomas. Literal interpretation of melan/oma is a _____ _____.
cancer (or carcinomas)	**12-38** A malignant melanoma, often shortened to melanoma, is a pigmented neoplasm that originates in the skin and is composed of melanocytes. It is highly metastatic, one of the most malignant of all skin cancers, and causes a high mortality rate in affected individuals. Figure 12-11 shows melanoma with two other common types of skin cancer. Squamous cell carcinoma, basal cell carcinoma, and malignant melanoma are all types of skin _____.

Solar keratoses, also called actinic keratoses, are premalignant lesions that are common in chronically sun-damaged skin. They are usually treated, because this type of keratosis can progress to squamous cell carcinoma. |
| **Kaposi's** | Kaposi's sarcoma is the most common malignancy associated with acquired immunodeficiency syndrome (AIDS). The lesions are small, purplish-brown papules that spread throughout the skin, the lymph nodes, and the internal organs. Other disorders associated with this lesion include diabetes and malignant lymphoma. The name of the lesion is _____ sarcoma (Figure 9-25). |
| **folliculitis** | **12-39** Chronic overexposure to sunlight is the major cause of skin cancer. Sunburn is a type of dermatitis that results from overexposure to the sun. Dermatitis is a very general term and applies to any type of inflammation of the skin, including skin infections.

Infections in intact skin often involve the hair follicles, where bacteria easily accumulate and grow well. Follicul/itis (fo-lik″u-li′tis) is a superficial bacterial infection involving the hair follicles, and uses *follicul(o),* which means follicle. Write the term that means inflammation of the hair follicles: _____.

Without treatment, folliculitis can progress to cellul/itis, a localized bacterial invasion of subcutaneous tissue. Cellulitis can also occur independently of folliculitis and is characterized by pain, heat, swelling, and redness. |

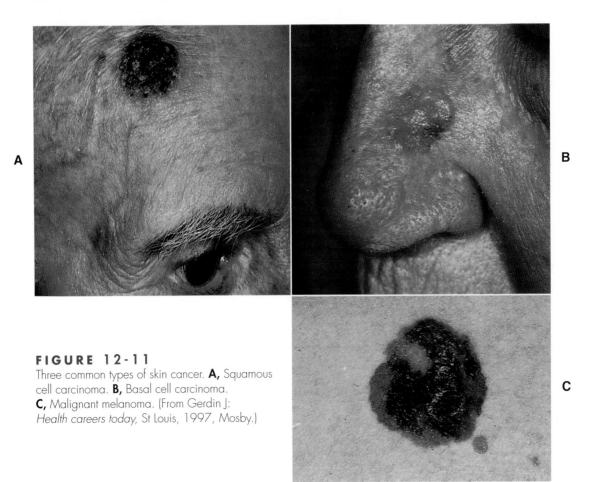

FIGURE 12-11
Three common types of skin cancer. **A,** Squamous
cell carcinoma. **B,** Basal cell carcinoma.
C, Malignant melanoma. (From Gerdin J:
Health careers today, St Louis, 1997, Mosby.)

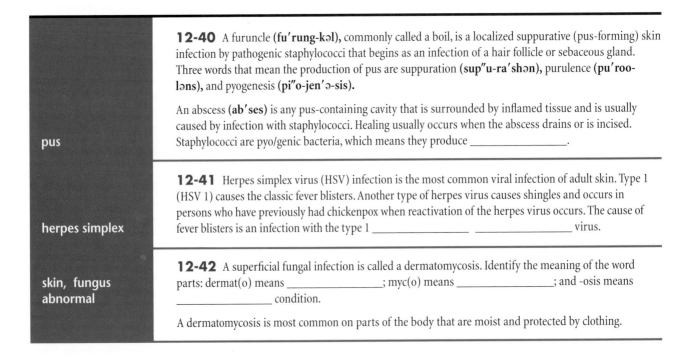

	12-40 A furuncle (**fu′rung-kəl**), commonly called a boil, is a localized suppurative (pus-forming) skin infection by pathogenic staphylococci that begins as an infection of a hair follicle or sebaceous gland. Three words that mean the production of pus are suppuration (**sup″u-ra′shən**), purulence (**pu′roo-ləns**), and pyogenesis (**pi″o-jen′ə-sis**).
pus	An abscess (**ab′ses**) is any pus-containing cavity that is surrounded by inflamed tissue and is usually caused by infection with staphylococci. Healing usually occurs when the abscess drains or is incised. Staphylococci are pyo/genic bacteria, which means they produce _____.
herpes simplex	**12-41** Herpes simplex virus (HSV) infection is the most common viral infection of adult skin. Type 1 (HSV 1) causes the classic fever blisters. Another type of herpes virus causes shingles and occurs in persons who have previously had chickenpox when reactivation of the herpes virus occurs. The cause of fever blisters is an infection with the type 1 _____ _____ virus.
skin, fungus abnormal	**12-42** A superficial fungal infection is called a dermatomycosis. Identify the meaning of the word parts: dermat(o) means _____; myc(o) means _____; and -osis means _____ condition. A dermatomycosis is most common on parts of the body that are moist and protected by clothing.

TABLE 12-2 Skin Eruptions Caused by Infectious Organisms*

BACTERIAL	FUNGAL	VIRAL
Erysipelas	Candidiasis	Herpes simplex type 1 fever blisters
Furuncles (boils) and carbuncles	Onychomycosis	Herpes zoster (shingles)
Impetigo	Tinea capitis (ringworm of scalp)	Rubella (German measles)
Leprosy	Tinea corporis (generalized)	Rubeola (measles)
Lyme disease	Tinea pedis (athlete's foot)	Varicella (chickenpox)
Meningococcal meningitis		Verrucae (warts)
Paronychia (infection of marginal structures around nail)		
Scarlet fever		
Syphilis		

*Sexually transmitted diseases are not included unless a generalized skin reaction is common. Complete definitions of the terms can be found in the Glossary/Index.

12-43 The skin serves as a protective barrier between the body's tissue and microorganisms most of the time. Trauma such as cuts, punctures, or burns expose the underlying tissue to infection. Climate, hygiene, and general health also play a part. Several skin eruptions caused by infectious microorganisms are presented in Table 12-2.

❑ SECTION C REVIEW *S*kin Lesions

This section review covers frames 12–30 through 12–43. Complete the table by writing a combining form in each blank.

Combining Form	Meaning
1. _____	follicle
2. _____	dry

(Use Appendix V to check your answers.)

*I*njuries to the Skin

The skin is subject to many injuries, since it serves as the external covering and the part of the body that is exposed to the external environment.

dryness

12-44 Xerosis is excessive _____ of the skin and can make it vulnerable to scaling, thinning, and injury. Xerosis is a minor irritation of the skin. Pruritus (**proo-ri′təs**) is an uncomfortable itching sensation that leads to the urge to scratch. If the skin is broken during scratching, the wound may become infected.

A wound is a physical injury involving a break in the skin, usually caused by an act or accident rather than a disease. The trauma to the skin and underlying tissues requires healing to repair the defect, whether the wound was created by a surgical incision or an accidental gunshot wound.

A surgical incision generally heals faster than other wounds because it is performed aseptically and minimal damage is done to the tissue by the sharp instrument. The combining forms *seps(o)* and *sept(o)* mean infection. A/septic means free of pathogenic organisms or _____ material. A laceration (**las″ər-a′shən**) is a torn, jagged wound. A puncture is a wound made by piercing. Skin is scraped or rubbed away by friction in an abrasion (**ə-bra′shən**). One type of injury, a contusion (**kən-too′zhən**), is caused by a blow to the body that does not disrupt the integrity of the skin. A contusion is called a bruise and is characterized by swelling, discoloration, and pain.

infected

laceration **puncture**	**12-45** A torn, jagged wound is called a _____, whereas a wound that is made by piercing is called a _____.
abrasion	When skin is scraped away by friction, it is called an _____.

12-46 Superficial wounds often heal without suturing. Deep wounds, those with gaping edges, or wounds located over joints where movement opens the cut edges are often sutured. Suturing stops the bleeding, holds the tissue together, and enhances the healing process. Dermabond is an adhesive spray that is used for closing certain wounds.

keloid

A mark that is left by healing of a lesion where excess collagen was produced to replace the injured tissue is called a scar. Excessive overgrowth of unsightly scar tissue, called a keloid (**ke′loid),** occurs in some individuals, especially blacks. Write the word that means overgrowth of scar tissue: _____.

12-47 Burns are tissue injuries resulting from excessive exposure to heat, electricity, chemicals, radiation, or gases in which the extent of the injury is determined by the amount of exposure and the nature of the agent that causes the burn. The magnitude of the injury is based on the depth and extent of the total body surface burn.

In the past, burns were classified into first-, second-, third-, and fourth-degree injuries. Today, the American Burn Association (ABA) advocates categorizing the burn injury according to the depth of tissue destruction as superficial-, partial-, full-, and deep full-thickness wounds (Figure 12-12).

full

In comparing a superficial partial-thickness burn and a full-thickness burn, the _____ -thickness burn destroys deeper layers of tissue.

epidermis

The superficial partial-thickness burn does not extend beyond which layer of skin? _____

dermis

In a deep partial-thickness burn, damage does not extend beyond which layer of skin? _____

subcutaneous

A full-thickness burn does not extend beyond the _____ fat layer.

deep
deep partial-
thickness

Muscle and bone are exposed in a _____ full-thickness burn.

Which type of burn is characterized by blisters? _____ _____

12-48 Burned tissue usually represents various levels of damage. In addition to the burn depth, burn severity takes into consideration factors such as the size and location of the burn, mechanism of injury, duration and intensity of the burn, and the age and health of the individual. The very young and older persons are most at risk.

Serious burn injuries can result in systemic disturbances, including fluid and protein losses, and abnormalities in many body systems. In addition, infection is a serious threat when the skin is destroyed and can no longer protect the underlying tissues from microorganisms.

without

12-49 Topical antimicrobial agents and dressings are applied to burned tissue to prevent infection, and aseptic procedures are followed. A/septic means _____ infection.

infection

You learned that both sept(o) and seps(o) mean infection. Sometimes sept(o) means septum. Asepsis means sterile, or the absence of _____.

Seps/is is a pathological state resulting from the presence of microorganisms or their toxins in the blood or other tissues. Sept/emia, also called septic/emia, is the presence of pathogenic microorganisms or their

blood

toxins in the _____.

Septicemia (**sep″tĭ-se′me-ə**) represents an overwhelming infection and can cause death. Anti/biotics are

against

given in septicemia to act _____ microorganisms.

Bacterio/static (**bak-tēr″e-o-stat′ik**) means inhibiting the growth of bacteria. Bacteri/cidal (**bak-tēr″ i-si′dəl**) means killing bacteria. Depending on the particular type, some agents prevent multiplication or growth of bacteria (bacteriostatic), whereas other agents actually kill bacteria (bactericidal). You learned earlier that bacteri(o) means bacteria; *bacter(i)* also means bacteria.

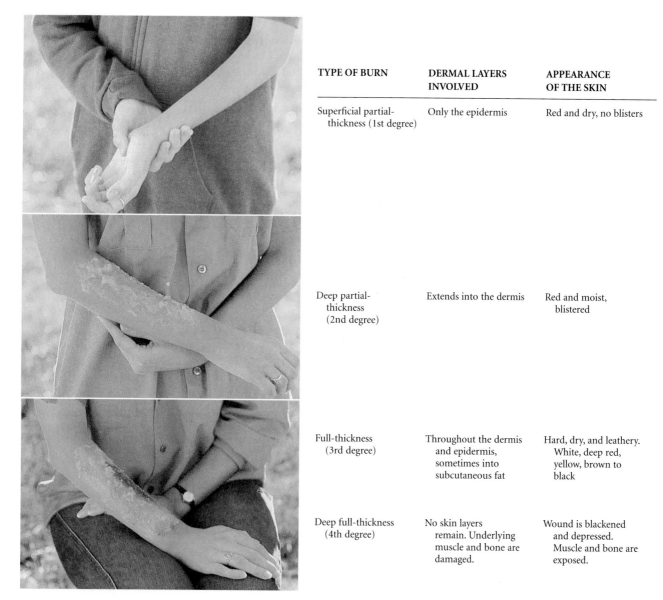

TYPE OF BURN	DERMAL LAYERS INVOLVED	APPEARANCE OF THE SKIN
Superficial partial-thickness (1st degree)	Only the epidermis	Red and dry, no blisters
Deep partial-thickness (2nd degree)	Extends into the dermis	Red and moist, blistered
Full-thickness (3rd degree)	Throughout the dermis and epidermis, sometimes into subcutaneous fat	Hard, dry, and leathery. White, deep red, yellow, brown to black
Deep full-thickness (4th degree)	No skin layers remain. Underlying muscle and bone are damaged.	Wound is blackened and depressed. Muscle and bone are exposed.

FIGURE 12-12
The tissues involved in burns of various depths. (From Judd RL, Ponsell PP: *Mosby's first responder,*
ed 2, St Louis, 1988, Mosby.)

12-50 Severe burns of the arms or legs can result in amputation. All depths of burns except the superficial partial-thickness burn may generally involve skin grafting. In a skin graft, skin is implanted to cover areas where skin has been lost. The graft is usually taken from the patient's own body to prevent rejection.

tissue

Histo/compatibility (**his″to-kəm-pat″ĭ-bil′ĭ-te**) is necessary for a successful transplant of any organ. Histo/compatibility means that the transplanted _____ is capable of surviving without ill effects. If the tissue is not compatible, this is called in/compatibility. The prefix ***in-*** means in, into, or not.

12-51 Frostbite is damage to skin, tissues and blood vessels as a result of prolonged exposure to cold. The extent of injury depends largely on the intensity and the duration of the exposure. Since injury is greater in hypoxic tissue, the individual's health is also involved. Hyp/oxia means a condition of inade-

oxygen

quate _____.

frostbite

Damage to tissue as a result of exposure to cold is called _____.

dead	**12-52** Necrosis (nə-kro′sis) is localized tissue death that occurs in response to disease or injury. When tissue is badly damaged, it becomes necro/tic (nə-krot′ik). The combining form ***necr(o)*** means dead or death. Necro/tic describes a characteristic of tissue that has been broken down. Necrotic tissue is _____ tissue.
debridement	Debridement (da-brēd′maw) is the removal of foreign material and dead or damaged tissue, especially in a wound. To debride is to remove by dissection. Write this word that means the removal of foreign material or damaged tissue by excision: _____.
necrosis	**12-53** Write a word that means dead condition: _____. This word means death of areas of tissue or bone surrounded by healthy parts.
dead	Necr/opsy (nek′rop-se) is examination of the _____ body. This is done to determine cause of death or pathological conditions. Another name for necropsy is autopsy.

❏ **SECTION D REVIEW**   *Injuries to the Skin*

This section review covers frames 12–44 through 12–53. Write the meaning for each combining form:

Combining Form	Meaning	Prefix	Meaning
1. bacter(i)	_____	5. _____	in, into, or not
2. necr(o)	_____		
3. seps(o)	_____		
4. sept(o)	_____		

(Use Appendix V to check your answers.)

Additional Pathology, Diagnosis, and Treatment of the Integumentary System

SECTION F

Skin changes may be related to specific skin diseases but also may reflect an underlying systemic disorder.

pale bluish red	**12-54** The skin is a reflection of the general health of a person. It is excessively red in hypertension and other conditions involving vasodilation. How might the skin appear in anemia? _____ Severe heart or lung disease may cause cyanosis, in which the skin would appear _____. Unusually yellow skin suggests the presence of greater than the normal amount of bile pigment in the blood (jaundice). What color are the palms in palmar erythema? _____ A partial or total absence of pigment in the skin, hair, and eyes is called albinism (al′bĭ-niz-əm). The combining forms ***alb(o)*** and ***albin(o)*** mean white.
white albino	**12-55** Albinism is present at birth. There is an absence of normal pigmentation owing to a defect in melanin precursors. In albinism, lack of pigmentation is implied by albin(o), which means _____. Sometimes the skin and eyes appear pinkish. An albin/o (al-bi′no) is a person affected with albinism. A person who lacks pigmentation in the skin, hair, and eyes is called an _____.

fish fish	**12-56** Ichthyosis (**ik″the-o′sis**) is a condition in which the skin is dry and scaly, resembling fish skin. The combining form ***ichthy(o)*** means fish. Ichthy/oid (**ik′the-oid**) means resembling a _____. Some forms of ichthyosis, but not all, are hereditary. Ichthy/osis is any of several generalized skin disorders marked by dryness and scaliness, resembling _____ skin.
dry skin xeroderma dry	**12-57** A mild, nonhereditary form of ichthyosis is called xeroderma (**zēr″o-der′mə**). Xero/derma literally means _____ _____. Mild ichthyosis, characterized by roughness and dryness of the skin, is called _____. Xer/ophthalm/ia (**zēr″of-thal′me-ə**) is a _____ condition of the eyeball resulting from vitamin A deficiency.
xerosis (zēr-o′sis) xeroradiography (zēr″o-ra″de-og′ rə-fe)	**12-58** Using -osis, write a word that means any dry condition: _____. This word may refer to abnormal dryness, as of the eye, skin, or mouth, but it is sometimes used to mean dry skin. There is a special type of radiography that uses a dry, photoelectric process rather than the usual x-ray film. This process permits visualization of the soft tissue and, for this reason, is most often used to detect lesions or calcifications in the breast. Using xer(o), write the name of this special type of radiography: _____.
hardened skin	**12-59** Scleroderma (**sklēr″o-der′mə**) is chronic hardening and thickening of the skin. The literal translation of sclero/derma is _____ _____.
lupus erythematosus	**12-60** Discoid lupus erythematosus (DLE) is primarily a disease of the skin. This chronic disorder is characterized by lesions that are covered with scales. The disorder was so named because of the reddish facial rash that appears in some patients, giving them a wolflike appearance. The combining form ***erythemat(o)*** means erythema, or redness. Erythema is redness (example, blushing) or inflammation of the skin (example, sunburn) or mucous membranes. This disorder is believed to be a problem of autoimmunity and is called discoid _____ _____.
pediculosis	**12-61** The skin can serve as a host to several parasitic diseases. Pediculosis (**pə-dik″u-lo′sis**) refers to infestation by human lice and is named for a genus of sucking lice, *Pediculus*. There are head lice, body lice, and pubic lice. Write the name of this disease that means infestation with lice: _____.
scabies	**12-62** Scabies is a contagious dermatitis caused by the itch mite and is transmitted by close contact. Write the name of this parasitic disease: _____.
treatment heliotherapy	**12-63** Ultraviolet light therapy is a common physical treatment for skin conditions. Ultraviolet radiation, the same energy as that of the sun, is more readily accessible and easier to control. Helio/therapy (**he″le-o-ther′ə-pe**) is _____ of disease by exposing the body to sun. The combining form ***heli(o)*** means the sun. Therapeutic use of the sun's rays is called _____.
water	**12-64** Certain wounds require the use of heat hydrotherapy. By its name, you know that heat hydro/therapy makes use of warm _____. The remaining types of physical therapy have to do with treatments of other parts of the body (for muscle pain, reduction of tissue swelling, increasing circulation to a part). The skin is involved in many cases, however, since the treatment is delivered through the skin.

sound	**12-65** Ultrasound is used therapeutically as a penetrating deep-heating agent for soft tissue. Ultrasound uses high-frequency _____ waves.
heat	Another method of generating heat in soft tissue is diathermy. Both diathermy and ultrasound are used to increase circulation to an inflamed area. Dia/therm/y (**di′ə-thər″me**) means passing high-frequency current through tissue to generate _____ in a particular part of the body.
	The prefix **dia-** means through. Dia/meter is a line passing through the center of a body or figure.
diathermy	Use of a high-frequency current to generate heat within some part of the body is called _____.
cryotherapy (kri″o-ther′ə-pe)	**12-66** Cryo/surgery (**kri″o-sər′jər-e**) is a technique of exposing tissues to extreme cold to produce well-defined areas of cell destruction.
	Remembering that *cry(o)* means cold, write a word that means treatment using cold temperatures: _____.
across, skin	**12-67** Various types of stimulation to the skin and subcutaneous tissue offer pain relief. Trans/cutaneous electrical nerve stimulation is one of these methods. Trans/cutaneous means that the electrical current is delivered _____ (or through) the _____. Electrodes are placed over the painful sites, and small amounts of electrical current are delivered to painful areas. This
transcutaneous	method is abbreviated TENS, which means _____ electrical nerve stimulation.
transdermal	**12-68** Transdermal drug delivery is a method of applying a drug to unbroken skin. The drug is absorbed through the skin and then enters the circulatory system. It is used particularly for estrogen, nicotine, and scopalomine (to prevent motion sickness). Not all medications can be administered in this way. Administration of a drug through unbroken skin is called _____ drug delivery.
placed feeling	**12-69** There are many methods for administering medications. Skin disorders, such as infections, irritations, or an allergic reaction, frequently require the use of a topical medication.
	Remember that top(o) means place; topical (**top′e-kəl**) medications are _____ directly on the skin. Topical an/esthetics are applied to produce a lack of _____.
air	**12-70** Topical medications may be found in many forms: aerosols, ointments, liquids, or creams. In aero/sols (**ār′o-solz**), the medicinal particles are suspended in _____ or gas.
topical	An ointment is a medicated, fatty, soft substance for external application to the body. In other words, an ointment is for what type of use? _____
mouth	**12-71** Oral medications are taken by _____. Aspirin is a well-known example of an oral medication.
beneath places it under the tongue	Sub/lingual (**səb-ling′gwəl**) medications are placed _____ the tongue and allowed to dissolve. Nitroglycerin, a drug used for certain types of heart disease, is often given sublingually. How does the patient take this medication? _____
beneath	**12-72** Parenteral (**pə-ren′tər-əl**) administration is injection through any route other than the alimentary canal. Some important forms of parenteral administration are intramuscular, subcutaneous, intradermal, and intravenous injections (Figure 12-13).
	A sub/cutaneous injection places a small amount of medication _____ the skin, into the subcutaneous tissue.

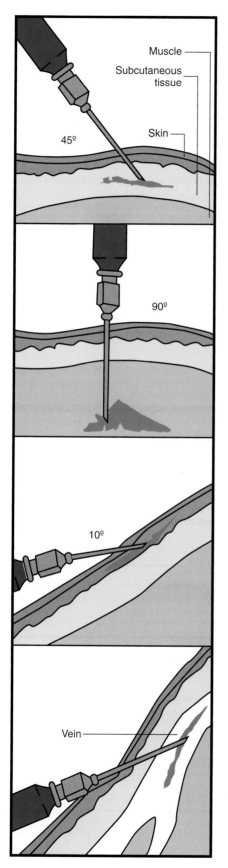

Subcutaneous

A subcutaneous injection places a small amount (0.5 to 2 ml) of medication below the skin layer into the subcutaneous tissue. The needle is inserted at a 45° angle.

Intramuscular

An intramuscular injection deposits medication into a muscular layer. As much as 3 to 5 ml may be administered in one injection, and depending on the size of the patient, a needle from 1 to 3 inches in length is used.

Intradermal

An intradermal injection places very small amounts (0.05 to 0.01 ml) of a drug into the outer layers of the skin with a very fine gauge, short needle. This type of injection is often used to test allergic reactions.

Intravenous

An intravenous injection is used to administer medications directly into the blood stream for immediate effect or to withdraw blood for testing purposes. A few milliliters of medication or much larger amounts (given over a long period of time) may be administered after venipuncture of the selected vein has been performed.

FIGURE 12-13
Needle insertion for types of injections. **A,** Subcutaneous; **B,** intramuscular; **C,** intradermal; **D,** intravenous. (From Kinn ME, Wood MA, Derge EF: *The medical assistant,* ed 7, Philadelphia, 1992, WB Saunders.)

into the muscle	**12-73** An intra/muscular (**in″trǝ-mus′ku-lǝr**) injection deposits medication _____.
into	An intra/dermal (**in″trǝ-dǝr′mǝl**) injection places very small amounts of medication _____ the outer layers of the skin.
into a vein	An intra/venous (**in″trǝ-ve′nǝs**) injection places medications _____.
Subcutaneous, intramuscular, and intravenous are abbreviated subq, IM, and IV, respectively.
	12-74 The skin continually serves as the protector of the inner organs from the external environment. An important characteristic of skin is its ability to communicate information to the trained observer.

❑ SECTION E REVIEW   𝒜dditional Pathology, Diagnosis, and Treatment of the Integumentary System

This section review covers frames 12–54 through 12–74. Write the meaning of each word part listed:

Combining Form	Meaning	Prefix	Meaning
1. albin(o)	_____	6. dia-	_____
2. alb(o)	_____		
3. erythemat(o)	_____		
4. heli(o)	_____		
5. ichthy(o)	_____		

(Use Appendix V to check your answers.)

𝒯erminology Challenge

This section challenges you to read, write, and understand new terms or concepts about the integumentary system.

hypodermic (hi″po-dǝr′mik)	**12-75** You learned several means of parenteral administration of drugs. Write an adjective that literally means "under the skin" to describe the type of needle used to give these types of injections: _____.
photodermatitis (fo″to-der″mǝ-ti′tis)

Literal translation is the recording instrument, not the film. | **12-76** Remembering that phot(o) means light, write a word that has a literal translation of inflammation of the skin due to light: _____.
Photodermatitis is an abnormal skin reaction to light.
Look at the term *photograph*, which we recognize as an image produed by light on film. Knowing the meaning of its parts, what is unusual about the term *photo/graph*? _____
Usage has changed the meaning of certain terms, such as photograph and radiograph. Radiogram and radiograph are both used to mean the film produced by radiography. |
| mycodermatitis (mi″ko-der″mǝ-ti′tis) | **12-77** Using photodermatitis as a model, write a word that means inflammation of the skin that is caused by a fungus: _____. |
| away | **12-78** You learned that ex- means out, without, or away from. Ex/foliation (**eks-fo″le-a′shǝn**) is a falling _____ of tissue in scales or layers. |

fatty	**12-79** The combining form *lip(o)* means fats. A lip/oma (**lip-o′məh**) is a common, benign _____ tumor that usually can be removed easily by excision.

It may seem natural to think of excision of a lipoma as lipectomy (**lĭ-pek′tə-me);** however, this is incorrect. Lipectomy originally meant excision of a mass of subcutaneous fat tissue, as from the abdominal wall. More recently the term has been extended to mean removal of fat from the neck, legs, arms, belly, and elsewhere by placing a narrow tube under the skin and applying a vacuum. The suction pulls the fat loose. This type of lipectomy is called liposuction, suction lipectomy, or suction-assisted lipectomy.

There is no review for this section.

Study the following list of selected abbreviations. Then read through the Chapter Pharmacology section and be sure you understand the effects and uses of the drug classes that are presented. When you are finished, work the Chapter Review. After completing the exercises, check your answers with the solutions in Appendix V.

You will find these items presented after the Chapter Review:

- Listing of Medical Terms
- Enhancing Spanish Communication

Selected Abbreviations

bx	biopsy	IM	intramuscular
DLE	discoid lupus erythematosus	IV	intravenous
EAHF	eczema, asthma, and hay fever	SG	skin graft
ECHO	(enteric cytopathogenic human orphan) virus	subq	subcutaneous
FB	foreign body	TENS	transcutaneous electrical nerve stimulation
HSV	herpes simplex virus	ung	ointment
HSV 1	herpes simplex virus type 1	UV	ultraviolet
I & D	incision and drainage	XP or XPD	xeroderma pigmentosum

Chapter Pharmacology

Class	Effect and Uses
Anesthetics, Local	**Relieve Superficial Pain**
benzocaine (Lanacaine)	Used to relieve pain and itching from various causes
lidocaine (Solarcaine)	Often used for sunburn pain
Antiacne Drugs, Topical	**Used to Treat Acne Vulgaris**
adapelene (Differin)	Retinoid-like action prevents blackheads
azelaic acid (Azelex)	Has activities similar to other drying antiacne drugs but also is antimicrobial for certain types of bacteria
benzoyl peroxide (Oxy10 Wash)	Produces a drying effect and is antimicrobial for the most prominent bacteria in sebaceous follicles
tazarotene (Tazorac)	Also used for the treatment of psoriasis
tetracyclines, topical (Topicycline)	Has local antiinfective effect
tretinoin (Retin-A)	Also used to improve photoaged skin, especially wrinkles and liver spots
Antihistamines, Topical	**Relieve Itching**
Benadryl	Produces local anesthetic activity

Continued

Chapter Pharmacology—cont'd

Class	Effect and Uses

(See pharmacology section of Chapter 3.)

Antiinfectives, Topical   **Inhibit the Growth of or Kill Microorganisms on the Skin**
Antibiotics   *Inhibit or destroy bacteria on the skin*
mupirocin (Bactroban) — Commonly used in impetigo
erythromycin (Akne-Mycin) — Used for acne vulgaris and as prophylaxis in wounds and burns
neomycin (Neomycin sulfate) — Prophylactic treatment of wounds or burns

Antifungals   *Inhibit the growth of fungi*
ciclopirox (Loprox) — Used for athlete's foot, jock itch, and ringworm
clotrimazole (Lotrimin) — Used for athlete's foot, ringworm, and other

Antivirals   *Have inhibitory effect on herpes simplex viruses type 1 and 2*
acyclovir (Zovirax) — Used to manage initial episodes of herpes genitalis and limited viral infections in immunocompromised patients
penciclovir (Denavir) — Used to treat cold sores on the lips

Anti–Poison Ivy Drugs   **Used to Prevent or Relieve the Symptoms Associated with Poison Ivy**
Rhuli cream — Relieves itching, pain, and discomfort of contact dermatoses
Calamatum — A spray that relieves itching and irritation
systemic prevention (poison ivy extract) — Recommended for prevention of poison ivy in hypersensitive individuals

Antipsoriatics   **Used to Treat Psoriasis**
anthralin (Anthra-Derm) — Ointment to treat the lesions of psoriasis
calcipotriene (Dovonex) — Topical use of synthetic vitamin D to heal the lesions of psoriasis
methotrexate (Methotrexate) — Systemic drug used for severe psoriasis only. Also used as antineoplastic agent and in rheumatoid arthritis

Antiseborrheic Drugs   **Reduce the Amount of Sebum Produced by the Sebaceous Glands**
selenium sulfide (Selsun Blue) — Used to treat dandruff and seborrheic dermatitis of the scalp
tar derivatives (Tegrin Medicated Shampoo) — Decrease epidermal proliferation and are antipruritic and antibacterial

Burn Preparations, Topical   **Used to Treat Burned Skin**
nitrofurazone (Furacin) — Antiinfective, also used on skin grafts
mafenide (Sulfamylon) — Bacteriostatic

Cauterizing agents   *Penetrate and destroy tissue*
Chloracetic acids — Used to destroy surface lesions that are not malignant

Corticosteroids, Topical   **Act Against Inflammation**
amcinonide (Cyclocort) — Relieves inflammation from various causes
hydrocortisone (Cort-Dome) — Relieves inflammation from various causes

Keratolytics   **Remove Warts, Calluses, and Corns**
salicylic acid (Compound W) — OTC solution for removing warts

Chapter Pharmacology—cont'd

Class	Effect and Uses
Scabicides/Pediculicides	**Kill Ectoparasites and Eggs**
lindane (Scabene)	Used for head lice, pubic lice, and body lice
Topical Drugs, Miscellaneous	
Fluorouracil (Efudex)	Used to treat multiple actinic or solar keratoses and superficial basal cell carcinomas
Minoxidil (Rogaine)	Stimulates growth of hair in certain types of male baldness

CHAPTER REVIEW 12

▶ **BASIC UNDERSTANDING**

REVIEWING WORD PARTS

I. Write a word (prefix, suffix, or combining form) for each clue.

CROSSWORD PUZZLE 12

Across

1 pus
2 poison
4 nature
6 fungus
8 pertaining to
9 hair
13 water
15 white
16 sebum
17 white
19 infection or septum
20 black
23 bacteria
25 hair
27 nail
28 fish
31 tumor
33 nail
34 skin
36 heat
38 horny
40 follicle
41 perspiration

Down

1 disease (combining form)
3 dry
5 into or not
7 cold
10 fat
11 fat
12 transmission
13 sun
14 skin
18 vessel
19 under
21 outside
22 armpit
24 redness
26 through
29 blue
30 wrinkle
32 to cause an action
34 killing
35 dead
37 middle
39 condition

MATCHING

II. Match modes of administration of medications in 1 through 4 with their descriptions in A through D.

_____ 1. intradermal

A. Administers medications directly into the blood stream

B. Deposits medication deeper than the other three that are listed

_____ 2. intramuscular

_____ 3. intravenous

_____ 4. subcutaneous

C. Places a small amount of drug into the outer layers of the skin

D. Places a small amount of medication below the skin

III. Match skin lesions in 1 through 8 with their characteristics (A-H):

_____ 1. bulla

_____ 2. cyst

_____ 3. fissure

_____ 4. macule

A. Blister, larger than 1 cm

B. Blister, smaller than 1 cm

C. Cracks in the skin

D. Discolored spot, not elevated

_____ 5. papule

_____ 6. pustule

_____ 7. scar

_____ 8. vesicle

E. Excess collagen production following injury

F. Fluid-filled sac containing pus

G. Sac filled with clear fluid

H. Solid elevation, less than 0.5 cm in diameter

LISTING

IV. Write five functions of the skin.

1. _____

2. _____

3. _____

4. _____

5. _____

MULTIPLE CHOICE

V. Select one answer (A–D) for each of the following multiple choice questions.

1. What does diaphoresis mean?
    A. breakdown of tissue by enzymes
    B. destruction by heat
    C. destruction of tissue by toxins
    D. excessive perspiration

2. Which of the following is an inflammatory skin disease that begins on the scalp but may involve other areas, particularly the eyebrows?
    A. acne vulgaris
    B. basal cell carcinoma
    C. seborrheic dermatitis
    D. trichorrhexis

3. To what does the term *cutaneous* pertain?
    A. fat
    B. sebum
    C. sweat
    D. skin

4. Cryosurgery destroys tissue using which of the following?
    A. cold temperature
    B. heat
    C. sunlight
    D. water

5. What is onychomycosis?
    A. a condition in which there is lack of nourishment for the nail bed
    B. a disease of the nails due to a fungus
    C. a morbid softening of the nails or the nail bed
    D. disturbance in the thermoregulatory system

6. What is removal of foreign material and dead or contaminated tissue from an infected or traumatic lesion until surrounding healthy tissue is exposed?
    A. debridement
    B. necrosis
    C. pyemia
    D. rhytidectomy

7. What is another term for ulceration of tissue?
    A. erosion
    B. macule
    C. vesicle
    D. wheal

8. What does trichoid mean?
    A. any disease of the hair
    B. appearing as a hairy heart
    C. breaking off of the hair
    D. resembling hair

9. Which of the following offers pain relief by delivering small amounts of current through an electrode placed over a painful site?
    A. hydrotherapy
    B. transcutaneous electrical nerve stimulation
    C. parenteral injection
    D. heliotherapy

10. What is pyodermatitis?
    A. a burning sensation of the skin
    B. a localized collection of pus
    C. a skin infection characterized by heat and redness
    D. inflammation of the skin caused by a pus-producing infection

FILL IN THE BLANKS

VI. Complete the sentences by writing a term in each blank space.

The outermost part of the skin, the (1) _____, consists of four to five layers of cells. These cells contain

(2) _____, which is a scleroprotein. The next layer of skin, the (3) _____, is also called the corium.

The deepest layer, called the subcutaneous (4) _____ tissue, serves as a cushion against shock and also provides

(5) _____.

    Sebum, an oily material that keeps hair and skin soft and pliable, is secreted by the (6) _____ glands. Sweat glands, also

called (7) _____ glands, produce perspiration, which helps cool the body.

WRITING TERMS

VII. Write words for the following:

1. death of tissue   _____
2. destruction by heat   _____
3. dry and scaly skin condition   _____
4. overgrowth of scar tissue   _____
5. pertaining to the armpit   _____

6. pertaining to the nail   _____
7. producing pus   _____
8. removal of a nail   _____
9. resembling hair   _____
10. tumor of a sweat gland   _____

▶ GREATER COMPREHENSION

SPELLING

VIII. Circle each misspelled term in this list and write the correct spelling.

    diathermy   heliotherapy   psoriasis   scleroderma   zerosis

MATCHING

IX. Match skin structures in the left column with their characteristics in the right column.

_____ 1. dermis
_____ 2. epidermis
_____ 3. sebaceous gland
_____ 4. sudoriferous gland
_____ 5. subcutaneous adipose tissue

A. Has cells that are constantly shed and replaced
B. Contains blood vessels and nerves
C. Secretes an oily material that protects the skin
D. Serves as insulation for the body
E. Helps regulate body temperature

X. Match the diseases or skin eruptions in 1 through 10 with their causative agent (bacteria, fungus, parasite, or virus) in the right column.

_____ 1. athlete's foot
_____ 2. fever blisters
_____ 3. furuncles
_____ 4. onychomycosis
_____ 5. pediculosis

_____ 6. rubella
_____ 7. scabies
_____ 8. scarlet fever
_____ 9. varicella
_____ 10. verrucae

A. bacteria
B. fungus
C. parasite
D. virus

INTERPRETING ABBREVIATIONS

XI. Write the meaning of each abbreviation:

1. bx _____
2. DLE _____
3. IM _____

4. SG _____
5. ung _____

PRONUNCIATION

XII. Pronunciation is shown for several medical terms. Indicate the primary accent in each term by marking it with a ′.

1. adipose (**ad ĭ pōs**)
2. cellulitis (**sel u li tis**)
3. dermabrasion (**dər mə bra shən**)
4. ichthyosis (**ik the o sis**)
5. nodule (**nod ūl**)

6. onychophagia (**on ĭ ko fa jə**)
7. papule (**pap ūl**)
8. pyogenesis (**pi o jen ə sis**)
9. subcutaneous (**sub ku ta ne əs**)
10. urticaria (**ur tĭ kar e ə**)

CATEGORIZING TERMS

XIII. Categorize each of the following terms as anatomical, diagnostic, radiological, surgical, or therapeutic by writing A, D, R, S, or T after each term.

1. abrasion _____
2. debridement _____
3. dermis _____
4. heliotherapy _____
5. ointment _____

6. palpation _____
7. petechiae _____
8. rhytidoplasty _____
9. seborrhea _____
10. xeroradiography _____

DRUG CLASSES

XIV. Match the drug classes in 1 through 7 with their uses in A through G.

_____ 1. antihistamines
_____ 2. antiinfectives
_____ 3. antiseborrheic drugs
_____ 4. cauterizing agents

A. Designed to act against inflammation
B. Destroy microorganisms
C. Penetrate and destroy tissue
D. Reduce the amount of sebum produced

_____ 5. corticosteroids
_____ 6. keratolytics
_____ 7. local anesthetics

E. Relieve itching
F. Relieve superficial pain
G. Remove warts, calluses, and corns

(Check your answers with the solutions in Appendix V.)

Listing of Medical Terms

abrasion	antipsoriatics	dermatologist	hidradenitis
abscess	apocrine gland	dermatomycosis	histocompatibility
acne vulgaris	asepsis	dermis	hydrotherapy
acrohypothermy	atrophy	diaphoresis	hyperthermia
adipose	axilla	diathermy	hypodermic
aerosol	axillary	discoid lupus erythematosus	hypopigmented
albinism	bactericidal	ecchymosis	hypothermia
albino	bacteriostatic	ectoderm	ichthyoid
alopecia	basal cell carcinoma	eczema	ichthyosis
anesthetic	bulla	electrodessication	incompatibility
antibacterial	cellulitis	electrolysis	integumentary
antifungal	contusion	endoderm	intradermal
antihistamine	corium	epidermis	intramuscular
antiinfective	corticosteroid	erosion	intravenous
antiinflammatory	cryosurgery	exfoliation	jaundice
antimycotic	cryotherapy	fissure	Kaposi's sarcoma
antiparasitic	cutaneous	folliculitis	keloid
antiperspirant	cyst	frostbite	keratin
antiseborrheic	debridement	fungicidal	keratogenesis
antisepsis	dermabrasion	furuncle	keratolytic
antiseptic	dermatitis	heliotherapy	keratoma

Listing of Medical Terms—cont'd

keratosis	onychomalacia	pyogenesis	topical medication
laceration	onychomycosis	pyrexia	transcutaneous electric nerve
lesion	onychopathy	retinoid	stimulator
lipectomy	onychophagia	rhytidoplasty	transdermal
lipoma	onychophagist	scabicide	trichoid
lunula	oral medication	scabies	trichopathy
macule	palmar erythema	scleroderma	trichophobia
melanoma	palpation	scleroprotein	trichosis
mesoderm	papule	sebaceous gland	ulcer
mycodermatitis	parenteral	seborrhea	ungual
necropsy	pediculicides	seborrheic dermatitis	urticaria
necrosis	pediculosis	seborrheic keratosis	verruca
necrotic	perspiration	sebum	vesicle
neoplasm	petechia	squamous cell carcinoma	wart
nevus	photodermatitis	subcutaneous	wheal
nodule	plaque	sublingual	xeroderma
ointment	pruritis	sudoriferous	xerophthalmia
onychectomy	psoriasis	thermoplegia	xeroradiography
onychoma	pustule	topical anesthetic	xerosis

Español Enhancing Spanish Communication

English	Spanish (pronunciation)	English	Spanish (pronunciation)
allergy	alergia (ah-LEHR-he-ah)	hives	roncha (RON-chah)
armpit	sobaco (so-BAH-co)	hypodermic	hipodérmico (e-po-DER-me-co)
biopsy	biopsia (be-OP-see-ah)	injection	inyección (in-yec-se-ON)
black	negro (NAY-gro)	injury	daño (DAH-nyo)
blue	azul (ah-SOOL)	nails	uñas (OO-nyahs)
body	cuerpo (coo-ERR-po)	perspiration	sudor (soo-DOR)
burn	quemadura (kay-mah-DOO-rah)	skin	piel (pe-EL)
dermatology	dermatología (der-mah-to-lo-HEE-ah)	sterile	estéril (es-TAY-reel)
eyebrow	ceja (SAY-hah)	ulcer	ulcera (OOL-say-rah)
eyelash	pestaña (pes-TAH-nyah)	wound	lesión (lay-se-ON)
gland	glándula (GLAN-doo-lah)	yellow	amarillo (ah-mah-REEL-lyo)
hair	pelo (PAY-lo)		

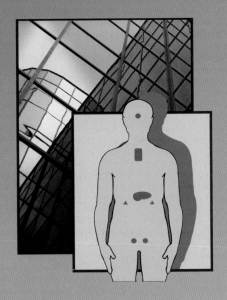

Endocrine System

13

Outline

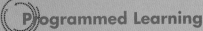
calc(i)	calcium
crin(o)	secrete
gigant(o)	large
gonad(o)	gonad
home(o)	sameness or constant
insulin(o)	insulin
iod(o)	iodine
mamm(o), mast(o)	breast
pancreat(o)	pancreas
parathyroid(o)	parathyroids
pituitar(o)	pituitary gland
thyr(o), thyroid(o)	thyroid gland
trop(o)	to stimulate

PREFIXES

exo-	outside or outward
pro-	before or for
tetra-	four
tri-	three

SUFFIXES

-physis	growth
-tropic	stimulate
-tropin	that which stimulates

Principal Word Parts

COMBINING FORMS

aden(o)	gland
adren(o), adrenal(o)	adrenal gland
andr(o)	male or masculine

Learning Goals

▶ BASIC UNDERSTANDING

In this chapter, you will learn to do the following:

1. Demonstrate a general understanding of the relationship between the nervous system and the endocrine system in maintaining homeostasis.
2. Name three mechanisms of hormonal regulation.
3. Recognize the hormones associated with the major endocrine organs and their target organs or functions.
4. Describe the relationship of the pancreas and diabetes mellitus.
5. Understand the meaning of endocrine versus exocrine glands.
6. Recognize structural and functional aspects of the breasts.
7. Write the meaning of word parts pertaining to the endocrine system, and use them to build and analyze medical terms.

▶ GREATER COMPREHENSION

8. Categorize the terms as anatomical, diagnostic, radiological, surgical, or therapeutic.
9. Spell the terms accurately.
10. Pronounce the terms correctly.
11. Know the meaning of the abbreviations.
12. Identify the effects or uses of the drug classes presented in this chapter.

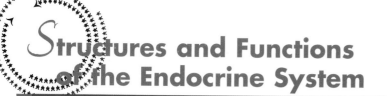

Structures and Functions of the Endocrine System

SECTION A

The endocrine system cooperates with the nervous system to regulate body activities. The endocrine system is composed of endocrine glands that secrete hormones.

	13-1 The endocrine (**en′do-krīn, en′do-krin**) and the nervous systems work together to maintain homeostasis (**ho″me-o-sta′sis**). The combining form *home(o)* means sameness or constant, and -stasis means stopping or controlling. Homeostasis is a relative constancy in the internal environment of the body.
homeostasis	The nervous system accomplishes regulation through electrical impulses and neurotransmitters. The endocrine system acts through chemical messengers called hormones. Working together, the nervous system and the endocrine system help maintain a constancy in the body that is called _____.
inside **secrete**	**13-2** The endocrine system is composed of the endocrine glands. Endo- means _____, and -crine means to _____. The locations of the major glands of the endocrine system are shown in Figure 13-1.
hormones	The secretions of endocrine glands are called hormones (**hor′mōnz**), chemical substances that are secreted into the blood and carried to another part of the body, where they exert specific physiological effects. The chemical secretions of endocrine glands are called _____.

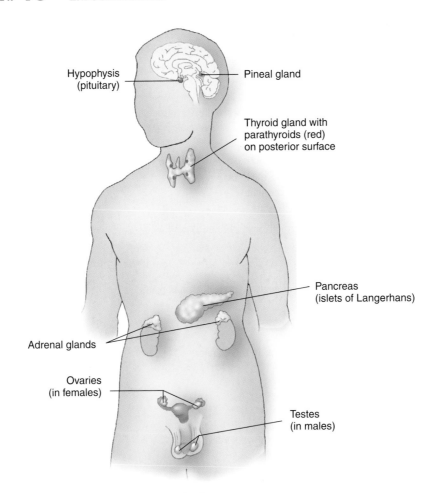

FIGURE 13-1
Location of major glands of the endocrine system.

---

blood (blood stream)

13-3 There are many glands in the body, and they are classified as either exo/crine or endo/crine glands. The prefix *exo-* means outside. Exocrine glands have ducts that enable them to empty secretions onto an external or an internal body surface. A sweat gland is an example of an exocrine gland. Endocrine glands are ductless and secrete their hormones into the _____, where they are carried to other parts of the body.

---

hypersecretion

13-4 Dysfunctions in hormone production fall into two categories, either a deficiency or an excess in secretion. A deficiency is called hypo/secretion. Excess secretion is called _____.

The organ or structure toward which the effects of a hormone are primarily directed is called the target organ. If a hormone has a specific effect on the thyroid, then the thyroid is the target organ. If a hormone has a specific effect on the ovaries, then the ovary is the _____ organ.

target

13-5 Hormones are either proteins or steroids. Most hormones in the human body are protein, with the exception of the sex hormones and those from the adrenal cortex. The significance of this is that proteins are quickly inactivated in the digestive tract, so these hormones are administered by injection if there is a deficiency. Sex hormones and other steroids can be taken orally.

gland	**13-6** The combining form *aden(o)* means gland, and most terms that use this word part refer to any gland, but there are a few exceptions. Aden/ectomy (**ad″ə-nek′tə-me**) means excision of any _____.
adenitis (ad″ə-ni′tis)	Write a term that means inflammation of a gland: _____.
adenopathy (ad″ə-nop′ə-the)	Write a term that has a literal translation of any disease of a gland: _____. This new term means any disease of a gland, especially the lymph nodes.
	An aden/oma (**ad″ə-no′mə**) is a benign tumor in which the cells are clearly derived from glandular tissue. In contrast, adenocarcinoma (**ad″ə-no-kahr″sĭ-no′mə**) is a malignant tumor derived from glandular tissue.

❑ SECTION A REVIEW   *S*tructures and Functions of the Endocrine System

This section review covers frames 13–1 through 13–6. Complete the table by writing the word part in the blank.

Combining Form	Meaning	Suffix	Meaning
1. _____	gland	3. exo-	_____
2. _____	sameness or constant		

(Use Appendix V to check your answers.)

*P*ituitary Gland: The "Master Gland"

A master endocrine gland, the pituitary, is located at the base of the brain and supplies numerous hormones that act directly on cells or stimulate other glands.

	13-7 Some hormones of the endocrine glands are released in response to the nervous system (i.e., the adrenal gland releases adrenaline in response to the sympathetic nervous system in stressful situations). Many endocrine glands, however, respond to hormones produced by the pituitary gland, which is nicknamed the "master gland" for this reason.
pituitary	The pituitary (**pĭ-too′ĭ-tar″e**) gland is a small, round structure about 1 cm (or ½ inch) in diameter that is attached by a stalk to the hypothalamus of the brain. The pituitary secretes a number of hormones that regulate various body processes. Write the name of this gland: _____.
under hypophysis	**13-8** The pituitary gland is also called the pituitary, the hypophysis cerebri, or simply the hypophysis (**hi-pof′ə-sis**). The suffix *-physis* means growth. The hypo/physis was so named because it grows _____ the cerebrum. The pituitary gland is called the pituitary or the _____.
gland	**13-9** Examine the diagram of the pituitary and its target organs in Figure 13-2. The pituitary is divided structurally and functionally into an anterior lobe and a posterior lobe. The anterior lobe of the pituitary is called the adenohypophysis. The word part *aden(o)* refers to a _____. This lobe is the glandular part of the hypophysis.

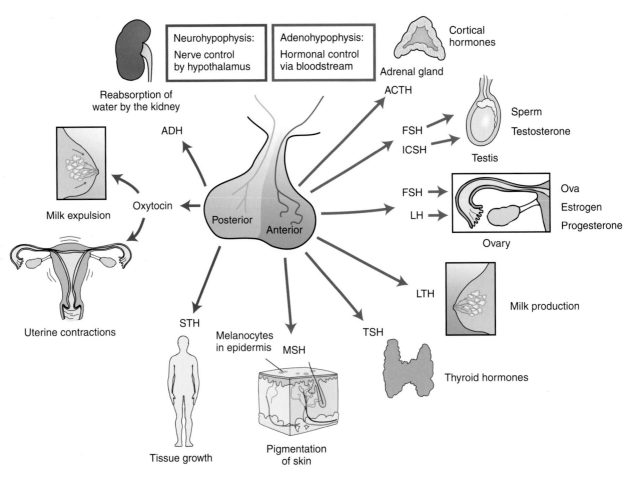

FIGURE 13-2

The pituitary, the master gland. The posterior pituitary lobe, shown on the left, is controlled by nervous stimulation by the hypothalamus and releases two hormones. In contrast, the anterior pituitary lobe is controlled by hypothalmic hormones brought by the blood stream and secretes many hormones.

anterior adenohypophysis	**13-10** The release of hormones from the adenohypophysis is controlled by regulating hormones produced by the hypothalamus. The adenohypophysis (**ad″ə-no-hi-pof′ĭ-sis**) is which lobe of the pituitary? _____ The name of the anterior lobe is formed by using aden(o) and hypophysis. Write this word: _____.
nerve neurohypophysis	**13-11** The posterior lobe of the pituitary is called the neurohypophysis (**noor″o-hi-pof′ə-sis**). The combining form neur(o) means _____. This lobe contains ends of neurons, the cell bodies of which are located in the hypothalamus. The hormones of the neurohypophysis are stored in the axon endings and are released when a nerve impulse travels down the axon. The portion of the pituitary that releases hormones when stimulated by nervous impulses from the hypothalamus is called the _____.

anterior	**13-12** Look again at Figure 13-2. Abbreviations such as ADH, STH, and MSH stand for pituitary hormones. The two hormones produced by the posterior lobe of the pituitary act directly on specific cells of the kidneys, the breasts, and the uterus. The anterior lobe of the pituitary produces many hormones, several of which act on other endocrine glands, causing them also to secrete hormones. The green labels in Figure 13-2 represent anterior pituitary hormones. Which lobe of the pituitary release the greater number of hormones? ________________ lobe

❑ SECTION B REVIEW *Pituitary Gland: The "Master Gland"*

This section review covers frames 13–7 through 13–12. Write the word part for the meaning that is listed.

Suffix	Meaning
1. ____________________	growth

(Use Appendix V to check your answer.)

SECTION C

Hormones of the Neurohypophysis

The hypothalamus plays an important role in hormonal regulation. The hormones of the neurohypophysis, antidiuretic hormone and oxytocin, are synthesized in the hypothalamus, then transported to the neurohypophysis for storage. They are released through nervous stimulation.

against diuretic	**13-13** The neurohypophysis does not synthesize hormones but stores two hormones that are produced by the hypothalamus. These two hormones are antidiuretic hormone and oxytocin. Antidiuretic **(an″tĭ-di″u-ret′ik)** hormone (ADH) affects the volume of urine excreted. The prefix *anti-* means ________________. Diuretic means increasing urine excretion or the amount of urine. It also means an agent that promotes urine excretion. Anti/diuretic hormone acts against a ________________. It acts in the kidneys to reabsorb water from the urine, producing a concentrated urine. Absence of this hormone produces diuresis, passage of large amounts of dilute urine.
increase decrease	**13-14** Some common substances such as tea, coffee, and water act as diuretics. Physicians also prescribe diuretic drugs to rid the body of excess fluid in patients with edema. Diuretics (increase or decrease) ________________ urination. Anti/diuretic hormone causes a(n) (increase or decrease) ________________ in the amount of water lost in urination.
oxytocin mammary	**13-15** The second hormone, oxytocin **(ok″sĭ-to′sin),** is released in large quantities just before a female gives birth. It causes uterine contractions, thus inducing childbirth. It also acts on the mammary glands to stimulate the release of milk. Write the name of the pituitary hormone that causes contraction of the uterus and acts on the mammary glands: ________________. The mammary **(mam′ər-e)** glands are the two glands of the female breasts that secrete milk. The combining form ***mamm(o)*** refers to the breast. The milk-producing glands of the female are called the ________________ glands.

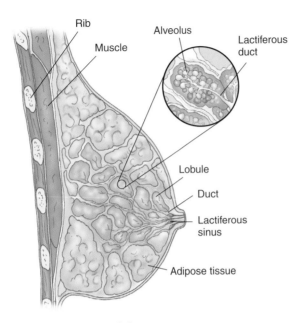

Lateral view

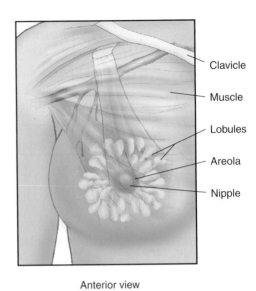

Anterior view

FIGURE 13-3

Structure of the adult female breast, lateral and anterior views. The breasts are mammary glands and function as part of both the endocrine and reproductive systems.

fatty

13-16 The female breasts are accessory reproductive organs. The breasts are located anterior to the chest muscles, and each breast contains 15 to 20 lobes of glandular tissue that radiate around the nipple.

Figure 13-3 shows the structural aspects of the breast. The circular pigmented area of skin surrounding the nipple is the areola. The lobes are separated by connective and adipose tissue. What type of tissue is adipose tissue? _____

The amount of adipose tissue determines the size of the breasts, but not the amount of milk that can be produced.

oxytocin

milk

13-17 During pregnancy, the mammary glands undergo changes that prepare them for production of milk. Each lobe is drained by its own lactiferous (**lak-tif′ər-əs**) duct, which has a dilated portion, called a sinus, that serves as a reservoir for milk. The nipple, located near the center, contains the openings of the milk ducts. The ejection of milk is brought about by the hormone released by the pituitary gland called

_____.

An interrelationship between the hypothalamus and the breast brings abut the release of oxytocin, which brings about the ejection of _____ by the breast (Figure 13-4).

production of milk

13-18 The secretion of milk is called lactation (**lak-ta′shən**). Lacto/genic means inducing the secretion of milk (lact[o] means milk).

Another hormone, pro/lactin, is the lacto/genic hormone. Although mentioned here, this hormone is secreted by the adenohypophysis. What is the function of prolactin (**pro-lak′tin**)?

_____

milk

production of milk

13-19 The prefix *pro-* means before or for. Pro/lactin (together with other hormones) is responsible for _____ production. Oxytocin causes the ejection of milk.

Lacto/genesis occurs after childbirth. Lacto/genesis (**lak″to-jen′ə-sis**) means

_____.

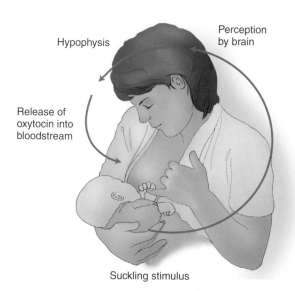

Hypophysis

Perception
by brain

Release of
oxytocin into
bloodstream

Suckling stimulus

FIGURE 13-4
Interrelationships of hypothalamus, neurohypophysis, and breast. Suckling by the infant stimulates nerve endings at the nipple. Impulses are carried to the hypothalamus, which causes the neurohypophysis to secrete oxytocin into the blood stream. The oxytocin is carried to the breast, where it causes milk to be expressed into the ducts. Milk begins to flow within 30 seconds to 1 minute after a baby begins to suckle.

breast mammogram (mam′ə-gram)	**13-20** You learned that mamm(o) means _____. Mammo/graphy is a diagnostic procedure that uses x-rays to study the breast. The roentgenogram produced in mammography (mə-mog′rə-fe) is called a _____. Figure 13-5 is a mammogram showing carcinoma of the breast.
	13-21 Excluding skin cancer, breast cancer has been the most common malignancy among women in the United States for many years. The cause of breast cancer is still unknown, but early detection through breast self-examination and mammography, and improved treatment have contributed to a slight decrease in mortality rates. Breast cancer in females is the second leading cause of cancer death, behind lung cancer. Treatment of breast cancer may require lumpectomy (removal of the lump or tumor), radiation therapy, chemotherapy, hormone manipulation, or mast/ectomy (surgical removal of the breast).
carcinoma of the breast mastalgia (mas-tal′jə) mastodynia (mas″to-din′e-ə) pain in the breast	**13-22** The combining form ***mast(o)*** also means breast. Masto/carcinoma (mas″to-kahr″sĭ-no′mə) is _____. Using mast(o) and the suffixes *-algia* and *-dynia*, write two words that mean pain in the breast: _____ and _____. Mamm/algia (mə-mal′jə) also means _____.
mastopexy (mas′to-pek-se) breast	**13-23** Write a word using mast(o) and the suffix *-pexy* that means surgical fixation of the breast: _____. Mastopexy is performed to correct a pendulous _____. (This is also called breast-lift.)

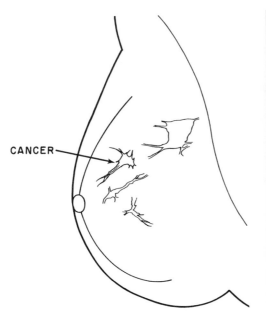 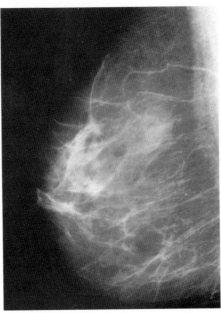

FIGURE 13-5
Mammogram, including a drawing, of cancer of the breast. The light areas indicate carcinoma. (From Svane G, Potchen EJ, Sierra A, Azavedo, E: *Screening mammography, breast cancer diagnosis in asymptomatic women,* St Louis, 1993, Mosby.)

mastitis (mas-ti′tis)	**13-24** Build words using mast(o) that mean inflammation of the breast _____.
mastectomy (mas-tek′tə-me)	removal of a breast (-ectomy means excision) _____.
mastoptosis (mas″to-to′sis)	sagging or prolapsed breast (-ptosis means prolapse) _____.
mastorrhagia (mas″to-ra′je-ə)	hemorrhage from the breast (-rrhagia means hemorrhage) _____.
between the breasts	Remembering that inter- means between, inter/mammary (in″ter mam′ah re) means situated _____.
behind	Remembering that retro- means behind, retro/mammary (ret″ro-mam′ər-e) means _____ the mammary gland, a milk-producing gland of the female breast.
plastic surgery of the breast	**13-25** Mammo/plasty (mam′o-plas″te) is _____.
breast **reduce**	Augmentation mammoplasty is plastic surgery to increase the size of the female _____. Reduction mammoplasty is plastic surgery to _____ the size of the breast.

❑ **SECTION C REVIEW**   *Hormones of the Neurohypophysis*

This section review covers frames 13–13 through 13–25. Complete the table by writing a word part or its meaning in each blank.

Combining Form	Meaning	Prefix	Meaning
1. mamm(o)	_____	3. _____	before or for
2. mast(o)	_____		

(Use Appendix V to check your answers.)

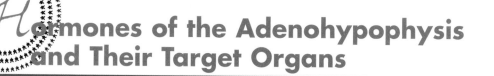

Hormones of the Adenohypophysis and Their Target Organs

The hypothalamus regulates the adenohypophysis by producing regulatory and inhibitory hormones, which stimulate or inhibit the secretion of its hormones. When the adenohypophysis secretes its hormones, they travel via the blood stream and bring about changes in other organs, often another endocrine gland. The parathyroid gland, an endocrine gland not directly controlled by the pituitary but closely linked with the thyroid gland, is also discussed.

stimulate **trop(o)**	**13-26** The adenohypophysis releases several hormones that regulate a large range of body activities. Look again at the target organs of these hormones (Figure 13-2). Most of these pituitary products stimulate other glands, and many of their names contain ***trop(o),*** which means to stimulate or turn. Tropic is an adjective that means to _____. The combining form that means to stimulate is _____. In endocrinology, ***-tropic*** generally means stimulate.
stimulates **somatotropin** (so″mə-to-tro′pin)	**13-27** Growth hormone (GH) is also called somato/tropic hormone (STH) or somatotropin. The suffix ***-tropin*** refers to that which stimulates. Somato/tropin is the hormone that _____ the body's growth. This hormone increases the rate of growth and maintains size once growth is attained. It is called the growth hormone or _____.
growth (or somatotropin)	**13-28** Insufficient growth hormone in childhood leads to dwarfism (**dwarf′iz-əm),** and the adult dwarf may be no more than 3 to 4 feet tall. Pituitary dwarfism is caused by a deficiency of which hormone? _____
decreased **hypopituitarism** **pituitary**	**13-29** The combining form ***pituitar(o)*** is used to build words that refer to the pituitary gland. Hypo/pituitar/ism (**hi″po-pĭ-too′ĭ-tə-riz″əm)** is _____ activity of the pituitary gland. Pituitary insufficiency in childhood has more drastic effects than the same disorder in adults. Because the pituitary produces many hormones, one or all may be altered. Only the more outstanding disorders are described. Pituitary insufficiency is called _____. Atrophy of the pituitary gland in an adult causes a state of ill health, malnutrition, and wasting known as pituitary cachexia (**kə-kek′se-ə).** Although cachexia may occur in many chronic diseases, pituitary cachexia is due to hyposecretion of the _____ gland.
hyperpituitarism (hi″per-pĭ-too′ĭ- tə-riz″əm) **somatotropin**	**13-30** Increased pituitary activity is _____. If this occurs during childhood, gigantism (***gigant[o]*** means large) may result, and the person will become much taller than normal. Overproduction of growth hormone before the epiphyses of the long bones close results in gigantism. Two opposite conditions, dwarfism and gigantism, are shown in Figure 13-6. Pituitary gigantism (**ji-gan′tiz-əm)** is caused by hypersecretion of which hormone? _____

FIGURE 13-6

Gigantism and dwarfism, resulting from abnormal secretions of growth hormone. Hypersecretion of growth hormone during the early years results in gigantism. The person usually has normal body proportions and normal sexual development. The same hypersecretion in an adult causes acromegaly. Hyposecretion of growth hormone during the early years produces a dwarf unless the child is treated with injections of growth hormone. (From Seely RR, Stephens TD, Tate P: *Anatomy and physiology*, ed 3, St Louis, 1995, Mosby.)

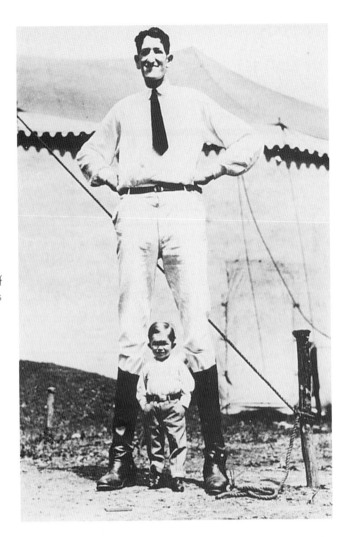

enlargement of the extremities	**13-31** The same excess of hormone in adults does not cause gigantism. Increased secretion of growth hormone in adults causes acromegaly (**ak″ro-meg′ə-le**). The name acromegaly denotes a typical feature of the disease (-megaly means enlargement). Acro/megaly means _____.
	Bones of the feet, hands, cheeks, and jaws thicken in this disease because of oversecretion of adenohypophyseal growth hormone (Figure 13-7).
	Hyperpituitarism almost always involves excessive secretion of growth hormone but may involve other pituitary hormones as well. The cause of excessive pituitary activity is often a tumor, especially a pituitary adenoma.
	Hypopituitarism results from congenital developmental defects (as in pituitary dwarfism), tumors that destroy the pituitary or the hypothalamus, or lack of blood circulation to the pituitary.
black	**13-32** Melanocyte-stimulating hormone (MSH) from the pituitary stimulates melanocytes distributed throughout the epidermis. MSH promotes pigmentation and controls the amount of melanin that melanocytes produce. The name *melanin* implies the color _____. Melanin is a black or dark brown pigment that occurs naturally in the hair, skin, and parts of the eye.
milk	**13-33** You read about the lactogenic hormone in the previous section. The lactogenic hormone (LTH), also called prolactin, is produced by the anterior pituitary and causes _____ production by the mammary glands.

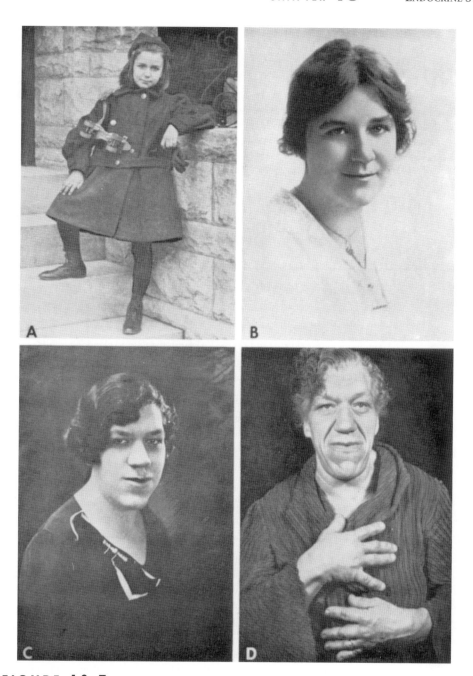

FIGURE 13-7
Progression of acromegaly. The patient is shown at age 9, age 16, age 33 with well-established acromegaly, and age 52 in the late stages of acromegaly. (From Ignatavicius DD, Workman ML, Mishler MA: *Medical-surgical nursing across the health care continuum*, ed 3, Philadelphia, 1999, WB Saunders.)

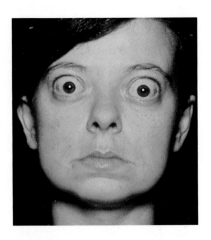

FIGURE 13-8
Graves' disease. Three important characteristics are hyperthyroidism, exophthalmos, and goiter. Exophthalmos is the result of fluid accumulation in the fat pads and muscles behind the eyeballs, which causes the eyes to protrude. A goiter is an enlarged thyroid gland, evidenced by the swelling in the neck. (From Stein JH, editor: *Internal medicine*, ed 4, St Louis, 1994, Mosby.)

inflammation of the thyroid gland	**13-34** Looking at Figure 13-2, you see that the pituitary secretes TSH that causes the glandular cells of the thyroid to produce thyroid hormones. TSH means thyroid-stimulating hormone, also called thyrotropin (**thi-rot′ro-pin**). The combining forms ***thyr(o)*** and ***thyroid(o)*** mean the thyroid gland. Thyroid/itis (**thi″roi-di′tis**) is _____.
excessive **eyes**	**13-35** Eu/thyroid means a normally funtioning thyroid, because eu- means good or normal. Hyper/thyroid/ism (**hi″pər-thi′ roid-iz-əm**) is a condition caused by _____ secretion of two hormones of the thyroid gland. This increases the metabolic rate, which then causes an increased demand for food to support this metabolic activity. The basal metabolic rate (BMR) is the energy used by a resting person to maintain vital functions. The patient with hyperthyroidism becomes excitable and nervous, exhibiting moist skin, rapid pulse, elevated metabolic rate, weight loss, and exophthalmos. In ex/ophthalmos (**ek″sof-thal′mos**), the _____ protrude outward. (One "o" is dropped to prevent double "o.")
thyrotoxicosis **excision of the thyroid**	**13-36** The most common form of hyperthyroidism is Graves' disease, believed to be an autoimmune disease. Three hallmarks of Graves' disease are hyperthyroidism, exophthalmos, and goiter (**goi″tər**). The patient shown in Figure 13-8 exhibits exophthalmos and goiter. A goiter is a description term that means an enlarged thyroid gland, usually evident as a pronounced swelling in the neck. It may be associated with hyperthyroidism, hypothyroidism, tumors, or thyroiditis. Thyrotoxicosis (**thi″ro-tok″sĭ-ko′sis**), also called thyroid storm, is a life-threatening event that is usually triggered by a major stressor, such as trauma or infection. Signs and symptoms result from a rapid increase in the metabolic rate and include fever, fast pulse, hypertension, gastrointestinal symptoms, agitation, and anxiety. A term for thyroid storm is _____. The treatment of hyperthyroidism is destruction of large amounts of the thyroid tissue by either surgery or radioactive materials or the use of anti/thyroid drugs to block the production of thyroid hormones. Thyroid/ectomy (**thi″roi-dek′tə-me**) is _____.
thyroid **iodine** **four**	**13-37** Thyro/xine (**thi-rok′sin**) is a hormone secreted by the gland for which it is named, the _____ gland. Thyroxine is tetra/iodo/thyro/nine (***tetra-*** means four; ***iod[o]*** means iodine) and is abbreviated T_4. Another hormone produced by the thyroid gland is tri/iodo/thyronine (**tri-i″o-do-thi′ro-nēn**), which is abbreviated T_3. Both of these hormones are synthesized by the thyroid using iodine. If there is a deficiency of _____ in the diet, the thyroid will not be able to produce sufficient T_3 and T_4 for metabolism. Both of these hormones control body metabolism. Thyroxine is also called tetra/iodo/thyronine, which means it has _____ iodine atoms in its chemical structure.

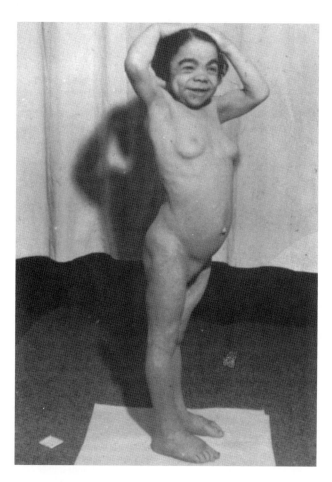

FIGURE 13-9

Cretinism. This 33-year-old untreated adult cretin exhibits characteristic features. She is only 44 inches tall, has under-developed breasts, protruding abdomen, umbilical hernia, widened facial features, and scant axillary and pubic hair. (From Ignatavicius DD, Workman ML, Mishler MA: *Medical-surgical nursing across the health care continuum,* ed 3, Philadelphia, 1999, WB Saunders.)

hypothyroidism (hi"po-thi'roid-iz-əm)	**13-38** Write a word that means decreased activity of the thyroid gland: _____. Hypothyroidism in childhood results in a condition called cretinism (**kre'tin-iz-əm**) and is due to insufficient thyroxine. The condition is characterized by arrested physical and mental development (Figure 13-9). Extreme inadequacy of thyroid function in childhood causes a condition called _____.
cretinism	Myxedema (**mik"sə-de'mə**) is caused by hyposecretion of thyroxine and T_3 during adulthood. The body retains water, and the resultant edema causes facial puffiness. This condition is caused by decreased secretion of the thyroid gland. Hormone therapy usually alleviates the symptoms.
hypothyroidism	**13-39** Because the thyroid gland absorbs iodine from the blood in order to synthesize T_3 and T_4, radio/iodine can be used to study the gland. Radioiodine, ^{131}I, like all radionuclides (radioisotopes), gives off radiation. The radioactive iodine uptake (RAIU) test measures the ability of the thyroid gland to trap and retain the ^{131}I after oral ingestion. A radiation counter determines the amount of ^{131}I uptake by the thyroid gland. If less than normal radioactive iodine is absorbed by the thyroid gland, which condition is expected, hypothyroidism or hyperthyroidism? _____
imaging **nuclear**	**13-40** Nuclear medicine is important in both the diagnosis and the treatment of disease. Imaging involves the production of a picture, image, or shadow that represents the object being studied. Nuclear medicine imaging or scans consist of administration of a radiopharmaceutical followed by the imaging of the spatial distribution of the radionuclide. Computed tomography and ultrasound techniques are other forms of _____, production of an image of the object being studied. Nuclear medicine imaging provides a high degree of contrast. Imaging of the spatial distribution of a radionuclide in a tissue is called _____ medicine imaging.

thyropathy (thi-rop′ə-the) **thyroid tumor**	**13-41** Using thyr(o), write a word that means any disease of the thyroid gland: _____. Thyr/oma (**thi-ro′mə**) is a _____ _____.
thyroid	**13-42** A third hormone produced by the thyroid gland is thyro/calcitonin (TCT, also called calcitonin). This hormone is involved in the homeostasis of the blood calcium level. Thyro/calcitonin (**thi″ro-kal″sĭ-to′nin**) is a hormone produced by the _____. The combining form *calc(i)* means calcium.
pertaining to the gonads **gonadotropic** **gonadotropin** (gon″ə-do-tro′pin) **gonads**	**13-43** The combining form *gonad(o)* means gonads (ovaries or testes). Gonad/al (**go′nad əl**) means _____. Gonado/tropic (**gon″ə-do-trop′ik**) hormones stimulate the ovaries of the female and the testes of the male. An adjective that means stimulating the gonads is _____. Follicle-stimulating hormone (FSH) and luteinizing (**loo′te-in-i″zing**) hormone (LH) are produced by the adenohypophysis. These two hormones have the gonads as target organs. Write a word that means a hormone that stimulates the gonads: _____. Hypo/gonad/ism (**hi″po-go′nad-iz-əm**) is decreased functional activity of the _____.
estrogen sperm progesterone testosterone	**13-44** FSH stimulates the ovaries to secrete estrogen and acts on the follicle, as its name implies. FSH stimulates production of sperm in the testes of the male. LH stimulates ovulation and production of progesterone in the female ovary. LH is often called interstitial cell-stimulating hormone (ISCH) in males because it promotes the growth of the interstitial cells of the testes and the secretion of testosterone. In summary, FSH stimulates the ovaries to produce the hormone _____. In males, FSH causes the production of _____. LH causes release of the ovum by the ovaries and production of the hormone _____. In males, LH causes the production of the hormone _____.
	13-45 The onset of puberty is triggered by the hypothalamus and the anterior pituitary. FSH and LH are gonadotropic hormones that act on the testes and ovaries. Male sex hormones are collectively called androgens, with testosterone being the most abundant. The period of life at which reproduction becomes possible is puberty. It is recognized by maturation of the genitals and appearance of secondary sex characteristics (Figure 13-10).
kidney **kidneys**	**13-46** The adrenal glands are target organs of another pituitary hormone. Since ren(o) means kidney, ad/ren/al (**ə-dre-nəl**) tells us that these glands are located near or toward the _____. An adrenal gland lies above each of the two kidneys. Supra/renal (**soo″prə-re′nəl**) means above the _____, and sometimes the adrenal glands are called the suprarenal glands.

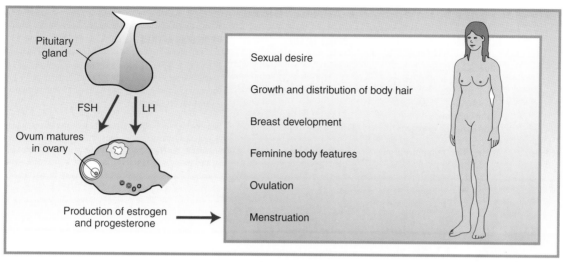

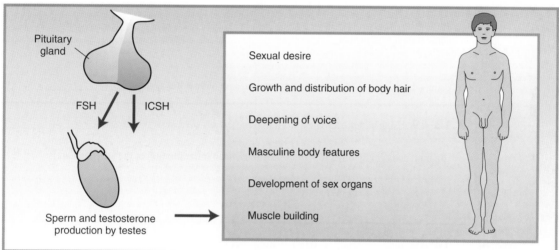

FIGURE 13-10
Secondary female and male sexual characteristics. The changes that occur at puberty are brought about by the hypothalamus and the anterior pituitary. Changes in the secretions of FSH and LH bring about changes in the ovaries and testes and the hormones they produce.

13-47 The outer cortex makes up the bulk of the gland, and the inner portion is called the medulla. Table 13-1 lists the important hormones produced by the adrenal glands.

The cortex and medulla of the adrenal gland are stimulated by different means, and they secrete different hormones. The hypothalamus influences both portions, but the medulla receives direct nervous stimulation, and the cortex is stimulated by adrenocorticotropic hormone brought by the circulating blood.

Write the names of the three general types of hormones secreted by the adrenal cortex:

mineralocorticoids, glucocorticoids, and androgens and estrogen

Mineralocorticoids (**min″ər-əl-o-kor′tĭ-koidz**) helps maintain water balance in the body. Glucocorticoids (**gloo″ko-kor′tĭ-koidz**) increase blood glucose and inhibit inflammation. Persons with severe inflammation, as in the joints, may receive injections of cortisone to relieve the pain and inflammation. Cortisone may also be included in topical creams and ointments to relieve skin inflammation.

TABLE 13-1   **Hormones Secreted by the Adrenal Gland**

GLAND	HORMONE	TARGET TISSUE	PRINCIPAL ACTION
Adrenal cortex	Mineralocorticoids (main one is aldosterone)	Kidney	Increases water retention by changing sodium and potassium reabsorption in the kidney tubules
	Glucocorticoids (main ones are cortisol and cortisone)	Most body tissue	Increases blood glucose levels; inhibits inflammation and the immune response
	Androgens and estrogens	Most body tissue	Secreted in such small amounts that the effect is generally masked by ovarian and testicular hormones
Adrenal medulla	Epinephrine, norepinephrine	Heart and blood vessels, liver, adipose	Increases heart rate and blood pressure, increases blood flow and blood glucose level, helps the body cope with stress

stimulates the adrenal glands

adrenalectomy (ə-dre″nəl-ek′to-me)

13-48   The hormone secreted by the adenohypophysis that stimulates the adrenal cortex is adreno/cortico/tropic (ə-dre″no-kor″tĭ-ko-trop′ik) hormone (ACTH). The combining forms *adren(o)* and *adrenal(o)* refer to the adrenal glands. Adreno/cortico/tropin (ə-dre″no-kor″tĭ-ko-trōp′in) is another name for a hormone that _____.

Using adrenal(o), write a word that means excision of an adrenal gland: _____.

adrenopathy (ad″rən-op′ə-the)
adrenitis (ad″rə-ni′tis)
adrenalitis (ə-dre″nəl-i′tis)

13-49   Using adren(o), write a word that means any disease of the adrenals: _____

Use both combining forms to write words that mean inflammation of the adrenal glands:
_____ and

_____.

enlargement

adrenals decreased adrenal activity

13-50   Adreno/megaly (ə-dre″no-meg′ə-le) is _____ of one or both adrenal glands.

Hyper/adrenal/ism (hi″pər-ə-dre′nəl-iz-əm) is increased secretory activity of the

_____.

Hypo/adrenal/ism (hi″po-ə-dre′nəl-iz-əm) is _____.

13-51   Hypersecretion of the adrenal cortex causes Cushing's syndrome. A syndrome is a set of symptoms that occur together and collectively characterize or indicate a particular disease or abnormal condition. Cushing's syndrome is characterized by elevated blood glucose levels, edema resulting from imbalance of water in the body, and masculinization in females.

Tumors that result in hypersecretion of androgens or estrogens before puberty usually have dramatic effects. This is called the adrenogenital (ə-dre″no-jen′ĭ təl) syndrome. There is a rapid onset of puberty and sex drive in males. Females develop the masculine distribution of body hair and the clitoris enlarges to look more like a penis.

masculine

hair

13-52   The combining form *andr(o),* means male or masculine. Testosterone is the most potent androgen and is produced in large quantities by the testes, making that produced by the adrenal glands insignificant in most cases. Andro/genic (an″dro-jen′ik) means producing _____ characteristics or masculinization. In females, the masculinization effect of androgen secretion may become evident after menopause unless replacement estrogen is taken. Excessive growth of body hair in the female is hirsutism (hir′soot-iz-əm). The Latin word *hirsutus* means shaggy. Hirsutism, however, means excessive growth of _____.

andropathy (an-drop'ə-the) **female breast condition**	**13-53** Write a word that means any disease peculiar to the male by joining andr(o) and the suffix for disease: _____. Occasionally an adrenal tumor secretes excess estrogens. When this occurs, the male patient develops gyneco/mast/ia, which translated literally means _____. Gynecomastia (**jin″ə-ko-mas′te-ə**) means excessive growth of the male mammary glands.
hyposecretion	**13-54** Hyposecretion of the adrenal cortex leads to Addison's disease. This life-threatening condition is characterized by dehydration, low blood glucose levels, bronzing of the skin and general ill health. Partial or complete failure of the adrenal gland can result from autoimmune processes, infection, tumors, or hemorrhage within the gland. Addison's disease results from _____ of the adrenal cortex.
epinephrine	**13-55** The adrenal medulla secretes two hormones, epinephrine (**ep″ĭ-nef′rin**), called also adrenaline (ə-**dren′ə-lin**), and norepinephrine (noradrenaline). The medulla mostly secretes epinephrine, which stimulates the heart. Norepinephrine causes blood vessels to constrict. Together they prepare the body for strenuous activity and are sometimes called the fight-or-flight hormones. The main fight-or-flight hormone is called _____. Hyposecretion of these two hormones produces no significant effect. Hypersecretion, usually from a tumor, puts the body in a prolonged or continual fight-or-flight mode.

❏ SECTION D REVIEW   𝓗ormones of the Adenohypophysis and Their Target Organs

This section review covers frames 13–26 through 13–55. Complete the table by writing a word part or its meaning in each blank.

Combining Form	Meaning	Prefix	Meaning
1. adren(o), adrenal(o)	_____	9. tetra-	_____
2. andr(o)	_____	**Suffix**	**Meaning**
3. gigant(o)	_____	10. _____	stimulate
4. gonad(o)	_____	11. _____	that which stimulates
5. _____	iodine		
6. _____	pituitary gland		
7. thyr(o), thyroid(o)	_____		
8. _____	to stimulate or turn		

(Use Appendix V to check your answers.)

Other Endocrine Tissues and Homeostasis

Three different mechanisms are used to regulate the secretion of hormones by endocrine tissues. In addition to the endocrine glands that have been studied in previous sections, the pancreas, the parathyroids, and the pineal gland are considered here along with a few other organs that have hormonal activity.

13-56 Strict regulation of hormonal secretion is important to maintain homeostasis. The body uses three different methods to regulate hormones: direct nervous stimulation, secretion of hormones in response to other hormones, and a negative feedback mechanism.

The adrenal medulla is an example of the first method, direct nervous stimulation. The adrenal medulla secretes epinephrine and norepinephrine in response to stimulation by sympathetic nerves.

Tropic hormones cause secretion of other hormones. For example, thyrotropin (TSH) from the anterior pituitary gland causes the thyroid gland to secrete the thyroid hormones.

The interaction between two important pancreatic hormones and the concentration of glucose in the blood is an example of a negative feedback system. In negative feedback, a gland is sensitive to the concentration of a substance that it regulates. Continue reading to see how this works.

islets

13-57 The pancreas has an exocrine portion that secretes digestive enzymes that are carried through a duct to the duodenum and an endocrine portion that secretes hormones into the blood. The endocrine portion consists of many small cell groups called islets of Langerhans. These cells secrete two hormones that have a role in regulating blood glucose levels. The endocrine portion of the pancreas is made up of many cell groups called _____ of Langerhans.

normal

The two hormones secreted by the islets of Langerhans are glucagon and insulin. The action of glucagon is to raise blood glucose levels. It is secreted in response to a low concentration of glucose in the blood. This mechanism prevents hypoglycemia (glyc[o] means sugar) from occurring between meals. Hypo/glyc/emia (**hi′po-gli-se′me-ə**) is less than _____ levels of glucose in the blood, since glucose is the type of sugar found in blood and is used by the body for energy. A person with hypoglycemia usually experiences weakness, headache, hunger, visual disturbances, and anxiety. If untreated, hypoglycemia can lead to coma and death. Treatment consists of administration of glucose in orange juice or other fluid, or intravenously if the person is unconscious. Write this term that means less than normal levels of glucose in

hypoglycemia

the blood: _____.

insulin

13-58 The action of insulin is opposite or antagonistic to glucagon. Insulin promotes the uptake and utilization of glucose for energy and is secreted in response to a high concentration of sugar in the blood. Insulin brings about a reduction in the blood glucose level.

Insufficient insulin activity may be caused by insufficient secretion or by insufficient or defective receptor sites on its target cells. These dysfunctions lead to diabetes mellitus (**di″ə-be′tēz mel′lə-təs),** which is characterized by abnormally high blood glucose levels. The combining form for insulin is *insulin(o).* Hypo/insulin/ism (**hi″po-in′su-lin-iz″əm**) is a deficient secretion of _____ by the pancreas.

excessive

13-59 Without insulin, glucose builds up in the blood and hyperglycemia results. Hyperglycemia causes serious fluid and electrolyte imbalances, ultimately resulting in the classic symptoms of diabetes: polyphagia, polyuria, and polydipsia. Polyphagia (**pol″e-fa′jə**) (poly, many and -phagia, eating) means excessive hunger and uncontrolled eating. Polyuria (**pol″e-u′re-ə**) (-uria, urination) means _____ urination. Polydipsia (**pol″ĭ-dip′se-ə**) (-dipsia, thirst) means excessive thirst.

When used alone, diabetes generally refers to diabetes mellitus (DM), but one should be aware that the term *diabetes* means excessive excretion of urine, and there is another unrelated type of diabetes.

TABLE 13-2 **Classification and Characteristics of Diabetes Mellitus**

TYPE OF DIABETES MELLITUS	CHARACTERISTICS
Type I diabetes	Absolute insulin deficiency Juvenile onset Ketosis sometimes occurs. Recessive gene puts one at risk.
Type II diabetes	Insulin resistance with deficient insulin secretion Most persons do not require insulin. Maturity onset Obesity is often involved.
Gestational diabetes	Carbohydrate intolerance is first recognized during pregnancy. High risk for developing diabetes several years later Children of affected mothers have increased risk of obesity and impaired glucose tolerance later in life.
Other types	Genetic defects Certain diseases such as pancreatitis and pancreatic tumors Endocrine diseases such as acromegaly, Cushing's disease, and hyperthyroidism Infections Induced by drugs or chemicals

diabetes mellitus

13-60 Broad classifications of diabetes mellitus are Type I, Type II, gestational, and other types (Table 13-2). Type I is genetically determined and results in absolute insulin deficiency; however, most people with this gene do not develop Type I diabetes, but 1 in 20 will. Persons with this particular gene are genetically susceptible and may or may not develop _____ _____.

The specific genetic link and development of Type II diabetes is unclear. Contributing factors may be genetic and environmental factors as well as the aging process and obesity. It is characterized by insulin resistance, rather than insufficient insulin secretion. This was formerly called non–insulin-dependent diabetes (NIDDM), but this was misleading, since some persons with Type II diabetes require insulin.

gestational

13-61 Gestational diabetes mellitus (GDM), first recognized during pregnancy, is a carbohydrate intolerance, usually caused by a deficiency of insulin. It disappears after delivery of the infant, but in a significant number of cases, returns years later. This type of diabetes is called _____ diabetes mellitus.

There are some other less common types of diabetes mellitus in addition to Type I, Type II, and gestational. An example is the type of DM associated with hyperthyroidism.

diuretic

13-62 One disorder that is also called diabetes but is not a disorder of carbohydrate metabolism is diabetes insipidus *(in-sip′ĭ-dəs)*. It is a disorder of water metabolism and is caused by a deficiency of ADH. ADH means anti-_____ hormone. Large quantities of dilute urine are excreted in diabetes insipidus, the characteristic for which it was named diabetes.

excessive
decreased

13-63 Hyper/insulin/ism (**hi″pər-in′sə-lin-iz″əm**) is _____ insulin in the blood. Hyperinsulinism results in hypo/glyc/emia, a _____ amount of glucose in the blood.

calcium

thyroid

13-64 Four small parathyroid glands, another type of endocrine gland, secrete parathyroid hormone (PTH) or parathormone (para- means near, beside, or abnormal). Parathyroid glands are located so near the thyroid (as the name implies) that they are embedded in its posterior surface. PTH increases the blood calcium levels and is regulated by a negative feedback mechanism. This means that PTH is secreted in response to low levels of _____ in the blood.

PTH has the opposite effect, or is antagonistic, to calcitonin secreted by the _____ gland.

TABLE 13-3 **Major endocrine glands and their secretions**

GLAND	PRIMARY SECRETIONS
Pituitary gland, anterior lobe	ACTH, FSH, GH, ICSH, LH, LTH, MSH, and TSH
Pituitary gland, posterior lobe	ADH and oxytocin
Adrenal glands, cortex	Aldosterone, cortisol, and androgens
Adrenal glands, medulla	Epinephrine and norepinephrine
Gonads, ovaries	Estrogen, progesterone, and HCG
Gonads, testes	Testosterone
Pancreas (islets of Langerhans)	Insulin and glucagon
Parathyroid glands	PTH
Thyroid gland	Thyroxine, triiodothyronine, and calcitonin
Pineal gland	Melatonin and serotonin
Thymus	Thymosin

---

hyperparathyroidism
(hi″pər par″ə-thi′roid-iz-əm)

13-65 The combining form **parathyroid(o)** means the parathyroids. Hypo/parathyroid/ism (hi″po-par″ə-thi′roid-iz-əm) is below normal functioning of the parathyroids. Write a word that means abnormally increased activity of the parathyroids: _____.

calcium

Hypoparathyroidism results in hypocalcemia (hi″po-kal-se′me-ə) (calc[i] means calcium), which is less than the normal level of _____ in the blood. Early surgeons learned the importance of calcium when they inadvertently removed the parathyroids while removing the thyroid. Hypocalcemia occurred 1 to 2 days after the surgery.

high blood calcium level

Hyperparathyroidism is abnormally increased activity of the parathyroid glands and causes hypercalcemia. Hyper/calc/emia (hi″per-kal-se′me-ə) is _____.

13-66 The pineal* (pi′ne-əl) gland, also called pineal body, is shaped like a pine cone and is attached to the posterior part of the brain. The exact functions of this gland have not been established, but there is evidence that it secretes the hormone melatonin (mel″-ə-to′nin). The pineal gland usually begins to diminish around the age of 7 years. If degeneration does not occur, the production of melatonin remains high and puberty may be delayed in females. This indicates that melatonin may inhibit the activities of the ovaries.

pineal

Melatonin is secreted by the _____ gland. In addition to a regulatory function in sexual development, functions of melatonin may include the sleepiness/wakefulness cycle, mood, and a decrease in skin pigmentation.

The major endocrine glands and their secretions are summarized in Table 13-3.

13-67 In addition to the endocrine glands you have studied, other organs that have some hormonal activity include the stomach, small intestines, thymus, heart, and placenta.

The lining of the stomach produces gastrin, which stimulates the production of hydrochloric acid, and the enzyme pepsin, all substances that are used in the digestion of food. The hormone gastrin (gastr[o] means stomach) is secreted in response to food in the stomach. Hormones secreted by the lining of the small intestine stimulate the pancreas and the gallbladder to produce substances that aid in digestion.

The thymus is located near the middle of the chest cavity behind the breast bone. It produces thymosin (thi′mo-sin), which assists in the development of lymphocytes, blood cells that function in immunity. The thymus, usually largest at puberty, diminishes in size as an individual reaches adulthood. The hormone produced by the thymus is called _____.

thymosin

Special cells in the atria, the upper chambers of the heart, produce a hormone (atriopeptin) that increases the loss of sodium and water in urine.

The placenta of a pregnant female produces human chorionic gonadotropin (HCG), estrogen, and progesterone, which function to maintain the uterine lining for pregnancy.

*Pineal (Latin: pineus, pine cone).

❑ SECTION E REVIEW   𝒪ther Endocrine Tissues and Homeostasis

This section review covers frames 13–56 through 13–67. Complete the table by writing a combining form in each blank.

Combining Form	Meaning	Combining Form	Meaning
1. _____	insulin	2. _____	parathyroids

(Use Appendix V to check your answers.)

𝒯erminology Challenge

This section contains additional information about the endocrine glands and may use word parts that were introduced in previous chapters or introduce terms that are somewhat more difficult to remember.

13-68 The mammary glands secrete a cloudy fluid called colostrum (kə-los′trəm) the first few days after a female gives birth. Owing to its high antibody and high protein content, colostrum serves adequately as food for the infant until the breasts begin to secrete milk, 2 to 3 days after parturition.

13-69 Fibro/cystic (fĭ″bro-sĭs′tĭk) breast disease is a disorder characterized by single or multiple benign tumors of the breast. This form of mammary dysplasia occurs as a result of cyclic breast changes that normally accompany the menstrual cycle.

fibrocystic

This disorder characterized by benign tumors of the breast is called _____ breast disease.

13-70 Prostaglandins (pros″tə-glan′dĭnz) are potent chemical regulators that are widely distributed in cells throughout the body. These hormonelike substances have a localized, immediate, and short-term effect on or near the cells where they are produced.

Prostaglandins have many effects, and the same substance sometimes has opposite effects on different tissues. Some of the effects include smooth muscle contraction, involvement in blood clotting, and many aspects of fever and pain. They are believed to be implicated in the symptoms of severe menstrual cramps, premenstrual syndrome, and premature labor. Write the name of these hormonelike substances:

prostaglandins

_____.

13-71 Antiinflammatory drugs are used pharmacologically to block or inhibit the synthesis of prostaglandins. Inhibiting their production reduces inflammation in a variety of inflammatory disorders, such as arthritis. Unfortunately, a side effect of this treatment makes an individual susceptible to ulcers, since prostaglandins inhibit production of hydrochloric acid in the stomach.

Study the following list of selected abbreviations. Then read through the Chapter Pharmacology section and be sure you understand the effects and uses of the drug classes that are presented. When you are finished, work the Chapter Review. After completing the exercises, check your answers with the solutions in Appendix V.

You will find these items presented after the Chapter Review:

• Listing of Medical Terms
• Enhancing Spanish Communication

Selected Abbreviations

ACTH	adrenocorticotropic hormone		LH	luteinizing hormone
ADA	American Diabetes Association		MSH	melanocyte-stimulating hormone
ADH	antidiuretic hormone		PRL	prolactin
BMR	basal metabolic rate		PTH	parathormone (parathyroid hormone)
DM	diabetes mellitus		RAIU	radioactive iodine uptake
FBS	fasting blood sugar		STH	somatotropic hormone
FSH	follicle-stimulating hormone		TSH	thyroid-stimulating hormone
GH	growth hormone		T_3	triiodothyronine
GTT	glucose tolerance test		T_4	thyroxine

Chapter Pharmacology

Class	Effect and Uses
Adrenal Cortical Steroids	**Used in Persons With Inadequate ACTH Secretion and to Treat Addison's Disease**
aminoglutethimide (Cytadren)	Used to treat Cushing's syndrome
cortisone	Used in Addison's disease
dexamethasone (Decadron)	Used to treat allergic disorders
fludrocortisone acetate (Florinef)	Used in Addison's disease
hydrocortisone (Cortef)	Used for allergic states, respiratory disease, osteoarthritis
methylprednisolone (Medrol)	Used in allergic states
prednisolone	Used in multiple sclerosis
prednisone (Deltasone)	Used in multiple sclerosis
triamcinolone (Aristocort)	Used in respiratory disease, bronchial asthma
Antidiabetic Drugs	
(See the pharmacology section in Chapter 7)	
Antiosteoporotics	**Used to Treat and Prevent Osteoporosis Especially in Postmenopausal Women**
alendronate (Fosamax)	Used to treat osteoporosis and Paget's disease
calcitonin-salmon (Miacalcin)	Used to treat Paget's disease, postmenopausal osteoporosis
Antithyroid Drugs	**Used to Treat Hyperthyroidism**
methimazole (Tapazole)	Used to treat hyperthyroidism and goiter
propylthiouracil (PTU)	Used to treat hyperthyroidism and goiter
Growth Hormone	**Used to Treat Growth Failure That May Result From Various Causes**
somatrem (Protropin)	Injections for children who have insufficient pituitary hormone.
Posterior Pituitary Hormones	**Used for Deficits in Oxytocin or ADH**
oxytocin (Pitocin)	Improves uterine contractions to achieve early vaginal delivery when needed or for expulsion of the placenta
vasopressin (Pitressin Synthetic)	Exerts an antidiuretic effect on the kidneys
Sex Hormones	
(See the pharmacology section in Chapter 9.)	
Thyroid Drugs	**Used to Treat Hypothyroidism, to Suppress TSH, and to Diagnose Thyroid Diseases**
thyroid	Used to treat hypothyroidism
levothyroxine (Synthroid)	Used to treat hypothyroidism
liotrix (Thyrolar)	Used to treat hypothyroidism

CHAPTER REVIEW 13

▶ **BASIC UNDERSTANDING**

REVIEWING WORD PARTS

I. Write a word (prefix, suffix, or combining form) for each clue.

CROSSWORD PUZZLE 13

Across

1 living
3 gland
4 pain
9 parathyroids
11 two, but not di-
13 iodine
14 outside or outward
15 large
18 four
20 below normal
21 secrete
22 gonad
24 before or for
27 breast, but not mamm(o)
28 calcium
30 one who
31 breast, but not mast(o)
33 milk
34 difficult or painful
36 excision
37 female
39 process of recording
42 change
43 origin
44 large
45 that which causes

Down

1 two
2 tumor
3 adrenal gland
5 nerve
6 pain
7 pancreas
8 growth
9 pituitary gland
10 insulin
12 sameness or constant
16 stimulate
17 poison
19 thyroid gland
23 male
25 near or beside
26 condition
27 black
29 medicine
32 against
35 controlling
36 swelling
37 a record
38 tumor
40 pertaining to
41 one who

MATCHING

II. Match each hormone with its target gland. (Some selections will be used more than once.)

_____ 1. antidiuretic hormone   **A.** Breasts
_____ 2. follicle-stimulating hormone   **B.** Gonads
_____ 3. luteinizing hormone   **C.** Kidneys
_____ 4. oxytocin   **D.** Thyroid gland
_____ 5. thyrotropin

III. Match hormones with the glands that secrete them.

_____ 1. adrenocorticotropin   **A.** Adrenals
_____ 2. antidiuretic hormone   **B.** Gonads
_____ 3. epinephrine   **C.** Pancreas
_____ 4. follicle-stimulating hormone   **D.** Pituitary
_____ 5. growth hormone   **E.** Thyroid
_____ 6. insulin
_____ 7. luteinizing hormone
_____ 8. melanocyte-stimulating hormone
_____ 9. oxytocin
_____ 10. testosterone
_____ 11. thyrocalcitonin
_____ 12. thyrotropin
_____ 13. thyroxine

IV. Match these hormones with their principal action.

_____ 1. calcitonin   **A.** Has antidiuretic effect
_____ 2. epinephrine   **B.** Decreases blood calcium level
_____ 3. insulin   **C.** Decreases blood glucose level
_____ 4. glucocorticoids   **D.** Increases blood calcium level
_____ 5. melanocyte-stimulating hormone   **E.** Increases blood glucose level
_____ 6. mineralocorticoids   **F.** Increases heart rate and blood pressure
_____ 7. parathormone   **G.** Promotes pigmentation of skin and hair

LISTING

V. Name three mechanisms of hormonal regulation.

1. _____
2. _____
3. _____

MULTIPLE CHOICE

VI. Select one answer (A-D) for each of the following multiple choice questions:

1. Which of the following is true of an exocrine gland?
   A. does not have ducts
   B. empties onto an internal or external surface
   C. secretes its hormones into the blood stream
   D. serves only as a storage reservoir for the hormone

2. What is the cause of thyrotoxicosis?
   A. exophthalmos
   B. goiter
   C. hyperthyroidism
   D. hypothyroidism

3. What is the expected result of increased secretion of growth hormone in adults?
   A. acromegaly
   B. cretinism
   C. gigantism
   D. gonadopathy

4. A goiter is enlargement of which of the following?
   A. gonads
   B. adrenals
   C. thyroid
   D. parathyroids

5. Which of the following is _not_ an endocrine gland?
   A. adrenal gland
   B. pancreas
   C. pituitary gland
   D. sweat gland

6. Which of the following hormones produce masculine sex characteristics?
   A. androgens
   B. prolactins
   C. estrogens
   D. triiodothyronines

7. What is another name for the lactogenic hormone?
   A. lactase
   B. lactose
   C. oxytocin
   D. prolactin

8. What is the name of the radiogram produced in a diagnostic procedure that uses x-ray to study the breast?
   A. mammogram
   B. mammography
   C. radioactive iodine uptake test
   D. reduction mammoplasty

9. What is the cause of Cushing's syndrome?
   A. hypersecretion of the adrenal cortex
   B. hypersecretion of the thyroid gland
   C. hyosecretion of the adrenal cortex
   D. hyposecretion of the thyroid gland

10. Addison's disease results from deficiency in the secretion
    of which hormone?
    A. androgenic hormone
    B. adrenocortical hormone
    C. thyrotropic hormone
    D. lactogenic hormone

11. Which statement is true regarding the endocrine and nervous systems?
    A. The endocrine system accomplishes regulation through neurotransmitters.
    B. The nervous system acts primarily through the use of hormones.
    C. The two systems act independent of nervous stimulation for regulating hormones in the body.
    D. The two systems work together to maintain homeostasis.

12. Which statement is true concerning the adult female breast?
    A. During pregnancy, mammary glands undergo changes in preparation for lactation.
    B. Ejection of milk is brought about by the lactogenic hormone.
    C. Having adipose tissue makes the breast part of the endocrine system.
    D. Milk is stored in the areola until it is ejected.

WRITING TERMS
VII. Write a term for each of the following:

1. abnormally low blood sugar   _____
2. decreased activity of the adrenal gland _____
3. deficiency of insulin   _____
4. excessive calcium in the blood   _____
5. increased activity of the thyroid gland _____
6. pertaining to the breast   _____
7. pertaining to the ovaries or testes   _____
8. producing masculine characteristics   _____
9. removal of a breast   _____
10. stability in the normal body state   _____

▶ **GREATER COMPREHENSION**

SPELLING
VIII. Circle each misspelled term in the following list and write its correct spelling:

adrenocorticotropic   dwarfism   hirsutism   mamoplasty   uthryoid

INTERPRETING ABBREVIATIONS

IX. Write the meaning of each abbreviation:

1. ACTH   _____
2. ADA   _____
3. BMR   _____
4. FSH   _____
5. PTH   _____

PRONUNCIATION

X. The pronunciation of several medical terms is shown. Indicate the primary accented syllable by marking it with a ′.

1. acromegaly (**ak ro meg ə le**)
2. adrenogenital (**ə dre no jen ĭ tal**)
3. andropathy (**an drop ə the**)
4. cachexia (**kə kek se ə**)
5. colostrum (**kə los trəm**)
6. ex/ophthalmos (**ek sof thal mos**)
7. homeo/stasis (**ho me o sta sis**)
8. hyper/calc/emia (**hi pər kal se me ə**)
9. hypophysis (**hi pof ə sis**)
10. lactiferous (**lak tif ər əs**)

CATEGORIZING TERMS

XI. Categorize each of the following terms as anatomical, diagnostic, radiological, or surgical by writing A, D, R, or S:

Category (A, D, R, or S)

1. adrenalectomy   _____
2. colostrum   _____
3. hypophysis   _____
4. hypopituitarism   _____
5. mammography   _____
6. mastopexy   _____
7. melatonin   _____
8. prostaglandin   _____
9. radioactive iodine uptake test   _____
10. thyroma   _____

DRUG CLASSES

XII. Write words in the blanks to complete the class of drugs in each sentence.

1. The class of drugs used to treat persons with inadequate ACTH secretion and to treat Addison's disease is _____ _____ steroids.

2. Anti-_____ drugs are prescribed when there is inadequate insulin.

3. The class of drugs that is used to treat growth failure is growth _____.

4. When there are deficits in oxytocin or ADH, _____ pituitary hormones are prescribed.

5. A class of drugs that is used to suppress TSH and to treat hypothyroidism is _____ drugs.

(Check your answers with the solutions in Appendix V.)

Listing of Medical Terms

acromegaly	endocrine	hypophysis	oxytocin
Addison's disease	epinephrine	hypopituitarism	pancreas
adenectomy	estrogen	hyposecretion	parathormone
adenitis	exocrine	hypothalamus	parathyroids
adenocarcinoma	exophthalmos	hypothyroidism	pineal gland
adenohypophysis	fibrocystic	insulin	pituitary cachexia
adenoma	follicle-stimulating hormone	intermammary	pituitary gland
adenopathy	gestational diabetes	islets of Langerhans	polydipsia
adrenal	gigantism	lactation	polyphagia
adrenal cortex	glucagon	lactiferous	polyuria
adrenal medulla	glucocorticoid	lactogenesis	progesterone
adrenalectomy	goiter	lactogenic hormone	prolactin
adrenaline	gonadal	lumpectomy	prostaglandin
adrenalitis	gonadotropic hormone	luteinizing hormone	retromammary
adrenitis	gonadotropin	mammalgia	somatotropic
adrenocorticotropic	gynecomastia	mammary gland	somatotropin
adrenocorticotropin	hirsutism	mammogram	suprarenal
adrenomegaly	homeostasis	mammography	target organ
adrenopathy	hormonal	mammoplasty	testosterone
aldosterone	hormone	mastalgia	tetraiodothyronine
androgen	human chorionic	mastectomy	thymosin
androgenic	gonadotropin	mastitis	thymus
adrenogenital	hyperadrenalism	mastocarcinoma	thyrocalcitonin
andropathy	hypercalcemia	mastodynia	thyroid
antidiuretic hormone	hyperglycemia	mastopexy	thyroidectomy
antiosteoporotic	hyperinsulinism	mastoptosis	thyroiditis
antithyroid	hyperparathyroidism	mastorrhagia	thyroma
cachexia	hyperpituitarism	medulla	thyropathy
colostrum	hypersecretion	melanin	thyrotoxicosis
cortex	hyperthyroidism	melanocyte-stimulating	thyrotropin
cortisone	hypoadrenalism	hormone	thyroxine
cretinism	hypocalcemia	melatonin	triiodothyronine
Cushing's syndrome	hypoglycemia	mineralocorticosteroid	trophic
diabetes insipidus	hypogonadism	myxedema	
diabetes mellitus	hypoinsulinism	neurohypophysis	
dwarfism	hypoparathyroidism	norepinephrine	

Español ## *Enhancing Spanish Communication*

English	Spanish (pronunciation)	English	Spanish (pronunciation)
adrenal	suprarenal (soo-prah-ray-NAHL)	growth	crecimiento (cray-se-me-EN-to)
adrenalin	adrenalina (ah-dray-nah-LEE-nah)	hormone	hormona (or-MOH-nah)
augmentation	aumento (ah-oo-MEN-to)	insulin	insulina (in-soo-LEE-nah)
beard	barba (BAR bah)	iodine	yodo (YO-do)
breasts	senos (SAY-nos)	masculine	masculino (mas-coo-LEE-no)
calcium	calcio (CAHL-se-o)	nipple	pezón (pay-SON)
diabetes	diabetes (de-ah-BAY-tes)	pancreas	páncreas (PAHN-cray-as)
dwarf	enano (AY-nah-no)	pituitary	pituitario (pe-too-e-TAH-re-o)
giant	gigante (he-GAHN-tay)	same	mismo (MEES-mo)
gland	glándula (GLAN-doo-lah)	synthesis	síntesis (SEEN-tay-sis)
glucose	glucosa (gloo-CO-sah)	thyroid	tiroides (te-RO-e-des)
goiter	papera (pah-PAY-rah)		

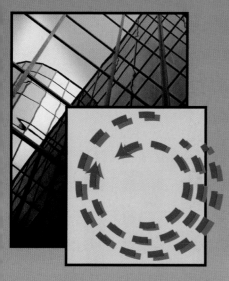

Basic Terminology: Review of Chapters 1 through 13

14

Learning Goals

After completing Chapters 1 through 13, you will be able to do the following:

1. Write or choose the correct meaning of more than 450 word parts.
2. Understand and write anatomical, diagnostic, radiological, surgical, and therapeutic terms.
3. Describe the major radiographic imaging techniques.
4. Demonstrate understanding of basic pharmacological terms.
5. Differentiate between the functions of the body systems and the major structures of those systems.

It is advisable to work all exercises in this chapter, including the crossword puzzle. It is an excellent test of memory of many word parts you have learned. It is preferable to work the entire review before checking your answers. Discuss the expected degree of accuracy with your instructor, but it should be quite high. It is suggested that you review all chapter reviews, including the Greater Comprehension sections.

REVIEWING WORD PARTS

I. Write a prefix, suffix, or combining form for each clue.

CROSSWORD PUZZLE 14

Across

1 hard
3 pus
4 without
7 sugar
9 milk
12 organs of reproduction
14 many
15 toward
18 white
19 vein
20 pain
21 away from
22 nail
26 behind
27 female
29 hair
31 incision (suffix)
34 lip
38 development
40 back
41 pain
42 carbon dioxide
43 yellow, fatty plaque
45 hardening
48 tumor
50 suture
53 enzyme

55 uterus
56 three
58 vagina
59 vomiting
60 air
61 brain
63 gums
64 condition
66 fungus
67 surgical puncture
69 softening
71 color
74 stiff
75 uterine tube
80 common bile duct
81 excision
83 inside
84 secrete (suffix)
85 feeling (combining form)
86 sensitivity to pain
88 kidney
89 head
90 cartilage
92 large intestine
94 ovary
95 narrowing
96 umbilicus

Down

2 starch
4 without
5 sameness
6 self
7 origin
8 skull
10 green
11 tooth
12 stomach
13 embryonic form
14 speech
16 tear
17 bile
19 after
23 equal
24 movement
25 against
26 digestion
28 irrigation
30 black
32 bad
33 killing
34 break
35 liver
36 ductus deferens
37 abdominal wall

39 mouth
41 joint
42 skin
44 normal
46 neck
47 red
49 beginning
50 rupture
51 chest
52 hemorrhage
54 upon
57 thirst
62 eyelid
65 blood
66 obsessive preoccupation
68 near
70 weakness
71 hidden
72 cancer
73 cramp
74 coal
76 eye
77 tongue
78 aged
79 heart
82 one
87 extremity
91 through

► CHAPTER 2

MATCHING

II. Match the specialists with the major area to which their practice is devoted.

_____ 1. endocrinologist	**A.**	Children
_____ 2. gerontologist	**B.**	Ear, nose, and throat
_____ 3. gynecologist	**C.**	Eye
_____ 4. ophthalmologist	**D.**	Females
_____ 5. otolaryngologist	**E.**	Heart
	F.	Hormonal system
	G.	Nervous system
	H.	Older persons
	I.	Radiant energy
	J.	Skin

MEDICAL SPECIALTIES

III. Write a medical term for each of the following definitions.

1. children's dental specialist _____
2. pertaining to the heart _____
3. pertaining to the mouth _____
4. subjective evidence of disease _____
5. the study of tumors _____

▶ CHAPTER 3

MATCHING
IV. Match each directional term with its meaning.

_____ 1. anterior   **A.** Above
_____ 2. dorsal   **B.** Back
_____ 3. lateral   **C.** Below
_____ 4. proximal   **D.** Far
_____ 5. superior   **E.** Front
               F. Middle
               G. Near
               H. Side

WRITING TERMS
V. Write a medical term for each of the following definitions.

1. cramping of the hand   _____
2. inflammation of the eye   _____
3. difficult movement   _____
4. incision of the eyelid   _____
5. lying face downward   _____

▶ CHAPTER 4

FILL IN THE BLANKS
VI. Write a letter in each blank to complete these sentences.

1. A pigment that is dark brown to black is __ __ __ __ __in.

2. Receiving a vaccination provides __ __ __ __ __ __ immunity.

3. The cell that transports oxygen is the __ __ __ __ __ __ __ cyte.

4. The degree of disease-causing capability of an organism is called v__ __ __ __ __ __ __ __ __.

5. The term a__ __ __ __ __ __ __ means having no tendency to repair itself or develop into new tissue.

WRITING TERMS
VII. Write a medical term for each of the following.

1. increase in the number of leukocytes   _____
2. irregularly shaped red blood cell   _____
3. red pigment of red blood cells   _____
4. resembling mucus   _____
5. within a cell   _____

▶ CHAPTER 5

FILL IN THE BLANKS
VIII. Write a letter in each blank to complete these sentences.

1. Blood vessels that supply blood to the heart are c__ __ __ __ __ __ __ arteries.

2. The heart and the blood vessels are c__ __ __ __ __ __ __ __ __ __ __ __ structures.

3. The largest artery is the a__ __ __ __.

4. The route that blood takes when it leaves the heart, travels throughout the body, and returns to the heart is the s__ __ __ __ __ __ __ circulation.

5. The thymus, the tonsils, vessels, nodes, and a special fluid make up the l__ __ __ __ __ __ __ __ system, which is part of the circulatory system.

WRITING TERMS
IX. Write a medical term for each of the following:

1. a tumor composed of lymph vessels   _____
2. absence of a heart beat   _____
3. decreased pulse   _____
4. increased blood pressure   _____
5. inner lining of the heart   _____

▶ CHAPTER 6

FILL IN THE BLANKS
X. Write a letter in each blank to complete these sentences.

1. A device that measures oxygen in the blood is called a pulse o__ __ __ __ __ __ __.

2. A condition of the lungs caused by inhalation of dust is pneum__ __ __ __ __ __ __ __ __.

3. A tumorlike growth that projects from a mucous membrane is a p__ __ __ __ __.

4. Rapid breathing is t__ __ __ __ __ __ __ __.

5. Effusion of fluid into the air spaces and tissues spaces of the lungs is pulmonary e__ __ __ __.

WRITING TERMS
XI. Write a medical term for each of the following.

1. air sacs of the lungs   _____
2. difficult breathing   _____
3. direct visualization of the bronchi   _____
4. inflammation of the nasal membranes   _____
5. within the windpipe   _____

▶ CHAPTER **7**

MATCHING

XII. Match terms in the left column with meanings in the right column.

_____ 1. fissure	**A.** Abnormal opening
_____ 2. fistula	**B.** Cracklike cleft or groove
_____ 3. hernia	**C.** Decay
_____ 4. lavage	**D.** Hemorrhage
_____ 5. ulcer	**E.** Irrigation of an organ
	F. Open sore or lesion
	G. Protrusion of an organ through the wall of a cavity
	H. Suture

WRITING TERMS

XIII. Write a medical term for each of the following.

1. enzyme that breaks down milk sugar   _____
2. excessive vomiting   _____
3. incision of the vagus nerve   _____
4. inflammation of the gallbladder   _____
5. visual inspection of the pylorus   _____

▶ CHAPTER **8**

FILL IN THE BLANKS

XIV. Write a letter in each blank to complete these sentences.

1. A toxic condition that occurs when the kidneys fail to function properly is u__ __ __ __ __.

2. Abnormal softening of the kidney is nephro__ __ __ __ __ __ __.

3. Inflammation of the renal pelvis is __ __ __ __ itis.

4. Surgical crushing of a stone is litho__ __ __ __ __ __.

5. The reservoir for urine until it is excreted is the b__ __ __ __ __ __.

WRITING TERMS

XV. Write a medical term for each of the following.

1. examination of the bladder interior   _____
2. functional unit of the kidney   _____
3. herniation of the urethra   _____
4. sugar in the urine   _____
5. ultrasound of the kidney   _____

▶ **CHAPTER 9**

MATCHING

XVI. Match terms in the left column with meanings in the right column. (Some choices will not be used, and some will be used more than once.)

_____ 1. ovary   **A.** A gamete

_____ 2. ovum   **B.** A gonad

_____ 3. spermatazoon   **C.** Normal site of implantation

_____ 4. testis   **D.** Product of fertilization

_____ 5. uterine tube   **E.** Receives the sperm during intercourse

_____ 6. zygote   **F.** Usual site of fertilization

WRITING TERMS

XVII. Write a medical term for each of the following.

1. a female pregnant for the first time   _____

2. a newborn child   _____

3. surgial fixation of the uterus   _____

4. the first occurrence of menstruation   _____

5. undescended testicle   _____

▶ **CHAPTER 10**

MATCHING

XVIII. Match the types of body movements with their meanings in the right column.

_____ 1. abduction   **A.** Circular movement of a limb

_____ 2. adduction   **B.** Movement of a bone around an axis

_____ 3. extension   **C.** Movement of the sole of the foot inward

_____ 4. flexion   **D.** Movement of the sole of the foot outward

_____ 5. inversion   **E.** Rotation that allows the palm of the hand to turn up

                     F. Rotation that turns the palm of the hand backward (down)

                     G. To bend

                     H. To bring together

                     I. To straighten

                     J. To take away

WRITING TERMS

XIX. Write a medical term for each of the following.

1. any disease of the joints   _____

2. deficiency of calcium in the body   _____

3. excision of the tailbone   _____

4. lateral curvature of the spine   _____

5. wrist bones   _____

► CHAPTER 11

FILL IN THE BLANKS
XX. Write a letter in each blank to complete the terms in the following.

1. The term for a cytoplasmic projection that carries impulses away from the body of the nerve cell is a__ __ __.

2. An irrational fear of heights is acro__ __ __ __ __ __ .

3. Membranes that cover the brain and spinal cord are m__ __ __ __ __ __ __.

4. The basic unit of the nervous system is the n__ __ __ __ __.

5. T__ __ __ __ __ receptors are capable of detecting changes in temperature.

WRITING TERMS
XXI. Write a medical term for each of the following.

1. excessive preoccupation with fire   _____
2. incision of the lacrimal sac   _____
3. paralysis of one side of the body   _____
4. surgical crushing of a nerve   _____
5. within the skull   _____

► CHAPTER 12

FILL IN THE BLANKS
XXII. Write a letter in each blank to complete the following.

1. A large blister is called a b__ __ __ __.

2. A nonelevated, discolored spot on the skin is a m__ __ __ __ __.

3. A term that means pertaining to the skin is c__ __ __ __ __ __ __ __.

4. Pertaining to fat is a__ __ __ __ __ __.

5. The oily material that keeps hair and skin soft is called s__ __ __ __.

WRITING TERMS
XXIII. Write a medical term for each of the following.

1. destruction of tissue using cold temperatures   _____
2. fungal disease of the nails   _____
3. inflammation of a sweat gland   _____
4. outermost layers of the skin   _____
5. resembling hair   _____

▶ **CHAPTER 13**

FILL IN THE BLANKS

XXIV. Write a letter in each blank to complete the terms in the following.

1. A relative constancy in the internal state of the body is h__ __ __ __ __ __ __ __ __ __.

2. Anti__ __ __ __ __ __ __ __ hormone causes resorption of water by the kidneys.

3. The gland that is called "the master gland" is the p__ __ __ __ __ __ __ __ __.

4. The breasts are the m__ __ __ __ __ __ glands.

5. The posterior lobe of the pituitary is called the neuro__ __ __ __ __ __ __ __ __ __ .

WRITING TERMS

XXV. Write a medical term for each of the following.

1. below normal blood sugar level   _____
2. cancerous tumor of a gland   _____
3. decreased parathyroid activity   _____
4. normal thyroid activity   _____
5. removal of the adrenal glands   _____

▶ **ALL CHAPTERS**

MATCHING

XXVI. Match body systems with their functions.

_____ 1. cardiovascular system   **A.** Acquires and provides nutrition
_____ 2. digestive system   **B.** Cooperates with the nervous system to provide movement; manufactures erythrocytes
_____ 3. endocrine system   **C.** Delivers oxygen and nutrients to all cells of the body
_____ 4. integumentary system   **D.** Filters the blood and excretes waste products
_____ 5. lymphatic system   **E.** Produces new individuals to assure continuation of the species
_____ 6. nervous system   **F.** Provides protection by covering the body
_____ 7. respiratory system   **G.** Provides homeostasis by cooperating with the nervous system through the use of hormones
_____ 8. reproductive system   **H.** Provides oxygen and expels waste carbon dioxide
_____ 9. skeletal system   **I.** Returns excess interstitial fluid to the bloodstream
_____ 10. urinary system   **J.** Serves as control center and communications network

XXVII. Match structures with the body system (A through J) that corresponds with their major function.

_____ 1. adrenal   _____ 12. prostate   **A.** Cardiovascular system
_____ 2. alveoli   _____ 13. sebaceous   **B.** Digestive system
_____ 3. aorta   gland   **C.** Endocrine system
_____ 4. axon   _____ 14. spleen   **D.** Integumentary system
_____ 5. cerebrum   _____ 15. stomach   **E.** Lymphatic system
_____ 6. cranium   _____ 16. trachea   **F.** Nervous system
_____ 7. epidermis   _____ 17. uterine   **G.** Reproductive system
_____ 8. gallbladder   tube   **H.** Respiratory system
_____ 9. heart   _____ 18. ureter   **I.** Skeletal system
_____ 10. patella   **J.** Urinary system
_____ 11. pituitary

(Check your answers with the solutions in Appendix V.)

Medical Abbreviations

AB	abortion
abd	abdomen, abdominal
ABO	blood groups
ac	before meals *(ante cibum)*
ACh	acetylcholine
ACTH	adrenocorticotropic hormone
AD	admitting diagnosis; right ear *(auris dextra)*
ADA	American Diabetes Association
ADD	attention deficit disorder
ADH	antidiuretic hormone
ADHD	attention-deficit hyperactivity disorder
ad lib.	freely as needed; at pleasure
ADL	activities of daily living
AFB	acid-fast bacillus
AFP	alpha-fetoprotein (abnormal finding in certain liver diseases or embryonic cells)
A/G	albumin/globulin ratio
AGN	acute glomerulonephritis
AHF	antihemophilic factor
AI	aortic insufficiency
AIDS	acquired immunodeficiency syndrome
ALL	acute lymphoblastic leukemia
ALP	alkaline phosphatase (liver function test)
ALS	amyotropic lateral sclerosis
AMA	American Medical Association
AML	acute myelogenous leukemia
ANA	antinuclear antibody
ANS	autonomic nervous system
AP	anteroposterior
aq	water *(aqua)*
ARC	AIDS-related complex
ARDS	adult respiratory distress syndrome
ARRT	American Registry of Radiologic Technologists
AS	left ear *(auris sinistra)*
ASD	atrial septal defect
ASHD	arteriosclerotic heart disease
ATS	anxiety tension state

AV, A-V	atrioventricular
BaE	barium enema
b.i.d.	twice a day *(bis in die)*
b.i.n.	twice a night *(bis in noctis)*
BK	below knee
BMR	basal metabolic rate
BP	blood pressure
BPH	benign prostatic hypertrophy
BSA	body surface area
BUN	blood urea nitrogen
BX	biopsy
C	Celsius; centigrade
C & S	culture and sensitivity
C-1, C-2, etc.	cervical vertebrae
Ca	calcium; cancer
CA	cancer; chronologic age
CABG	coronary atery bypass graft
CAD	coronary artery disease
CAL	chronic airflow limitation
CBC	complete blood count
CCU	critical care unit
CDC	Centers for Disease Control and Prevention
CGN	chronic glomerulonephritis
CHD	coronary heart disease
CHF	congestive heart failure
CK (CPK)	creatine kinase (formerly called creatine phosphokinase), enzyme released by damaged heart or other skeletal muscle)
CNS	central nervous system
COLD	chronic obstructive lung disease
COPD	chronic obstructive pulmonary disease
CPD	cephalopelvic disproportion
CPR	cardiopulmonary resuscitation
CRF	chronic renal failure
CS	central service or central supply; cesarean section
C-section	cesarean section
CSF	cerebrospinal fluid
CSM	cerebrospinal meningitis
CT, CAT	computed tomography
CTS	carpal tunnel syndrome
CUG	cystourethrogram
CVA	costovertebral angle; cerebrovascular accident
CVOD	cerebrovascular obstructive disease
Cx	cervix
CXR	chest x-ray
cysto	cytoscopic examination
D	dose; right *(dexter)*
D & C	dilatation and curettage (dilation and curettage)
DES	diethylstilbestrol (a synthetic estrogen; females who are exposed in utero are subject to increased risk of vaginal or cervical carcinomas)
diff	differential count (WBCs)
DIC	disseminated intravascular coagulation
DIP	distal interphalangeal
DIPJ	distal interphalangeal joint
DJD	degenerative joint disease
DLE	discoid lupus erythematosus
DM	diabetes mellitus
DMARDs	disease-modifying antirheumatic drugs

DOA	dead on arrival
DOB	date of birth
DSM	Diagnostic and Statistical Manual of Mental Disorders
DT	delirium tremens
DTR	deep tendon reflex
Dx	diagnosis
EAHF	eczema, asthma, and hay fever
ECG, EKG	electrocardiogram
ECHO	(enteric cytopathogenic human orphan) virus
EDD	expected delivery date
EEG	electroencephalogram
EFM	electronic fetal monitor (embryonic cells)
ELISA	enzyme-linked immunosorbent assay (commonly used in AIDS diagnosis)
EMG	electromyogram
EMI	electrical and musical induction (brain scanner)
ENT	ear, nose, and throat
EOM	extraocular movements
ER	emergency room
ESR	erythrocyte sedimentation rate
ESWL	extracorporeal shockwave lithotripsy
ET	endotracheal
F	Fahrenheit
FANA	fluorescent antinuclear antibody
FB	foreign body
FBS	fasting blood sugar
FHR	fetal heart rate
FHS	fetal heart sound
FHT	fetal heart tone
FSH	follicle-stimulating hormone
fx	fracture
G	gravida (pregnant)
GA	gastric analysis
GB	gallbladder
GC	gonococcus
GFR	glomerular filtration rate
GI	gastrointestinal
GP	general practice or practitioner
GTT	glucose tolerance test
GU	genitourinary
Gyn	gynecology
Hb, Hgb	hemoglobin
HBV	hepatitis B virus
HCG	human chorionic gonadotropin
HCT	hematocrit
HCV	hepatitis C virus
HDV	hepatitis D virus
HgA, HgC, HgE, HgF, HgS	hemoglobins A, C, E, F, and S
HGH	human growth hormone
HIV	human immunodeficiency virus
h/o	history of
HPF	high power field
HPV	human papillomavirus
HSV	herpes simplex virus
HSV 1	herpes simplex virus type 1 (oral herpes)
HSV 2	herpes simplex virus type 2 (genital herpes)
H/U	history of
Hx	history
IC	irritable colon

ICP	intracranial pressure
ICU	intensive care unit
IDDM	insulin-dependent diabetes mellitus
IgA, IgD, IgG, IgM, IgE	immunoglobulins
I & D	incision and drainage
I & O	intake and output
IBD	inflammatory bowel disease
IM	intramuscular
IRDS	infant respiratory distress syndrome
IU	international unit
IUD	intrauterine device
IV	intravenous
IVC	intravenous cholangiogram
IVP	intravenous pyelogram
jt	joint
KJ	knee jerk
KUB	kidney, ureter, bladder
L-1, L-2, etc.	lumbar vertebrae
LA	left atrium
lat.	lateral
LCA	left coronary artery
LDH	lactate dehydrogenase (enzyme elevated after MI)
LE	lupus erythematosus
LH	luteinizing hormone
lig	ligament
LLL	left lower lobe
LLQ	left lower quadrant
LMP	last menstrual period
LPF	low power field
LPN	licensed practical nurse
LUL	left upper lobe
LUQ	left upper quadrant
LS	lumbosacral
LV	left ventricle
LVN	licensed vocational nurse
MA	mental age
MCA	middle cerebral artery
MCH	mean corpuscular hemoglobin (amount of Hb in each RBC)
MCHC	mean corpuscular hemoglobin concentration (amount of Hb per unit of blood)
MCV	mean corpuscular volume (size of individual RBC)
MI	myocardial infarction
MMPI	Minnesota Multiphasic Personality Inventory
MRI or RI	magnetic resonance imaging
MS	multiple sclerosis
MSH	melanocyte-stimulating hormone
MVP	mitral valve prolapse
NB	newborn
NG tube	nasogastric tube
NGU	nongonococcal urethritis
NIDDM	noninsulin-dependent diabetes mellitus
noct	night
NPO, npo	nothing by mouth *(non per os)*
NSAID	nonsteroidal antiinflammatory drugs
OA	occipital artery
OB	obstetrics
OB-GYN	obstetrics and gynecology
OCG	oral cholangiogram
OD	right eye *(oculus dexter);* overdose

omn hor	every hour (*omni hora*)
OPS	outpatient service
OR	operating room
OT	occupational therapy
OTC	over the counter (drug that can be obtained without a prescription)
PA	posteroanterior or physician assistant
pH	potential of hydrogen
PaO_2	partial pressure of arterial oxygen
Pap	Papanicolaou smear, stain, or test
PAT	paroxysmal atrial tachycardia
path	pathology
PCV	packed cell volume
PE	physical examination
PEG	pneumoencephalography
PET	positron emission tomography
PFT	pulmonary function test
PKU	phenylketonuria
PMN	polymorphonuclear
PMS	premenstrual syndrome
PNS	peripheral nervous system
po	by mouth (*per os*)
PP	after meals (*postprandial*)
PRL	prolactin
p.r.n.	as the occasion arises, as needed (*pro re nata*)
Pt	patient
PT	physical therapy; prothrombin time
PTA	percutaneous transluminal angioplasty
PTCA	percutaneous transluminal coronary angioplasty
PTH	parathormone
PTT	partial thromboplastin time
PU	peptic ulcer
PVC	premature ventricular contractions
Px	physical examination
q.d.	every day (*quaque die*)
q.h.	every hour (*quaque hora*)
q.i.d.	four times a day (*quantum in die*)
R	radiology; roentgen; respiration
RA	rheumatoid arthritis; right atrium
rad	radiation absorbed dose
RAIU	radioactive iodine uptake
RBC	red blood cell; red blood cell count
RCA	right coronary artery
RDAs	recommended dietary/daily allowances
RDS	respiratory distress syndrome
REM	rapid eye movement
RES	reticuloendothelial system
RF	rheumatoid factor
Rh	rhesus factor in blood
RLL	right lower lobe
RLQ	right lower quadrant
RN	registered nurse
ROM	range of motion
RP	retrograde pyelogram
RUL	right upper lobe
RUQ	right upper quadrant
RV	right ventricle

Rx	prescription
SA	sinoatrial
SaO$_2$	arterial oxygen saturation
SCI	spinal cord injury
segs	segmented neutrophils
SG	skin graft
SGOT, SGPT	enzyme tests of liver function
SI	sacroiliac
SIDS	sudden infant death syndrome
SLE	systemic lupus erythematosus
SLR	straight leg raising
SNS	somatic nervous system
SOB	shortness of breath
stat	immediately *(statim)*
STD	sexually transmitted disease
STH	somatotropic hormone
subq	subcutaneous
Sx	symptom
T-1, T-2, etc.	thoracic vertebrae
T$_3$	triiodothyronine
T$_4$	thyroxine
T & A	tonsillectomy and adenoidectomy
TAH	total abdominal hysterectomy
TB	tuberculosis
TENS	transcutaneous electrical nerve stimulator
TIA	transient ischemic attack
t.i.d.	three times a day *(ter in die)*
TMJ	temporomandibular joint
TPN	total parenteral nutrition
TSH	thyroid-stimulating hormone
TTO	transtracheal oxygen
TUR, TURP	transurethral resection of the prostate
Tx	traction or treatment
U/A	urinalysis
UGI	upper gastrointestinal
ung	ointment
URI	upper respiratory tract infection
UTI	urinary tract infection
UV	ultraviolet
VCUG	voiding cystourethrogram
VC	vital capacity
VD	venereal disease
VDRL	Venereal Disease Research Laboratory (also test for syphilis)
VS, v.s.	vital signs
WBC	white blood cells or count
WNL	within normal limits
XP or XPD	xeroderma pigmentosum

English-Spanish Translation of Selected Terms

APPENDIX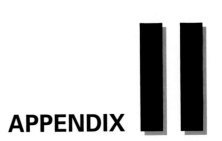

II

English	Spanish (pronunciation)
abdomen	abdomen (ab-DOH-men), vientre (ve-EN-tray)
acidity	acidez (ah-se-DES)
acute	agudo (ah-GOO-do)
adrenal	suprarenal (soo-prah-ray-NAHL)
adrenaline	adrenalina (ah-dray-nah-LEE-nah)
aged	envejecido (en-vay-hay-SEE-do)
allergy	alergia (ah-LEHR-he-ah)
augmentation	aumento (ah-oo-MEN-to)
anemia	anemia (ah-NAY-me-ah)
anesthesia	anestesia (ah-nes-TAY-se-ah)
anesthetic	anestésico (ah-nes-TAY-se-co)
ankle	tobillo (to-BEEL-lyo)
antibiotic	antibiótico (an-te-be-O-te-co)
anxiety	ansiedad (an-se-ay-DAHD)
appendix	apéndice (ah-PEN-de-say)
appetite	apetito (ah-pay-TEE-to)
arm	brazo (BRAH-so)
armpit	sobaco (so-BAH-co)
artery	arteria (ar-TAY-re-ah)
asphyxia	asfixia (as-FEEC-se-ah)
asthma	asma (AHS-mah)
augmentation	aumento (ah-oo-MEN-to)
back	espalda (es-PAHL-dah)
beard	barba (BAR-bah)
belch	eructo (ay-ROOK-to)
belly	barriga (bar-REE-gah)
benign	benigno (bay-NEEG-no)
biopsy	biopsia (be-OP-see-ah)
birth	nacimiento (nah-se-me-EN-to)
black	negro (NAY-gro)
bladder	vejiga (vah-HEE-gah)
blood	sangre (SAHN-gray)
blood pressure	presión sanguínea (pray-se-ON san-GEE-nay-ah)
blood sample	muestra de sangre (moo-AYS-tah de SAHN-gray)
blue	azul (ah-SOOL)

English	Spanish (pronunciation)
body	cuerpo (coo-ERR-po)
bone	hueso (oo-AY-so)
brain	cerebro (say-RAY-bro)
breasts	senos (SAY-nos)
breathe	alentar (ah-len-TAR), respirar (res-pe-RAR)
breathing	respiración (res-pe-rah-se-ON)
burn	quemadura (kay-mah-DOO-rah)
calcium	calcio (CAHL-se-o)
calculus	cálculo (CAHL-coo-lo)
cancer	cáncer (CAHN-ser)
capillary	capilar (cah-pe-LAR)
cartilage	cartílago (car-TEE-lah-go)
catheter	catéter (cah-TAY-ter)
cheek	mejilla (may-HEEL-lyah)
chest	pecho (PAY-cho)
chew, to	masticar (mas-te-CAR)
child	niña (NEE-nya), niño (NEE-nyo)
childbirth	parto (PAR-to)
cholesterol	cholesterol (co-les-tay-ROL)
chronic	crónico (CRO-ne-co)
circumcision	circumcisión (ser-coon-se-se-ON)
clot	coágulo (co-AH-goo-lo)
collarbone	clavícula (clah-VEE-coo-lah)
conception	concepción (con-sep-se-ON)
concussion	concusión (con-coo-se-ON)
condom	condón (con-DON)
conscious	consciente (cons-se-EN-tay)
consciousness	conciencia (con-se-EN-se-ah)
constipation	estreñimiento (es-tray-nye-me-EN-to)
contraception	contracepción (con-trah-cep-se-ON)
convulsion	convulsión (con-vool-se-ON)
cough	tos (tos)
cranium	cráneo (CRAH-nay-o)
cream	crema (CRAY-mah)
cry, to	llorar (lyo-RAR)
defecate	evacuar (ay-vah-coo-AR)
dentist	dentista (den-TEES-tah)
dermatology	dermatología (der-mah-to-lo-HEE-ah)
destruction	destrucción (des-trooc-se-ON)
diabetes	diabetes (de-ah-BAY-tes)
diagnosis	diagnosis (de-ag-NO-ses)
diagnostic	diagnóstico (de-ag-NOS-te-co)
dialysis	diálisis (de-AH-le-sis)
diaphragm	diafragma (de-ah-FRAHG-mah)
diarrhea	diarrea (de-ar-RAY-ah)
digestion	digestión (de-hes-te-ON)
disease	enfermedad (en-fer-may-DAHD)
dizziness	vértigo (VERR-te-go)
dwarf	enano (ay-NAH-no)
ear	oreja (o-RAY-hah)
edema	hidropesía (e-dro-pay-SEE-ah)
elbow	codo (CO-do)
electricity	electricidad (ay-lec-tre-se-DAHD)
enzyme	enzima (en-SEE-mah)
epilepsy	epilepsia (ay-pe-LEP-se-ah)

English	Spanish (pronunciation)
erect, straight	derecho (day-RAY-cho)
erection	erección (ay-rec-se-ON)
esophagus	esófago (ay-SO-fah-go)
excretion	excreción (ex-cray-se-ON)
extremity	extremidad (ex-tray-me-DAHD)
eye	ojo (O-ho)
eyeball	globo del ojo (GLO-bo del O-ho)
eyebrow	ceja (SAY-hah)
eyelash	pestaña (pes-TAH-nyah)
eyelid	párpado (PAR-pah-do)
face	cara (CAH-rah)
fainting	languidez (lan-gee-DES), desmayo (des-MAH-yo)
fatigue	fatiga (fah-TEE-gah)
fear	miedo (me-AY-do)
feces	excremento (ex-cray-MEN-to)
feminine	femenina (fay-may-NEE-na)
fetus	feto (FAY-to)
fever	fiebre (fe-AY-bray)
fiber	fibra (FEE-brah)
finger	dedo (DAY-do)
fingerprint	impresión digital (im-pray-se-ON de-he-TAHL)
fire	fuego (foo-AY-go)
fluid	fluido (floo-EE-do)
foam	espuma (es-POO-mah)
foot (pl., feet)	pie (PE-ay), pies (PE-ays)
forearm	antebrazo (an-tay-BRAH-so)
fracture	fractura (frac-TOO-rah)
gallbladder	vesícula biliar (vay-SEE-coo-la be-le-AR)
gallstone	cálculo biliar (CAHL-coo-lo be-le-AR)
giant	gigante (he-GAHN-tay)
gland	glándula (GLAN-doo-lah)
goiter	papera (pah-PAY-rah)
glucose	glucosa (gloo-CO-sah)
gray	gris (grees)
green	verde (VERR-day)
growth	crecimiento (cray-se-me-EN-to)
gum, gingiva	encía (en-SEE-ah)
gynecology	ginecología (he-nay-co-lo-HEE-ah)
hair	pelo (PAY-lo)
hand	mano (MAH-no)
head	cabeza (cah-BAY-sah)
headache	dolor de cabeza (do-LOR day cah-BAY-sa)
heart	corazón (co-rah-SON)
heat	calor (cah-LOR)
heel	talón (tah-LON)
hemorrhage	hemorragia (ay-mor-RAH-he-ah)
hernia	hernia (AYR-ne-ah), quebradura (kay-brah-DOO-rah)
high blood pressure	hipertensión, presión alta (e-per-ten-se-ON, pray-se-ON AHL-tah)
hip	cadera (cah-DAY-rah)
hives	roncha (RON-chah)
hormone	hormona (or-MOH-nah)
hunger	hambre (AHM-bray)
hypodermic	hipodérmico (e-po-DER-me-co)
imperfect	imperfecto (im-per-FEC-to)

English	Spanish (pronunciation)
impotency	impotencia (im-po-TEN-se-ah)
inflammation	inflamación (in-flah-mah-se-ON)
influenza	gripe (GREE-pay)
injection	inyección (in-yec-se-ON)
injury	daño (DAH-nyo)
instrument	instrumento (ins-troo-MEN-to)
insulin	insulina (in-soo-LEE-nah)
intercourse, sexual	cópula (CO-poo-lah)
intestine	intestino (in-tes-TEE-no)
iodine	yodo (YO-do)
jaw	mandíbula (man-DEE-boo-lah)
joint	articulación (ar-te-coo-lah-se-ON), coyuntura (co-yoon-TOO-rah)
kidney	riñón (ree-NYON)
knee	rodilla (ro-DEEL-lyah)
kneecap	rótula (RO-too-lah)
laxative	purgante (poor-GAHN-tay)
leg	pierna (pe-ERR-nah)
leukemia	leucemia (lay-oo-SAY-me-ah)
life	vida (VEE-dah)
ligament	ligamento (le-gah-MEN-to)
light	luz (loos)
lips	labios (LAH-be-os)
liver	hígado (EE-ga-do)
lobe	lóbulo (LO-boo-lo)
lung	pulmón (pool-MON)
lymph	linfa (LEEN-fah)
lymphatic	linfático (lin-FAH-te-co)
malignant	maligno (mah-LEEG-no)
masculine	masculino (mas-coo-LEE-no)
membrane	membrana (mem-BRAH-nah)
menopause	menopausia (may-no-PAH-oo-se-ah)
menstruation	menstruación (mens-troo-ah-se-ON)
microscope	microscopio (me-cros-CO-pe-o)
milk	leche (LAY-chay)
mind	mente (MEN-te)
mouth	boca (BO-cah)
movement	movimiento (mo-ve-me-EN-to)
mucus	moco (MO-co)
murmur	murmullo (moor-MOOL-lyo)
muscle	músculo (MOOS-coo-lo)
nails	uñas (OO-nyahs)
narcotic	narcótico (nar-CO-te-co)
narrow	estrecho (es-TRAY-cho)
navel	ombligo (om-BLEE-go)
neck	cuello (coo-EL-lyo)
nerve	nervio (NERR-ve-o)
nervous	nervioso (ner-ve-O-so)
neurology	neurología (nay-oo-ro-lo-HEE-ah)
newborn	recién nacida (ray-se-EN nah-SEE-dah)
nipple	pezón (pay-SON)
nose	nariz (nah-REES)
nostril	orificio de la nariz (or-e-FEE-se-o day lah nah-REES)
nutrition	nutrición (noo-tre-se-ON)
obstruction	obstrucción (obs-trooc-se-ON)

English	Spanish (pronunciation)
optic	óptico (OP-te-co)
optician	óptico (OP-te-co)
orange (color)	anaranjado (ah-nah-ran-HAH-do), naranjado (nah-ran-HAH-do)
orthodontist	ortodóntico (or-to-DON-te-co)
ovarian	ovárico (o-VAH-re-co)
ovary	ovario (o-VAH-re-o)
oxygen	oxígeno (ok-SEE-hay-no)
pain	dolor (do-LOR)
painful	doloroso (do-lo-RO-so)
palm	palma (PAHL-mah)
pancreas	páncreas (PAHN-cray-as)
paralysis	parálisis (pah-RAH-le-sis)
parasite	parásito (pah-RAH-se-to)
parturition	parto (PAR-to)
pathology	patología (pah-to-lo-HEE-ah)
penis	pene (PAY-nay)
perspiration	sudor (soo-DOR)
phalanges	falanges (fah-LAHN-hays)
phosphorus	fósforo (FOS-fo-ro)
physical examination	examen físico (ek-SAH-men FEE-se-co)
pink	rosa (RO-sah)
pituitary	pituitario (pe-too-e-TAH-re-o)
pneumonia	neumonía (nay-oo-mo-NEE-ah), pulmonía (pool-mo-NEE-ah)
pregnancy	embarazo (em-bah-RAH-so)
pregnant	embarazada (em-bah-rah-SAH-dah)
prolapse	prolapso (pro-LAHP-so)
prostate	próstata (PROS-ta-tah)
prostatic	prostático (pros-TAH-te-co)
prostatitis	prostatitis (pros-ta-TEE-tis)
protection	protección (pro-tec-se-ON)
psychiatry	psiquiatría (se-ke-ah-TREE-ah)
psychology	psicología (se-co-lo-HEE-ah)
pulse	pulso (POOL-so)
radiation	radiación (rah-de-ah-se-ON)
rectum	recto (REK-to)
red	rojo (ROH-ho)
reduction	reducción (ray-dooc-se-ON)
renal artery	arteria renal (ar-TAY-re-ah ray-NAHL)
renal calculus	cálculo renal (CAHL-coo-lo ray-NAHL)
reproduction	reproducción (ray-pro-dooc-se-ON)
respiration	respiración (res-pe-rah-se-ON)
rhythm	ritmo (REET-mo)
rhythm method	método de ritmo (MAY-to-do day REET-mo)
rib	costilla (cos-TEEL-lyah)
ringing	zumbido (zoom-BEE-do)
rupture	ruptura (roop-TOO-rah)
sacrum	hueso sacro (oo-AY-so SAH-cro)
saliva	saliva (sah-LEE-vah)
same	mismo (MEES-mo)
seizure	ataque (ah-TAH-kay)
sensation	sensación (sen-sah-se-ON)
sexual	sexual (sex-soo-AHL)
shoulder	hombro (OM-bro)
shoulder blade	espaldilla (es-pal-DEEL-lyah)

English	Spanish (pronunciation)
skeleton	esqueleto (es-kay-LAY-to)
skin	piel (pe-EL)
skull	cráneo (CRAH-nay-o)
sleep	sueño (soo-AY-nyo)
sole	planta (PLAHN-tah)
sound	sonido (so-NEE-do)
spasm	espasmo (es-PAHS-mo)
spinal column	columna vertebral (co-LOOM-nah ver-tay-BRAHL)
spine	espinazo (es-pe-NAH-so)
spiral	espiral (es-pe-RAHL)
spleen	bazo (BAH-so)
sprain, to	torcer (tor-SERR)
starch	almidón (al-me-DON)
sterile	estéril (es-TAY-reel)
sternum	esternón (es-ter-NON)
stiff	tieso (te-AY-so)
stomach	estómago (es-TOH-mah-go)
stone	cálculo (CAHL-coo-lo)
stroke	ataque de apoplejía (ah-TAH-kay de ah-po-play-HEE-ah)
support	sustento (sus-TEN-to)
surgeon	cirujano(a) (se-roo-HAH-no) (na)
surgery	cirugía (se-roo-HEE-ah)
suture	sutura (soo-TOO-rah)
swallow	tragar (trah-GAR)
sweat	sudor (soo-DOR)
swelling (to swell)	hinchar (in-CHAR)
symptom	síntoma (SEEN-to-mah)
synthesis	síntesis (SEEN-tay-sis)
tears	lágrimas (LAH-gre-mahs)
temperature	temperatura (tem-pay-rah-TOO-rah)
temple	sien (se-AN)
tendon	tendón (ten-DON)
testicle	testículo (tes-TEE-coo-lo)
tests	pruebas (proo-AY-bahs)
therapy	tratamiento (trah-tah-me-EN-to)
thigh	muslo (MOOS-lo)
thirst	sed (sayd)
throat	garganta (gar-GAHN-tah)
thumb	pulgar (pool-GAR)
thyroid	tiroides (te-RO-e-des)
toe	dedo del pie (DAY-do del PE-ay)
tongue	lengua (LEN-goo-ah)
tonsil	tonsila (ton-SEE-lah), amígdala (ah-MEEG-dah-lah)
tooth (pl., teeth)	diente (de-AYN-tay), dientes (de-AYN-tays)
trachea	tráquea (TRAH-kay-ah)
transfusion	transfusión (trans-foo-se-ON)
trauma	daño (DAH-nyo), herida (ay-REE-dah)
treatment	tratamiento (trah-tah-me-EN-to)
ulcer	ulcera (OOL-say-rah)
urea	urea (oo-RAY-ah)
urinalysis	urinálisis (oo-re-NAH-le-sis)
urinary	urinario (oo-re-NAH-re-o)
urinary system	sistema urinario (sis-TAY-mah oo-re-NAH-re-o)
urinate	orinar (o-re-NAR)

English	Spanish (pronunciation)
urination	urinación (oo-re-nah-se-ON)
urine	orina (o-REE-nah)
urology	urología (oo-ro-lo-HEE-ah)
uterus	útero (OO-tay-ro)
vagina	vagina (vah-HEE-nah)
varicose veins	venas varicosas (VAY-nahs vah-re-CO-sas)
vein	vena (VAY-nah)
vertebral column	columna vertebral (co-LOOM-nah ver-tay-BRAHL)
vessel	vaso (VAH-so)
vision	visión (ve-se-ON)
voice	voz (vos)
voiding	urinar (oo-re-NAR)
vomiting	vómito (VOH-mee-toh)
water	agua (AH-goo-ah)
weakness	debilidad (day-be-le-DAHD)
white	blanco (BLAHN-co)
wound	lesión (lay-se-ON)
wrist	muñeca (moo-NYAY-cah)
x-ray	radiografía (rah-de-o-grah-FEE-ah)
yellow	amarillo (ah-mah-REEL-lyo)

Spanish-English Translation of Selected Terms

APPENDIX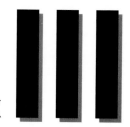

Spanish	English	Spanish	English
acidez	acidity	cadera	hip
adrenalina	adrenaline	calcio	calcium
agua	water	cálculo	calculus, stone
agudo	acute	cálculo biliar	gallstone
alentar	breathe	cálculo renal	renal calculus
alergia	allergy	calor	heat
almidón	starch	cáncer	cancer
amarillo	yellow	capilar	capillary
amígdala	tonsil	cara	face
anaranjado	orange-colored	cartílago	cartilage
anemia	anemia	catéter	catheter
anestesia	anesthesia	ceja	eyebrow
anestésico	anesthetic	cerebro	brain
ansiedad	anxiety	circuncisión	circumcision
antebrazo	forearm	cirugía	surgery
antibiótico	antibiotic	cirujano(a)	surgeon
apéndice	appendix	clavícula	collarbone
apetito	appetite	coágulo	clot
arteria	artery	codo	elbow
articulación	joint	colesterol	cholesterol
asfixia	asphyxia	columna vertebral	spinal column, vertebral column
asma	asthma		
ataque	seizure	concepción	conception
ataque de apoplejía	stroke	conciencia	consciousness
aumento	augmentation	concusión	concussion
azul	blue	condón	condom
barba	beard	consciente	conscious
barriga	belly	contracepción	contraception
bazo	spleen	convulsión	convulsion
benigno	benign	cópula	sexual intercourse
biopsia	biopsy	corazón	heart
blanco	white	costilla	rib
boca	mouth	coyuntura	joint
brazo	arm	cráneo	cranium, skull
cabeza	head	crecimiento	growth

Spanish	English	Spanish	English
crema	cream	impresión digital	fingerprint
crónico	chronic	fuego	fire
cuello	neck	fluido	fluid
cuerpo	body	espuma	foam
daño	trauma, injury	fósforo	phosphorus
debilidad	weakness	fractura	fracture
dedo del pie	toe	garganta	throat
dentista	dentist	gigante	giant
derecho	erect, straight	ginecología	gynecology
dermatología	dermatology	glándula	gland
desmayo	fainting	globo del ojo	eyeball
destrucción	destruction	glucosa	glucose
diafragma	diaphragm	gripe	influenza
diagnóstico	diagnostic	gris	gray
diálisis	dialysis	hambre	hunger
diarrea	diarrhea	hemorragia	hemorrhage
diente, dientes	tooth (pl., teeth)	hidropesía	edema
dolor	pain	hígado	liver
dolor de cabeza	headache	hinchar	swelling, to swell
doloroso	painful	hipertensión	high blood pressure
electricidad	electricity	hipodérmico	hypodermic
embarazada	pregnant	hombro	shoulder
embarazo	pregnancy	hormona	hormone
enano	dwarf	hueso	bone
encía	gum, gingiva	hueso sacro	sacrum
envejecido	aged	imperfecto	imperfect
enzima	enzyme	impotencia	impotency
epilepsia	epilepsy	inflamación	inflammation
erección	erection	instrumento	instrument
eructo	belch	insulina	insulin
esófago	esophagus	intestino	intestine
espalda	back	inyección	injection
espaldilla	shoulder blade	labios	lips
espasmo	spasm	lágrimas	tears
espinazo	spine	languidez	fainting
espiral	spiral	leche	milk
esqueleto	skeleton	lengua	tongue
estéril	sterile	lesión	wound
esternón	sternum	leucemia	leukemia
estómago	stomach	ligamento	ligament
estrecho	narrow	linfa	lymph
estreñimiento	constipation	linfático	lymphatic
evacuar	defecate	llorar	to cry
examen físico	physical examination	lóbulo	lobe
excreción	excretion	luz	light
excremento	feces	maligno	malignant
extremidad	extremity	mandíbula	jaw
falanges	phalanges	mano	hand
fatiga	fatigue	masculino	masculine
femenina	feminine	masticar	to chew
feto	fetus	mejilla	cheek
fibra	fiber	membrana	membrane
fiebre	fever	menopausia	menopause
dedo	finger	menstruación	menstruation

Spanish	English	Spanish	English
mente	mind	presión sanguínea	blood pressure
método de ritmo	rhythm method	prolapso	prolapse
microscopio	microscope	próstata	prostate
miedo	fear	prostático	prostatic
mismo	same	prostatitis	prostatitis
moco	mucus	protección	protection
movimiento	movement	pruebas	tests
muestra de sangre	blood sample	psicología	psychology
muñeca	wrist	psiquiatría	psychiatry
murmullo	murmur	pulgar	thumb
músculo	muscle	pulmón	lung
muslo	thigh	pulmonía	pneumonia
nacimiento	birth	pulso	pulse
naranjado	orange-colored	purgante	laxative
narcótico	narcotic	quebradura	hernia
nariz	nose	quemadura	burn
negro	black	radiación	radiation
nervio	nerve	radiografía	x-ray
nervioso	nervous	recién nacida	newborn
neumonía	pneumonia	recto	rectum
neurología	neurology	reducción	reduction
niño (a)	child	reproducción	reproduction
nutrición	nutrition	respiración	breathing, respiration
obstrucción	obstruction	respirar	breathe
ojo	eye	riñón	kidney
ombligo	navel	ritmo	rhythm
óptico	optician, optic	rodilla	knee
oreja	ear	rojo	red
orificio de la nariz	nostril	roncha	hives
orina	urine	rosa	pink
orinar	urinate	rótula	kneecap
ortodóntico	orthodontist	ruptura	rupture
ovárico	ovarian	sangre	blood
ovario	ovary	sed	thirst
oxígeno	oxygen	senos	breasts
palma	palm	sensación	sensation
páncreas	pancreas	sien	temple
papera	goiter	síntesis	synthesis
parálisis	paralysis	síntoma	symptom
parásito	parasite	sistema urinario	urinary system
parpado	eyelid	sobaco	armpit
parto	childbirth, parturition	sonido	sound
patología	pathology	sudor	sweat, perspiration
pecho	chest	sueño	sleep
pelo	hair	suprarenal	adrenal
pene	penis	sustento	support
pestaña	eyelash	sutura	suture
pezón	nipple	talón	heel
pie (pl., pies)	foot (pl., feet)	temperatura	temperature
piel	skin	tendón	tendon
pierna	leg	testículo	testicle
pituitario	pituitary	tieso	stiff
planta	sole	tiroides	thyroid
presión alta	high blood pressure	tobillo	ankle

Spanish	English	Spanish	English
tonsila	tonsil	vaso	vessel
torcer	to sprain	vejiga	bladder
tos	cough	vena	vein
tragar	swallow	venas varicosas	varicose veins
transfusión	transfusion	verde	green
tráquea	trachea	vértigo	dizziness
tratamiento	treatment, therapy	vesícula biliar	gallbladder
ulcera	ulcer	vida	life
uñas	nails	vientre	abdomen
urinación	urination	visión	vision
urinálisis	urinalysis	vómito	vomiting
urinar	voiding	voz	voice
urinario	urinary	yodo	iodine
urología	urology	zumbido	ringing
útero	uterus		

Conversion Tables

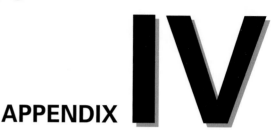

APPENDIX **IV**

WEIGHT EQUIVALENTS

1 lb = 453.6 g = 0.4536 kg = 16 oz
1 oz = 38.35 g
1 kg = 1,000 g = 2.2046 lb
1 g   = 1,000 mg
1 mg = 1,000 μg = 0.001 g
1 μg = 0.001 mg = 0.000001 g
1 μg/g or 1 mg/kg is the same as ppm

CONVERSION FACTORS

1 milligram	= 1/65	grain	(1/60)
1 gram	= 15.43	grains	(15)
1 kilogram	= 2.20	pounds	(avoirdupois)
	2.68	pounds	(Troy)
1 milliliter	= 16.23	minims	(15)
1 liter	= 1.06	quarts	(1+)
	33.80	fluid ounces	(34)
1 gram	= 0.065	gm	(60 mg)
1 dram	= 3.9	gm	(4)
1 ounce	= 31.1	gm	(30+)
1 minim	= 0.062	ml	(0.06)
1 fluid dram	= 3.7	ml	(4)
1 fluid ounce	= 29.57	ml	(30)
1 pint	= 473.2	ml	(500−)
1 quart	= 946.4	ml	(1000−)

Figures in parentheses are commonly employed approximate values.

TEMPERATURE CONVERSION

°Celsius to °Fahrenheit: $(°C)\left(\dfrac{9}{5}\right) + 32°$

°Fahrenheit to °Celsius: $(°F - 32°)\left(\dfrac{5}{9}\right)$

WEIGHT—UNIT CONVERSION FACTORS

Units Given	Units Wanted	For Conversion Multiply By
lb	g	453.6
lb	kg	0.4536
oz	g	28.35
kg	lb	2.2046
kg	mg	1,000,000.
kg	g	1,000.
g	mg	1,000.
g	μg	1,000,000.
mg	μg	1,000.
mg/g	mg/lb	453.6
mg/kg	mg/lb	0.4536
μg/kg	μg/lb	0.4536
Mcal	kcal	1,000.
kcal/kg	kcal/lb	0.4536
kcal/lb	kcal/kg	2.2046
ppm	μg/g	1.
ppm	mg/kg	1.
ppm	mg/lb	0.4536
mg/kg	%	0.0001
ppm	%	0.0001
mg/g	%	0.1
g/kg	%	0.1

VOLUME EQUIVALENTS

Household	Metric
1 drop (gt)	= 0.06 milliliter (ml)
15 drops (gtt)	= 1 ml (1 cc)
1 teaspoon (tsp)	= 5 (4) ml
1 tablespoon (tbs)	= 15 ml
2 tablespoons	= 30 ml
1 ounce (oz)	= 30 ml
1 teacup	= 180 ml (6 oz)
1 glass	= 240 ml (8 oz)
1 measuring cup	= 240 ml (½ pint)
2 measuring cups	= 500 ml (1 pint)

All tables from Appendix IV are from Kirk RW, and Bistner SI: *Handbook of Veterinary Procedures and Emergency Treatment*, 3rd ed, Philadelphia, WB Saunders Company, 1981.

Solutions to Chapter Reviews

APPENDIX V

CHAPTER 1

ANSWERS FOR SECTION REVIEWS

A.

1. two
2. Write more than two words.

B.

1. Each chapter uses terms you learned in previous chapters.
2. Word building is a system of learning word parts to understand and write terms.

C.

1. CF
2. CF
3. WR
4. CF
5. WR
6. WR
7. CF
8. WR
9. WR
10. CF
11. adenopathy
12. biliary
13. cyanosis
14. dermal
15. duodenostomy
16. electrode
17. glossopathy
18. hematology
19. spirometry
20. tomography
21. P
22. S
23. P
24. S
25. CF
26. S
27. P
28. CF
29. S
30. P
31. S
32. S
33. S
34. P
35. S
36. P
37. P
38. P

D.

1. CF
2. CF
3. S
4. P
5. P
6. P
7. S
8. P
9. P
10. CF
11. acidosis
12. acromegaly
13. antiemesis
14. bronchoscopy
15. dysphagia
16. hypothyroidism
17. leukocytosis
18. malabsorption
19. myometrium
20. thrombophlebitis

E.

1. Pronunciation is shown when new terms are introduced and in the index/glossary.
2. six

3. se
4. hi
5. "i" of hi, "e" of se, "e" of me

F.

1. capsules
2. cataracts
3. calculi
4. cortices
5. diagnoses
6. neuroses
7. protozoa
8. viruses
9. appendix
10. fungus
11. larynx
12. prognosis
13. sarcoma
14. spermatozoon

ANSWERS FOR CHAPTER REVIEW

I.

```
B A C I L L I     F
      A     B R O N C H I
      T           A
  C A R C I N O M A               V
  O       N       E               A
  M     A   P             V   P   R
  B A C T E R I A     S   O   H   I
  I       R   E       L   W   A   C
  N     R I       F       V E R T E B R A E
  I   I L E A   I   E   C   L   Y   S   P
  N         X   F   C   O   N     R
  G R E E K     I   O   M   G     I
    O         P R I M A R Y   E   M
T H O R A X                 S E P T A
    T                             R
                                  Y
```

II.

1. CF
2. CF
3. S
4. CF
5. S
6. P
7. P
8. S
9. S
10. CF

III.

1. alkalosis
2. cardiomegaly

3. bradypnea
4. bronchoscope
5. dysphonia
6. hypodermic
7. leukemia
8. melanoid
9. myocardial
10. thrombosis

IV.

1. (correct)
2. (correct)
3. costectomy
4. (correct)
5. (correct)

6. humeroscapular
7. (correct)
8. (correct)
9. (correct)
10. (correct)

V.

1. kal-<u>ka</u>′ne-əl
2. di″əg-<u>no</u>′sis
3. gas″tro-<u>meg</u>′ə-le
4. lap″ə-<u>ros</u>′kə-pe
5. <u>mi</u>′o-plas″te
6. o-<u>tal</u>′je-ə
7. <u>fren</u>′ik
8. sklə-<u>rot</u>′ik

9. tri-<u>ko</u>′sis
10. u-<u>re</u>′ter

VI.

1. adductors
2. alveolus
3. appendix
4. bursae
5. capillaries
6. cortices
7. diagnoses
8. ovaries
9. phalanx
10. thorax

CHAPTER 2

ANSWERS FOR SECTION REVIEWS

A.
1. life or living
2. tissue
3. nerve or nervous system
4. disease
5. nature
6. to cut
7. up or again
8. pertaining to
9. pertaining to
10. one who
11. one who studies
12. study or science of
13. to view
14. incision (cutting)

B.
1. tooth
2. feeling
3. tooth
4. mouth
5. straight
6. child or foot
7. repair
8. foot
9. not or without
10. inside
11. foot
12. condition
13. foot

C.
1. heart
2. secrete
3. skin
4. aged or elderly
5. aged or elderly
6. female
7. immune
8. larynx
9. midwife
10. tumor
11. eye
12. ear
13. mind
14. radius or radiant energy
15. rheumatism
16. nose
17. urine or urinary tract
18. pertaining to
19. secrete
20. one who
21. practitioner
22. medicine
23. medicine
24. condition, theory, or process

D.
1. sensitivity to pain
2. vision
3. drugs
4. drugs
5. treatment
6. poison

ANSWERS FOR CHAPTER REVIEW

I.

II.
1. I
2. J
3. A
4. D
5. E
6. F
7. G
8. H
9. B
10. C

III.
1. H
2. E
3. A
4. J
5. D
6. G
7. C
8. B
9. F
10. I

IV.
1. E
2. J
3. F

4. H
5. D
6. G
7. C
8. B
9. A
10. I

V.
1. anesthesia
2. anatomy
3. dermatology
4. endocrine
5. geriatrics
6. orthopedist
7. otic
8. pharmacologist
9. therapeutic
10. urology

VI.
1. B
2. A
3. D
4. C
5. A
6. D
7. C

8. C
9. D
10. B

VII.
1. pedodontics
2. subnormal
3. gerontal
4. ophthalmic
5. therapeutic
6. gastroenterologist
7. toxic
8. analgesic
9. biopsy
10. pathology

VIII.
cardiac, psychiatry

IX.
1. freely as desired (at pleasure)
2. biopsy
3. diagnosis
4. history
5. intake and output
6. night
7. nothing by mouth

8. over the counter
9. every day
10. four times a day

X.
1. D
2. E
3. B
4. C
5. A

XI.
1. generic
2. effects (or uses)
3. reactions
4. malignancies
5. analgesics
6. anesthetics
7. radiopharmaceuticals
8. blocking
9. parenteral

XII.
1. (an es the ze ol′ə je)
2. (gas tro en tər ol′ə je)
3. (his tol′ə je)
4. (or tho don′iks)
5. (ra de o loj′ik)

CHAPTER 3

ANSWERS FOR SECTION REVIEWS

A.
1. front, anterior
2. tail or lower part of body, caudal
3. head, cephalad
4. distant (or far), distal
5. back side, dorsal
6. situated below, inferior
7. side, lateral
8. middle, medial or median
9. behind (toward the back), posterior
10. near, proximal
11. uppermost, superior
12. belly, ventral

13. two
14. one
15. toward

B.
1. chest (or thorax)
2. pain

C.
1. abdomen
2. cranium (skull)
3. pelvis
4. peritoneum
5. spine
6. pertaining to

D.
1. extremity
2. hand
3. blue
4. digit
5. electricity
6. to print or record
7. muscle
8. instrument that records
9. process of recording
10. condition, disease, or abnormal increase
11. surgical repair
12. cramp or twitching

E.
1. eyelid
2. brain

3. giant
4. movement
5. umbilicus
6. body
7. body
8. against
9. slow
10. bad or difficult
11. in or inside
12. large
13. fast
14. inflammation
15. enlarged
16. disease
17. breathing

ANSWERS FOR CHAPTER REVIEW

I.

```
C X R                    A                A B D
Y                    D E N T O            A
A S                      I          A D C T
N                    O S I S        Y   T Y
T O M Y     A            T   P E L V I N   L
    E       C H I R O    A     A   I   O
    G       R            S   T H O R A C O
C A U D O       P   B M R     M
    L           E A L     C   P     E
    Y           A   E N C E P H A L O
          L     N       P     A   E     P
    B S A T A C H Y     H   L C   O R T H O
          I     A   P A   O R T H O   S
          E     K   R     L       R   T
          P R O X I M O   S O M A T O   E
          O     N       U     N     O R
                E       P     T       O
          P L A S T Y   E   P E D O
E E G             I     R     R
          C R A N I O   D O R S O
```

II.
1. cranial
2. spinal
3. thoracic
4. abdominal
5. pelvic

III.
1. RUQ
2. RLQ
3. LUQ
4. LLQ

IV.
1. frontal
2. midsagittal
3. transverse
4. anterior, ventral
5. posterior, dorsal
6. lateral

V.
1. E
2. D
3. B
4. C
5. H
6. F
7. G
8. B
9. A
10. E

VI.
1. B
2. D
3. A
4. B
5. D
6. C
7. C
8. C
9. B
10. B

VII.
1. bradypnea
2. ophthalmopathy
3. myospasm
4. blepharotomy
5. omphalitis
6. dermatitis
7. abdominopelvic
8. thoracic
9. traumatic
10. electroencephalography

VIII.
blepharal, midsagittal, superficial

IX.
1. B
2. H
3. C
4. I
5. F
6. A
7. G
8. D
9. E

X.
1. abdomen or abdominal
2. basal metabolic rate
3. chest x-ray
4. electrocardiogram
5. lateral
6. left upper quadrant
7. posteroanterior
8. symptom
9. vital signs
10. within normal limits

XI.
amebicides, antibacterials, antifungals, antihelmintics, antimalarials, antituberculars antivirals

XII.
1. (bi lat′ər əl)
2. (kahr de op′ə the)
3. (sə fal′ik)
4. (dər′mə to plas te)
5. (lum′bar)
6. (mi og′rə fe)
7. (om fal′ik)
8. (pos tər o soo pēr′e or)
9. (soo pĭ na′shən)
10. (vis′ər əl)

CHAPTER 4

ANSWERS FOR SECTION REVIEWS

A.
1. coagulation
2. little cell or compartment
3. cell
4. red
5. blood
6. white
7. words or study
8. vessel
9. outside
10. between
11. within
12. that which causes
13. pertaining to
14. to cause an action or the result of an action
15. cell
16. production
17. that which causes production

B.
1. nucleus
2. destruction (or dissolving)
3. shape (or form)
4. nucleus
5. attraction
6. thrombus (or clot)
7. many
8. excision; surgical removal
9. blood
10. substance that dissolves or destroys
11. destruction or dissolving
12. capable of dissolving
13. like or resembling
14. decreased or deficient
15. pertaining to

C.
1. color
2. hemoglobin
3. equal
4. large or enlarged
5. large or enlarged
6. small
7. normal
8. irregular
9. to view or examine
10. round
11. no, not, or without
12. excessive or more than normal
13. beneath or below normal
14. instrument used to view or examine
15. viewing

D.
1. fibrin
2. across or through

E.
1. to eat
2. protection

F.
1. air or gas
2. green
3. water
4. black
5. mucus
6. yellow
7. vision
8. pertaining to (or characterized by)
9. state (or condition)

ANSWERS FOR CHAPTER REVIEW

I.

II.
1. A
2. C
3. B
4. C
5. B

III.
1. A
2. C
3. D
4. B

IV.
1. D
2. C
3. A
4. D
5. B
6. D
7. D
8. C
9. A
10. C
11. B
12. D
13. A
14. C
15. C

V.
1. polyuria
2. poikilocyte
3. leukocytosis
4. thrombocyte
5. coagulopathy
6. toxicosis
7. coagulation
8. thrombolysis
9. intercellular
10. cytology

VI.
agglutination
anaerobic
fibrinolysis
polymorphonuclear
toxicity
vaccination
xanthochromia

VII.
1. T
2. T
3. F
4. F
5. T

VIII.
1. T
2. F
3. F
4. F
5. F

IX.
1. A
2. E
3. B
4. F

X.
1-5 (any of these, no particular order) barriers, complement, interferon, phagocytes, inflammation

XI.
1-2 (no particular order) cell-mediated immunity and antibody-mediated immunity

XII.
1. anti-hemophilic factor
2. enzyme-linked immunosorbent assay
3. hematocrit
4. hemoglobin

5. hemoglobin S
6. immunoglobulin G
7. polymorphonuclear
8. prothrombin time
9. rhesus factor in blood
10. white blood cell

XIII.
1. (ə rith ro poi e′sis)
2. (fi brĭ nol′ə sis)
3. (hem ə to′mə)
4. (hi po kro′mik)
5. (tok sis′ĭ te)

XIV.
1. A
2. D
3. S
4. A
5. D
6. D
7. D

XV.
1. C
2. B
3. A
4. E
5. F
6. D

CHAPTER 5

ANSWERS FOR SECTION REVIEWS

A.
1. artery
2. arteriole
3. vein
4. lung
5. vein
6. vein
7. venule
8. pertaining to
9. little

7. septum
8. sinus
9. valve
10. valve
11. ventricle
12. above or upon
13. around
14. three
15. membrane

B.
1. atrium
2. crown
3. endocardium
4. mediastinum
5. myocardium
6. pericardium

C.
1. aneurysm
2. vessel
3. aorta
4. yellowish, fatty plaque
5. light
6. hard, hardening

7. vessel
8. tumor; swelling
9. abnormal hardening
10. artificial opening
11. cutting instrument

D.
1. sound
2. oxygen
3. rhythm
4. sound
5. chest
6. down; from; reversing
7. instrument used to measure
8. process of measuring

9. abnormal fear
10. narrowing; stricture

E.
1. gland
2. adenoid
3. cancer
4. cancer
5. lymph
6. lymph node
7. lymph vessel
8. lymphatics
9. spleen
10. thymus
11. tonsil
12. swelling

Answers for Chapter Review

I.

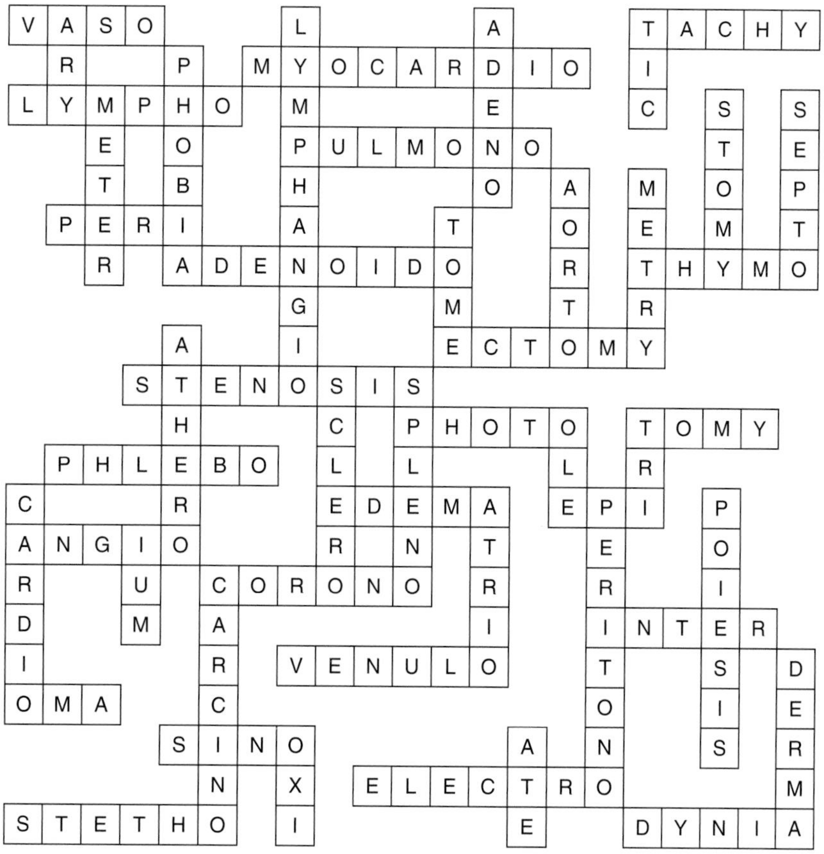

(Crossword puzzle grid with answers)

II.

1. lymphangi(o)
2. arter(o), arteri(o)
3. arteriol(o)
4. phleb(o), ven(i), ven(o)
5. venul(o)

10. A
11. D
12. A
13. B
14. A
15. B

III.

1-3 (no particular order)
1. returns excess fluid to the bloodstream
2. absorbs fats and fat-soluble vitamins from small intestine
3. body defense

IV.

1. B
2. C
3. D
4. C
5. C
6. C
7. C
8. B
9. B

V.

1. systemic
2. pulmonary
3. cardiovascular
4. arteries
5. capillaries
6. aorta
7. myocardium
8. atria, ventricles
9. coronary
10. lymphatic

VI.

1. aortopathy
2. lymphadenitis
3. occlusion
4. asystole
5. endocardium
6. extravascular

7. carcinoma
8. tonsillectomy
9. bradycardia
10. lymphedema

VII.

1. axillary nodes
2. inguinal nodes
3. palatine tonsil
4. cervical nodes
5. thymus
6. spleen

VIII.

atherosclerosis, ischemia

IX.

1. vena cavae
2. atrium
3. right ventricle
4. lungs
5. left atrium
6. bicuspid (or mitral)
7. aorta
8. arterioles
9. capillaries

10. veins
11. lymphatic
12. lymph
13. veins
14. systemic

X.

(No particular order)
1. increased cardiac output
2. increased blood viscosity
3. increased blood volume
4. decreased elasticity of arterial walls

XI.

1. arteriosclerotic heart disease
2. atrioventricular
3. carcinoma
4. coronary artery bypass graft
5. coronary artery disease
6. cardiopulmonary resuscitation
7. left ventricle
8. myocardial infarction

9. right atrium (also rheumatoid arthritis)
10. ventricular septal defect

XII.
1. congestive heart failure
2. chest x-ray
3. pertaining to difficult breathing
4. the abnormal accumulation of fluid in the interstitial spaces of tissues

5. Use nasal prongs to deliver oxygen at a setting of 4 L per min.
Take 40 milligrams of Lasix each day by mouth.
Take 5 milligrams of Vasotec each day by mouth.

XIII.
1. (kar de o mi op′ə the)
2. (lim fad ə nop′ə the)
3. (lim fog′rə fe)
4. (per ĭ kahr′de əl)
5. (vas o di la′shən)

XIV.
1. R
2. D
3. S
4. D
5. D
6. D
7. R
8. S
9. D
10. A

XV.
1. D
2. A
3. B
4. C

CHAPTER 6

ANSWERS FOR SECTION REVIEWS

A.
1. acid
2. alkaline, basic
3. to breathe; spiral
4. in-
5. ex-
6. -ation
7. -capnia

B.
1. alveoli
2. bronchi
3. bronchiole
4. pharynx
5. paralysis

6. phren(o)
7. trache(o)
8. paralysis
9. prolapse

C.
1. epiglottis
2. gen(o)
3. lith(o)
4. nose
5. palat(o)
6. above or upon
7. pain
8. origin or beginning

9. condition
10. stone or calculus
11. -rrhea

D.
1. fibr(o)
2. lob(o)
3. pleur(o)
4. lungs or air
5. lungs
6. lungs
7. surgical puncture
8. stretching or dilation

E.
1. anthrac(o)
2. atel(o)
3. coni(o)
4. embol(o)
5. malac(o)
6. phas(o)
7. phon(o)
8. plas(o)
9. meta-
10. sym- or syn-
11. -malacia
12. -plasia
13. -ptysis
14. -stasis

ANSWERS FOR CHAPTER REVIEW

I.

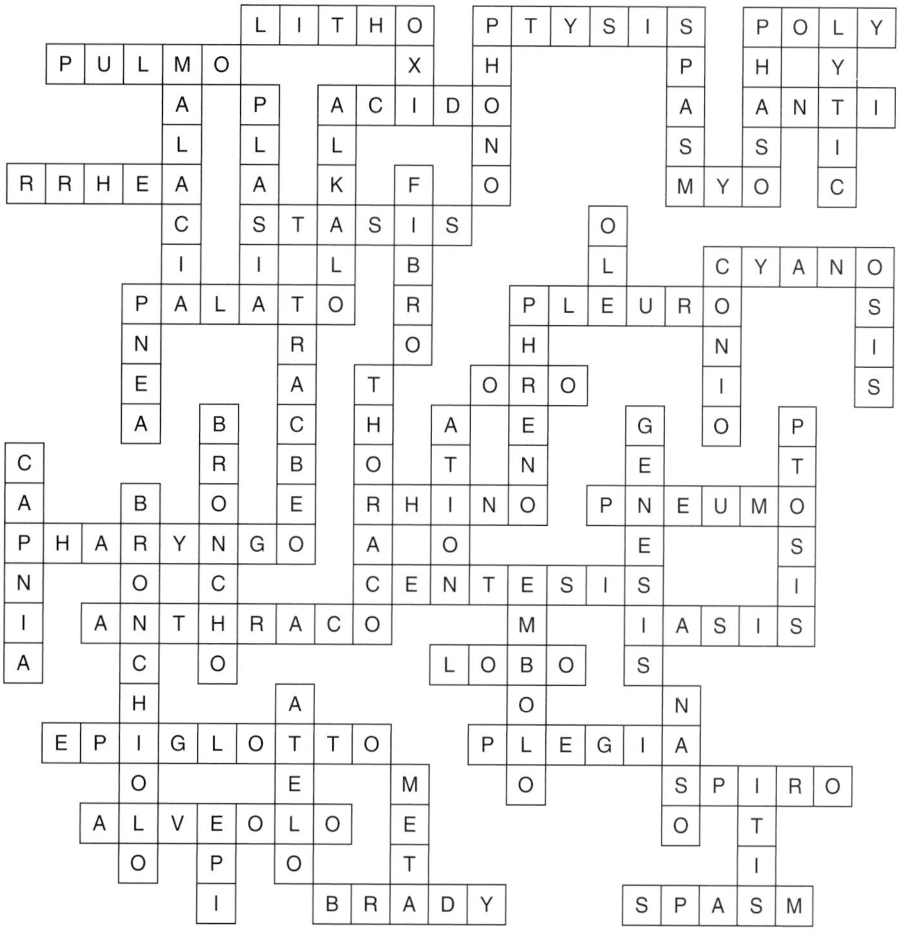

(Crossword puzzle grid)

Across/down answers include: LITHO, PTYSIS, POLY, PULMO, ACIDO, ANTI, RRHEA, STASIS, MYO, CYANO, PALATO, PLEURO, ORO, RHINO, PNEUMO, PHARYNGO, CENTESIS, ANTHRACO, IASIS, LOBO, EPIGLOTTO, PLEGIA, SPIRO, ALVEOLO, BRADY, SPASM

II.

1. G
2. A
3. B
4. F
5. D
6. E
7. C

III.

1. H
2. B
3. C
4. F
5. G
6. E

IV.

1. sin(o)
2. nas(o), rhin(o)
3. pharyng(o)
4. laryng(o)
5. trache(o)
6. bronch(o), bronchi(o)
7. phren(o)
8. alveol(o)
9. bronchiol(o)

V.

Sequence: 1, 5, 3, 2, 4, 7, 6

VI.

(any five, no particular order)
provide oxygen,
eliminate carbon dioxide,
maintain acid-base balance, produce speech,
facilitate smell,
maintain body's heat and water balance

VII.

1. A
2. A
3. C
4. D
5. C
6. B
7. B
8. B
9. A
10. C
11. B
12. D
13. A
14. C
15. D

VIII.

1. hypocapnia
2. laryngectomy
3. fibrothorax
4. bronchiolitis
5. nasoseptoplasty
6. carcinogenesis
7. alveolar
8. pharyngeal
9. bronchoplasty
10. phrenoptosis
11. tachypnea
12. embolectomy
13. rhinorrhea
14. pneumomalacia
15. palatoplasty

IX.

auscultation, hemoptysis

X.

1. endotracheal
2. pulmonary function test
3. right lower lobe
4. transtracheal oxygen
5. upper respiratory infection

XI.
1. C
2. B
3. A
4. C
5. C

XII.
1. (as fik′se ə)
2. (noo mo mə la′shə)
3. (pəl mon′ik)
4. (ri no lĭ thi′ə sis)
5. (spi rom′ə ter)

XIII.
1. D
2. D
3. R
4. D
5. T
6. S
7. D
8. A

9. S
10. A

XIV.
1. A
2. D
3. C
4. B

CHAPTER 7

Answers for Section Reviews

A.
1. starch
2. thirst
3. fruct(o)
4. glyc(o) or glycos(o)
5. intestines
6. milk
7. fats
8. protein
9. normal, well, or good
10. outside or outward
11. bad
12. near, beside, or abnormal
13. -ase
14. vomiting
15. -ose
16. -pepsia
17. eat or swallow
18. eating or swallowing

B.
1. anus
2. colon; large intestine
3. intestines; small intestine
4. esophag(o)
5. gastr(o)
6. mouth
7. contraction

C.
1. lip
2. teeth
3. fungus
4. gingiv(o)
5. tongue
6. tongue
7. mandible
8. fungus

9. maxilla
10. pus

D.
1. pylor(o)
2. vag(o)
3. surgical fixation
4. -cele
5. -pexy

E.
1. appendix
2. cec(o)
3. colon; large intestine
4. diverticul(o)
5. duodenum
6. ileum
7. jejun(o)
8. proct(o)
9. rectum

10. sigmoid(o)
11. place or position
12. virus
13. virus
14. -clysis

F.
1. bile
2. bile
3. gallbladder
4. choledoch(o)
5. cyst(o)
6. liver
7. pancreat(o)
8. saliva or salivary gland
9. salivary gland
10. below or under
11. structure; having the shape of

ANSWERS FOR CHAPTER REVIEW

I.

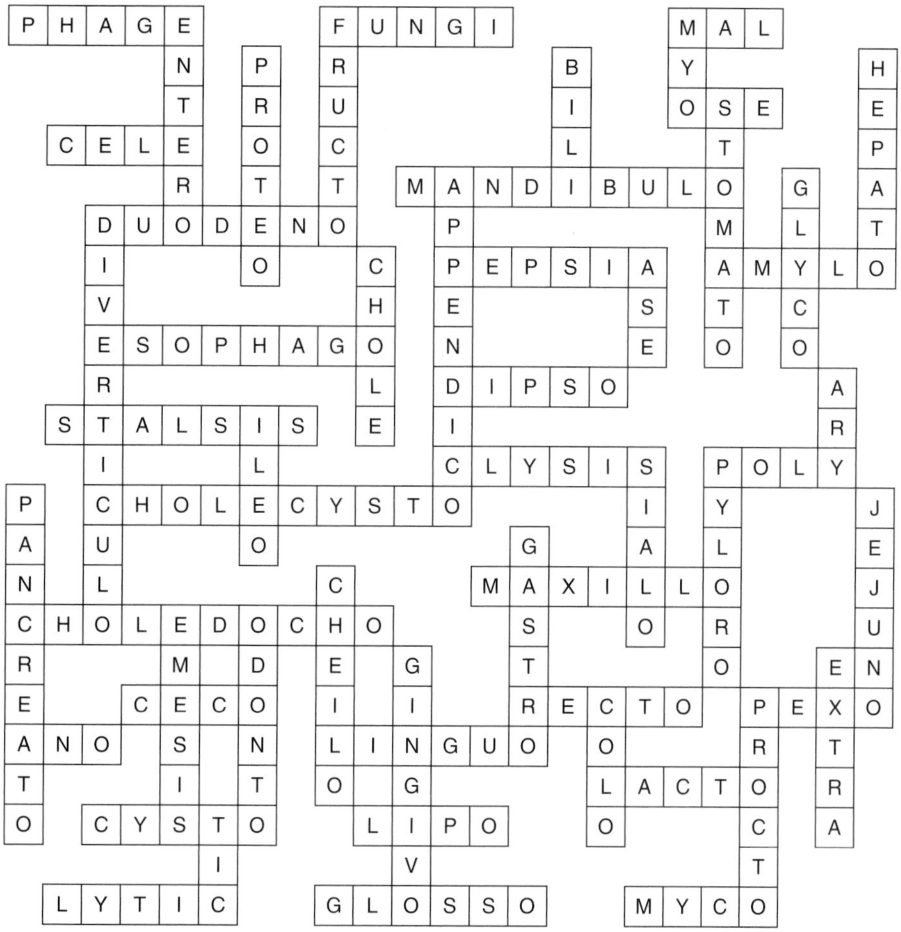

(crossword grid)

```
P H A G E       F U N G I       M A L
    N   P   R           B   Y O S E       H
    T   R   U           I   T             E
C E L E   R   T     M A N D I B U L O   G P
    R   T   T         P       O M     L   A
D U O D E N O   C   P E P S I A   A M Y L O
I       O   H   E       S   T O   C
V       L   E   N   D I P S O       O       A
E S O P H A G O   I               A
R       L   E   C L Y S I S   P O L Y       J
S T A L S I S   E       I   Y   L           E
I       L           G       A   L           J
P   C H O L E C Y S T O   M A X I L L O     U
A   U       O           S         O R       N
N   L       C           T         O     E
C H O L E D O C H O   I   R E C T O   P E X O
R   M   D   E   G     L                 R
E   C E C O   I   I   I N G U O   O     R
A N O   S   N   L I N G U O   O   L A C T O   R
T       I   T   O   G         O       C     A
O   C Y S T O   L I P O           C
    I           V                 T
L Y T I C   G L O S S O   M Y C O
```

II.
1. A
2. B
3. E
4. C
5. D

III.
1. C
2. B
3. A
4. H
5. D
6. F
7. E
8. G

IV.
1. pharyng(o)
2. sial(o), sialaden(o)
3. hepat(o)
4. cholecyst(o)
5. duoden(o)
6. or(o), stomat(o)
7. esophag(o)
8. gastr(o)
9. pancreat(o)
10. jejun(o)
11. ile(o)
12. col(o)
13. an(o)

V.
1. incisor
2. cuspid
3. bicuspid
4. molar

VI.
1. A
2. B
3. A
4. C
5. D
6. C
7. B
8. D
9. B
10. B
11. A
12. A
13. D
14. A
15. D
16. D
17. B
18. C
19. A
20. B

VII.
1. D
2. A
3. D
4. C
5. D

VIII.
1. teeth
2. bolus
3. esophagus
4. cardiac sphincter
5. rugae
6. chyme
7. pyloric sphincter
8. absorption
9. villi
10. large intestine

IX.
1. hepatopathy
2. stomatomycosis
3. lactase
4. polyphagia
5. vagotomy
6. hyperlipemia or hyperlipidemia
7. sialadenitis
8. colitis
9. pyloroscopy
10. enteroplegia
11. choledochal
12. gingival
13. esophagoptosis
14. colopexy
15. glossoplasty

X.

denture, gastric, lipopenia,

XI.

1. gallbladder
2. gastrointestinal
3. intravenous cholangiogram
4. nothing by mouth
5. total parenteral nutrition

XII.

1. (ko le sis to gas′trik)
2. (ko led′ə kəl)
3. (ko le lĭ thi′ah sis)
4. (ko lek ta′zhə)
5. (fis′tu lə)
6. (hep ə to meg′ə le)
7. (jĕ joo no il e os′to me)
8. (prok tos′kə pe)

9. (sig moi′do skōp)
10. (səb ling′gwəl)

XIII.

1. D
2. T
3. S
4. S
5. R
6. S

7. D
8. R
9. D
10. A

XIV.

1. D
2. A
3. C
4. B

CHAPTER 8

ANSWERS FOR SECTION REVIEWS

A.

1. kidney
2. kidney
3. ureter(o)
4. urethr(o)
5. urin(o), sometimes ur(o)

B.

1. glomerul(o)
2. py(o)
3. pyel(o)
4. -cele
5. -tripsy

C.

1. new
2. hemorrhage

3. suture
4. flow or discharge
5. rupture

D.

1. double
2. genitals or reproduction
3. disease
4. grapelike cluster; uvula
5. twisted

E.

1. albumin
2. sugar or sweet
3. ketone body
4. few
5. night
6. night

ANSWERS FOR CHAPTER REVIEW

I.

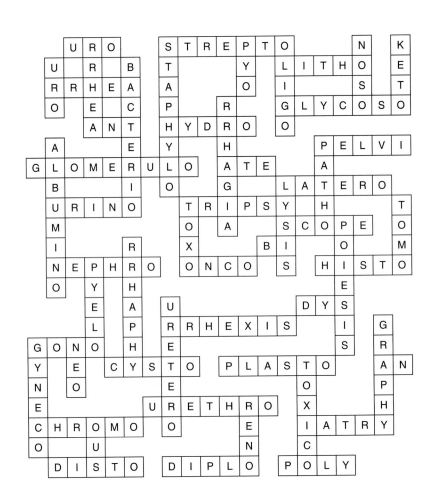

II.
1. E
2. D
3. A
4. C
5. B

III.
1. nephr(o), ren(o)
2. ureter(o)
3. cyst(o)
4. urethr(o)

IV.
1. T
2. T
3. T
4. T
5. F
6. T
7. T

V.
1. D
2. B
3. C
4. D
5. B
6. C
7. B
8. A
9. B

10. A
11. C
12. C
13. B
14. A
15. D
16. D
17. D
18. C
19. B
20. C

VI.
1. nephromalacia
2. uropathy
3. interrenal
4. cystostomy
5. urethrorrhagia
6. pyelitis
7. ketonuria
8. nosocomial
9. renal
10. ureterolithiasis
11. cystorrhexis
12. glycosuria
13. lithotripsy
14. urethrorrhaphy
15. cystoscopy

VII.
1. glomerulus
2. proximal convoluted tubule

3. Bowman's capsule
4. distal convoluted tubule
5. collecting duct

VIII.
cardionephric, hematuria, polycystic, urethrorectal

IX.
1. abdominal
2. glomerulus
3. Bowman's capsule
4. reabsorption
5. urine
6. pelvis

X.
1. blood urea nitrogen
2. chronic glomerulonephritis
3. chronic renal failure
4. extracorporeal shockwave lithotripsy
5. glomerular filtration rate
6. genitourinary
7. intake and output
8. intravenous pyelogram
9. low-power field
10. voiding cystourethrogram

XI.
1. B
2. A

3. B
4. B
5. one dose taken 30 minutes before penicillin injection
6. anti-infectives

XII.
1. (sis to lǐ thek′tə me)
2. (di u re′sis)
3. (glo mer′u li)
4. (he mo di al′ə sis)
5. (lith′o trip se)
6. (nef ro lǐ thi′ah sis)
7. (nef ro so nog′rah fe)
8. (pi′ě lo gram)
9. (pi o nə fro′sis)
10. (u rog′rə fe)

XIII.
1. A
2. S
3. S
4. T
5. D
6. D
7. D
8. A
9. R
10. S

CHAPTER 9

ANSWERS FOR SECTION REVIEWS

A.
1. cervic(o)
2. vagina
3. organs of reproduction
4. uterus
5. measure of uterine tissue
6. ovary
7. ovary
8. perine(o)
9. salping(o)
10. uterus
11. vagina
12. vulv(o)
13. pertaining to

B.
1. amnion
2. chorion

3. month
4. ovum (or egg)
5. spermatozoa
6. spermatozoa
7. symptom
8. heat
9. against
10. embryonic form
11. killing
12. origin or beginning

C.
1. fet(o)
2. nat(o)
3. par(o)
4. ecto-
5. multi- (or poly)
6. before
7. new

8. none
9. after or behind
10. first
11. false
12. four
13. pregnancy
14. pregnant female
15. woman who has given birth

D.
1. cold
2. formation or development
3. treatment

E.
1. epididymis
2. testis

3. penis
4. prostat(o)
5. scrot(o)
6. testis
7. vessel; ductus deferens

F.
1. hidden
2. epididymis
3. testis
4. penis
5. scrotum
6. semen
7. testis

G.
1. varicose vein

ANSWERS FOR CHAPTER REVIEW

I.

(Completed crossword puzzle — words filled in the grid include:)

PRE, SEMINO, VARICO, PRIM, SCT, QU, ME, ME, G, PERI, THERMO, ANTE, NT, ANTI, AD, COLPO, LAPARO, O, MULTI, IT, DA, ORCHIDO, SE, CHORIO, GRAPH, NULLI, CYESIS, CO, STR, SPV, H, PR, PENO, DYS, BLAST, EPIDIDYMO, NC, SST, CYTE, EXT, TOXO, MY, OOPHORO, SART, SPERMATO, OO, INTRA, NEO, VAS, THEV, NTER, SOMA, SC, GRAVIDA, ENDO, CONCP, FE, UL, SYMPTO, VARIO, POLY, UTERO, VAGINO, MUCO

II.
1. A
2. B
3. C

III.
1. B
2. A
3. A
4. B
5. C
6. F
7. E
8. D

IV.
1. C, D
2. B, C
3. C, E, F
4. A, C, E, F

V.
1. oophor(o)
2. salping(o)
3. hyster(o)
4. cervic(o)
5. colp(o)

VI.
1. vas(o)
2. urethr(o)
3. pen(o)
4. prostat(o)
5. epididym(o)
6. orchi(o)
7. scrot(o)

VII.
1. A
2. B
3. C

4. A
5. C
6. C
7. A
8. D
9. B
10. C
11. B
12. A
13. C
14. D
15. B
16. B
17. A
18. B
19. D
20. C
21. A
22. C
23. B
24. A
25. B

VIII.
1. ovarian
2. ovulation
3. estrogen
4. uterine
5. menses (or menstruation)

IX.
1. vasectomy
2. colposcope
3. dilation, curettage
4. prostatectomy
5. I

X.
1. parturition
2. vulva

3. salpingitis
4. epididymitis
5. dysmenorrhea
6. ovulation
7. oophorectomy
8. amniorrhexis
9. vasorrhaphy
10. leukorrhea

XI.
1. anteversion
2. retroversion
3. anteflexion
4. retroflexion

XII.
dysplasia, ectopic, salpingocele

XIII.
1. benign prostatic hypertrophy
2. cervix
3. expected delivery date
4. electronic fetal monitor
5. fetal heart rate
6. follicle-stimulating hormone
7. hepatitis B virus
8. luteinizing hormone
9. newborn
10. transurethral resection of the prostate

XIV.
1. (am ne o kor′e al)
2. (klit′ə ris)
3. (kol po ser′vĭ kəl)
4. (kol′po plas te)
5. (krip tor′kĭ diz əm)
6. (fe tos′kə pe)
7. (mi o mə tri′tis)
8. (ne′o nāt)
9. (fi mo′sis)
10. (u nip′ə rə)

XV.
1. D
2. S
3. A

4. T
5. R
6. S
7. A
8. D
9. D
10. S

XVI.
1. F
2. C
3. E
4. D
5. A
6. B

CHAPTER 10

ANSWERS FOR SECTION REVIEWS

A.
1. calcium
2. bone
3. spinal cord or bone marrow
4. nutrition
5. nutrition

B.
1. coccyx
2. cost(o)
3. lumbar (or lower back)
4. spine
5. sacr(o)
6. vertebra (spine)

7. stern(o)
8. vertebra
9. split

C.
1. calcane(o)
2. carp(o)
3. clavicul(o)
4. femor(o)
5. fibul(o)
6. humer(o)
7. ili(o)
8. ischi(o)
9. patell(o)
10. phalang(o)
11. pub(o)

12. radi(o)
13. scapul(o)
14. tars(o)
15. tibi(o)
16. uln(o)

D.
1. ankyl(o)
2. joint
3. joint or articulation
4. burs(o)
5. chondr(o)
6. synovial membrane
7. tendon
8. -clasia
9. -desis

E.
1. blast(o)
2. fasci(o)
3. muscle
4. viscer(o)
5. away from
6. toward
7. weakness

F.
1. situated below
2. retro-
3. super-
4. supra-
5. malignant tumor from connective tissue

ANSWERS FOR CHAPTER REVIEW

I.

```
T A R S O        C           S C H I S I S
R       M   M Y E L O        T         F
O       A     A     F I B U L O   T       E
P E R I   B U R S O   A   C   C H O N D R O   M
H   N E O     I     S   A   A     O       R
O   T       M A L A C I A   L   L         O
                  I   S   C O C C Y G O
M E T R Y   R A C H I   O   T   I   A
A   O     R     P   H   I   A   N K Y L O   P
L   M E G A   T R O P H Y   E   M   E       U
E   E   S   H   A   N   M     A       B
C     R E T R O   C L A V I C U L O   C Y T O
O   A     O     A   A   S     E
  D E S I S   C R A N I O   S C A P U L O   S Y N
S     A     G   U       T   D E
U   U V E R T E B R O   L   S   O
P E L V I   C   L   S P O N D Y L O   O
E N   S   C A R P O   A   N
R O   C   M   S   T   O S T E O
  T   E A B   T   H U M E R O   V
  I N F R A     I     L   O R T H O
  B   O   P   L     L   M   A
  I   O   I S C H I O   E E D E M A N
  O   L   U   O     S   T   I     N
    S T O M Y   M   A U T O   S A C R O   A T E
```

II.
1. A
2. B
3. E
4. C
5. D

III.
1. J
2. H
3. A
4. D
5. I
6. G
7. C
8. F
9. B
10. E

IV.
1. clavicul(o)
2. stern(o)
3. cost(o)
4. ili(o)
5. pub(o)
6. ischi(o)
7. crani(o)
8. scapul(o)
9. humer(o)
10. radi(o)
11. uln(o)
12. carp(o)
13. femor(o)
14. patell(o)
15. tibi(o)
16. fibul(o)
17. tars(o)
18. phalang(o)

V.
1. J
2. D
3. H
4. I
5. F
6. E
7. B
8. G
9. C
10. A

VI.

cervical #1, coccygeal #5,
lumbar #3, sacral #4,
thoracic #2

VII.
1. A
2. B

3. D
4. A
5. C
6. D
7. A
8. A
9. A
10. A
11. C
12. A
13. D
14. D
15. C
16. C
17. A
18. C
19. C
20. C

VIII.
1. periosteum
2. calcipenia
3. articulation
4. tendons
5. rheumatoid
6. lupus erythematosus
7. ankylosing
8. circumduction
9. scoliosis
10. intrathecal

IX.
1. osteoblast
2. dislocation
3. chondrectomy
4. sternotomy
5. bursitis
6. myelitis
7. myomalacia
8. calcaneodynia
9. clavicular
10. arthroplasty

X.
carpectomy, myelosuppression, spondylitis

XI.
1. axial
2. appendicular
3. diaphysis
4. epiphyses
5. cranial
6. true
7. sternum
8. false
9. floating
10. yellow
11. red

XII.
1. skeletal
2. visceral
3. myocardium
4. connective

5. cartilage
6. bursae
7. osteoarthritis
8. gout

XIII.
1. carpal tunnel syndrome
2. distal interphalangeal
3. erythrocyte sedimenta-tion rate
4. range of motion
5. first thoracic vertebra

XIV.
1. (ar thro kla′zhə)
2. (ar thros′kə pe)
3. (kon dro sar ko′mə)
4. (fash′e ə)
5. (lum′bar)
6. (mi al′jə)
7. (mi əs the′ne ə)

8. (os te o pə ro′sis)
9. (stər no kos′təl)
10. (tib e o fem′ər əl)

XV.
1. S
2. R
3. A
4. S
5. D
6. D
7. S
8. D
9. D
10. A

XVI.
1. C
2. B
3. A

CHAPTER 11

ANSWERS FOR SECTION REVIEWS

A.
1. tree
2. neuroglia or sticky substance

B.
1. arachn(o)
2. cerebell(o)
3. cerebr(o)

4. mening(o)
5. one
6. narc(o)
7. twice
8. half
9. half or partly
10. -lepsy
11. -kinesia

C.
1. sensitivity to pain
2. hearing
3. chem(o)
4. tear
5. iris
6. iris
7. cornea; hard or horny
8. tear

9. eye
10. against
11. sensation or perception

D.
1. mind
2. fire
3. split
4. excessive preoccupation

ANSWERS FOR CHAPTER REVIEW

I.

```
L E P S Y     M A N I A     M         O
      S             U E      P
    P Y R O         T        N    I         M O N O
T       C     M     C O N T R A         E        K
R R H E A     Y     E       O           I D I O
I       O     N E U R O     A       N        N
P       L     L     E     C     R     G      E
S     K E R A T O     B L E P H A R O            S
Y       C           R     R     C           I
    D A C R Y O     O     E S T H E S I A
        I           B     N           N
  S P A S M         O     E     O     T
    E       O P H T H A L M O     C H E M O
    M       L       P     R     C
O I D     A L G E S I O     T     P     U
U       U     C     I     L     L
S     Q U A D R I     H     C     N A R C O
      I     O I R I D O     S
D E N D R O     Z     T
I       P H O B I A     M Y O
```

II.
1. A
2. B
3. B
4. B
5. A

III.
1. A
2. D
3. E
4. C
5. B

IV.
1. D
2. A
3. A
4. B
5. B
6. C
7. C
8. A
9. A
10. B
11. B
12. A
13. B
14. C
15. C
16. D
17. D
18. D
19. A
20. D

V.
1. botulism
2. epilepsy
3. paraplegia
4. otorrhea
5. schizophrenia

VI.
1. meninges
2. cerebrum
3. cerebrospinal
4. neuron
5. neuroglia (or glial)
6. axon
7. dendrite
8. neurotransmitter
9. sensory
10. somatic
11. autonomic

VII.
1. pyrophobia
2. intercerebral
3. neurolysis
4. hyperalgesia
5. cerebellitis
6. audiometry
7. neural
8. lacrimal
9. myelography
10. intracranial

VIII.
1. myelin
2. neuromuscular
3. acetylcholine
4. synapse
5. stem
6. diencephalon
7. cerebrum
8. epinephrine
9. acetylcholine
10. motor

IX.
1. attention deficit disorder
2. amyotrophic lateral sclerosis
3. central nervous system
4. cerebrospinal fluid
5. cerebrovascular accident or costovertebral angle
6. Diagnostic and Statistical Manual of Mental Disorders
7. electroencephalogram
8. intracranial pressure
9. multiple sclerosis
10. transient ischemic attack

X.
1. (aw de om′ə ter)
2. (ser ə bel′ər)
3. (ser e bro spi′nəl)
4. (en sef′ə lo sel)

5. (mon o ple′jə)
6. (noor ar throp′ə the)
7. (noo rog′le ə)
8. (noo rol′ə sis)
9. (fag o ma′ne ə)
10. (ri no dak′re o lith)

XI.
1. A
2. A
3. A
4. R
5. D
6. S

7. D
8. D
9. D
10. D

XII.
dementia, pyrophobia

XIII.
1. analgesics
2. anesthetics
3. anxiety
4. anticonvulsants
5. vomiting (or nausea)
6. psychotic
7. emetics

CHAPTER 12

ANSWERS FOR SECTION REVIEWS

A.
1. fat
2. skin
3. cornea; hard or horny
4. wrinkle
5. sebum
6. meso-
7. skin or germ layer

B.
1. axilla (armpit)
2. sweat
3. nail
4. hair
5. hair
6. nail
7. transmission

C.
1. follicul(o)
2. xer(o)

D.
1. bacteria
2. dead
3. infection
4. infection or septum
5. in-

E.
1. white
2. white
3. erythema or redness
4. sun
5. fish
6. through

ANSWERS FOR CHAPTER REVIEW
I.

P	Y	O		T	O	X	I	C	O			P	H	Y	S	I	O	
A						E			M	Y	C	O					N	
T	I	C				R			R									
H		P	I	L	O				Y				A		P			
O			I			H	Y	D	R	O			D		H			
	D		P			E			A	L	B	I	N	O				
S	E	B	O		A	L	B	O				P		R				
V		R				I			S	E	P	T	O		E			
A		M	E	L	A	N	O		U						S			
S		C			X			B	A	C	T	E	R	I				
C		T	R	I	C	H	O		D			R		S				
U	N	G	U	O				I	C	H	T	H	Y	O				
L			L		C		R		A			T						
O	M	A		O	N	Y	C	H	O		C	U	T	A	N	E	O	
T				A		Y	T		I			M						
E		N		N		T	I	D	K	E	R	A	T	O				
T	H	E	R	M	O	I	D	A	T									
	C		E	S	D	A	T											
	R		F	O	L	L	I	C	U	L	O							
H	I	D	R	O							S							

II.
1. C
2. B
3. A
4. D

III.
1. A
2. G
3. C
4. D
5. H
6. F
7. E
8. B

IV.
(any five, no particular order)
1. protective covering
2. water balance
3. temperature regulation
4. sensory reception
5. vitamin D synthesis
6. psychosocial function

V.
1. D
2. C
3. D
4. A
5. B

6. A
7. A
8. D
9. B
10. D

VI.
1. epidermis
2. keratin
3. dermis
4. fat (or adipose)
5. insulation
6. sebaceous
7. sudoriferous

VII.
1. necrosis
2. thermolysis
3. ichthyosis
4. keloid
5. axillary
6. ungual
7. pyogenic
8. onychectomy
9. trichoid
10. hidradenoma

VIII.
xerosis

IX.
1. B
2. A
3. C
4. E
5. D

X.
1. B
2. D
3. A
4. B
5. C
6. D
7. C
8. A
9. D
10. D

XI.
1. biopsy
2. discoid lupus erythematosus
3. intramuscular
4. skin graft
5. ointment

XII.
1. (ad′ĭ pōs)
2. (sel u li′tis)

3. (dər mə bra′shən)
4. (ik the o′sis)
5. (nod′ūl)
6. (on i ko fa′jə)
7. (pap′ūl)
8. (pi o jen′ə sis)
9. (sub ku ta′ne əs)
10. (ur ti kar′e ə)

XIII.
1. D
2. S
3. A
4. T
5. T
6. D
7. D
8. S
9. D
10. R

XIV.
1. E
2. B
3. D
4. C
5. A
6. G
7. F

CHAPTER 13

ANSWERS FOR SECTION REVIEWS

A.
1. aden(o)
2. home(o)
3. outside

B:
1. -physis

C.
1. breast
2. breast
3. pro-

D.
1. adrenal glands
2. male or masculine
3. large
4. gonads
5. iod(o)
6. pituitar(o)
7. thyroid gland

8. trop(o)
9. four
10. -tropic
11. -tropin

E.
1. insulin(o)
2. parathyroid(o)

ANSWERS FOR CHAPTER REVIEW

I.

B	I	O					A	D	E	N	O			D	Y	N	I	A				
I		M		P		P		D								E		U		L		
	P	A	R	A	T	H	Y	R	O	I	D	O				U		R		G		
B		N		N		Y		E		N		H			I	O	D	O		I		
T		C		S		E		N		S		U				M		O		A		
U		R		I		S		O		U					E	X	O					
I		E		S		A		L		L			G	I	G	A	N	T	O		T	
T		A			T	E	T	R	A		N				R		H	Y	P	O		
C	R	I	N	O		H		G	O	N	A	D	O						P	R	O	X
O						Y				D			I			P	R	O				I
		P			R		I				S		R		C	A	L	C	I	O		C
	M	A	S	T	O		S		M	A	M	M	O						A			O
	E	R						D	Y	S									T			
	L	A	C	T	O		E	C	T	O	M	Y							R			
G	Y	N	E	C	O		D		I				G	R	A	P	H	Y				I
R		O		N			E		E					S								S
A				C		M	E	T	A		G	E	N	I	C			S	A	N	T	
M	E	G	A	L	O		A		L					S								

II.
1. C
2. B
3. B
4. A
5. D

III.
1. D
2. D
3. A
4. D
5. D
6. C
7. D
8. D
9. D
10. B
11. E
12. D
13. E

IV.
1. B
2. F
3. C
4. E
5. G
6. A
7. D

V.
(no particular order)
1. nervous stimulation
2. secretion of hormones in response to other hormones
3. negative feedback mechanism

VI.
1. B
2. C
3. A
4. C
5. D
6. A
7. D
8. A
9. A
10. B
11. D
12. A

VII.
1. hypoglycemia
2. hypoadrenalism
3. hypoinsulinism
4. hypercalcemia
5. hyperthyroidism
6. mammary
7. gonadal
8. androgenic
9. mastectomy
10. homeostasis

VIII.
mammoplasty, euthyroid

IX.
1. adrenocorticotropic hormone
2. American Diabetes Association
3. basal metabolic rate
4. follicle-stimulating hormone
5. parathormone

X.
1. (ak″ro meg′ə le)
2. (ə dre no jen′i tal)
3. (an drop′ə the)
4. (kə kek′se ə)
5. (cə los′trəm)
6. (ek sof thal′mos)
7. (ho″me o sta′ sis)
8. (hi″pər kal se′me ə)
9. (hi pof′ə sis)
10. (lak tif′ər əs)

XI.
1. S
2. D
3. A
4. D
5. R
6. S
7. D
8. D
9. R
10. D

XII.
1. adrenal cortical
2. diabetic
3. hormone
4. posterior
5. thyroid

CHAPTER 14

I.

```
K E R A T O     P Y O       A       H       A     G L Y C O     L A C T O
        M                 G E N I T O       U       E       R       B       H       D
P O L Y     A D     C       A               M       T       N       A   L   A L B O   O   N T
H       L       A   H       S       P H L E B O           D Y N I A           O           T
A B   O N Y C H O   T       O           O           I           S       R           T
S       I       R   L       R       S   K       C           P O S T E R O           O
O       S       G Y N E C O       T R I C H O       M       E
    T O M Y       O       L       C       N       N       E       P       C H E I L O
H       A       O       V       Y       I       E       T       L       S       A               L
E       P L A S I A   S   D O R S O       R       A   I       A   A L G I A       P
P       T       S   I       A   I   C A P N I A       S       I       T       A
A T H E R O       O   S C L E R O       U       O           I       T   O M A   R
T       U   M       E       R       T   G   R R H A P H Y       R       E       O
O       T       A   R       R   Y       A S E R       R       R   E       O
    H Y S T E R O   V   T R I   N       N   H   D   C O L P O
        O       O   H       I       H       E   E M E S I S       I
A E R O       A       C E R E B R O   O   L       I   X   P
    A   G I N G I V O   O           L       I A S I S   O           H
M Y C O       I               C E N T E S I S   O       P   E
A       O   M A L A C I A   P       S       C H R O M O   R   A
N       C   S       S   H   A N K Y L O       R   O   A
I   S A L P I N G O   T   A   N   T           G   G   P   I   O
A   R   A   P   H   T           G   G   P   I   O
    C   C   S   C H O L E D O C H O   L   E C T O M Y   U
    A   I   M   T   N   R       O   R   O   I N
C R I N E   E S T H E S I O   A L G E S I O           I
    D   O       A   A   A   C       S   N E P H R O
    I   C E P H A L O   C H O N D R O   T
C O L O       M   B   R       I   O O P H O R O
        S T E N O S I S   O M P H A L O
```

II.
1. F
2. H
3. D
4. C
5. B

III.
1. pedodontist
2. cardiac
3. oral
4. symptom
5. oncology

IV.
1. E
2. B
3. H
4. G
5. A

V.
1. chirospasm
2. ophthalmitis
3. dyskinesia
4. blepharotomy
5. prone

VI.
1. melan(in)
2. active
3. erythro(cyte)
4. (v)irulence
5. (a)plastic

VII.
1. leukocytosis
2. poikilocyte
3. hemoglobin
4. mucoid or mucous
5. intracellular

VIII.
1. (c)oronary
2. (c)ardiovascular
3. (a)orta
4. (s)ystemic
5. (l)ymphatic

IX.
1. lymphangioma
2. asystole
3. bradycardia
4. hypertension
5. endocardium

X.
1. (o)ximeter
2. (pneum)oconiosis
3. (p)olyp
4. (t)achypnea
5. (e)dema

XI.
1. alveoli
2. dyspnea
3. bronchoscopy
4. rhinitis
5. endotracheal

XII.
1. B
2. A
3. G
4. E
5. F

XIII.
1. lactase
2. hyperemesis
3. vagotomy
4. cholecystitis
5. pyloroscopy

XIV.
1. (u)remia
2. (nephro)malacia
3. pyel(itis)
4. (litho)tripsy
5. (b)ladder

XV.
1. cystoscopy
2. nephron
3. urethrocele
4. glycosuria
5. nephrosonography

XVI.
1. B
2. A

3. A
4. B
5. F
6. D

XVII.
1. primigravida
2. neonate
3. hysteropexy
4. menarche
5. cryptorchidism

XVIII.
1. J
2. H
3. I
4. G
5. C

XIX.
1. arthropathy
2. calcipenia
3. coccygectomy
4. scoliosis
5. carpals

XX.
1. (a)xon
2. (acro)phobia
3. (m)eninges
4. (n)euron
5. (t)hermo(receptors)

XXI.
1. pyromania
2. dacryocystotomy
3. hemiplegia
4. neurotripsy
5. intracranial

XXII.
1. (b)ulla
2. (m)acule
3. (c)utaneous
4. (a)dipose
5. (s)ebum

XXIII.
1. cryosurgery
2. onychomycosis
3. hidradenitis

4. epidermis
5. trichoid

XXIV.
1. (h)omeostasis
2. (anti)diuretic
3. (p)ituitary
4. (m)ammary
5. (neuro)hypophysis

XXV.
1. hypoglycemia
2. adenocarcinoma
3. hypoparathyroidism
4. euthyroid
5. adrenalectomy

XXVI.
1. C
2. A
3. G
4. F
5. I
6. J
7. H
8. E
9. B
10. D

XXVII.
1. C
2. H
3. A
4. F
5. F
6. I
7. D
8. B
9. A
10. I
11. C
12. G
13. D
14. E
15. B
16. H
17. G
18. J

Word Parts

I. ENGLISH—GREEK OR LATIN

Meaning	Combining Form, Prefix, or Suffix
abdomen	abdomin(o)
abdominal wall	lapar(o)
abnormal	par-, para-
above	epi-
acid	acid(o)
across	trans-
adenoids	adenoid(o)
adrenalin	adrenalin(o)
adrenals	adren(o), adrenal(o)
after	post-
again	ana-
against	anti-, contra-
air	aer(o), pneum(o)
air sac	alveol(o)
albumin	albumin(o)
alkaline	alkal(o)
alveolus	alveol(o)
amnion	amni(o)
aneurysm	aneurysm(o)
ankle bone	tars(o)
anus	an(o)
anus and rectum	proct(o)
aorta	aort(o)
appendix	append(o), appendic(o)
arachnoid	arachn(o)
armpit	axill(o)
arms and legs	acr(o)
around	peri-
arteriole	arteriol(o)
artery	arter(o), arteri(o)
atrium	atri(o)
attraction	phil(o)
auditory tube	salping(o)
away from	ab-, ex-

Meaning	Combining Form, Prefix, or Suffix
back	dors(o)
backward	retr(o)
bacteria	bacter(i), bacteri(o)
bad	dys-, mal-
before	ante-, pre-, pro-
beginning	gen(o), -gen, -genic, -genesis, -genous
behind	poster(o), post-, retr(o)
belly side	ventr(o)
below or beneath	hypo-, sub-
below normal	hypo-
beside	par-, para-
between	inter-
beyond	supra-
bile	bil(i), chol(e)
binding	-desis
birth	nat(o)
birth (give birth)	par(o)
woman who has given birth	-para
black	melan(o)
bladder	cyst(o)
blood	hem(a), hem(o), hemat(o), -emia
blue	cyan(o)
body	som(a), somat(o)
bone	oste(o)
bone marrow	myel(o)
brain	cerebr(o), encephal(o)
break	-clasia
breast	mamm(o), mast(o)
breast bone	stern(o)
breathe, breathing	-pnea, spir(o)
bronchi	bronch(o), bronchi(o)
bronchiole	bronchiol(o)

Meaning	Combining Form, Prefix, or Suffix	Meaning	Combining Form, Prefix, or Suffix
bursa	burs(o)	digit	dactyl(o)
calcaneus	calcane(o)	dilation	-ectasia, -ectasis
calcium	calc(i)	discharge	-rrhea
calculus	lith(o), -lith	disease	nos(o), path(o),
cancer	cancer(o), carcin(o)		-osis, -pathy
carbon dioxide	-capnia	dissolving	lys(o)
carpus	carp(o)	distant	dist(o), tel(e)
cartilage	chondr(o)	diverticula	diverticul(o)
cecum	cec(o)	double	dipl(o)
cell	cyt(o), -cyte	down	de-
cerebellum	cerebell(o)	drooping	-ptosis
cerebrum	cerebr(o)	drugs	pharmac(o),
cervix uteri	cervic(o)		pharmaceut(o)
change	meta-	dry	xer(o)
chemical	chem(o)	duct	vas(o)
chest	steth(o), thorac(o)	ductus deferens	vas(o)
child	ped(o)	(vas deferens)	
chorion	chori(o)	duodenum	duoden(o)
clavicle	clavicul(o)	dust	coni(o)
clot (thrombus)	thromb(o)	ear	ot(o)
cluster	staphyl(o)	eat	phag(o)
coagulation	coagul(o)	edge of eyelid	tars(o)
coal	anthrac(o)	egg	o(o)
coccyx	coccyg(o)	electricity	electr(o)
cold	cry(o)	embolus	embol(o)
collarbone	clavicul(o)	embryonic form	-blast, blast(o)
colon	col(o)	endocardium	endocardi(o)
color	chrom(o)	enzyme	-ase
common bile duct	choledoch(o)	epididymis	epididym(o)
compartment	cellul(o)	epiglottis	epiglott(o)
condition	-ia, -iasis, -ism, -osis, -y	equal	is(o)
constant	home(o)	erythema	erythemat(o)
controlling	-stasis	esophagus	esophag(o)
cornea	kerat(o)	examine	scop(o)
cramp	-spasm	instrument used	-scope
cranium	crani(o)	process of	-scopy
crown	coron(o)	examining	
cut (to cut)	tom(o)	excessive	hyper-
incision or cutting	-tomy	excision	-ectomy
instrument used	-tome	extremities	acr(o)
to cut		eye	ocul(o), ophthalm(o)
cyst	cyst(o)	eyelid	blephar(o)
death	necr(o)	false	pseud(o)
decreased or		far	dist(o)
deficient	-penia	fascia	fasci(o)
destruction	lys(o)	fast	tachy-
that which destroys	-lysin	fat	adip(o), lip(o)
process of	-lysis	fear (abnormal)	-phobia
destroying		feeling	esthesi(o), -esthesia
capable of	-lytic	female	gynec(o)
destroying		femur	femor(o)
development	plas(o), -plasia	fetus	fet(o)
diaphragm	-phren(o)	few	olig(o)
difficult	dys-	fiber, fibrous	fibr(o)
digestion	-pepsia	fibula	fibul(o)

Meaning	Combining Form, Prefix, or Suffix	Meaning	Combining Form, Prefix, or Suffix
fingers or toes	dactyl(o)	inferior	infer(o)
fire	pyr(o)	inflammation	-itis
first	primi-	ingest	phag(o)
fish	ichthy(o)	inside	in-, en-, end-, endo-
flow	-rrhea	insulin	insulin(o)
follicle	follicul(o)	intestine	enter(o), intestin(o)
foot	ped(o), pod(o), pes-, -pod	iodine	iod(o)
for	pro-	iris	ir(o), irid(o)
form	morph(o)	irregular	poikil(o)
formation	plas(o), -plasia	irrigation	-clysis
formation of an opening	-stomy	ischium	ischi(o)
four	quadri-, tetra-	jejunum	jejun(o)
from	de-	joined together	syn-, sym-
front	anter(o)	joint	arthr(o)
fruit	fruct(o)	ketone bodies	ket(o), keton(o)
fungus	fung(i), myc(o)	kidney	nephr(o), ren(o)
fusion	-desis	killing	-cidal
gall	chol(e)	kneecap	patell(o)
gallbladder	cholecyst(o)	large	gigant(o), macr(o), megal(o), -megaly
gland	aden(o)	large intestine	col(o)
glomerulus	glomerul(o)	larynx	laryng(o)
gonads (ovaries and testes)	gonad(o)	life	bi(o)
good	eu-	light	phot(o)
green	chlor(o)	lip	cheil(o)
growth	-physis	liver	hepat(o)
gums	gingiv(o)	living	bi(o)
hair	pil(o), trich(o)	lobe	lob(o)
half	hemi-, semi-	location	top(o)
hand	chir(o)	lower back	lumb(o)
hard	kerat(o), scler(o)	lung	pneum(o), pneumon(o), pulm(o), pulmon(o)
hardening	scler(o), -sclerosis	lymph	lymph(o)
head	cephal(o)	lymph node	lymphaden(o)
hearing	audi(o)	lymph vessel	lymphangi(o)
heart	cardi(o)	lymphatics	lymph(o), lymphat(o)
heat	therm(o)	male	andr(o)
heel bone	calcane(o)	mandible	mandibul(o)
hemoglobin	hemoglobin(o)	many	multi-, poly-
hemorrhage	-rrhagia	masculine	andr(o)
hernia	-cele	maxilla	maxill(o)
hidden	crypt(o)	measure	metr(o)
horny	kerat(o)	instrument used	-meter
humerus	humer(o)	process	-metry
ileum	ile(o)	mediastinum	mediastin(o)
ilium	ili(o)	medicine	-iatrics, -iatry, pharmac(o)
immune	immun(o)	membrane	-eum, -ium
imperfect	atel(o)	meninges	mening(o)
incision	tom(o), -tomy	middle	medi(o), meso-
instrument used	-tome	midwife	obstetr(o)
incomplete	atel(o)	milk	lact(o)
increase	-osis	mind	ment(o), phren(o), psych(o)
individual	idio-		
infection	seps(o), sept(o)	month	men(o)

Meaning	Combining Form, Prefix, or Suffix	Meaning	Combining Form, Prefix, or Suffix
more than normal	hyper-	pituitary gland	pituitar(o)
mouth	or(o), stomat(o)	place (position)	top(o)
movement	kinesi(o), -kinesia	pleura	pleur(o)
mucus	muc(o)	poison	tox(o), toxic(o)
muscle	muscul(o), my(o)	practitioner	-iatrician
myocardium	myocardi(o)	pregnant female	-gravida
nail	onych(o), ungu(o)	pregnancy	-cyesis
narrowing	-stenosis	preoccupation	
nature	physi(o)	(excessive)	-mania
near	par-, para-, proxim(o)	production	-poiesis
neck	cervic(o)	prolapse	-ptosis
nerve	neur(o), nerv(o)	process	-ation
neuroglia	gli(o)	production cause	-poietin
new	neo-	prostate gland	prostat(o)
new opening	-stomy	protection	-phylaxis
next (as in a series)	meta-	protein	prote(o)
no	a-, an-	pubis	pub(o)
none	nulli-	pus	py(o)
normal	norm(o), eu-	pylorus	pylor(o)
nose	nas(o), rhin(o)	radiant energy	radi(o)
not	a-, an- in-	radius	radi(o)
nucleus	kary(o), nucle(o)	record (the record)	-gram
nutrition	troph(o), -trophy	to record	gram(o)
obsessive		recording	
preoccupation	-mania	instrument	-graph
old, elderly	ger(a), ger(o),	rectum	rect(o)
geront(o)		red, redness	erythr(o),
one	uni-, mon(o)	erythemat(o)	
one who	-er, -ist	removal	-ectomy
one who studies	-logist	renal pelvis	pyel(o)
organs of		reproduction	gon(o)
reproduction	genit(o), gon(o)	resembling	-oid
origin	gen(o), -gen, -genic,	reversing	de-
	-genesis, -genous	rheumatism	rheumat(o)
out	ex-	ribs	cost(o)
outside	ecto-, exo-, extra-	round	spher(o)
outward	exo-	rupture	-rrhexis
ovary	oophor(o)	sac	cyst(o)
oxygen	ox(i)	sacrum	sacr(o)
pain	-algia, -dynia	sag	-ptosis
painful	dys-	saliva	sial(o)
palate	palat(o)	salivary gland	sialaden(o)
pancreas	pancreat(o)	sameness	home(o)
paralysis	pleg(o), -plegia	scapula	
parathyroid gland	parathyroid(o)	(shoulder blade)	scapul(o)
patella (kneecap)	patell(o)	scrotum	scrot(o)
pelvis	pelv(i)	sebum	seb(o)
penis	pen(o)	secrete	crin(o), -crine
pericardium	pericardi(o)	seizure	-lepsy
perineum	perine(o)	self	aut(o)
peritoneum	periton(o)	semen	semin(o)
perspiration	hidr(o)	sensation	esthesi(o)
pertaining to	-ac, -al, -eal, -ic, -ous,	sensitivity to pain	algesi(o)
	-ary, -tic	septum	sept(o)
phalanges	phalang(o)	shape	morph(o)
pharynx	pharyng(o)	shoulder blade	scapul(o)

Meaning	Combining Form, Prefix, or Suffix	Meaning	Combining Form, Prefix, or Suffix
side	later(o)	tail	caud(o)
sigmoid colon	sigmoid(o)	tail bone	coccyg(o)
single	mon(o)	tarsals (ankle bones)	tars(o)
sinus	sin(o)	tear (crying)	dacry(o), lacrim(o)
situated above	super(o), super-,	teeth	dent(i), dent(o),
supra-			odont(o)
situated below	infer(o), infra-	tendon	ten(o), tend(o),
skin	cutane(o), derm(a),		tendin(o)
	dermat(o)	testis, testicle	orchi(o), orchid(o),
skull	crani(o)		test(o)
sleep	narc(o)	thirst	dips(o)
slow	brady-	thorny	spin(o)
small	micr(o), -ole	three	tri-
small intestine	enter(o)	throat	pharyng(o)
soft, softening	malac(o), -malacia	thrombus	thromb(o)
sound	ech(o), son(o)	through	dia-, trans-
specialist	-ist	thymus	thym(o)
speech	phas(o)	thyroid gland	thyr(o), thryoid(o)
sperm, spermatozoa	spermat(o), sperm(o)	tibia	tibi(o)
spider	arachn(o)	tissue	hist(o)
spinal cord	myel(o)	together	sym-
spine	rach(i), rachi(o),	tongue	gloss(o), lungu(o)
	spondyl(o), spin(o)	tonsil	tonsill(o)
spitting	-ptysis	toward	ad-, -ad
spiral	spir(o)	trachea	trache(o)
spleen	splen(o)	transmission	phoresis
split	schist(o), schiz(o),	treatment	therapeut(o), -therapy
	-schisis	tree	dendr(o)
star	astr(o)	tumor	onc(o), -oma
starch	amyl(o)	turn	trop(o)
sternum (breast		twice	di-
bone)	stern(o)	twisted	strept(o)
sticky substance	gli(o)	twitching	-spasm
stiff	ankyl(o)	two	bi-, di-
stimulate	trop(o), -tropic	ulna	uln(o)
that which		umbilicus	omphal(o)
stimulates	-tropin	under	sub-
stomach	gastr(o)	up	ana-
stone	lith(o), -lith	upon	epi-
stopping	-stasis	uppermost	super(o)
straight	orth(o)	ureter	ureter(o)
stretching	-ectasia, ectasis	urethra	urethr(o)
stricture	-stenosis	urinary tract	ur(o)
structure	-id	urination	urin(o)
study or science of	-logy	urine	ur(o), urin(o)
sugar	glyc(o), glycos(o), -ose	uterine tissue	metr(o)
sun	heli(o)	uterine tube	salping(o)
surgical crushing	-tripsy	uterus	hyster(o), uter(o)
surgical fixation	pex(o), -pexy	uvula	staphyl(o)
surgical puncture	-centesis	vagina	colp(o), vagin(o)
surgical repair	-plasty	vagus nerve	vag(o)
suture	-rrhaphy	valve	valv(o), valvul(o)
sweat	hidr(o)	varicose vein	varic(o)
swelling	-edema	vein	phleb(o), ven(o),
symptom	sympt(o)		ven(i)
synovial membrane	synov(o), synovi(o)	ventral	ventr(o)

Meaning	Combining Form, Prefix, or Suffix	Meaning	Combining Form, Prefix, or Suffix
ventricle	ventricul(o)	water	hydr(o)
venule	venul(o)	weakness	-asthenia
vertebra	spondyl(o), vertebr(o)	white	alb(o), albin(o),
vessel	angi(o), vas(o),		leuk(o)
	vascul(o)	windpipe	trache(o)
view	-opsy	within	intra-
viscera	viscer(o)	without	a-, an-, ex-
vision	opt(o), optic(o)	wrinkle	rhytid(o)
voice	phon(o)	wrist bone	carp(o)
vomiting	-emesis	yellow	xanth(o)
vulva	vulv(o)	yellow, fatty plaque	ather(o)
washing out	-clysis		

II. WORD PARTS—ENGLISH

Combining Form, Prefix, or Suffix	Meaning	Combining Form, Prefix, or Suffix	Meaning
a-	no; not; without	append(o),	
ab-	away from	appendic(o)	appendix
abdomin(o)	abdomen	arachn(o)	arachnoid; spider
-ac	pertaining to	arter(o),	
acid(o)	acid	arteri(o)	artery
acr(o)	extremities; arms or	arteriol(o)	arteriole
legs		arthr(o)	joint
ad-	toward	-ary	pertaining to
-ad	toward	-ase	enzyme
aden(o)	gland	-asthenia	weakness
adenoid(o)	adenoids	astr(o)	star
adip(o)	fat	-ate	cause or result of an
adren(o),			action
adrenal(o)	adrenal glands	atel(o)	imperfect or
adrenalin(o)	adrenalin		incomplete
aer(o)	air or gas	ather(o)	yellow, fatty plaque
-al, -an	pertaining to	-ation	process
alb(o),		atri(o)	atrium
albin(o)	white	audi(o)	hearing
albumin(o)	albumin	aut(o)	self
algesi(o)	sensitivity to pain	axill(o)	armpit
-algia	pain	bacter(i),	
alkal(o)	alkaline; basic	bacteri(o)	bacteria
alveol(o)	alveolus; air sac	bi-	two
amni(o)	amnion	bi(o)	life; living
amyl(o)	starch	bil(i)	bile
an-	no; without	-blast,	
an(o)	anus	blast(o)	embryonic form
ana-	up or again	blephar(o)	eyelid
andr(o)	male or masculine	brady-	slow
aneurysm(o)	aneurysm	bronch(o),	
angi(o)	vessel	bronchi(o)	bronchi
ankyl(o)	stiff	bronchiol(o)	bronchiole
-ant	that which causes	burs(o)	bursa
ante-	before	calc(i)	calcium
anter(o),	front	calcane(o)	calcaneus (heel bone)
anthrac(o)	coal	cancer(o),	
anti-	against	carcin(o)	cancer
aort(o)	aorta	-capnia	carbon dioxide

Combining Form, Prefix, or Suffix	Meaning	Combining Form, Prefix, or Suffix	Meaning
cardi(o)	heart	dia-	through
carp(o)	carpus (wrist bone)	dipl(o)	double
caud(o)	tail	dips(o)	thirst
cec(o)	cecum	dist(o)	distant; far
-cele	hernia	diverticul(o)	diverticula
cellul(o)	little cell or	dors(o)	back
	compartment	duoden(o)	duodenum
-centesis	surgical puncture	-dynia	pain
cephal(o)	head	dys-	bad; difficult; painful
cerebell(o)	cerebellum	-eal	pertaining to
cerebr(o)	cerebrum; brain	ech(o)	sound
cervic(o)	neck; cervix uteri	-ectasia,	
cheil(o)	lip	-ectasis	stretching, dilation
chem(o)	chemical	ecto-	situated on or outisde
chir(o)	hand	-ectomy	excision; removal
chlor(o)	green	-edema	swelling
chol(e)	gall; bile	electr(o)	electricity
cholecyst(o)	gallbladder	embol(o)	embolus
choledoch(o)	common bile duct	-emesis	vomiting
chondr(o)	cartilage	-emia	blood
chori(o)	chorion	enter(o)	intestine; small
chrom(o)	color		intestine
-cidal	killing	epi-	above; upon
-clasia	break	epididym(o)	epididymis
clavicul(o)	clavicle (collar bone)	en-	inside
-clysis	irrigation; washing out	encephal(o)	brain
coagul(o)	coagulation	end-,	
coccyg(o)	coccyx (tail bone)	endo-	inside
col(o)	colon; large intestine	endocardi(o)	endocardium
colp(o)	vagina	epiglott(o)	epiglottis
coni(o)	dust	-er	one who
contra-	against	erythr(o)	red
coron(o)	crown	erythemat(o)	erythema or redness
cost(o)	ribs	esophag(o)	esophagus
crani(o)	cranium; skull	esthesi(o)	feeling
crin(o),		-esthesia	feeling
-crine	secrete	eu-	good; normal
cry(o)	cold	-eum	membrane
crypt(o)	hidden	ex-	out; without; away from
cutane(o)	skin	exo-	outside; outward
cyan(o)	blue	extra-	outside
-cyesis	pregnancy	fasci(o)	fascia
cyst(o)	bladder; cyst; sac	femor(o)	femur
cyt(o),		fet(o)	fetus
-cyte	cell	fibr(o)	fiber; fibrous
dacry(o)	tear	fibrin(o)	fibrin
dactyl(o)	digits; fingers or toes	fibul(o)	fibula
de-	down; from; reversing	follicul(o)	follicle
dendr(o)	tree	fruct(o)	fruit
dent(i),		fung(i)	fungus
dent(o)	teeth	gastr(o)	stomach
-derm,		gen(o),	
derm(a),		-gen,	
dermat(o)	skin	-genic,	
-desis	binding, fusion	-genesis,	
di-	twice; two	-genous	beginning; origin

Combining Form, Prefix, or Suffix	Meaning	Combining Form, Prefix, or Suffix	Meaning
genit(o)	organs of reproduction	inter-	between
ger(a),		intestin(o)	intestines
ger(o),	old; elderly	intra-	within
geront(o)		iod(o)	iodine
gigant(o)	large	ir(o), irid(o)	iris
gingiv(o)	gums	is(o)	equal
gli(o)	neuroglia or a sticky substance	ischi(o)	ischium
		-ist	one who
glomerul(o)	glomerulus	-itis	inflammation
gloss(o)	tongue	-ium	membrane
glyc(o),		jejun(o)	jejunum
glycos(o)	sugar	kary(o)	nucleus
gon(o)	genitals; reproduction	kerat(o)	cornea; horny; hard
gonad(o)	gonads (ovaries or testes)	ket(o), keton(o)	ketone bodies
		kinesi(o),	
-gram	a record	-kinesia	movement
gram(o)	to record	lacrim(o)	tear
-graph	instrument for recording	lact(o)	milk
		lapar(o)	abdominal wall
-graphy	process of recording	laryng(o)	larynx
-gravida	pregnant female	later(o)	side
gynec(o)	female	-lepsy	seizure
heli(o)	sun	leuk(o)	white
hem(a),		lingu(o)	tongue
hem(o),		lip(o)	fat
hemat(o)	blood	lith(o),	
hemi-	half	-lith	stone; calculus
hemoglobin(o)	hemoglobin	lob(o)	lobe
hepat(o)	liver	-logist	one who studies
hidr(o)	sweat; perspiration	-logy	study or science of
hist(o)	tissue	lumb(o)	lower back
home(o)	constant; sameness	lymph(o)	lymph; lymphatics
humer(o)	humerus (upper arm bone)	lymphaden(o)	lymph node
		lymphangi(o)	lymph vessel
hydr(o)	water	lymphat(o)	lymphatics
hyper-	excessive; more than normal	lys(o)	destruction; dissolving
		-lysin	that which destroys
hypo-	beneath; below normal	-lysis	process of destroying
hyster(o)	uterus	-lytic	capable of destroying
-ia,		macr(o)	large
-iasis	condition	mal-	bad
-iatrician	practitioner	malac(o)	soft; softening
-iatrics,		-malacia	softness
-iatry	medicine	mamm(o)	breast
-ic	pertaining to	-mania	excessive preoccupation
ichthy(o)	fish		
-id	structure; having the shape of	mast(o)	breast
		mandibul(o)	mandible
idio-	individual	maxill(o)	maxilla
ile(o)	ileum	medi(o)	middle
ili(o)	ilium	mediastin(o)	mediastinum
immun(o)	immune	mega(o)	large
in-	not; inside	megal(o)	large; enlarged
infer(o)	inferior; situated below	-megaly	enlargement
infra-	below	melan(o)	black
insulin(o)	insulin	men(o)	month

Combining Form, Prefix, or Suffix	Meaning	Combining Form, Prefix, or Suffix	Meaning
mening(o)	meninges	oste(o)	bone
ment(o)	mind	ot(o)	ear
meso-	middle	-ous	pertaining to or characterized by
meta-	change; next, as in a series	ox(i)	oxygen
metr(o)	measure; uterine tissue	palat(o)	palate
-meter	instrument used to measure	pancreat(o)	pancreas
		par-,	
-metry	process of measuring	para-	near; beside; abnormal
micro-	small	-para	woman who has given birth
mon(o)	one or single		
morph(o)	form; shape	par(o)	to give birth
muc(o)	mucus	parathyroid(o)	parathyroid gland
multi-	many	patell(o)	patella (kneecap)
muscul(o)	muscle	path(o),	
my(o),		-pathy	disease
myocardi(o)	myocardium	ped(o)	child; foot
myc(o)	fungus	pelv(i)	pelvis
myel(o)	bone marrow; spinal cord	pen(o)	penis
		-penia	deficient; decreased
narc(o)	sleep	-pepsia	digestion
nas(o)	nose	peri-	around
nat(o)	birth	pericardi(o)	pericardium
necr(o)	death	perine(o)	perineum
neo-	new	periton(o)	peritoneum
nephr(o)	kidney	pes-	foot
neur(o)	nerve	pex(o),	
norm(o)	normal	-pexy	surgical fixation
nos(o)	disease	phag(o)	eat; ingest
nucle(o)	nucleus	phalang(o)	phalanges (finger and toe bones)
nulli-	none		
o(o)	egg	pharmac(o)	drugs; medicine
obstetr(o)	midwife	pharmaceut(o)	drugs
ocul(o)	eye	pharyng(o)	throat; pharynx
odont(o)	teeth	phas(o)	speech
-oid	resembling	phil(o)	attraction
-ole	small	phleb(o)	vein
olig(o)	few	-phobia	abnormal fear
-oma	tumor	phon(o)	voice
omphal(o)	umbilicus (navel)	-phoresis	transmission
onc(o)	tumor	phot(o)	light
onych(o)	nail	phren(o)	diaphragm; mind
oophor(o)	ovary	-phylaxis	protection
ophthalm(o)	eye	physi(o)	nature
-opia	vision	-physis	growth
-opsy	to view	pil(o)	hair
opt(o),		pituitar(o)	pituitary gland
optic(o)	vision	plas(o),	
or(o)	mouth	-plasia	formation; development
orchi(o),		plast(o)	repair
orchid(o)	testis	-plasty	surgical repair
orth(o)	straight	pleg(o),	
-ose	sugar	-plegia	paralysis
-osis	condition; disease; increase	pleur(o)	pleura
		-pnea	breathing

Combining Form, Prefix, or Suffix	Meaning	Combining Form, Prefix, or Suffix	Meaning
pneum(o)	air; lung	-scope	instrument used for viewing
pneumon(o)	lung	-scopy	process of visually examining
-pod, pod(o)	foot	scrot(o)	scrotum
-poiesis	production	seb(o)	sebum
-poietin	substance that causes production	semi-	half
poikil(o)	irregular	semin(o)	semen
poly-	many	seps(o)	infection
post-	after; behind	sept(o)	infection; septum
poster(o)	behind	sial(o)	saliva; salivary glands
pre-	before	sialaden(o)	salivary gland
primi-	first	sigmoid(o)	sigmoid colon
pro-	before; for	sin(o)	sinus
proct(o)	anus; rectum	som(a), somat(o)	body
prostat(o)	prostate gland	son(o)	sound
prote(o)	protein	-spasm	cramp; twitching
proxim(o)	near	sperm(o), spermat(o)	spermatozoa
pseud(o)	false	spher(o)	round
psych(o)	mind	spin(o)	spine or thorny
-ptosis	sag; prolapse	spir(o)	to breathe; spiral
-ptysis	spitting	splen(o)	spleen
pub(o)	pubis	spondyl(o)	vertebrae (spine)
pulm(o), pulmon(o)	lungs	-stalsis	contraction
py(o)	pus	staphyl(o)	cluster; uvula
pyel(o)	renal pelvis	-stasis	stopping; controlling
pylor(o)	pylorus	-stenosis	stricture; narrowing
pyr(o)	fire	stern(o)	sternum (breast bone)
quadri-	four	steth(o)	chest
rach(i), rachi(o)	spine	stomat(o)	mouth
radi(o)	radius; radiant energy	-stomy	formation of an opening
rect(o)	rectum	strept(o)	twisted
ren(o)	kidney	sub-	below; under
retro-	behind; backward	super(o)	situated above or uppermost
rheumat(o)	rheumatism	super-	above or excess
rhin(o)	nose	supra-	above; beyond
rhytid(o)	wrinkle	sym-, syn-	joined; together
-rrhagia	hemorrhage	sympt(o)	symptom
-rrhaphy	suture	synov(o), synovi(o)	synovial membrane
-rrhea	flow; discharge	tachy-	fast
-rrhexis	rupture	tars(o)	tarsals; edge of eyelid
sacr(o)	sacrum	tel(e)	distant
salping(o)	uterine tubes; auditory tube	ten(o), tend(o), tendin(o)	tendon
-sarcoma	malignant tumor from connective tissue	test(o)	testes
scapul(o)	scapula (shoulder blade)	tetra-	four
-schisis, schist(o), schiz(o)	split	therapeut(o)	treatment
scler(o)	hard; hardening	therm(o)	heat
-sclerosis	abnormal hardening	thorac(o)	chest
scop(o)	examine; to view	thromb(o)	clot or thrombus
		thym(o)	thymus

Combining Form, Prefix, or Suffix	Meaning	Combining Form, Prefix, or Suffix	Meaning
thyr(o)	thyroid gland	ur(o)	urine; urinary tract
thyroid(o)		ureter(o)	ureter
tibi(o)	tibia	urethr(o)	urethra
-tic	pertaining to	urin(o)	urine or urination
tom(o)	to cut	uter(o)	uterus
-tome	instrument used in cutting	vag(o)	vagus nerve
		vagin(o)	vagina
-tomy	incision, cutting	valv(o)	valve
tonsill(o)	tonsil	valvul(o)	
top(o)	place; position	varic(o)	varicose vein
tox(o),		vas(o)	vessel; duct; vas deferens
toxic(o)	poison	vascul(o)	vessel
trache(o)	trachea (windpipe)	ven(i),	
trans-	through; across	ven(o)	vein
tri-	three	ventr(o)	ventral; belly side
trich(o)	hair	ventricul(o)	ventricle of brain or heart
-tripsy	surgical crushing		
trop(o)	to stimulate or turn	venul(o)	venule
troph(o),		vertebr(o)	vertebrae
-trophy	nutrition	viscer(o)	viscera
-tropic	stimulate	vulv(o)	vulva
-tropin	that which stimulates	xanth(o)	yellow
uln(o)	ulna	xer(o)	dry
ungu(o)	nail	-y	condition or state
uni-	one		

Bibliography

American Cancer Society: *Ca—A Cancer Journal for Clinicians—* Vol 50, No 1, Atlanta, GA, 2000.

Applegate EJ: *The anatomy and physiology learning system: textbook,* Philadelphia, 2000, WB Saunders.

Bedolla M: *Essential Spanish for health care,* New York, 1997, Living Language, A Random House Company.

Bonewit K: *Clinical procedures for medical assistants,* ed 3, Philadelphia, 1990, WB Saunders.

Dorland's Illustrated Medical Dictionary, ed 29, Philadelphia, 1994, WB Saunders.

Dunmore CW, Fleischer RM: *Medical terminology, exercises in etymology,* ed 2, Philadelphia, 1985, FA Davis.

Frederick PM, Kinn ME: *Medical office assistant,* ed 5, Philadelphia, 1981, WB Saunders.

Fuller JR: *Surgical technology principles and practices,* ed 2, Philadelphia, 1986, WB Saunders.

Ignatavicius DD, Workman ML, Mishler MA: *Medical-surgical nursing across the health care continuum,* Philadelphia, 1991, WB Saunders.

Joyce EV, Villanueva ME: *Say it in Spanish: a guide for health care professionals,* Philadelphia, 1996, WB Saunders.

Miller BF, Keane CB: *Encyclopedia and dictionary of medicine, nursing, and allied health,* ed 4, Philadelphia, 1987, WB Saunders.

Mosby's medical, nursing, and allied health dictionary, St Louis, 1998, Mosby.

Polaski AL, Tatro SE: *Luckmann's core principles and practice of medical-surgical nursing,* Philadelphia, 1996, WB Saunders.

Sloane SB: *The medical word book,* ed 3, Philadelphia, 1991, WB Saunders.

Thomas CL (editor): *Taber's cyclopedic medical dictionary,* ed 17, Philadelphia, 1993, FA Davis.

Velasquez M: *Velasquez Spanish and English dictionary,* Clinton, NJ, 1985, New Win Publishing.

Index/Glossary

NOTE: Page numbers followed by the letter f refer to figures; those followed by the letter t refer to tables.

558

aerobic (ār-o′bik) having molecular oxygen present; growing, living, or occurring in the presence of molecular oxygen; requiring oxygen for respiration; designed to increase oxygen consumption by the body. 93, 271

aerosol (ār′o-sol) a suspension of fine particles in air or gas. 456

afebrile (a-feb′ril) without fever. 61

afferent (af′ər-ənt) conducting or conveying toward a center. 391

agglutination (ə-gloo″tĭ-na′shən) aggregation of suspended cells into clumps or masses; also the process of union in wound healing. 88

agoraphobia (ag″o-rə-fo′be-ə) intense, irrational fear of open spaces, characterized by marked fear of being alone or of being in public places where escape would be difficult or help might be unavailable. 421

AIDS see acquired immunodeficiency syndrome.

albinism (al′bĭ-niz-əm) congenital absence of pigment in the skin, hair, and eyes, owing to absence or defect of tyrosinase, an enzyme that catalyzes the oxidation of tyrosine, a precursor of melanin. 454

albino (al-bi′no) a person affected with a congenital absence of normal pigmentation in the body owing to a defect in melanin precursors. 454

albumin (al-bu′min) a protein found in animal tissue and the major serum protein. 269

albuminuria (al″bu-mĭ-nu′re-ə) the presence of albumin in the urine. 269

aldosterone (al-dos′tər-ōn) the principal electrolyte-regulating steroid hormone secreted by the adrenal cortex. 482t

algesia (al-je′zhə) sensitivity to pain; hyperesthesia. 418

alimentary tract (al″ə-men′tər-e trakt) the part of the digestive structures formed by the esophagus, stomach, and the intestines; digestive tract. 196

alimentation (al″ə-men-ta′shən) the act of giving or receiving nutriment. 198

alkalemia (al″kə-le′me-ə) increased pH (abnormal increased alkaline condition) of the blood. 157, 158t

alkaline (al′kə-līn, -lin) having the reactions of an alkali, any of a class of compounds that form soluble soaps with fatty acids, turn red litmus blue, and form soluble carbonates. 157

alkalosis increased alkaline nature of body fluids owing to accumulation of base or loss of acid. 156

allergen (al′ər-jen) an antigenic substance capable of producing immediate-type hypersensitivity (allergy). 91

allergy (al′ər-je) a hypersensitive state acquired through exposure to a particular allergen. 91

alopecia (al″o-pe′she-ə) baldness; absence of hair from skin areas where it is normally present. 440

alveolar (al-ve′ə-lər) pertaining to the alveoli. 162

alveolus (al-ve′ə-ləs) a small saclike dilatation. 162

    pulmonary a. (pool′mo-nar′e) one of a cluster of small outpocketings at the end of the bronchioles through which the exchange of carbon dioxide and oxygen takes place between alveolar air and capillary blood. 162

Alzheimer's disease (awltz′hi-marz dĭ-zēz′) a progressive degenerative disease of the brain of unknown cause and characterized by diffuse atrophy throughout the cerebral cortex with distinctive histopathologic changes; sometimes called primary degenerative dementia. 403

ambulation (am″bu-la′shən) the act of walking. 60

amenorrhea (ə-men″o-re′ə) absence or abnormal stoppage of the menses. 307

amniocentesis (am″ne-o-sen-te′sis) percutaneous transabdominal puncture of the amnion for the purpose of removing amniotic fluid. 296

amniochorial, amniochorionic (am″ne-o-kor′e-əl, am″ne-o-kor″e-on′ik) relating to both amnion and chorion. 291

amnion (am′ne-on) the thin membrane that lines the chorion and contains the fetus and the amniotic fluid around it. 291

amniorrhea (am″ne-o-re′ə) escape of the amniotic fluid. 291

amniorrhexis (am″ne-o-rek′sis) rupture of the amnion. 291

amniotic (am″ne-ot′ik) pertaining to or developing an amnion. 291

    a. fluid (floo′id), the liquid or albuminous fluid contained in the amnion. 291

amniotomy (am″ne-ot′ə-me) deliberate rupture of the fetal membranes to induce labor. 291

amylase (am′ə-lās) an enzyme that breaks down starch. 199

amylolysis (am″ə̄-lol′ə̄-sis) the breaking down of starch, or its conversion to sugar. 198

amyotrophic lateral sclerosis (a-mi″o-trof′ik lat′ər-əl sklə-ro′sis) (ALS) a motor neuron disease marked by progressive muscular weakness and atrophy with spasticity and exaggerated reflexes, caused by degeneration of motor neurons of the spinal cord, medulla, and cortex; also called Lou Gehrig's disease. 408

anaerobic (an″ə-ro′bik) thriving best without oxygen. 271

anal (a′nəl) pertaining to the anus. 203, 223

    a. canal (kə-nal′) the terminal portion of the digestive tract. 223

    a. fissure (fish′ər) a linear ulcer at the margin of the anus. 224

analgesic (an″əl-je′zik) relieving pain; a medication that relieves pain. 30, 418

anaphylactic (an″ə-fə-lak′tik) pertaining to anaphylaxis. 91

anaphylaxis (an″ə-fə-lak′sis) a manifestation of immediate hypersensitivity in which exposure of a sensitized individual to a specific antigen or hapten results in urticaria, pruritis, and angioedema, followed by vascular collapse and shock and often accompanied by life-threatening respiratory distress; a general term originally applied to the situation in which exposure to a toxin resulted not in development of immunity (prophylaxis) but in hypersensitivity. 91

anastomosis (ə-nas″tə-mo′sis) an opening created by surgical, traumatic, or pathological means between two normally distinct organs or spaces; a communication between two vessels by collateral channels. 219, 220f

anatomic (an″ə-tom′ik) pertaining to anatomy or to the structure of the body. 43

    a. position (pə-zish′ən), the position in which the body is erect, facing forward with the arms at the sides and the palms toward the front. 43

anatomical (an″ə-tom′ĭkəl) pertaining to anatomy or the structure of the organism. 48

    a. plane (plăn) points of reference by which imaginary dissecting lines are drawn through the body to describe locations. 48

anatomist (ə-nat′ə-mist) a specialist in anatomy. 19

anatomy (ə-nat′ə-me) the science of the structure of living organisms. 17

androgen (an′dro-jen) any substance that possesses masculinizing activities, such as the testicular hormone, testosterone. 482

androgenic (an″dro-jen′ik) producing masculine characteristics. 482

andropathy (an′drop′ə- the) any disease peculiar to males. 483

anemia (ə-ne′me-ə) a condition in which the blood is deficient in red blood cells, hemoglobin, or both. 79, 80, 84, 85f

    aplastic a. (ə-plas′tik), anemia caused by a disease of the bone marrow, characterized by absence of regeneration of red blood cells. 86

    sickle cell a. (sik′əl sel), a genetically caused defect of hemoglobin synthesis, occurring almost exclusively in blacks, characterized by the presence of sickle-shaped erythrocytes in the blood and homozygosity for S hemoglobin. Other symptoms include arthralgia, acute abdominal pain, and ulcerations of the legs. 84

anesthesia (an″es-the′zhə) having no feeling or sensation. 23

anesthesiologist (an″əs-the″ze-ol′ə-jist) a physician who specializes in the administration of anesthetics during surgery. 23

anesthesiology (an″əs-the″ze-ol′ə-je) that branch of medicine that studies anesthesia and anesthetics. 23

anesthetic (an″ə-thet′ik) pertaining to or producing anesthesia; an agent that produces anesthesia. 23

anesthetist (ə-nes′thə-tist) a nurse or technician trained to administer anesthetics. 23

aneurysm (an′u-rizm) a sac formed by localized dilation of an artery or vein, or of the heart. 122, 403

aneurysmal (an″u-riz′məl) pertaining to or resembling an aneurysm.

aneurysmectomy (an″u-riz-mek′to-me) surgical removal of the sac of an aneurysm. 404

angiectasis (an″je-ek′tə-sis) the dilatation of a blood vessel. 142

angiectomy (an″je-ek′tə-me) removal or resection of a vessel. 124

angina pectoris (an-ji′nə, an′jə-nə pek′to-ris) severe pain and constriction about the heart caused by an insufficient supply of blood to the heart itself. 48, 135

angiocardiography (an″je-o-kahr″de-og′rə-fe) radiography of the heart and major vessels after injection of a radiopaque contrast medium into a blood vessel or one of the cardiac chambers. 132

angiocarditis (an″je-o-kahr-di′tis) inflammation of the heart and great blood vessels. 118

angiogram (an′je-o-gram″) a radiograph of blood vessels filled with a contrast medium. 131

angiography (an″je-og′rə-fe) radiographic visualization of vessels of the body. 131

angioma (an″je-o′mə) a tumor the cells of which tend to form or are made up of blood or lymph vessels. 124

angiopathy (an-je-op′ə-the) any disease of the vessels. 118

angioplasty (an′je-o-plas″te) surgical repair of the blood vessels. 118

    percutaneous transluminal a. (per″ku-ta′ne-əs trans-loo′mĭ-nəl) compression of fatty deposits of plaque in a blood vessel by an inflated balloon on the end of a catheter; balloon catheter dilation. 132

angiorrhaphy (an″je-or′ə-fe) suture of a vessel or vessels. 143

angiospasm (an′je-o-spaz″əm) spasmodic contraction of the blood vessels. 118

angiostenosis (an″je-o-stə-no′sis) narrowing of the caliber of a vessel. 131

angiostomy (an″je-os′tə-me) surgical formation of a new opening into a blood vessel. 124

angiotomy (an″je-ot′ə-me) incision or severing of a blood or lymph vessel. 124

anhydrous (an-hi′drəs) lacking water. 97

anisocytosis (an-i″so-si-to′sis) a condition in which erythrocytes are not of equal size. 83, 85f

ankylosed (ang′kə-lōzd) stiffened or fused, as a joint. 361

ankylosing spondylitis (ang″kə-lo′sing spon″də-li′tis) inflammation of the spine marked by stiffening of the spinal joints and ligaments, so that movement becomes increasingly painful and difficult. It is a form of rheumatoid arthritis that affects the spine, and affects males almost exclusively. 358, 359t

ankylosis (ang″kə-lo′sis) immobility of a joint. 358

anodontia (an″o-don′shə) congenital absence of the teeth; may involve all or only some of the teeth. 235

anomaly (ə-nom′ə-le) marked deviation from the normal standard, especially as a result of congenital defects. 377

anorchidism (an-or′kĭ-diz″əm) absence of testes. 320

anorchism (an-or′kiz-əm) congenital absence of the testis, either unilaterally or bilaterally. 320

anorexia (an″o-rek′se-ə) lack or loss of appetite for food. 197

　a. nervosa (ner-vo′sə) a mental disorder occurring predominantly in females, having onset usually in adolescence, and characterized by refusal to maintain a normal minimal body weight, intense fear of becoming obese that is undiminished by weight loss, disturbance of body image resulting in a feeling of being fat even when extremely emaciated, and amenorrhea (in females). 197

anorexiant (an″o-rek′se-ənt) causing anorexia or loss of appetite. 200, 237

anotia (an-o′shə) congenital absence of the external ear(s). 423

anoxia (ə-nok′se-ə) a total lack of oxygen; often used interchangeably with *hypoxia* to mean a reduced supply of oxygen to the tissues. 182

antacid (ant-as′id) 1. counteracting acidity. 2. a substance that counteracts or neutralizes acidity, usually of the stomach. 215

antagonist (an-tag′ə-nist) a muscle the action of which is the direct opposite of that of another muscle; a substance that tends to nullify the action of another; a tooth in one jaw that articulates with a tooth in the other jaw. 362

　opioid a. (o′pe-oid), a drug that counteracts the effects of opium or opioid drugs. 37

antarthritic (ant″ahr-thrit′ik) 1. alleviating arthritis. 2. an agent that alleviates arthritis. 379

anteflexion (an-te-flek′shən) 1. forward curvature of an organ or part. 2. the forward curvature of the uterus. 310

antenatal (an″te-na′təl) occurring or formed before birth; prenatal. 301

antepartum (an″te-pahr′təm) in obstetrics, before the onset of labor, with reference to the mother. 301

anterior (an-tēr′e-ər) situated in front or in the forward part of an organism. 43

anterolateral (an″tər-o-lat′ər-əl) situated anteriorly and to one side. 45

anteromedial (an″tər-o-me′de-əl) situated anteriorly and to the medial side. 46

anteromedian (an″tər-o-me′de-ən) situated anteriorly toward the median plane. 43

anteroposterior (an″tər-o-pos-tēr′e-ər) from front to back of the body, such as the direction of a radiographic projection. 44

anterosuperior (an″tər-o-soo-pēr′e-ər) situated anteriorly and superiorly. 46

anteversion (an″te-vər′zhən) the forward tipping or tilting of an organ; displacement in which the uterus is tipped forward, but is not bent at an angle. 310

anthracosis (an-thrə-ko′sis) a usually asymptomatic form of pneumoconiosis caused by deposition of coal dust in the lungs. 177

antianginal (an″te-an-ji′nəl) preventing or alleviating angina; an agent that prevents or alleviates angina. 145

antianxiety (an″te-ang-zi′ə-te) reducing anxiety. 424

antiarrhythmic (an″te-ə-rith-mik) preventing or alleviating cardiac arrhythmia; an agent that prevents or alleviates arrhythmia. 145

antiarthritic (an″te-ahr-thrit′ik) an agent that alleviates arthritis; alleviating arthritis. 379

antiasthmatic (an″te-az-mat′ik) alleviating asthma; a drug that alleviates asthma. 186

antibacterial (an″tĭ-bak-te′re-əl) destroying or suppressing the growth or reproduction of bacteria; a substance that destroys bacteria or suppresses their growth or reproduction. 63

antibiotic (an″tĭ-bi-ot′ik) destructive of life; a chemical substance produced by a microorganism that inhibits the growth of or kills other microorganisms. 460

antibody (an′tĭ-bod″e) an immunoglobulin that interacts only with the antigen that induced its synthesis or with an antigen closely related to it. 89

anticancer (an″tĭ-kan′sər) against cancer; a drug used to treat cancer. 181

anti–canker sore (an″tĭ–kang′kər sor) against canker sores; a drug used to treat canker sores. 237

anticholinergic (an″tĭ-ko″lin-ər′jik) blocking the passage of impulses through the parasympathetic nerves; an agent that blocks the parasympathetic nerves. 186

anticoagulant (an″tĭ-ko-ag′u-lənt) preventing blood clotting; any substance that prevents blood clotting. 75, 76, 99

anticonvulsant (an″tĭ-kən-vul′sənt) preventing or relieving convulsions; an agent that prevents or relieves convulsions. 425

anti–cystic fibrosis (an″tĭ–sis′tik fi-bro′sis) against cystic fibrosis; an agent used to treat cystic fibrosis. 186

antidepressant (an″tĭ-de-pres′ənt) preventing or relieving depression; an agent that is used to treat the symptoms of depression. 420

antidiabetic (an″tĭ-di″ə-bet′ik) preventing or alleviating diabetes; an agent that prevents or alleviates diabetes. 237

antidiarrheal (an″tĭ-di″ə-re′əl) counteracting diarrhea; an agent that is effective in combating diarrhea. 216, 237

antidiuretic (an″tĭ-di″u-ret′ik) suppressing the rate of urine formation; an agent that suppresses urine formation. 471

　a. hormone (hor′mōn), a hormone produced by the hypothalamus that decreases the amount of water lost in urination. 471

antiemetic (an″te-ə-met′ik) preventing or alleviating nausea and vomiting; an agent that prevents or alleviates nausea and vomiting. 237

antifebrile (an″tĭ-feb′ril) relieving or reducing fever; an agent that relieves or reduces fever. 61

antiflatulent (an″tĭ-flat′u-lənt) relieving or preventing excessive gas in the stomach or intestine; an agent that relieves excessive gas in the stomach or intestine. 238

antifungal (an″tĭ-fung′gəl) destructive to fungi, or suppressing their reproduction or growth; an agent that is effective against fungal infections. 63, 460

antigen (an′tĭ-jən) any substance that is capable, under appropriate conditions, of inducing a specific immune response and of reacting with the products of that response. 91

antihelmintic (an″tĭ-hel-min′tik) destructive to parasitic worms; an agent that is effective against infections with parasitic worms. 63

antihistamine (an″tĭ-his′tə-mēn) a drug that counteracts the action of histamine. 91, 99, 179, 187

antihypertensive (an″tĭ-hi″pər-ten′siv) counteracting high blood pressure; an agent that reduces high blood pressure. 126, 144

antiinfective (an″te-in-fek′tiv) capable of killing or preventing the multiplication of infectious agents; an agent that so acts. 60, 63, 272

antiinflammatory (an″te-in-flam′ə-to″re) counteracting or suppressing inflammation; an agent that counteracts or suppresses the inflammatory process. 61, 356

antimalarial (an″tĭ-mə-lar′e-əl) therapeutically effective against malaria; an agent that is therapeutically effective against malaria. 63

antimicrobial (an″tĭ-mi-kro′be-əl) killing microorganisms or suppressing their multiplication or growth; an agent that kills microorganisms or suppresses their multiplication or growth. 61, 63

antimycotic (an″tĭ-mi-kot′ik) suppressing the growth of fungi. 464

antineoplastic (an″tĭ-ne″o-plas′tik) inhibiting or preventing the development of neoplasms; checking the maturation and proliferation of malignant cells; an agent having such properties. 36, 181

antiodontalgic (an″tĭ-o″don-tal′jik) relieving toothache. 235

antiosteoporotic (an″tĭ-os″te-o-pə-rot′ik) against osteoporosis; a drug used to treat osteoporosis. 488

antiparasitic (an″tĭ-par″ə-sit′ik) acting against parasites; an agent that is used to treat parasitic infections. 464

antiperspirant (an″tĭ-pər′spər-ant″) inhibiting or preventing perspiration; an agent that inhibits or prevents perspiration. 442

antiplatelet (an″tĭ-plāt′lət) directed against or destructive to blood platelets. 99

antipsychotic (an″tĭ-si-kot′ik) drugs that are effective in the treatment of psychosis. 420, 426

antipyretic (an″tĭ-pi-ret′ik) relieving or reducing fever; an agent that relieves or reduces fever. 61, 64

antisepsis (an″tĭ-sep′sis) the prevention of sepsis; any procedure that significantly reduces the microbial flora of skin or mucous membranes. 464

antiseptic (an″tĭ-sep′tik) pertaining to asepsis; a substance that inhibits the growth and development of microorganisms without necessarily killing them. 464

antispasmodic (an″tĭ-spaz-mod′ik) relieving spasm, usually of smooth muscle; an agent that relieves muscle spasms. 237

antitoxin (an″tĭ-tok′sin) antibody against a toxin; a purified antiserum from animals that is administered as a passive immunizing agent.

antitubercular (an″tĭ-too-bər′ku-lor) therapeutically effective against tuberculosis; an agent that is therapeutically effective against tuberculosis. 64

antitussive (an″tĭ-tus′iv) relieving or preventing cough; an agent that relieves or prevents cough. 179, 187

antiviral (an″tĭ-vi′rəl) destroying or suppressing viruses; an agent that destroys viruses or suppresses their replication. 64, 460

anuria (an-u′re-ə) complete suppression of urinary secretion by the kidneys. 97, 270

anuric (an-u′rik) pertaining to or characterized by lack of secretion of urine. 270

anus (a′nəs) the distal or terminal opening of the alimentary canal. 203

aorta (a-or′tə) the main trunk from which the systemic arterial system proceeds. 108, 115, 119, 120f, 121f

　abdominal a. (ab-dom′ĭ-nəl), continuation of the thoracic aorta. 119, 121f

　arch of a., the continuation of the ascending aorta that gives rise to the descending aorta. 119, 121f

　ascending a. (ə-send′ing), the proximal portion of the aorta arising from the left ventricle, giving origin to the right and left coronary arteries before continuing as the arch of the aorta. 119, 121f

　descending a. (de-send′ing), the continuation of the aorta from the arch of the aorta, in the thorax, to the point of its division into the common iliac arteries. 119, 121f

　thoracic a. (thə-ras′ik), the proximal portion of the descending aorta. 119, 121f

aortic (a-or′tik) of or pertaining to the aorta. 119

aortitis (a″or-ti′tis) inflammation of the aorta. 119

aortogram (a-or′to-gram) the radiographic record resulting from aortography. 122

aortography (a″or-tog′rə-fe) radiography of the aorta after the injection of an opaque medium. 122

aortopathy (a″or-top′ə-the) any disease of the aorta. 119

aortosclerosis (a-or″to-sklə-ro′sis) abnormal hardening of the aorta. 119

aphagia (ə-fa′jə) refusal or loss of the ability to swallow. 197

aphasia (ə-fa′zhə) defect or loss of the power of expression by speech, writing, or signs, or of comprehending spoken or written language, due to injury or disease of the brain. 183

aphasic (ə-fa′zik) pertaining to or affected with aphasia; a person affected with aphasia. 183

aphonia (a-fo′ne-ə) loss of voice. 182

aplasia (ə-pla′zhə) lack of development of an organ or tissue. 183

aplastic (ə-plas′tik) pertaining to or characterized by aplasia. 86

apnea (ap′ne-ə) cessation of breathing. 156

appendectomy (ap″en-dek′tə-me) surgical removal of the vermiform appendix. 222

appendicitis (ə-pen″dĭ-si′tis) inflammation of the vermiform appendix. 222

appendicular (ap″en-dik′u-lər) pertaining to the vermiform appendix; pertaining to an appendage. 343, 349

appendix (ə-pen′diks) a general term used to designate a supplementary, accessory, or dependent part attached to a main structure; also called appendage. It is frequently used alone to refer to the appendix vermiformis. 222

approximate (ə-prok′sĭ-māt″) to bring close together. 213

approximation (ə-prok″sĭ-ma′shən) the act or process of bringing closer. 213

arachnoid (ə-rak′noid) resembling a spider's web; the middle of the three meninges. 395

arrhythmia (ə-rith′me-ə) any variation from the normal rhythm of the heartbeat. 128

arterial (ahr-tēr′e-əl) pertaining to an artery or to the arteries. 108, 118

arteriectasis (ahr″tə-re-ek′tə-sis) dilatation of an artery. 142

arteriogram (ahr-ter′e-o-gram) a radiograph of an artery after injection of a radiopaque medium. 118

arteriograph (ahr-tēr′e-o-graf) a film produced by arteriography. 118

arteriography (ahr-tēr′e-og′rə-fe) radiography of arteries after injection of radiopaque material into the blood stream. 118

arteriole (ahr-tēr′e-ōl) a minute arterial branch, especially one just proximal to a capillary. 108

arteriolitis (ahr-tēr″e-o-li′tis) inflammation of the arterioles. 122

arteriopathy (ahr-tēr″e-op′ə-the) any arterial disease. 118

arteriorrhagia (ahr-tēr″e-o-ra′je-ə) hemorrhage from an artery. 143

arteriorrhexis (ahr-tēr″e-o-rek′sis) rupture of an artery. 143

arteriosclerosis (ahr-tēr″e-o-sklə-ro′sis) a group of diseases characterized by thickening and loss of elasticity of arterial walls. 125

arteriosclerotic (ahr-tēr″e-o-sklə-rot′ik) pertaining to or affected with arteriosclerosis. 125

arteriovenous (ahr-tēr″e-o-ve′nəs) pertaining to or affecting an artery and a vein. 122

arteritis (ahr″tə-ri′tis) inflammation of an artery. 118

artery (ahr′tər-e) a vessel through which the blood passes away from the heart to the various parts of the body. 108

arthralgia (ahr-thral′jə) pain in a joint. 359

arthrectomy (ahr-threk′to-me) the excision of a joint. 360

arthritis (ahr-thri′tis) inflammation of joints. 357

rheumatoid a. (roo″mə-toid), a chronic systemic disease primarily of the joints, marked by inflammatory changes in the synovial membranes and articular structures and by muscle atrophy and rarefaction of the bones. In late stages deformity and ankylosis develop. 357, 359t

arthrocentesis (ahr″thro-sen-te′sis) puncture and aspiration of a joint. 360

arthrochondritis (ahr″thro-kon-dri′tis) inflammation of the cartilage of a joint. 361

arthroclasia (ahr″thro-kla′zhə) the surgical breaking down of an ankylosed joint. 361

arthrodesis (ahr″thro-de′sis) the surgical fixation of a joint. 360

arthrodynia (ahr″thro-din′e-ə) pain in a joint. 359

arthrogram (ahr′thro-gram) a radiographic record after introduction of opaque contrast material into a joint. 360

arthrography (ahr-throg′rə-fe) radiography of a joint after injection of opaque contrast material. 360

arthrolysis (ahr-throl′ə-sis) destruction of a joint; the operative loosening of adhesions in an ankylosed joint. 361

arthropathy (ahr-throp′ə-the) any joint disease. 359

arthroplasty (ahr′thro-plas″te) plastic surgery of a joint or of joints. 356, 360

arthrosclerosis (ahr″thro-sklə-ro′sis) hardening of the joints. 360

arthroscope (ahr′thro-skōp) an endoscope for examining the interior of a joint and for carrying out diagnostic and therapeutic procedures within the joint. 360

arthroscopy (ahr-thros′kə-pe) examination of the interior of a joint with an arthroscope. 360

arthrotomy (ahr-throt′ə-me) surgical incision of a joint. 360

articular (ahr-tik′u-lər) of or pertaining to a joint. 355

articulation (ahr-tik″u-la′shən) the place of union or junction between two or more bones of the skeleton; a joint; the enunciation of words and sentences. 355

asbestosis (as″bes-to′sis) a form of lung disease caused by inhaling fibers of asbestos. 177

ascending (ə-send′ing) having an upward course. 221

a. colon (ko′lon), the first part of the large intestine beginning at the cecum. 221f

ascites (ə-si′tēz) effusion and accumulation of serous fluid in the abdominal cavity. 52

asepsis (a-sep′sis) free from infection. 453

aspermatogenesis (a-spər″mə-to-jen′ə-sis) absence of development of spermatozoa. 292

aspermia (ə-spər′me-ə) failure of formation or emission of semen. 292

asphyxia (as-fik′se-ə) pathological changes caused by lack of oxygen in respired air. 156

asphyxiation (as-fik″se-a′shən) the causing of or state of asphyxia; suffocation. 156

aspiration (as″pĭ-ra′shən) the removal of fluids or gases from a cavity by the application of suction; drawing in or out as by suction. 169, 341

asthma (az′mə) a condition marked by recurrent attacks of paroxysmal dyspnea, with wheezing due to spasmodic contraction of the bronchi. 178t

asthmatic (az-mat′ik) pertaining to or affected with asthma. 192

astigmatism (ə-stig′mə-tiz-əm) unequal curvature of the refractive surfaces of the eye. 415, 416f

asymptomatic (a″simp-to-mat′ik) showing or causing no symptoms. 34

asystole (a-sis′to-le) cardiac arrest; absence of a heartbeat. 129

atelectasis (at″ə-lek′tə-sis) incomplete expansion of a lung or a portion of a lung; airlessness or collapse of a lung that had once been expanded. 178t

atherosclerosis (ath″ər-o-sklə-ro′sis) a common form of arteriosclerosis in which deposits of yellowish plaques are formed within the arteries. 125

atraumatic (a″traw-mat′ik) not causing damage or injury. 61

atrial (a′tre-əl) pertaining to an atrium. 114

a. septal defect (sep′təl de′fekt), a congenital heart defect in which there is an opening between the atria. 129

atriomegaly (a″tre-o-meg′ə-le) abnormal dilatation or enlargement of an atrium of the heart. 129

atrioseptoplasty (a″tre-o-sep″to-plas′te) plastic repair to correct an abnormal opening between the atria. 129

atrioventricular (a″tre-o-ven-trik′u-lər) pertaining to an atrium of the heart and to a ventricle. 115

a. node (nōd), specialized heart muscle fibers that receive impulses from the sinoatrial node and transmit them to the bundle of His. 117

atrium (a′tre-əm) a chamber; used in anatomy to designate a chamber affording entrance to another structure or organ. Usually used alone to designate an atrium of the heart. 114

atrophy (at′rə-fe) a wasting away; a diminution in the size of a cell, tissue, organ, or part. 358, 367, 445

audiologist (aw″de-ol′ə-jist) a person skilled in audiology, including diagnostic testing and the rehabilitation of those whose impaired hearing cannot be improved by medical or surgical means. 418

audiology (aw″de-ol′ə-je) the science of hearing, particularly diagnostic testing and the study of impaired hearing that cannot be improved by medication or surgical therapy. 418

audiometer (aw″de-om′ə-tər) an electronic device that produces acoustic stimuli of known frequency and intensity for the measurement of hearing. 418

auditory (aw′dĭ-tor″e) pertaining to the sense of hearing. 167

a. tube (tōōb), the narrow channel connecting the middle ear and the nasopharynx. Formerly called the eustachian tube. 167

auscultation (aws″kəl-ta′shən) the act of listening for sounds within the body, chiefly for ascertaining the condition of the lungs, heart, pleura, abdomen, and other organs, and for the detection of pregnancy. 182

autism (aw′tiz-əm) preoccupation with inner thoughts, daydreams, fantasies, delusions, and hallucinations; egocentric, subjective thinking lacking objectivity and connection with reality. 420

autoimmune (aw″to-ĭ-mūn′) pertaining to autoimmunity, a condition characterized by a specific humoral or cell-mediated immune response against constituents of the body's own tissues. 357

autologous (aw-tol′ə-gəs) related to self; originating within an organism itself. 97

autonomic (aw″to-nom′ik) self-controlling; functionally independent. 409

a. nervous system (ner′vəs sis′təm), the part of the nervous system related to involuntary body functions. 409

autopsy (aw′top-se) the postmortem examination of a body. 34

axial (ak′se-əl) of or pertaining to the axis of a structure or part, as the long axis of a tooth. 342f, 343

axilla (ak-sil′ə) the armpit. 439

axillary (ak′sĭ-lar″e) pertaining to the axilla. 136, 439

a. nodes (nōdz), lymph nodes located in the axilla. 136

axon (ak′son) the nerve process by which impulses travel away from the cell body of a neuron. 392

bacilli (bə-sil′i) rod-shaped bacteria. 264

bactericidal (bak-ter″ĭ-si′dəl) capable of killing bacteria. 453

bacteriophage (bak-tēr′e-o-fāj″) a virus that lyses bacteria. 197

bacteriostatic (bak-tēr″e-o-stat′ik) inhibiting the growth or multiplication of bacteria; an agent that inhibits the growth or multiplication of bacteria. 453

bacterium (bak-tēr′e-əm) in general, any of the unicellular prokaryotic microorganisms that commonly multiply by cell division (fission) and the cell of which is typically contained within a cell wall. 264

balanitis (bal″ə-ni′tis) inflammation of the glans penis. 325

barium (bar′e-əm) a pale yellow metallic element belonging to the alkaline earths. 217

    b. enema (en′ə-mə), use of barium sulfate as an enema in x-ray and fluoroscopic examination of the colon; lower gastrointestinal series. 212

    b. meal (mēl), use of ingested barium sulfate to make the outline of the esophagus, stomach, and small intestines more visible during x-ray or fluoroscopic examination; upper gastrointestinal series. 212

    b. swallow (swahl′o), roentgenography of the esophagus after ingestion of barium sulfate; esophagram. 210

Bartholin's gland (bahr′to-linz gland) one of two small mucous glands located one in each lateral wall of the vestibule of the vagina, near the vaginal opening. 284

basal (ba′səl) pertaining to or situated near a base. 478

    b. cell carcinoma (sel kahr″sĭ-no′mə), an epithelial tumor of the skin originating from neoplastic differentiation of basal cells, rarely metastatic but locally invasive and aggressive. 449, 450f

base (bās) a substance that combines with acids to form salts. 157

basophil (ba′so-fil) a granular leukocyte that has cytoplasm that contains coarse bluish black granules of variable size. 77f

benign (bə-nīn′) not malignant; not recurrent; favorable for recovery. 142

biceps (bi′seps) a muscle having two heads. 362

biconcave (bi′kon′kāv) having two concave surfaces. 60

bicuspid (bi-kus′pid) having two cusps; a mitral valve; a premolar tooth. 115

    b. valve (valv), mitral valve. 115

bifurcate (bi-fər′kāt) forked; divided into two branches. 60

bilateral (bi-lat′ər-əl) having two sides, or pertaining to both sides. 45

    b. nephromegaly (nef″ro-meg′ə-le), enlargement of both kidneys. 249

bile (bīl) a fluid secreted by the liver and poured into the small intestine. Important constituents are conjugated bile salts, cholesterol, phospholipid, bilirubin diglucuronide, and electrolytes. 217

biliary (bil′e-ar-e) pertaining to bile, to bile ducts, or to the gallbladder. 229

biochemist (bi″o-kem′ist) one who specializes in the chemistry of living organisms and of vital processes. 19

biohazard (bi′o-haz″ərd) a potentially dangerous infectious agent such as may be found in a clinical microbiology laboratory or used in experimental studies on genetic recombination. 34

biologic, biological (bi-o-loj′ik, bi-o-loj′ĭ-kəl) pertaining to biology or the study of life and living organisms. 33

biologist (bi-ol′ə-jist) an expert in biology. 19

biology (bi-ol′ə-je) the science that deals with the phenomena of life and living organisms in general. 17

biopsy (bi′ŏp-se) removal and examination, usually microscopic, of tissue from the living body. A biopsy is performed to establish precise diagnosis. 17

bipara (bip′ə-rə) a female who has borne two children. 298

bladder (blad′ər) a membranous sac serving as a receptacle for a secretion, especially the urinary bladder, which serves as a reservoir for urine. 259

blepharal (blef′ə-ral) pertaining to the eyelid. 58

blepharedema (blef″ar-ə-de′mə) swelling of the eyelids. 62, 414

blepharitis (blef″ə-ri′tis) inflammation of the eyelid. 58

blepharoplasty (blef′ə-ro-plas″te) plastic surgery of the eyelid. 58, 414

blepharoplegia (blef″ə-ro-ple′je-ə) paralysis of an eyelid or of both muscles of the eyelid. 62

blepharoptosis (blef″ə-rop-to′sis) drooping of an upper eyelid; ptosis. 62, 414, 415f

blepharospasm (blef′ə-ro-spaz″əm) twitching of the eyelid. 58

blepharotomy (blef″ə-rot′ə-me) surgical incision of an eyelid. 58

block (blok) an obstruction or stoppage; regional anesthesia. 128

    heart b. (hahrt), impairment of conduction of an impulse in heart excitation, either permanent or transient and due to anatomical or functional impairment. 128

blood (blud) the fluid that circulates through the heart and blood vessels, carrying nutrient and oxygen to the body cells. 73

    b. cells (selz), red and white corpuscles. 76, 77

    b. pressure (presh′ər), the pressure existing in the large arteries at the height of the pulse wave. 126, 127f, 128f

    b. vessels (ves′əlz), the arteries, veins, and capillaries. 108, 109f, 110f, 118

bolus (bo′ləs) a rounded mass of food or a pharmaceutical preparation ready to swallow, or such a mass passing through the gastrointestinal tract. 201

bone (bōn) the rigid connective tissue constituting most of the skeleton of vertebrates. 338, 339f

    b. marrow (mar′o), the soft material filling the cavities of bones. 338, 341, 345

botulism (boch′u-liz-əm) a type of food poisoning caused by a neurotoxin produced by the growth of *Clostridium botulinum* in improperly canned or preserved foods. 408

Bowman's capsule (bo′mənz cap′səl) part of the kidney that functions as a filter in the formation of urine. 254

bradycardia (brad″e-kahr′de-ə) slow heartbeat, as evidenced by slowing of the pulse rate to less than 60. 128

bradykinesia (brad″e kĭ-ne′zhə) slow movement; sluggishness of physical or mental responses. 60, 403

bradypepsia (brad″e pep′se-ə) abnormally slow digestion. 199

bradyphasia (brad″e fa′ze ah) slow speech. 183

bradypnea (brad″e-ne′ə, brad-ip′ne-ə) abnormal slowness of breathing. 59, 160

brain (brān) that part of the central nervous system contained within the cranium, consisting of the cerebrum, cerebellum, pons, medulla oblongata, and midbrain. 397, 398f

    b. stem (stem), the stemlike portion of the brain connecting the cerebral hemispheres with the spinal cord and constituting the pons, medulla oblongata, and mesencephalon. 397, 398f

breast (brest) the anterior aspect of the chest; mammary gland. 412

    b. augmentation (awg″men-ta′shən) insertion of an implant behind the breast to increase its size. 474

    b. reduction (re-duk′shən) surgical removal of excess breast and skin tissue. 474

Bright's disease (brīts dĭ-zēz′) a vague term for kidney disease, usually referring to degenerative kidney disease. 251

bronchiectasis (brong″ke-ek′tə-sis) chronic dilatation of the bronchi. 171, 172

bronchiole (brong′ke-ōl) one of the fine divisions of the bronchial tree. 162, 163

bronchiolectasis (brong″ke-o-lek′tə-sis) dilation of the bronchioles. 172

bronchiolitis (brong″ke-o-li′tis) inflammation of the bronchioles; bronchopneumonia. 172

bronchitis (brong-ki′tis) inflammation of the bronchi. 171

bronchoalveolar (brong″ko-al-ve′ə-lər) pertaining to a bronchus and alveoli. 172

bronchoconstriction (bron″ko-kən-strik′shən) the act or process of decreasing the caliber of a bronchus; bronchostenosis. 171

bronchodilator (brong″ko-di-la′tor) stretching or expanding the air passages; an agent that causes dilation of the bronchi. 171, 186

bronchogenic (brong-ko-jen′ik) originating in a bronchus. 171

bronchogram (brong′ko-gram) the record obtained by bronchography. 171

bronchography (brong-kog′rə-fe) radiography of the bronchial tree after injection of an opaque solution. 171

broncholithiasis (brong″ko-lĭ-thi′ə-sis) a condition in which calculi are present within the lumen of the tracheobronchial tree. 171

bronchopathy (brong kop′ə-the) any disease of the bronchi. 171

bronchoplasty (brong′ko-plas″te) plastic surgery of the bronchus. 171

bronchopneumonia (brong″ko-nōō-mo′ne-ə) a name given to an inflammation of the lungs that usually begins in the terminal bronchioles. These become clogged with a mucopurulent exudate forming consolidated patches in adjacent lobules. 171

bronchopulmonary (brong″ko-pul′mə-nar″e) pertaining to the lungs and their air passages; both bronchial and pulmonary. 171

bronchoscope (brong′ko-skōp) instrument for viewing the bronchi. 171

bronchoscopic (brong″ko-skop′ik) pertaining to either bronchoscopy or the bronchoscope. 171

bronchoscopy (brong-kos′kə-pe) examination of the bronchi through a bronchoscope. 171

bronchospasm (brong′ko-spaz″əm) spasmodic contraction of the smooth muscle of the bronchi, as occurs in asthma. 171

bronchus (brong′kəs) either of the two main branches of the trachea. 171

bulbourethral glands (bul″bo-u-re′thrəl glandz) Cowper′s glands; two small glands, one on each side of the prostate gland. They secrete a viscid fluid that forms part of the seminal fluid. 312

bulimia (bu-lim′e-ə) a mental disorder occurring predominantly in females, with onset usually in adolescence or early adulthood, characterized by episodes of binge eating that continue until terminated by abdominal pain, sleep, or self-induced vomiting; by awareness that the binges are abnormal. 197

bulla (bul′ə) a large vesicle, more than 1 cm in circumference, containing fluid. 444

burn (bərn) injury to tissues caused by contact with dry heat (fire), moist heat (steam or hot liquid), chemicals (e.g., corrosive substances), electricity (current or lightning), friction, or radiant and electromagnetic energy. 452, 453f

    first degree b., a burn in which damage is limited to the epidermis. 452

    second degree b., one in which damage extends through the epidermis and into the dermis. 452

    third degree b., one in which the epidermis and dermis are destroyed and damage extends into the underlying tissue. 452

bursa (bər′sə) a sac or saclike cavity filled with a viscid fluid and situated at places in the tissues at which friction would otherwise develop. 355

dialysis (di-al′ə-sis) the diffusion and ultrafiltration of blood across a semipermeable membrane in order to remove toxic materials and maintain proper balance of fluid and blood electrolytes, and so forth, in cases of improper kidney function; hemodialysis. 37, 250

  peritoneal d. (per″ĭ-to-ne′əl), dialysis in which the lining of the peritoneal cavity is used as the dialysis membrane. 250

diaphoresis (di″ə-fo-re′sis) sweating or perspiration, especially profuse perspiration. 442

diaphragm (di′ə-fram) the muscular partition that separates the chest and abdominal cavities and serves as the major inspiratory muscle; a contraceptive device of rubber or soft plastic material that is placed over the cervix before intercourse. 51, 162

diaphragma (di″ə-frag′mə) the diaphragm. 162

diaphysis (di-af′ə-sis) the elongated, cylindrical portion (shaft) of a long bone. 338, 339f

diarrhea (di″ə-re′ə) abnormal frequency and softness of fecal discharge. 216

diastole (di-as′to-le) the relaxation or the period of relaxation of the heart, especially of the ventricles. 126

diastolic (di″ə-stol′ik) pertaining to diastole. 126

diathermy (di′ə-thər″me) a treatment in which heat is passed through body tissues. 456

diencephalon (di″ən-sef′ə-lon) the portion of the brain that consists of the hypothalamus and thalamus. 397, 398f

digestion (di-jes′chən) the process or act of converting food into chemical substances that can be absorbed and assimilated; the subjection of a body to prolonged heat and moisture, so as to disintegrate and soften it. 201

digit (dij′it) a finger or toe. 54

dilatation (dil″ə-ta′shən) the condition of being dilated or stretched beyond normal dimensions. 119, 299

dilation (di-la′shən) the act of stretching. 119, 299

dilation and curettage (di-la′shən and ku″rə-tahzh′) (D&C) a surgical procedure that expands the opening into the uterus so that the surface of the uterine wall can be scraped. 306

dilator (di-la′tər) an instrument used in enlarging an orifice or canal by stretching; a general term for a muscle that dilates. 119

diplegia (di-ple′je-ə) paralysis affecting like parts on both sides of the body. 407

diplococci (dip″lo-kok′si) a pair of spherical bacteria, resulting from incomplete separation after cell division; plural of diplococcus. 265, 266f, 267f

disease (dĭ-zēz′) any deviation from or interruption of the normal structure or function of any part, organ, or system of the body that is manifested by a characteristic set of symptoms and signs. 135

disk (disk) a circular or rounded flat plate. 375

  herniated d. (hər′ne-āt″əd), rupture of an intervertebral disk. 375

dislocation (dis″lo-ka′shən) displacement of a bone from a joint. 369, 370f

disorder (dis-or′dər) a derangement or abnormality of function; a morbid physical or mental state. 135

dissection (dĭ-sek′shən) cutting to separate and expose, such as for the anatomical study of a cadaver; a part of an organism prepared by dissecting.

distal (dis′təl) far or distant from the origin or point of attachment. 47

diuresis (di″u-re′sis) increased urination. 270

diuretic (di″u-ret′ik) increasing urination or an agent that increases urination. 270, 471

diverticulectomy (di″vər-tik″u-lek′tə-me) excision of a diverticulum. 222

diverticulitis (di″vər-tik″u-li′tis) inflammation of a diverticulum, especially related to colonic diverticula. 222

diverticulosis (di″vər-tik″u-lo′sis) the presence of diverticula in the absence of inflammation. 222

diverticulum (di″vər-tik′u-ləm) a circumscribed pouch of variable size occurring normally or created by herniation of the lining through a defect in the muscular coat of a tubular organ. 222

dopamine (do′pə-mēn) an intermediate product in the synthesis of norepinephrine that acts as a neurotransmitter in the central nervous system. It also acts on peripheral receptors, e.g., in blood vessels. 393, 413

dorsal (dor′səl) pertaining to the back; denoting a position more toward the back surface than some other object of reference. 44

  d. cavity (kav′ĭ-te), the body cavity located near the posterior surface of the body. It is further divided into the cranial cavity and the vertebral canal. 51

dorsalgia (dor-sal′jə) pain in the back. 359

dorsocephalad (dor″so-sef′ə-lad) toward the back of the head. 47

dorsodynia (dor″so-din′e-ə) pain in the back. 59

dorsolateral (dor″so-lat′ər-əl) pertaining to the back and the side. 44

dorsoventral (dor″so-ven′trəl) pertaining to the back and belly surfaces; passing from the back to the belly surface. 44

Down syndrome (doun sin′drōm) a chromosome disorder characterized by a small flattened skull, short, flat-bridge nose, epicanthal fold, short phalanges, widened spaces between the first and second digits of hands and feet, and moderate to severe mental retardation. Called also trisomy 21 and nondisjunction; formerly called mongolism. 296

duct (dukt) a passage with well-defined walls. 202f

  hepatic d. (hə-pat′ik), duct that carries bile from the liver. 202f, 229

  lactiferous d. (lak-tif′ər-əs), duct that drains the lobe of a mammary gland.

  nasolacrimal d. (na″zo-lak′rĭ-məl), duct that conveys tears from the lacrimal sac to the nasal cavity. 165

ductus (duk′təs) a general term for a passage with well-defined walls; a duct. 312

  d. deferens, (def′ər-enz) the excretory duct of the testis; vas deferens. 312, 313

duodenal (doo″o-de-nəl) pertaining to the duodenum. 218

  d. ulcer (ul′sər), an ulcer on the mucosa of the duodenum. 215

  d. carcinoma (kahr″sĭ-no′mə), cancer of the duodenum. 218

duodenitis (doo″o-də-ni′tis) inflammation of the duodenum. 218

duodenography (doo″o-de-nog′rə-fe) roentgenographic examination of the duodenum. 218

duodenoscope (doo″o-de′no-skōp) an endoscope for examination of the duodenum. 219

duodenoscopy (doo″o-də-nos′kə-pe) endoscopic examination of the duodenum. 219

duodenostomy (doo″o-də-nos′tə-me) formation of a new opening into the duodenum. 218

duodenotomy (doo″o-də-not′ə-me) incision into the duodenum. 218

duodenum (doo″o-de′nəm) the part of the small intestine that connects with the stomach. 218

Dupuytren's contracture (doo-pwe-trahz′kən-trak′chər) contracture of the palmar fascia causing the ring and little fingers to bend into the palm so that they cannot be extended. 375

dura mater (doo′rə ma′tər) the outermost and toughest of the three membranes of the brain and spinal cord. 395

dwarfism (dworf′iz-əm) a disease in which the person is much smaller than the normal size of humans. The condition is due to insufficient growth hormone in childhood. 475, 476f

dyscrasia (dis-kra′zhə) an abnormal state or condition. 60, 86

dysentery (dis′ən-ter″e) any of a number of disorders marked by inflammation of the intestine, especially the large intestine, with abdominal pain and frequent stools. 234

dysfunction (dis-funk′shən) any abnormality of the functioning of an organ. 60, 126

dyskinesia (dis″kĭ-ne′zhə) difficult movement. 60

dyslexia (dis-lek′se-ə) inability to read, spell, and write words, despite the ability to see and recognize letters. 408

dysmenorrhea (dis″men-ə-re′ə) painful menstruation. 307

dyspepsia (dis-pep′se-ə) poor digestion. 199

dysphagia (dis-fa′je-ə) difficulty in swallowing. 197

dysphasia (dis-fa′zhə) speech impairment. 183

dysphonia (dis-fo′ne-ə) difficulty in speaking or weak voice. 182

dysplasia (dis-pla′zhə) abnormality of development; in pathology, alteration in size, shape, and organization of adult cells. 303

dyspnea (disp′ne-ə) difficult breathing. 156

dyspneic (disp-ne′ik) referring to or characterized by difficult breathing. 156

dysrhythmia (dis-rith′me-ə) disturbance of rhythm. 128

dystocia (dis-to′shə) abnormal or difficult labor. 324

dystrophy (dis′trə-fe) faulty nutrition. 378

dysuria (dis-u′re-ə) difficult or painful urination. 261

ecchymosis (ek″ĭ-mo′sis) a small hemorrhagic spot, larger than a petechia, in the skin or mucous membrane forming a nonelevated, rounded or irregular, blue or purplish patch. 445, 446f, 448f

echocardiogram (ek″o-kahr′de-o-gram″) the record produced by echocardiography. 133

echocardiography (ek″o-kahr″de-og′rə-fe) recording of the heart walls or internal structures of the heart and neighboring tissue by the echo obtained from beams of ultrasonic waves directed through the chest wall. 133

echoencephalogram (ek″o-en-sef′ə-lo-gram″) the record produced by echoencephalography. 401

echoencephalography (ek″o-en-sef″ə-log′rə-fe) a diagnostic technique in which ultrasonic waves are beamed through the head from both sides, and echoes are recorded as graphic tracings. 401

echogram (ek′o-gram) the record made by echography. 133

echography (ə-kog′rə-fe) a diagnostic aid in which ultrasonic waves are directed at the tissues, and a record is made of the sound waves reflected back through the tissues to differentiate structures. 133

eclampsia (ə-klamp′se-ə) convulsions occurring in a pregnant woman with hypertension, proteinuria, and/or edema. 297

ectoderm (ek′to-dərm) in embryology, the outermost layer of cells in the blastoderm. 438

ectopic (ek-top′ik) out of the usual place. 296

  e. pregnancy (preg′nən-se), the implantation of a fertilized egg in any place other than the uterus. 296, 297

eczema (ek′zə-mə) a dermatitis occurring as a reaction to many endogenous and exogenous agents, characterized in the acute stage by erythema, edema associated with a serous exudate oozing and vesiculation, and crusting and scaling. 449

edema (ə-de′mə) an abnormal accumulation of fluid in intercellular spaces in the tissues. 135, 138
  pulmonary e. (pool′mo-nar″e), abnormal diffuse, extravascular accumulation of fluid in the pulmonary tissues. 175

effacement (ə-fās′mənt) the taking up or obliteration of the cervix in labor when it is so changed that only the thin external os remains. 299

efferent (ef′ər-ənt) conveying away from a center. 391

effusion (ə-fu′zhən) the escape of fluid into a part or tissue; an effused material. 113
  pleural e. (ploor′əl), presence of liquid in the pleural space. 172

ejaculation (e-jak″u-la′shən) a sudden act of expulsion, as of the semen. 312

ejaculatory (e-jak′u-lə-to″re) pertaining to ejaculation. 312

electrocardiogram (e-lek″tro-kahr′de-o-gram″) a tracing produced by the electrical impulses of the heart. 19, 55, 134

electrocardiograph (e-lek′tro-kahr′de-o-graf″) an instrument used to record the electrical current produced by the heart contractions. 55, 134

electrocardiography (e-lek″tro-kahr″de-og′rə-fe) recording the electrical currents of the heart muscle. 55, 133, 134

electrodesiccation (e-lek″tro-des″ĭ-ka′shən) dehydration of tissue by the use of a high frequency electric current. 445

electroencephalogram (e-lek″tro-en-sef′ə-lo-gram″) a record produced by the electrical impulses of the brain. 56

electroencephalograph (e-lek′tro-en-sef′ə-lo′graf″) a machine used to record the electrical impulses of the brain. 56, 402, 423

electroencephalography (e-lek″tro-en-sef″ə-log′rə-fe) the recording of the electrical currents of the brain by means of electrodes applied to the scalp, to the surface of the brain, or placed within the substance of the brain. 56, 402, 423

electrogram (e-lek′tro-gram) any record showing changes in electrical current. 55

electrolysis (e″lek-trol′ə-sis) destruction by passage of a galvanic electrical current, as in removal of excessive hair from the body. 439

electromyogram (e-lek″tro-mi′o-gram) the record obtained by electromyography. 367

electromyography (e-lek″tro-mi-og′rə-fe) the recording and study of the intrinsic electrical properties of skeletal muscle. 367

electrophoresis (e-lek″tro-fə-re′sis) the separation of ionic solutes in a liquid under the influence of an applied electric field. 86
  hemoglobin e. (he′mo-glo″bin), electrophoresis of blood to determine the type of hemoglobin present. 86

elephantiasis (el″ə-fən-ti′ə-sis) a disease caused by a parasitic infestation and characterized by inflammation and obstruction of the lymphatics and increased size of nearby tissue. 138

elimination (e-lim″ĭ-na′shən) the act of expulsion or of extrusion, especially of expulsion from the body; omission or exclusion, as in an elimination diet. 73, 201, 202t, 442

emaciation (e-ma″she-a′shən) excessive leanness; a wasted condition of the body. 225

embolectomy (em″bə-lek′tə-me) surgical removal of an embolus from a blood vessel where it has lodged. 176

embolism (em′bə-liz-əm) the sudden blocking of a vessel by a clot or foreign material that has been brought to its site of lodgment by the blood stream. 175, 176
  coronary e. (kor′ə-nar″e), embolism of one of the coronary arteries. 130

embolus (em′bo-ləs) a clot or other plug brought by the blood stream and forced into a smaller vessel where it lodges, thus obstructing circulation. 175, 176t, 403

embryo (em′bre-o) derivatives of the fertilized ovum that eventually become the offspring. 291

embryologist (em″bre-ol′ə-jist) an expert in embryology. 19

embryology (em″bre-ol′ə-je) the science of the development of the individual during the early stages of life. 16-17

emesis (em′ə-sis) vomiting; an act of vomiting. 197

emetics (ə-met′iks) agents that cause vomiting. 197

emphysema (em″fə-se′mə) an accumulation of air in tissues or organs; pulmonary disease characterized by destruction of many of the alveolar walls. 178t

empyema (em″pi-e′mə) accumulation of pus in a cavity of the body. If used without a descriptive qualifier, it refers to thoracic empyema. 172

enamel (ə-nam′əl) the hard substance covering the dentin of the crown of a tooth. 208f

encephalitis (en-sef″ə-li′tis) inflammation of the brain. 57, 58, 403

encephalography (en-sef″ə-log′rə-fe) radiography of the brain. 401

encephalomalacia (en-sef″ə-lo-mə-la′shə) softening of the brain. 407

encephalomeningitis (en-sef″ə-lo-men″in-ji′tis) inflammation of the brain and its membranes. 403

encephalomyelitis (en-sef″ə-lo-mi″ə-li′tis) inflammation involving both the brain and the spinal cord. 403

encephalomyelopathy (en-sef″ə-lo-mi″əl-op′ə-the) a disease involving the brain and the spinal cord. 407

encephalopathy (en-sef″ə-lop′ə-the) any disease of the brain. 57

encephalosclerosis (en-sef″ə-lo-sklə-ro′sis) hardening of the brain. 407

endarterectomy (end-ahr″tər-ek′tə-me) excision of the atheromatous tunica intima of an artery. 125

endocardial (en″do-kahr′de-əl) pertaining to the endocardium; situated or occurring within the heart. 113

endocarditis (en″do-kahr-di′tis) inflammation of the inner lining of the heart. 113

endocardium (en″do-kahr-de-um) the membrane lining the inner surface of the heart. 112f, 113

endocrine (en′do-krīn, en′do-krin) secreting internally; applied to organs that secrete hormones into the blood stream. 29

endocrinologist (en″do-krĭ-nol′ə-jist) a physician who treats diseases arising from disordered internal secretions. 29

endocrinology (en″do-krĭ-nol′ə-je) the science that studies the endocrine glands and the hormones they produce. 29

endocrinotherapy (en″do-krĭ″no-ther′ə-pe) treatment of disease by the use of endocrine preparations; hormonotherapy. 34

endoderm (en′do-dərm) the innermost of the three primary germ layers of the embryo. 438

endodontics (en″do-don-tiks) the branch of dentistry concerned with the cause, prevention, diagnosis, and treatment of conditions that affect the tooth pulp, root, and periapical tissues. 22

endodontist (en″do-don′tist) a dentist who specializes in prevention and treatment of conditions that affect the tooth pulp, root, and periapical tissues. 22, 208

endodontitis (en″do-don-ti′tis) inflammation of the dental pulp. 206

endodontium (en″do-don′she-əm) dental pulp. 206

endogastric (en″do-gas′trik) pertaining to the interior of the stomach. 210

endogenous (en-doj′ə-nəs) produced within or caused by factors within an organism. 34, 197

endometriosis (en″do-me″tre-o′sis) ectopic endometrium located in various places, usually in the pelvic cavity. 324, 325f

endometritis (en″do-me-tri′tis) inflammation of the lining of the uterus. 324

endometrium (en″do-me′tre-əm) the membrane that lines the cavity of the uterus. 286

endonasal (en″do′na′zəl) within the nose. 164

endorphin (en-dor′fin, en′dor-fin) any of three amino acid residues that bind to opioid receptors in the brain and have potent analgesic activity. 393

endoscope (en′do-skōp) an instrument for the examination of the interior of a hollow viscus. 219

endoscopy (en-dos′ko-pe) visual inspection of any cavity of the body by means of an endoscope. 219

endotracheal (en″do-tra′ke-əl) within the trachea. 170
  e. intubation (in″too-ba′shən), a procedure in which a tube is placed through the nose or mouth into the trachea in order to establish an airway. 170

enteral, enteric (en′tər-əl, en-ter′ik) pertaining to the small intestine. 200

enteritis (en″tər-i′tis) inflammation of the intestine, especially the small intestine. 217

enterocele (en′tər-o-sēl″) any hernia of the intestine.

enteroclysis (en″tər-ok′lə-sis) irrigation of the intestine. 217

enterocolitis (en″tər-o-ko-li′tis) inflammation involving both the small intestine and the colon. 203

enterodynia (en″tər-o-din′e-ə) intestinal pain. 217

enteroplegia (en″tər-o-ple′jə) paralysis of the intestine. 223

enterostasis (en″tər-o-sta′sis) the stopping of food in its passage through the intestine. 217

enuresis (en″u-re′sis) involuntary discharge of urine after the age at which urinary control should have been achieved; often used with specific reference to involuntary discharge of urine occurring during sleep at night (bed-wetting). 270

eosinophil (e″o-sin′o-fil) a granular leukocyte with a nucleus that usually has two lobes and cytoplasm containing coarse, round granules that are readily stained by eosin. 77f

epicardium (ep″ĭ-kahr′de-um) the layer of serous pericardium on the surface of the heart. 112f, 113

epidemiologist (ep″ĭ-de″me-ol′o-jist) a specialist in epidemiology. 28

epidemiology (ep″ĭ-de″me-ol′o-je) the study of the relationships of factors determining the frequency and distribution of diseases in the human community; the field of medicine dealing with the determination of causes of localized outbreaks of infection or other disease of recognized cause. 28

epidermis (ep″ĭ-dər′mis) the outermost, nonvascular layer in the skin. 435, 436f

epididymis (ep″ĭ-did′ə-mis) the elongated cordlike structure along the posterior border of the testis that provides for storage, transit, and maturation of spermatozoa and is continuous with the ductus deferens. 312

epididymitis (ep″ĭ-did″ə-mi′tis) inflammation of the epididymis. 312

epidural (ep″ĭ-doo′rəl) situated on or outside of the dura mater. 396

epigastric (ep″ĭ-gas′trik) pertaining to the epigastrium, or upper middle region of the abdomen. 49

epiglottiditis, epiglottitis (ep″ĭ-glot″ĭ-di′tis, ep′ĭ-glō-ti′tis) inflammation of the epiglottis. 30

epiglottis (ep″ĭ-glot′is) the lidlike structure composed of cartilage that covers the larynx during swallowing. 168

fibrothorax (fi″bro-thor′aks) a condition characterized by adhesions of the two layers of pleura, resulting in the lung being covered by a thick layer of fibrous tissue. 172

fibrotic (fi-brot′ik) referring to or characterized by fibrosis. 172

fibrous (fi′brəs) composed of or containing fiber. 355

fibula (fib′u-lə) the smaller of the two lower leg bones. 343

fibular (fib′u-lər) pertaining to the fibula, a bone in the lower leg. 352

fimbria (fim′bre-ə) any structure that resembles a fringe or border, such as the long fringelike extension of a uterine tube that lies close to the ovary. 282

fissure (fish′ər) a split; a cleft or groove. 224, 445

fistula (fis′tu-lə) an abnormal communication between two internal organs, or from an internal organ to the body surface. 223, 311f

flatulence (flat′u-ləns) the presence of excessive amounts of air or gases in the stomach or intestine, leading to distention of the organs. 212

flexion (flek′shən) the act of bending; being bent. 363, 366f

flexor (flek′sor) any muscle that flexes a joint. 363

fluoroscopy (floo-ros′kə-pe) examination by means of a fluoroscope, a device that allows both structural and functional visualization of internal structures. 210, 217

follicle (fol′ĭ-kəl) a sac or pouchlike depression or cavity. 287

    graafian f. (graf′e-ən), a mature vesicular follicle of the ovary. 334

    f. stimulating hormone (stim′u-lā-ting hor′mōn) (FSH), one of the gonadotropic hormones of the anterior pituitary that stimulates the growth and maturation of ovarian follicles, stimulates estrogen secretion, and promotes endometrial changes. This hormone also stimulates spermatogenesis in the male. 287, 315, 316f

follicular (fo-lik′u-lər) of or pertaining to a follicle or follicles. 287

folliculitis (fo-lik″u-li′tis) inflammation of a follicle or follicles; used ordinarily in reference to hair follicles but sometimes in relation to follicles of other kinds. 449

foramen magnum (fo′ra-men mag′nəm) the opening in the occipital bone through which the spinal cord passes from the brain. 397

foreskin (for′skin) the prepuce, the loose skin covering the end of the penis. 312

fracture (frak′chər) a break or rupture in a bone; the breaking of a part, especially a bone. 369, 370f

    closed f. (klōzd), one that does not produce an open wound in the skin. 369

    comminuted f. (kom′ĭ-noōt′əd), one in which the bone is crushed or splintered. 369, 370f

    compound f. (kom′pound), open fracture. 369

    greenstick f. (grēn′stik), one in which only one side of a bone is broken. 369

    impacted f. (im-pak′təd), one in which one fragment is firmly driven into the other. 369, 370f

    oblique f. (o-blēk′), one that is slanted, between the direction of and at a right angle to the axis of the bone. 369

    open f. (o′pən), one in which a wound through the overlying or adjacent soft tissues communicates with the site of the break. 369

    simple f. (sim′pəl), closed fracture. 369

    transverse f. (trans-vərs′), one at right angles to the axis of the bone. 369, 370f

frontal (frun′təl) pertaining to the forehead; a plane that divides the body into anterior and posterior portions. 44, 48, 397

frostbite (fros′bīt) damage to tissues as the result of exposure to low environmental temperatures. 453

fructase (frook′tās) an enzyme that breaks down fructose. 245

fructose (frook′tōs) a sugar that occurs in honey and many sweet fruits. 198

fundus (fun′dəs) the bottom or base of anything. 210

fungal (fun′gəl) pertaining to a fungus. 204

fungicidal (fun″jĭ-si′dəl) destroying fungi. 464

fungus (fun′gəs) a general term used to denote a group of microorganisms that includes mushrooms, yeasts, rusts, molds, and smuts. 204

furuncle (fu′rung-kəl) a painful nodule formed in the skin by circumscribed inflammation enclosing a core; a boil. 450

gallbladder (gawl′blad′ər) the reservoir for bile on the posteroinferior surface of the liver. 201, 202f

gallstone (gawl′stōn) a calculus formed in the gallbladder or bile duct. 228

gamete (gam′ēt) a male or female reproductive cell; spermatozoon or ovum. 290

ganglion (gang′gle-on) a general term for a group of nerve cell bodies located outside the central nervous system; a benign cystic tumor occurring commonly on the wrist and consisting of a thin fibrous capsule enclosing a clear mucinous fluid. 375

gastralgia (gas-tral′jə) pain of the stomach; stomachache. 210, 212

gastrectasia, gastrectasis (gas-trek-ta′zhə, gas-trek′tə-sis) stretching of the stomach. 212

gastrectomy (gas-trek′tə-me) removal of all or part of the stomach. 215

gastric (gas′trik) pertaining to the stomach. 203

    g. carcinoma (kakr″sĭ-no′mə), cancer of the stomach. 210

    g. hypertrophy (hi-pər′tro-fe), enlarged stomach. 212

    g. lavage (lah-vahzh′), washing out of the stomach. 215

gastritis (gas-tri′tis) inflammation of the stomach. 212

gastrocele (gas′tro-sēl) hernia of the stomach. 213

gastroduodenal (gas″tro-doo″o-de′nəl) pertaining to or communicating with the stomach and duodenum. 220

    g. anastomosis (ə-nas′tə-mo′sis), surgical connection of the stomach and duodenum after removal of a portion of either of the two structures. 220

gastroduodenitis (gas″tro-doo-ad″ə-n′tis) inflammation of the stomach and duodenum. 218

gastroduodenostomy (gas″tro-doo″o-də-nos′tə-me) formation of a new opening between the stomach and the duodenum. 220

gastrodynia (gas″tro-din′e-ə) pain in the stomach. 212

gastroenteritis (gas″tro-en″tər′i′tis) inflammation of the stomach and intestines. 216

gastroenterocolitis (gas″tro-en″tər-o-ko-li′tis) inflammation of the stomach, small intestine, and colon. 221

gastroenterologist (gas″tro-en″tər-ol′ə-jist) a physician who specializes in the stomach and intestines and their diseases. 28

gastroenterology (gas″tro-en″tər-ol′ə-je) the study of the stomach and intestines and associated diseases. 28, 216

gastroenterostomy (gas″tro-en-tər-os′tə-me) surgical creation of an artificial passage between the stomach and intestines, usually the jejunum. 220

gastroesophageal reflux disease (gas″tro-ĕ-sof″ə-je′əl re′flăks dĭ-zēz′) any condition noted clinically or histopathologically resulting from gastroesophageal reflux. 214

gastrointestinal (gas″tro-in-tes′tĭ-nəl) pertaining to the stomach and the intestines. 196

gastrojejunostomy (gas″tro-jə-joo-nos′tə-me) surgical creation of an anastomosis between the stomach and the jejunum; also, the anastomosis so established. 219, 220

gastromalacia (gas″tro-mə-la′shə) abnormal softening of the stomach. 212

gastromegaly (gas″tro-meg′ə-le) enlargement of the stomach. 212

gastropathy (gas-trop′ə-the) any disease of the stomach. 212

gastropexy (gas′tro-pek″se) surgical fixation of the stomach to the abdominal wall. 212

gastroplasty (gas′tro-plas″te) plastic surgery of the stomach. 212

gastroptosis (gas″trop-to′sis) sagging of the stomach. 212

gastropulmonary (gas″tro-pul′mo-nar-e) pertaining to the stomach and lungs. 212

gastrorrhaphy (gas-tror′ə-fe) suture of the stomach. 234

gastrorrhexis (gas″tro-rek′sis) rupture of the stomach.

gastroscope (gas′tro-skōp) instrument for viewing inside the stomach. 212

gastroscopy (gas-tros′kə-pe) inspection of the interior of the stomach by means of the gastroscope. 219

gastrostomy (gas-tros′tə-me) the creation of a new opening into the stomach. 212

general practitioner (jen′ər-əl prak-tish′ən-er) a physician who treats people of all ages for many types of disorders. Also known as a family doctor. 24

general surgery (jen′ər-əl sur′jər-e) the medical specialty that deals with many types of surgery rather than specializing in only one area. 21

genital (jen′ĭ-təl) pertaining to the genitals. In its plural form, genitals refers to the reproductive organs. 281

    g. herpes (hər′pēz), herpes genitalis; herpetic lesions on the male or female genitalia. 321

    g. warts (worts), condyloma acuminatum; venereal warts, papillomas occurring on the genitalia, caused by an infectious virus. 322t, 323

genitalia (jen″ĭ-tāl′e-ə) the reproductive organs. 281

genitourinary (jen″ĭ-to-u′rĭ-nar-e) pertaining to the genital and urinary organs; urogenital. 263

geriatrics (jer″e-at′riks) the branch of medicine that deals with problems and diseases of old age. 26, 27

gerodontics (jer″o-don′tiks) dentistry dealing with dental problems of older people. 27

gerodontist (jer″o-don′tist) a dentist specializing in dental problems of older people. 27

gerontal (jer-on′təl) pertaining to old age. 27

gerontologist (jer″on-tol′ə-jist) a specialist in diseases of old age. 26

gerontology (jer″on-tol′ə-je) the branch of science that deals with the problems of aging in all of its aspects. 26

gestation (jes-ta′shən) pregnancy. 293

gestational (jes-ta′shən-əl) pertaining to pregnancy or the period of development of the young in viviparous animals, from the time of fertilization of the ovum until birth. 293

    g. diabetes (di″ə-be′tēz), carbohydrate intolerance with onset or first recognition during pregnancy. 485

gigantism (ji-gan′tiz-əm, ji′gən-tiz-əm) a condition in which a person reaches an abnormal stature, owing to excessive growth hormone during childhood. 57, 475, 476f

gingiva (jin′jĭ-və, jin-ji′və) the gum; the mucous membrane with supporting and fibrous tissue that covers the toothbearing border of the jaw. 205

gingival (jin′jĭ-vəl) pertaining to the gums. 205

gingivalgia (jin″jĭ-val′jə) pain in the gums. 205

gingivectomy (jin″jĭ-vek′tə-me) cutting away part of the gums. 205

gingivitis (jin″jĭ-vi′tis) inflammation of the gum. 205

gingivoglossitis (jin″jĭ-vo-glos-i′tis) inflammation of the gums and tongue. 205

hemocyte (he′mo-sīt) a blood cell. 76

hemodialysis (he″mo-di-al′ə-sis) the process of diffusing blood through a semipermeable membrane for the purpose of removing toxic materials and maintaining acid-base balance in cases of impaired kidney function. 250

hemoglobin (he′mo-glo″bin) the oxygen-carrying red pigment of red blood cells. 79, 83, 86

    h. A, normal adult hemoglobin, composed of two alpha and two beta chains. 86

hemoglobinopathy (he″mo glo″bin-op′ə-the) a hematologic disorder caused by genetically determined abnormal hemoglobin. 86

hemolysin (he-mol′ə-sin) a substance that causes destruction of red blood cells. 79

hemolysis (he-mol′ə-sis) destruction of red blood cells that results in the liberation of hemoglobin. 79

hemolytic (he″mo-lit′ik) pertaining to, characterized by, or producing hemolysis. 84

hemolyze (he′mo-līz) to subject to or to undergo hemolysis. 86

hemopericardium (he″mo-per″ĭ-kahr′de-əm) an effusion of blood within the pericardium. 113

hemophilia (he″mo-fil′e-ə) a hereditary hemorrhagic disorder caused by deficiency of antihemophilic factor VIII or IX. 80, 86t

hemoptysis (he-mop′tĭ-sis) the spitting of blood or blood-stained sputum. 179

hemorrhage (hem′ə-rəj) bleeding; the escape of blood from the vessels. 263

hemorrhoid (hem′ə-roid) a varicose dilation of a vein of the anal canal inside or just outside the rectum that causes pain, itching, and bleeding. 224

hemorrhoidectomy (hem″ə-roid-ek′tə-me) excision of hemorrhoids. 224

hemostasis (he″mo-sta′sis, he-mos′tə-sis) the checking of the flow of blood either by coagulation or surgical means; interruption of blood flow through any vessel or to any part of the body. 87

hemostatic (he″mo-stat′ik) checking the flow of blood, an agent that arrests the flow of blood. 99

hemotherapy (he″mo-ther′ə-pe) treatment of disease by the administration of blood or blood products. 341

hemothorax (he″mo-thor′aks) a collection of blood in the chest cavity. 48, 94, 176, 177f

hepatectomy (hep′ə-tek′tə-me) excision of part of the liver. 228

hepatic (hə-pat′ik) pertaining to the liver. 228

hepatitis (hep″ə-ti′tis) inflammation of the liver. 227, 322t, 323

hepatocyte (hep′ə-to-sīt) a parenchymal liver cell. 228

hepatolith (hep′ə-to-lith″) a gallstone. 228

hepatolytic (hep″ə-to-lit′ik) destructive to the liver; hepatotoxic. 229

hepatoma (hep″ə-to′mə) a tumor of the liver, especially hepatocellular carcinoma. 228

hepatomegaly (hep″ə-to-meg′ə-le) enlargement of the liver. 229

hepatopathy (hep″ə-top′ə-the) any disease of the liver. 228

hepatorrhagia (hep″ə-to-ra′jə) hemorrhage from the liver. 143

hepatosplenomegaly (hep″ə-to-sple″no-meg′ə-le) enlargement of the liver and spleen. 228

hepatotomy (hep″ə-tot′ə-me) surgical incision of the liver. 228

hepatotoxic (hep″ə-to-tok′sik) toxic to liver cells. 229

hernia (hər′ne-ə) protrusion of an organ or part of it through the wall of the cavity that contains the organ. 213, 214

    femoral h. (fem′or-əl), hernia into the femoral canal. 213

    hiatal h. (hi-a′təl), protrusion of any structure through the esophageal hiatus of the diaphragm. 213

    umbilical h. (əm-bil′ĭ-kəl), protrusion of part of the intestine at the umbilicus, the defect in the abdominal wall and protruding bowel being covered with skin and subcutaneous tissue. 213

herniated disk (hər′ne-āt″əd disk) herniation of an intervertebral disk. 375

herpes (hər′pēz) a word that at one time was used to indicate any inflammatory skin disease marked by small vesicles in clusters and caused by a virus. Its use as a single word is imprecise but often refers to the condition of cold sores or fever blisters. 450

    h. genitalis (jen″ĭ-tal′is), herpetic blisters on the male or female genitalia. 321, 322t

    h. simplex type 1, fever blister; a reddish raised fluid-filled vesicle that develops on the skin or mucous membrane in nongenital areas of the body. 450

    h. zoster (zos′tər), an acute infectious, usually self-limited disease believed to represent activation of latent varicella-zoster virus in those who have been rendered partially immune after a previous attack of chickenpox; also called shingles. 451t

hiatal (hi-a′təl) affecting or pertaining to a hiatus. 213

hiatus (hi-a′təs) general term for a gap or opening. 213

hidradenitis (hi″drad-ə-ni′tis) inflammation of a sweat gland. 442

hidradenoma (hi″drad-ə-no′mə) tumor of a sweat gland.

hidrosis (hi-dro′sis) formation and excretion of sweat; excessive sweating.

hirsutism (hir′soot-iz-əm) abnormal hairiness, especially an adult male pattern of hair distribution in women. 482

histamine (his′tə-mēn) a substance present in the body that has known pharmacological action when released from injured cells. Histamine can also be produced synthetically. 91

histocompatibility (his″to-kəm-pat″ĭ-bil′ĭ-te) the ability of donor tissue to survive after a transplant, rather than being rejected by the immune system of the patient who receives the tissue. 453

histologist (his-tol′ə-jist) one who studies tissue. 19

histology (his-tol′ə-je) study of the minute structure, composition, and function of tissues. 17, 19

histolysis (his-tol′ə-sis) the destruction of tissue.

histolytic (his″to-lit′ik) pertaining to or characterized by the breaking down or dissolution of tissue.

historrhexis (his″to-rek′sis) the breaking down of tissues.

hives (hīvz) urticaria. 444

holistic (ho-lis′tik) considering a person as a functioning whole. 18

homeostasis (ho″me-o-sta′sis) sameness or stability in the normal body state of an organism. 390, 467

homologous (ho-mol′o-gəs) corresponding in structure, position, origin, etc.; denoting individuals of the same species but antigenically distinct; pertaining to an antibody and the antigen that elicited its production. 97

hormone (hor′mōn) a chemical substance produced in the body that has a specific effect on the activity of certain cells or organs. 29, 467

humeral (hu′mər-əl) pertaining to the humerus, the upper arm bone. 350

humeroradial (hu″mər-o-ra′de-əl) pertaining to the humerus and radius. 351

humeroscapular (hu″mər-o-skap′u-lər) pertaining to the upper arm bone and the shoulder blade. 350

humeroulnar (hu″mər-o-ul′nər) pertaining to the humerus and ulna. 351

humerus (hu′mər-əs) the bone of the upper arm, extending from shoulder to elbow. 343

Huntington's disease (hunt′ing-tənz dĭ-zēz′) an autosomal dominant disease characterized by chronic, progressive, complex, jerky movements and mental deterioration terminating in dementia. 403

hydrocele (hi′dro-sēl) a circumscribed collection of fluid, especially pertaining to fluid collection in the scrotum. 319

hydrocelectomy (hi″dro-se-lek′tə-me) excision of a hydrocele. 334

hydrocephaly, hydrocephalus (hi″dro-sef′ə-le, hi″dro-sef′ə-ləs) a condition characterized by abnormal accumulation of cerebrospinal fluid within the skull, with enlargement of the head, atrophy of the brain, mental retardation, and convulsions. 93, 94f, 398

hydronephrosis (hi″dro-nə-fro′sis) distention of the kidney with urine, as a result of obstruction of the ureter. 254, 257, 258f

hydrophobia (hi″dro-fo′be-ə) rabies, a viral disease transmitted to a human by the bite of an infected animal. 423

hydrotherapy (hi″dro-ther′ə-pe) treatment using water. 97, 455

hydrothorax (hi″dro-thor′aks) a collection of water fluid in the pleural cavity. 172

hydroureter (hi″dro-u-re′tər) abnormal distention of the ureter owing to obstruction from any cause. 257, 258f

hypalgesia (hi″pal-je′ze-ə) descreased sensitivity to pain. 418

hyperacidity (hi″pər-ə-sid′ĭ-te) an excessive amount of acid. 215

hyperadrenalism (hi″pər-ə-dre′nəl-iz-əm) increased activity of the adrenal glands. 482

hyperalgesia (hi″pər-al-je′ze-ə) excessive sensitivity to pain. 418

hyperalgia (hi-pər-al′jə) excessive sensitivity to pain. 185

hyperalimentation (hi″pər-al″ĭ-men-ta′shən) the intravenous infusion of a hypertonic solution that contains sufficient nutrients to sustain life. 200

hypercalcemia (hi″pər-kal-se′me-ə) an increased level of calcium in the blood. 486

hypercalciuria (hi″pər-kal″se-u′re-ə) excessive calcium in the urine. 340

hypercapnia (hi″pər-kap′ne-ə) excessive carbon dioxide in the blood. 157

hyperchromia (hi″pər-kro-me-ə) excessive pigmentation, especially as related to the hemoglobin content of erythrocytes. 84

hyperchromic (hi″pər-kro′mik) highly or excessively stained or colored. 84

hyperemesis (hi″pər-em-ə-sis) excessive vomiting. 197

hyperemia (hi″pər-e′me-ə) excessive blood flow to a part of the body. 142

hyperesthesia (hi″pər-es-the″zhə) increased sensitivity to pain. 185, 418

hyperextension (hi″pər-ək-sten′shən) extreme or excessive extension of a limb or part. 405, 406f

hyperflexion (hi″pər-flek′shən) overflexion of a limb or part owing to force. 405, 406f

hyperglycemia (hi″pər-gli-se′me-ə) an increased amount of sugar in the blood. 198

hyperinsulinism (hi″pər-in′sə-lin-iz″əm) excessive secretion of insulin by the pancreas, resulting in an increased level of insulin in the blood and hypoglycemia. 485

hyperkinesia, hyperkinesis (hi″pər-kĭ-ne′zhə, hi″pər-kĭ-ne′sis) abnormally increased muscular function or activity. 420

hyperlipemia (hi″pər-li-pe′me-ə) An increased amount of fat in the blood. 199

hyperlipidemia (hi″pər-lip″ĭ-de′me-ə) a general term for elevated concentrations of any or all of the lipids in the plasma. 199

hyperopia (hi″pər-o′pe-ə) an error of refraction in which rays of light entering the eye are brought to a focus behind the retina; called also farsightedness. 415, 416f

hyperoxemia (hi″pər ok′se′me-ə) increased amount of oxygen in the blood. 182

hyperparathyroidism (hi″pər-par″ə-thi′roid-iz-əm) increased secretion of hormone by the parathyroids. 486

hyperpituitarism (hi″pər-pĭ-too′ĭ-tə-riz″əm) increased secretion by the pituitary gland. 475, 476

hyperplasia (hi″pər-pla′zhə) abnormal increase in the number of normal cells in a tissue. 318, 367

hyperpnea (hi″pərp-ne′ə) an abnormal increase in depth and rate of respiration. 156

hyperpyrexia (hi″pər-pi-rek′se-ə) a highly elevated body temperature of around 105° F or above. 61

hyperpyrexial (hi″pər-pi-rek′se-əl) pertaining to an elevated body temperature. 61

hypersecretion (hi″pər-se-kre′shən) excessive secretion. 482

hypersensitivity (hi″pər-sen″sĭ-tiv′ĭ-te) a state in which the body reacts with an exaggerated response to a foreign agent. 91

hypertension (hi″pər-ten′shən) increased blood pressure. 126

hyperthermia (hi″pər-ther′me-ə) greatly increased body temperature. 442

hyperthyroidism (hi″pər-thi′roid-iz-əm) increased activity of the thyroid gland. 478

hypertrophy (hi-pər′tro-fe) enlargement of an organ owing to an increase in the size of preexisting cells. 318, 367

hyperventilation (hi″pər-ven″tĭ-la′shən) abnormally increased pulmonary ventilation, resulting in greater than normal loss of carbon dioxide, which, if prolonged, may lead to alkalosis. 156

hypesthesia (hĭp″əs-the′zhə) decreased sensitivity, particularly to touch; hypoesthesia. 418

hypnotic (hip-not′ik) inducing sleep; pertaining to or of the nature of hypnotism; a drug that acts to induce sleep.

hypoacidity (hi″po-ə-sid′ĭ-te) less than normal amount of acid.

hypoadrenalism (hi″po-ə-dre′nəl-iz-əm) decreased activity of the adrenal glands. 482

hypoalgesia (hi″po-al-je′se-ə) decreased sensitivity to pain. 418

hypocalcemia (hi″po-kal-se′me-ə) decreased amount of calcium in the blood. 486

hypocapnia (hi″po-kap′ne-ə) deficiency of carbon dioxide in the blood resulting from hyperventilation and eventually leading to alkalosis. 157

hypochondriac (hi″po-kon′dre-ak) pertaining to the hypochondrium; a person who has morbid anxiety about his or her health but has no attributable cause. 49, 51

hypochromia (hi″po-kro′me-ə) abnormal decrease in the hemoglobin content of the erythrocytes. 84

hypochromic (hi″po-kro′mik) pertaining to or marked by hypochromia. 84

hypodermic (hi″po-dər′mik) applied or administered beneath the skin. 458

hypoesthesia (hi″po-es-the′zhə) abnormal decrease in sensitivity to stimuli. 418

hypogastric (hi″po-gas′trik) situated below the stomach; pertaining to the hypogastrium. 49

hypoglossal (hi″po-glos′əl) beneath the tongue. 205

hypoglycemia (hi″po-gli-se′me-ə) an abnormally low concentration of glucose in the blood. 198, 232, 484

hypogonadism (hi″po-go′nad-iz-əm) decreased functional activity of the gonads, with retardation of sexual development. 480

hypoinsulinism (hi″po-in′su-lin-iz″əm) deficient secretion of insulin by the pancreas. 484

hypoparathyroidism (hi″po-par″ə-thi′roid-iz-əm) decreased secretion of hormone by the parathyroids. 486

hypopharynx (hi″po-far′inks) that portion of the pharynx below the upper edge of the epiglottis, opening into the larynx and esophagus. 193

hypophysis (hi-pof′ə-sis) the pituitary gland. 468f, 469

hypopituitarism (hi″po-pĭ-too′ĭ-tə-riz″əm) decreased activity of the pituitary gland. 475, 476

hyposecretion (hi″po-se-kre′shən) diminished secretion as of a gland. 468

hypotension (hi″po-ten′shən) decreased blood pressure. 126

hypothalamus (hi″po-thal′ə-məs) the part of the brain most concerned with moderating behavior related to internal physiological states. 397, 398f, 472, 473f

hypothermia (hi″po-thər′me-ə) low body temperature. 442

hypothyroidism (hi″po-thi′roid-iz-əm) decreased activity of the thyroid gland. 479

hypoxemia (hi″pok-se′me-ə) deficient oxygen in the blood. 158, 182

hypoxia (hi-pok′se-ə) a condition of decreased oxygen. 158

hysterectomy (his″tər-ek′tə-me) removal of the uterus. 282, 304

    abdominal h. (ab-dom′ĭ-nəl), a hysterectomy performed through an incision in the abdominal wall. 304

    vaginal h. (vaj′ĭ-nəl), a hysterectomy performed through the vagina. 304

hysteropathy (his″tə-rop′ə-the) any uterine disease or disorder. 309

hysteropexy (his″tər-o-pek-se) surgical fixation of the uterus. 309

hysteroptosis (his″tər-op-to′sis) falling or prolapse of the uterus. 309

hysterosalpingogram (his″tər-o-sal″ping′go-gram) the record produced by x-ray examination of the uterus and uterine tubes after the injection of opaque material. 309

hysterosalpingography (his″tər-o-sal″ping-gog′rə-fe) roentgenography of the uterus and uterine tubes after injection of opaque material. 309

hysterosalpingo-oophorectomy (his″tər-o-sal-pin″go-o-of″ə-rek′tə-me) excision of the uterus, uterine tubes, and ovaries. 304

hysteroscopy (his″tər-os′kə-pe) inspection of the interior of the uterus with an endoscope. 309

ichthyoid (ik′the-oid) resembling a fish. 455

ichthyosis (ik″the-o′sis) any of several generalized skin disorders marked by dryness and scaliness, resembling fish skin. 455

idiopathic (id″e-o-path′ik) occurring without known cause, self-originated.

ileitis (il″e-i′tis) inflammation of the ileum. 221

ileocecal (il″e-o-se′kəl) pertaining to the ileum and cecum. 222

    i. valve (valv), the valve that regulates the passage of contents of the small intestine into the cecum, the first part of the large intestine. 222

ileostomy (il″e-os′tə-me) surgical creation of an opening into the ileum, usually by establishing a stoma on the abdominal wall. 221

ileum (il′e-əm) the distal portion of the small intestine, which extends from the jejunum to the cecum. 201, 202f, 219

iliac (il′e-ak) pertaining to the ilium, a bone of the pelvis. 49, 349

    i. artery (ahr′tər-e), one of several arteries that supply blood to the lower extremities. 109f

    i. vein (vān), one of several large veins that return blood from the lower extremities. 109f

iliofemoral (il″e-o-fem′or-əl) pertaining to the ilium and the femur. 352

iliopubic (il″e-o-pu′bik) pertaining to the ilium and the pubis, two bones of the pelvis. 349

ilium (il′e-əm) the lateral flaring portion of the hip bone. 343

imaging (im′ə-jing) the production of images, especially in radiological and ultrasound images. 479

    nuclear medicine i. (noo′kle-ər med′ĭ-sin), administration of a radiopharmaceutical followed by the imaging of the spatial distribution of the radionuclide. 479

immunity (ĭ-mu′nĭ-te) being immune; security against a particular disease; nonsusceptibility to the invasive or pathogenic effects of certain antigens. 89, 91, 92f, 96

immunocompromised (im″u-no-kom′prə-mīzd) having the immune response attenuated by administration of immunosuppressive drugs, by irradiation, by malnutrition, or by some disease processes. 92

immunodeficiency (im″u-no-də-fish-ən-se) a deficiency in immune response. 323

immunoglobulin (im″u-no-glob′u-lin) a protein of animal origin that has known antibody activity. 89

immunologist (im″u-nol′o-jist) a person who makes a special study of immunology. 27

immunology (im″u-nol′o-je) the branch of medical science concerned with the response of the organism to antigenic challenge, recognition of self from nonself, and all of the aspects of immune phenomena. 27

immunosuppressant, immunosuppressive (im″u-no-sə-pres′ənt, im″u-no-sə-pres′iv) pertaining to or inducing immunosuppression. 92

impacted (im-pak′təd) driven firmly in; closely or firmly lodged in position. 225

    i. fracture (frak′chər), the breaking of a bone in which one fragment is firmly driven into the other. 369, 370f

impaction (im-pak′shən) the condition of being firmly lodged or wedged. 225

    fecal i. (fe′kəl), a collection of puttylike or hardened feces in the rectum or sigmoid. 225

impetigo (im″pə-ti′go) an inflammatory, contagious skin disease marked by isolated pustules and usually caused by staphyloccal or streptococcal infection. 451t

implantation (im″plan-ta′shən) attachment of the fertilized egg to the epithelial lining of the uterus and its embedding in the compact layer of the endometrium. 289, 290f

impotence (im′pə-təns) inability of the male to achieve or maintain an erection. 317

incise (in-sīz′) to cut into. 17

incision (in-sizh′ən) a cut or wound produced by a sharp instrument; the act of cutting. 17

incisor (in-si′zor) any of the four anterior teeth in either jaw. 207

incompatibility (in″kəm-pat″ĭ-bil′ĭ-te) the unsuitability of one thing to another. 453

incontinence (in-kon′tĭ-nəns) inability to control excretory functions. 270

infarct (in′fahrkt) an area of necrosis in a tissue caused by local ischemia resulting from obstruction of circulation to the area. 130

infarction (in-fahrk′shən) the formation of a localized area of necrosis owing to insufficient blood supply, produced by an occlusion. 130

    myocardial i. (mi″o-kahr′de-əl), death of an area of the heart muscle, occurring as a result of oxygen deprivation. 130

infection (in-fek′shən) invasion and multiplication of microorganisms in body tissues. 60, 61, 81

    nosocomial i. (nos″o-ko′me-əl), infection acquired while one is hospitalized. 267

    opportunistic i. (op″ər-too-nis′tik), infection with any organism that occurs because of the opportunity afforded by the altered physiological state of the host. 322t

infectious (in-fek′shəs) capable of being transmitted; pertaining to a disease caused by a microorganism; producing infection. 60, 97

    i. mononucleosis (mon″o-noo″kle-o′sis), an acute infectious disease that primarily affects lymphoid tissue. The cause of most cases of infectious mononucleosis is the Epstein-Barr virus. 97

inferior (in-fēr′e-ər) situated below or directed downward; in anatomy it is used in reference to the lower surface of a structure or to the lower of two or more similar structures. 46

inferomedian (in″fər-o-me′de-ən) situated in the middle of the underside. 46

inflammation (in″flə-ma′shən) a localized protective response elicited by injury or destruction of tissues. 58, 81

influenza (in″floo-en′zə) an acute viral infection involving the respiratory tract. 178t

infraclavicular (in″frə-klə-vik′u-lər) below the collarbone. 376

infracostal (in″frə-kos′təl) below a rib. 376

infrapatellar (in″frə-pə-tel′ər) beneath the kneecap. 376

infrascapular (in″frə-skap′u-lər) beneath the shoulder blade. 376

infrasternal (in″frə-stər′nəl) beneath the breastbone. 376

ingestion (in-jes′chən) the act of taking food, medicines, etc., into the body by mouth. 197

inguinal (ing′gwĭ-nəl) pertaining to the inguen, or groin. 49, 213

i. node (nōd), one of several lymph nodes located in the groin. 136

inhalation (in″hə-la′shən) drawing air or other substances into the nasal or oral respiratory route; any drug administered by the respiratory route. 155

inject (in-jekt′) to force a fluid into a part or organ. 456

injection (in-jek′shən) the forcing of a liquid into a part; a substance that is injected. 456-458

intradermal i. (in″trə-dər′məl), placement of a small amount of a drug into the outer layers of the skin with a very fine gauge, short needle. 457f, 458

intramuscular i. (in″trə-mus′ku-lər), the deposition of medication into a muscular layer, usually in the anterior thigh, deltoid, or one of the buttocks. 457f, 458

intravenous i. (in″trə-ve′nəs), injection into a vein. 457f, 458

subcutaneous i. (sub″ku-ta′ne-əs), injection of a small amount of medication below the skin layer into the subcutaneous tissue. 456, 457f, 458

inspiration (in″spĭ-ra′shən) the drawing of air into the lungs. 155, 163f

insulin (in′sə-lin) a hormone secreted by the beta cells of the islets of Langerhans of the pancreas into the blood. 232, 484

integumentary (in-teg′u-men′tar-e) pertaining to, composed of, or serving as skin. 435

interalveolar (in″tər-al-ve′o-lər) between the alveoli. 185

intercellular (in″tər-sel′u-lər) situated between the cells of a structure. 97

intercerebral (in″tər-ser′ə-brəl) between the two cerebral hemispheres. 432

interchondral (in″tər-kon′drəl) between two or more cartilages. 361

intercostal (in″tər-kos′təl) between the ribs. 346

i. muscles (mus′əls), the muscles that move the ribs when breathing. 346

interdental (in″tər-den′təl) between the teeth. 206

interferon (in″tər-fēr′on) any of a family of glycoproteins that exert nonspecific antiviral activity, have immunoregulatory functions, and can inhibit the growth of nonviral intracellular parasites. 89

intermammary (in″tər-mam′ə-re) between the breasts. 474

internal medicine (in-ter′nel med′ĭ-sin) the branch of medicine that treats diseases of the internal organs by other than surgical means. 27

internist (in-ter′nist) a specialist in internal medicine. 27

interocular (in″tər-ok′u-lər) between the eyes. 411

interpubic (in″tər-pu′bik) between the pubic bones. 349

interrenal (in″tə-re′nəl) situated between the kidneys. 271

interscapular (in″tər-skap′u-lər) between the shoulder blades. 349

interstitial (in″tər-stish′əl) pertaining to or situated between parts or in the interspaces of a tissue.

i. cells of Leydig (li′dig), cells in the testes that are responsible for the production of testosterone.

i. fluid (floo′id), tissue fluid or fluid occupying spaces between tissue cells. 73

intervertebral (in″tər-ver′tə-brəl) between two contiguous vertebrae. 348

i. disk (disk), the layer of fibrocartilage between the bodies of adjoining vertebrae. 348

intestinal (in-tes′tĭ-nəl) pertaining to the intestine. 203

intestine (in-tes′tin) The portion of the alimentary canal that extends from the pyloric opening of the stomach to the anus. 216

intraarterial (in″trə-ahr-tēr′e-əl) within an artery or arteries. 132

intraarticular (in″trə-ahr′tik′u-lər) within a joint. 360

intracellular (in″trə-sel′u-lər) within a cell. 73

intracerebral (in″trə-ser′ə-brəl) within the cerebrum. 396

intracranial (in″trə-kra′ne-əl) within the skull. 392

intradermal (in″trə-dər′məl) situated within the skin. 457f, 458

intramuscular (in″trə-mus′ku-lər) situated in the muscle. 457f, 458

intraocular (in″trə-ok′u-lər) situated within the eye. 411

intrasternal (in″trə-stər′nəl) within the sternum. 344

intrathecal (in″trə-the′kəl) within a sheath or within the spinal canal. 377

intrauterine device (in″trə-u′tər-in də-vīs′) (IUD) a contraceptive device inserted into the uterine cavity. 293

intravascular (in″trə-vas′ku-lər) within a vessel or vessels. 73, 131

intravenous (in″trə-ve′nəs) situated within the vein. 257

i. pyelogram (pi′ə-lo-gram), roentgenogram of the ureter and renal pelvis after intravenous injection of a radiopaque material. 257

intubation (in″too-ba′shən) insertion of a tube into a body canal or organ. 170f

endotracheal i. (en″do-tra′ke-əl), insertion of a tube into the trachea. 170f

nasotracheal i. (na″zo-tra′ke-əl), insertion of a tube through the nose into the trachea to serve as an airway. 170f

orotracheal i. (or″o-tra′ke-əl), insertion of a tube through the mouth into the trachea to serve as an airway. 170f

inversion (in-vər′zhən) a turning inward, inside out, upside down, or other reversal of the normal relation of a part. 366f, 367

in vitro (in ve′tro) in an artificial environment or within a test tube. 75

in vivo (in ve′vo) within the living body. 75

involuntary (in-vol′ən-tar″e) not done willingly. 362

iritis (i-ri′tis) inflammation of the iris, usually marked by pain, congestion in the ciliary region, photophobia, contraction of the pupil, and discoloration of the iris. 412

ischemia (is-ke′me-ə) deficiency of blood owing to functional constriction or actual obstruction of a blood vessel. 130

myocardial i. (mi″o-kahr′de-əl), deficiency of blood supply to the heart muscle owing to obstruction or constriction of the coronary arteries. 130

ischial (is′ke-əl) pertaining to the ischium, a bone of the pelvis. 349

ischialgia (is″ke-al′jə) pain in the ischium. 349

ischiococcygeal (is″ke-o-kok′sij′e-əl) pertaining to the ischium and the coccyx (tailbone). 349

ischiodynia (is″ke-o-din′e-ə) pain in the ischium. 349

ischiofemoral (is″ke-o-fem′o-rəl) pertaining to the ischium and the femur. 352

ischiopubic (is″ke-o-pu′bik) pertaining to the ischium and pubic region. 349

ischium (is′ke-əm) the inferior, dorsal portion of the hip bone. 343

islets of Langerhans (i′lets of lahng′ər-hahnz) irregular microscopic structures scattered throughout the pancreas and constituting the endocrine portion. In humans they are composed of at least three types of cells that secrete insulin, glucagon, and somatostatin. 484

isocytosis (i″so-si-to′sis) a condition in which the cells are the same size, especially red blood cells. 83

isotonic (i″so-ton′ik) equal tension; denoting a solution in which body cells can be placed without net flow of water across the cell's semipermeable membrane; denoting a solution that has the same tonicity as another solution with which it is compared. 84

jaundice (jawn′dis) yellowness of the skin, sclerae, and excretions because of increased bilirubin in the blood and deposition of bile pigments. 95, 228

jejunoileostomy (jə-joo″no-il″e-os′tə-me) formation of a new opening between the jejunum and the ileum. 220

jejunotomy (jə″joo-not′ə-me) surgical incision of the jejunum. 219

jejunum (jə-joo′nəm) that portion of the small intestine that extends from the duodenum to the ileum. 219, 220f

joint (joint) the site of junction or union between two or more bones. 355, 356f

synovial j. (sĭ-no′ve-əl), a general classification of joints that have a cavity between articulating bones and are freely movable. 355, 356f

Kaposi's sarcoma (kah′po-shēz, kap′o-sēz sahr-ko′mə) a malignant neoplastic proliferation characterized by the development of bluish-red cutaneous nodules, usually on the lower extremities, that slowly increase in size and number and spread to more proximal sites. 323f, 449

karyomegaly (kar″e-o-meg′ə-le) abnormal enlargement of the cell nucleus. 81

keloid (ke′loid) a sharply elevated, irregularly shaped, progressively enlarging scar resulting from formation of excessive amounts of collagen in the dermis during connective tissue repair. 452

keratin (ker′ə-tin) a protein that forms the epidermis, hair, and all horny tissue. 435

keratitis (ker″ə-ti′tis) inflammation of the cornea. 412

keratogenesis (ker″ə-to-jen′ə-sis) the formation of horny material. 435

keratolytic (ker″ə-to-lit′ik) pertaining to, characterized by, or producing keratolysis, dissolving of the horny layer of epidermis; an agent that promotes keratolysis. 460

keratoma (ker″ə-to′mə) a horny tumor; a tumor composed of keratin. 435

keratosis (ker″ə-to′sis) any horny growth; a condition of the skin characterized by the formation of horny growths or excessive development of the horny growth. 436, 437f

actinic k. (ak-tin′ik), a sharply outlined, red or skin-colored growth that usually affects the middle-aged or elderly and may give rise to a squamous cell carcinoma. 436, 449

seborrheic k. (seb″o-re′ik), a common benign, noninvasive tumor of the skin characterized by soft, crumbly plaques, varying in pigmentation, and occurring most often on the face, trunk, and extremities usually in middle life. 436, 437f

lobule (lob′ūl) a small lobe. 314
>*hepatic l.* (hə-pat′ik), the small functional unit of the liver.

loop of Henle (lo͞op əv hen′le) a long, U-shaped part of the renal tubule, extending through the medulla from the end of the proximal convoluted tubule to the beginning of the distal convoluted tubule. 255

lordosis (lor-do′sis) the anterior concavity in the curvature of the lumbar and cervical spine as viewed from the side. The term is used to refer to abnormally increased curvature (swayback) and to the normal curvature (normal lordosis). 371, 372f

lumbar (lum′bahr) pertaining to the lower back. 49, 346

lumpectomy (ləm-pek′tə-me) surgical excision of only the palpable lesion in carcinoma of the breast; surgical removal of a mass. 473

lunula (loo′nu-lə) a small crescent or moon-shaped area. 443

lupus erythematosus (loo′pəs er″ə-the″mə-to′sis) (LE) a group of connective tissue disorders primarily affecting women aged 20 to 40 years, comprising a spectrum of clinical forms in which cutaneous disease may occur with or without systemic involvement. 357, 358f
>*cutaneous l. e.* (ku′ta′ne-əs), a form of lupus erythematosus in which the skin may be the only organ involved, or it may precede the involvement of other systems. 357
>*discoid l. e.* (dis′koid) (DLE), a chronic form of cutaneous lupus erythematosus in which the skin lesions mimic those of the systemic form but systemic signs are rare, although multisystem manifestations may develop after many years. 357, 358f, 455

luteal (loo′te-əl) pertaining to or having the properties of the corpus luteum or its active principle. 287

luteinizing hormone (loo′te-in-ī″zing hor′mōn) a hormone secreted by the anterior lobe of the hypophysis that stimulates development of the corpus luteum. 287, 315, 316f, 480

Lyme disease (līm dǐ-zez′) a recurrent multisystemic disorder, beginning with a rash and followed by arthritis of the large joints, myalgia, malaise, and neurologic and cardiac manifestations. It is caused by the bacteria *Borrelia burgdorferi,* carried by the deer tick *Ixodes dammini.* 359t

lymph (limf) a transparent fluid that is found in lymphatic vessels that consists of a liquid portion and of cells that are mostly lymphocytes. 136
>*l. nodes* (nōdz), small knots of lymphatic tissue found at intervals along the course of the lymphatic vessels. 136

lymphadenitis (lim-fad″ə-ni′tis) inflammation of a lymph node. 140

lymphadenoma (lim-fad″ə-no′mə) enlargement of the lymph nodes. 140

lymphadenopathy (lim-fad-ə-nop′ə-the) any disease of the lymph nodes. 140, 321

lymphangiography (lim-fan″je-og′rə-fe) roentgenography of the lymphatic vessels after the injection of contrast medium. 139

lymphangioma (lim-fan″je-o′mə) a tumor composed of newly formed lymph channels. 124, 139

lymphangitis (lim″fan-ji′tis) inflammation of a lymphatic vessel. 139

lymphatics (lim-fat′iks) a system of vessels that collects tissue fluids from all parts of the body and returns the fluids to the blood circulation. 136, 137f

lymphatology (lim″fə-tol′ə-je) the study of the lymph and lymphatic system. 136

lymphatolysis (lim″fə-tol′ə-sis) destruction of lymphatic tissue. 136

lymphedema (lim″fə-de′mə) chronic edema of an extremity because of obstruction within the lymph vessels or the lymph nodes, resulting in accumulation of interstitial fluid. 138, 139f

lymphocyte (lim′fo-sīt) any of the mononuclear leukocytes found in the blood, lymph, and lymphoid tissues that are responsible for humoral and cellular immunity. 77f, 138

lymphogenous (lim-foj′ə-nəs) producing lymph; produced from lymph or in the lymphatics. 143

lymphogram (lim′fo-gram) a roentgenogram of the lymphatic vessels and lymph nodes. 138

lymphography (lim-fog′rə-fe) roentgenography of the lymphatic vessels and nodes after injection of radiopaque material. 138

lymphoma (lim-fo′mə) a lymphatic tumor; any neoplastic disorder of lymphoid tissue. 139

lymphostasis (lim-fos′tə-sis) stoppage of lymph flow. 138

macrocephaly (mak″ro-sef′ə-le) excessive size of the head. 62

macrocyte (mak′ro-sīt) a very large cell, usually referring to a very large red blood cell. 83, 85f

macrocytosis (mak″ro-si-to′sis) an increase in the number of large red blood cells. 83

macrodontia (mak″ro-don′shə) a developmental disorder characterized by increase in the size of the teeth that may affect a single tooth or all of the teeth. 235

macrophage (mak′ro-fāj) any of the mononuclear phagocytes found in the walls of blood vessels and in loose connective tissue. 89

macropodia (mak″ro-po′de-ə) increased size of the foot. 62

macroscopy (mə-kros′kə-pe) examination with the naked eye; macroscopic examination. 83

macule (mak′ūl) a discolored spot on the skin that is not elevated above the surface. 444

magnetic resonance imaging or scan, resonance imaging (MRI) a noninvasive method of creating images of body parts based on the magnetic properties of chemical elements within the body. 401

malabsorption (mal″əb-sorp′shən) faulty nutritive absorption. 197

malacia (mə-la′shə) a morbid softness or softening of a tissue or part. 177

malaise (mah-lāz′) a general feeling of ill health. 234

malaria (mə-lar′e-ə) an infectious disease mainly found in parts of Africa, Asia, Turkey, the West Indies, Central and South America, and Oceania, caused by intracellular protozoa of the genus *Plasmodium* and usually transmitted by the bites of infected mosquitoes. 86t

malignant (mə-lig′nənt) tending to grow worse and threatening to result in death. 180

malleus (mal′e-əs) the outermost of the auditory ossicles and the one attached to the membrana tympani. 344t

malnutrition (mal″noo-trish′ən) poor nutrition. 197

malocclusion (mal″o-kloo′zhən) improper position of the teeth resulting in the faulty meeting of the teeth or jaws. 208

malposition (mal″pə-zizh′ən) an abnormal position. 208

mammalgia (mə-mal′jə) painful breast. 473

mammary (mam′ər-e) pertaining to the breast. 471

mammogram (mam′ə-gram) a roentgenogram of the breast. 473, 474

mammography (mə-mog′rə-fe) the use of x-ray examination to diagnose diseases of the breast. 473

mammoplasty (mam′o-plas″te) surgical repair of the breast. 474
>*augmentation m.* (awg-men-ta′shən), plastic surgery to increase the size of the female breast. 474
>*reduction m.* (re-duk′shən), plastic surgery to reduce the size of the female breast. 474

mandible (man′dǐ-bəl) the bone of the lower jaw. 208

mandibular (man-dib′u-lər) pertaining to the lower jaw bone, or mandible. 208

mania (ma′ne-ə) a phase of bipolar disorder characterized by expansiveness, elation, agitation, hyperexcitability, hyperactivity, and increased speed of thought and speech (flight of ideas); called also manic syndrome; as a combining form, it signifies obsessive preoccupation. 421

marrow (mar′o) the soft material that fills the cavities of bones. 338, 341, 345

mastalgia (mas-tal′jə) pain in the breast. 473

mastectomy (mas-tek′tə-me) surgical removal of a breast. 474

mastitis (mas-ti′tis) inflammation of the breast. 474

mastocarcinoma (mas″to-kahr″sǐ no′mə) cancerous tumor of the breast. 473

mastodynia (mas″to-din′e-ə) painful breast. 473

mastoiditis (mas″toid-i′tis) inflammation of the mastoid antrum and cells. 415

mastopexy (mas′to-pek″se) plastic surgery to correct a pendulous breast. 473

mastoptosis (mas″to-to′sis) sagging breasts. 474

mastorrhagia (mas″to-ra′je-ə) hemorrhage from a breast. 474

matrix (ma′triks) the intracellular substance of a tissue or the tissue from which a structure develops. 443

maxilla (mak-sil′ə) the irregularly shaped bone that helps form the upper jaw. 208

maxillary (mak′sǐ-lar″e) pertaining to the maxilla. 208

mechanoreceptor (mek″ə-no-re-sep′tor) a receptor that is excited by mechanical pressures or distortions, as those responding to sound, touch, and muscular contractions. 411

medial, median (me′de-əl, me′de-ən) pertaining to the middle or midline of a body or structure; pertaining to the middle layer of structures. 46

mediastinoscope (me″de-ə-sti′no-skōp) an endoscope used to examine the mediastinum. 111

mediastinoscopy (me″de-as″tǐ-nos′kə-pe) examination of the mediastinum using an endoscope inserted through an anterior midline incision just above the thoracic inlet. 111

mediastinum (me″de-əs-ti′nəm) a median partition; an area in the middle of the chest that contains the heart and its large vessels, trachea, esophagus, thymus, and lymph nodes. 111

medical (med′ǐ-kəl) pertaining to medicine. 31
>*m. laboratory* (lab′rə-tor″e), a place equipped for performing tests on patients for the purpose of diagnosis and monitoring of health. 31
>*m. laboratory assistant* (ə-sis′tənt), one who has received limited training in clinical laboratory techniques. 31
>*m. records* (rek′ordz), transcripts of information obtained from a patient, guardian, or professionals and presented in tabular, outline, or written form; a department in the hospital where such records are kept. 31
>*m. technician* (tek-nish′ən), one who has received formal training in laboratory techniques in a 2-year associate degree program at a community college, a vocational technical school, or a private school. 31
>*m. technologist* (tek-nol′ə-jist), one who is skilled in the performance of clinical laboratory procedures used in the diagnosis of disease and evaluation of patient progress. In general, the technologist has completed 4 years of specialized education in medical technology. 31

m. transcription (trans-krip′shən), the production of typed medical reports from dictated messages by physicians. 31

medicine (med′ĭ-sin) a drug or remedy; the science of diagnosis and treatment of disease and the maintenance of health; the nonsurgical treatment of disease. 18, 30

emergency room m. (e-mər′jen-se rōōm), the medical specialty that deals with acutely ill or injured patients who require immediate medical attention. 27

internal m. (in-tər′nəl), a branch of medicine that deals specifically with diagnosis and medical treatment of diseases and disorders of internal structures of the body. 27

nuclear m. (noo′kle-ər), the branch of medicine concerned with the diagnostic, therapeutic, and investigative use of radionuclides. 479

rehabilitation m. (re″hə-bil″ĭ-ta′shən), the branch of medicine that deals with restoring a person′s ability to live and work as normally as possible after a disabling injury or illness. 31

mediolateral (me″de-o-lat′ər-əl) pertaining to the middle and to one side. 46

medulla (mə-dul′ə) the innermost part of an organ or structure. 397, 398f

adrenal m. (ə-dre′nəl), the inner portion of the adrenal gland, which secretes epinephrine. 481, 484

megalocyte (meg′ə-lo-sīt″) an extremely large red blood cell. 83

megalogastria (meg″ə-lo-gas′tre-ə) enlargement or abnormally large size of the stomach; gastric hypertrophy. 212

megalomania (meg″ə-lo-ma′ne-ə) a disordered mental state characterized by delusions of grandeur. 421

melancholy (mel′ən-kol″e) a depressed and painful emotional state. 95

melanin (mel′ə-nin) the dark pigment of the skin, hair, eye, and certain tumors. 95, 476

melanocyte (mel′ə-no-sīt, mə-lan′o-sīt) a black cell; a cell that produces melanin. 95

melanoderma (mel″ə-no-der′mə) an abnormal deposit of melanin in the skin due to an increase in production of melanin by the melanocytes or to an increase in the number of melanocytes. 96

melanoid (mel′ə-noid) resembling something black or dark; resembling melanin. 95

melanoma (mel″ə-no′mə) a tumor arising from the melanocytic system of the skin and other organs. When used alone, the term refers to malignant melanoma. 95, 142, 179, 449

malignant m. (mə-lig′nənt), a malignant neoplasm of melanocytes that occurs most often in the skin but also may occur elsewhere. 95

melatonin (mel″ə-to′nin) a hormone synthesized by the pineal gland the secretion of which increases during exposure to light; in mammals it influences hormone production and in many species regulates seasonal changes such as reproductive pattern and fur color. In humans it is implicated in the regulation of sleep, mood, puberty, and ovarian cycles. 486

menarche (mə-nahr′ke) the beginning of the menstrual function. 287

Meniere′s disease (men″e-ārz′dĭ-zēz′) hearing loss, tinnitus, and vertigo resulting from noninfectious disease of the ear. 418

meningeal (mə-nin′je-əl) of or pertaining to the meninges. 396

meninges (mə-nin′jēz) the three membranes covering the brain and the spinal cord: dura mater, arachnoid, and pia mater. 395f, 396

meningitis (men″in-ji′tis) inflammation of the meninges, the membranes that cover the brain and the spinal cord. Meningitis is caused by a variety of infectious microorganisms. 403

cerebral m. (sə-re′brəl), inflammation of the membranes of the brain. 403

meningococcal m. (mə-ning″go-kok′əl), meningitis caused by *Neisseria meningitidis.* 451t

spinal m. (spi′nəl), inflammation of the membranes of the spinal cord. 403

meningocele (mə-ning′go-sēl″) a hernial protrusion of meninges through a defect in the skull or vertebral column. 408

meningomyelocele (mə-ning″go-mi′ə-lo-sēl″) hernial protrusion of the spinal cord and the meninges, through a defect in the spine. 408

menopause (men′o-pawz) that period in a female′s life when menstruation ceases. 287

menorrhagia (men″o-ra′jə) abnormally profuse menstruation. 307

menorrhea (men″o-re′ə) menstruation; too profuse menstruation. 307

menses (men′sēz) menstruation, the monthly flow of blood from the female genital tract. 289

menstrual (men′stroo-əl) pertaining to the menses. 289

menstruation (men″stroo-a′shən) the cyclic, physiologic discharge through the vagina of blood and mucosal tissues from the nonpregnant uterus. 287

mental (men′təl) pertaining to the mind. 420

m. retardation (re″tahr-da′shən), abnormally low intellectual functioning. 420

mesenteric (mez″ən-ter′ik) pertaining to the mesentery, a fold of the peritoneum. 109f, 120f

mesoderm (mez′o-dərm) in embryology the middle layer of cells in the blastoderm. 438

mesonasal (mez″o-na′zəl) situated in the middle of the nose.

metabolism (mə-tab′ə-liz″əm) the sum of all the physical and chemical processes by which living organized substance is produced and maintained (anabolism), and also the transformation by which energy is made available for the uses of the organism (catabolism). 198

metacarpal (met″ə-kahr′pəl) pertaining to the metacarpus, the part of the hand between the wrist and fingers; one of the bones of the metacarpus. 352

metastasis (mə-tas′tə-sis) a growth of pathogenic microorganisms or of abnormal cells distant from the site primarily involved by the morbid process.180

metastatic (met″ə-stat′ik) pertaining to or of the nature of metastasis. 180

metatarsal (met″ə-tahr′səl) pertaining to the metatarsus; a bone of the metatarsus. 354

metatarsophalangeal (met″ə-tahr″so-fə-lan′je-əl) pertaining to the metatarsus and the phalanges of the toes. 375

metritis (mə-tri′tis) inflammation of uterine tissue. 286

metrorrhagia (me″tro-ra′je-ə) uterine bleeding, usually of normal amount, occurring at completely irregular intervals, the period of flow sometimes being prolonged. 307

microbiology (mi″kro-bi-ol′ə-je) the science that deals with the study of microorganisms. 268

microcardia (mi″kro-kahr′de-ə) smallness of the heart. 131

microcephaly (mi″kro-sef′ə-le) abnormal smallness of the head. 62

microcyte (mi′kro-sīt) an abnormally small erythrocyte, 5 microns or less in diameter. 83, 85f

microcytosis (mi″kro-si-to′sis) an increase in the number of undersized red blood cells. 83

microorganism (mi″kro-or′gən-iz-əm) a minute living organism, usually microscopic, including bacteria, rickettsiae, viruses, molds, yeasts, and protozoa. 268

microscope (mi′kro-skōp) an instrument for viewing small objects that must be magnified in order to be seen. 17, 33, 83

microscopy (mi-kros′kə-pe) viewing things with a microscope. 83

microsurgery (mi″kro-sər″jər-e) dissection of minute structures of the body using a microscope. 33

microtia (mi-kro′shə) severe hypoplasia or aplasia of the pinna of the ear, with a blind or absent external auditory meatus. 62

microtome (mi′kro-tōm) an instrument used to cut thin sections for microscopic study.

midbrain (mid′brān″) the part of the brain that connects the pons and the cerebellum with the hemispheres of the cerebrum; mesencephalon. 397, 398f

midsagittal (mid-saj′ĭ-təl) the plane vertically dividing the body through the midline into right and left halves. 44, 48

migraine (mi′grān) an often familial symptom complex of periodic attacks of vascular headache, usually temporal and unilateral in onset, commonly associated with irritability, nausea, vomiting, constipation or diarrhea, and often photophobia. 400f, 402

mineral (min′ər-əl) a nonorganic homogenous solid substance, usually a constituent of the earth′s crust. 64, 338

mineralocorticoid (min″ər-əl-o-kor′tĭ-koid) any of the group of corticosteroids, principally aldosterone, predominantly involved in the regulation of electrolyte and water balance in the body. 481, 482t

mitral (mi′trəl) pertaining to the mitral or bicuspid valve; shaped like a miter. 115

mittelschmerz (mit′əl-shmertz) pain associated with ovulation, usually occurring in the middle of the menstrual cycle. 324

molar (mo′lər) a posterior tooth that is used for grinding food and acts as a major jaw support in the dental arch. 207, 208f

monocyte (mon′o-sīt) a mononuclear phagocytic leukocyte that is 13 to 25 microns in diameter and has an ovoid or kidney-shaped nucleus and abundant gray-blue cytoplasm. 77f

mononucleosis (mon″o-noo″kle-o′sis) an excessive number of monocytes in the blood; the term also refers to infectious mononucleosis. 97

monoplegia (mon″o-ple′jə) paralysis of a limb. 407

mons (monz) a general term for an elevation, or eminence. 284

m. pubis (pu′bis), the rounded fleshy prominence over the symphysis pubis. 284

mucoid (mu′koid) resembling mucus. 93, 204

mucolytic (mu″ko-lit′ik) dissolving mucus; an agent that dissolves or destroys mucus. 178

mucosa (mu-ko′sə) mucous membrane. 204

mucous (mu′kəs) pertaining or relating to, or resembling mucus; mucoid; covered with mucus; secreting, producing, or containing mucus. 204

mucus (mu′kəs) the free slime of the mucous membranes, composed of secretion of the glands, various salts, desquamated cells, and leukocytes. 204

multigravida (mul″tĭ-grav′ĭ-də) a woman who has been pregnant several times, or at least twice, before. 298

multinuclear, multinucleate (mul″tĭ-noo′kle-ər, mul″tĭ-noo′kle-āt) having several nuclei.

multipara (məl-tip′ə-rə) a female who has borne more than one viable child. 299

multiple sclerosis (mul′tĭ-pəl sklə-ro′sis) a chronic disease of the central nervous system in which there is development of disseminated demyelinated glial patches called plaques. 408

murmur (mur′mər) an auscultatory sound, particularly a periodic sound of short duration of cardiac or vascular origin. 127

muscle (mus′əl) an organ that produces movement of an animal by contraction. 362

m. relaxant (re-lak′sənt), an agent that causes the muscles to relax. 367

muscular (mus′ku-lər) pertaining to or composing muscle; having a well-developed musculature. 367

   m. dystrophy (dis′trə-fe), a genetically determined myopathy characterized by atrophy and wasting away of muscles. 378

musculoskeletal (mus″ku-lo-skel′ə-təl) pertaining to or comprising the skeleton and the muscles, as musculoskeletal system. 368

myalgia (mi-al′jə) pain in a muscle or muscles. 368

myasthenia (mi″əs-the′ne-ə) muscle weakness. 367

   m. gravis (grav′is), a disease characterized by muscle weakness, owing to a functional abnormality. 367, 418

mycodermatitis (mi″ko-der″mə-ti′tis) inflammation of the skin owing to a fungus. 458

mycologist (mi-kol′ə-jist) a specialist in the study of fungi; one who studies fungi.

mycosis (mi-ko′sis) any condition caused by fungi. 204

myelencephalitis (mi″əl-en-sef″ə-li′tis) inflammation of the brain and the spinal cord; myeloencephalitis. 341

myelin sheath (mi′ə-lin shēth) the sheath surrounding the axon of some (the myelinated) nerve cells. 392

myelitis (mi″ə-li′tis) inflammation of the bone marrow; inflammation of the spinal cord. 341

myeloblast (mi′ə-lo-blast) embryonic form of blood cell found in the bone marrow. 341

myelocyte (mi′ə-lo-sīt) a cell found in the bone marrow. 341

myeloencephalitis (mi″ə-lo-en-sef″ə-li′tis) inflammation of the brain and the spinal cord. 341

myelogram (mi′ə-lo-gram) X-ray film of the spinal cord. 407

myelography (mi″ə-log′rə-fe) roentgenography of the spinal cord after injection of a contrast medium into the subarachnoid space. 407

myelomalacia (mi″ə-lo-mə-la′shə) morbid softening of the spinal cord. 407

myelosuppression (mi″ə-lo-sə-presh′ən) inhibition of bone marrow activity. 341

myelosuppressive (mi″ə-lo-sə-pres′iv) inhibiting bone marrow activity; an agent that inhibits bone marrow activity. 341

myoblast (mi′o-blast) embryonic cell that becomes a cell of the muscle fiber. 368

myocardial (mi″o-kahr′de-əl) pertaining to the muscular tissue of the heart. 113

   m. infarction (in-fahrk′shən), development of an infarct in the myocardium, usually the result of ischemia after occlusion of a coronary artery. 130

myocarditis (mi″o-kahr-di′tis) inflammation of the heart muscle. 113

myocardium (mi″o-kahr′de-əm) the middle and thickest layer of the heart wall, made up of cardiac muscle. 111, 112f, 113

myocele (mi′o-sēl) hernia of the muscle. 368

myocellulitis (mi″o-sel″u-li′tis) inflammation of cellular tissue and muscle. 368

myodynia (mi″o-din′e-ə) pain in a muscle. 368

myofascial (mi″o-fash′e-əl) pertaining to or involving the fascia surrounding and associated with muscle tissue. 378

myofibril (mi″o-fi′bril) one of the slender threads of a muscle fiber, composed of numerous myofilaments. 387

myofibroma (mi″o-fi-bro′mə) a tumor composed of muscular and fibrous elements. 368

myofibrosis (mi″o-fi-bro′sis) replacement of muscle tissue by fibrous tissue. 368

myogram (mi′o-gram) the record or tracing produced by muscle contraction. 55

myograph (mi′o-graf) the instrument used to record muscle contraction. 55

myography (mi-og′rə-fe) the use of a myograph to record muscle contractions. 55

myolysis (mi-ol′ĭ-sis) destruction of muscle tissue. 368

myomalacia (mi″o-mə-la′shə) morbid softening of muscle. 368

myometritis (mi″o-mə-tri′tis) inflammation of the myometrium, the muscular substance of the uterus. 286

myometrium (mi-o-me′tre-əm) the smooth muscle of the uterus. 286

myopathy (mi op′ə the) any disease of muscle. 368

myopia (mi-o′pe-ə) the error of refraction in which rays of light entering the eye are brought to a focus in front of the retina; also called nearsightedness. 415, 416f

myoplasty (mi′o-plas″te) surgical repair of a muscle. 368

myorrhaphy (mi-or′ə-fe) suture of divided muscle. 368

myospasm (mi′o-spaz-əm) cramping of a muscle. 55, 393

myxedema (mik″sə-de′mə) a condition resulting from hypothyroidism characterized by dry, waxy swelling of the skin. 479

narcolepsy (nahr′ko-lep″se) recurrent, uncontrollable brief episodes of sleep. 402

narcotic (nahr-kot′ik) pertaining to or producing narcosis, nonspecific and reversible depression of function of the central nervous system marked by stupor or insensibility produced by drugs; an agent that produces insensibility or stupor, applied especially to the opioids. 36, 420

nares (na′rēz) the nostrils, the external opening of the nose. 164

nasal (na′zəl) pertaining to the nose. 164

nasogastric (na″zo-gas′trik) pertaining to the nose and stomach. 236

nasolacrimal (na″zo-lak′rĭ-məl) pertaining to the nose and lacrimal apparatus. 165

   n. duct (dukt), a tubular passage that carries tears from the eye to the nose. 165

nasopharyngeal (na″zo-fə-rin′je-əl) pertaining to the nasopharynx. 167

nasopharyngitis (na″zo-far″in-ji′tis) inflammation of the nasopharynx. 167

nasopharynx (na″zo-far′inks) the upper part of the pharynx, continuous with the nasal passages. 167

nasoscope (na′zo-skōp) instrument for examining inside the nose. 165

nasoseptoplasty (na″zo-sep′to-plas″te) surgical repair of the nasal septum. 164

nasotracheal (na″zo-tra′ke-əl) pertaining to the nose and trachea. 170

natal (na′təl) pertaining to birth. 6

necrophobia (nek″ro-fo′be-ə) fear of death or dead bodies.

necropsy (nek′rop-se) examination of a dead body; autopsy. 454

necrosis (nə-kro′sis) death of tissue. 454

necrotic (nə-krot′ik) pertaining to or characterized by necrosis. 454

neonatal (ne″o-na′təl) pertaining to a newborn child, usually designating the first 4 weeks after birth. 301

neonate (ne′o-nāt) a newborn child. 301

neonatologist (ne″o-na-tol′ə-jist) a physician who specializes in care of the newborn. 33, 301

neonatology (ne″o-na-tol′ə-je) the branch of medicine dealing with treatment of the newborn infant. 33, 301

neoplasia (ne″o-pla′zhə) the formation of a neoplasm or the progressive multiplication of cells for no known cause. 235

neoplasm (ne′o-plaz-əm) tumor; any new and abnormal growth. Neoplasms may be benign or malignant. 181, 235

neoplastic (ne″o-plas′tik) tending to produce neoplasms. 235

nephrectomy (nə-frek′tə-me) surgical excision of a kidney. 249

nephritis (nə-fri′tis) inflammation of the kidney. 251

nephrocele (nef′ro-sēl) hernia of the kidney. 259

nephrolith (nef′ro-lith) a kidney stone. 252

nephrolithiasis (nef″ro-lĭ-thi′ə-sis) a condition marked by the presence of kidney stones. 252

nephrolithotomy (nef″ro-lĭ-thot′ə-me) removal of renal calculi by cutting into the kidney. 253

nephrolysis (nə-frol′ə-sis) destruction of kidney tissue; freeing of a kidney from adhesions. 251

nephromalacia (nef″ro-mə-la′shə) softening of the kidney. 251

nephromegaly (nef″ro-meg′ə-le) enlargement of the kidney. 249

nephron (nef′ron) the structural and functional unit of the kidney. 254, 256f

nephropexy (nef′ro-pek″se) surgical fixation of a floating kidney. 251

nephroptosis (nef″rop-to′sis) downward displacement of the kidney; floating kidney. 251, 252t

nephropyosis (nef″ro-pi-o′sis) suppuration of the kidney. 271

nephrorrhaphy (nef-ror′ə-fe) suture of the kidney. 263

nephrosclerosis (nef″ro-sklə-ro′sis) hardening of the kidney due to renovascular disease. 252

nephroscope (nef′ro-skōp) an instrument inserted into an incision in the renal pelvis for viewing the interior of the kidney. 253

nephroscopy (nə-fros′kə-pe) visualization of the kidney using a nephroscope. 253

nephrosis (nĕ-fro′sis) any disease of the kidney, especially a noninflammatory one characterized by purely degenerative lesions of the renal tubules. 252

nephrosonography (nef″ro-so-nog′rə-fe) ultrasonic scanning of the kidney. 251

nephrostomy (nə-fros′tə-me) the creation of a fistula leading directly into the renal pelvis. 254, 258f

   percutaneous catheter n. (per″ku-ta′ne-əs kath′ə-tər), placement of a catheter into the kidney through the skin, providing for diversion of the renal output, certain surgical procedures, including biopsies, and infusion of substances to dissolve calculi. 254

nephrotic syndrome (nə-frot′ik sin′drōm) a clinical classification that includes all diseases of the kidney characterized by chronic loss of protein in the urine and subsequent depletion of body protein. 252t

nephrotomogram (nef″ro-to′mo-gram) a sectional radiograph of the kidney obtained by nephrotomography. 251

nephrotomography (nef″ro-to-mog′rə-fe) radiologic visualization of the kidney by tomography after intravenous introduction of contrast medium. 251

nephrotoxic (nef″ro-tok′sik) destructive to kidney cells. 251

nephroureterectomy (nef″ro-u″rə-tər-ek′tə-me) excision of a kidney and a whole or part of the ureter. 259

neural (noor′əl) pertaining to a nerve or connected with the nervous system. 393

neuralgia (nōō-ral′jə) pain of a nerve. 407

neurasthenia (noor″əs-the′ne-ə) a nervous condition characterized by chronic weakness, easy fatigability, and sometimes exhaustion. 421

neurectomy (nōō-rek′to-me) excision of a part of a nerve. 419

neuritis (nōō-ri′tis) inflammation of a nerve. 58

neuroarthropathy (noor″o-ahr-throp′ə-the) any disease of joint structures associated with diseases of the central or peripheral nervous system. 407

neurogenic (nōōr″o-jen′ik) originating in the nervous system. 419

neuroglia (nōō-rog′le-ə) the supporting structure of nervous tissue. 391, 392

orally (o′rəl-le) by mouth.

orchialgia (or″ke-al′jə) pain in a testis. 319

orchidalgia (or″kĭ-dal′jə) pain in a testis. 319

orchidectomy (or″kĭ-dek′tə-me) excision of a testicle.

orchiditis (or″kĭ-di′tis) inflammation of a testicle. 320

orchidopexy (or′kĭ-do-pek″se) orchiopexy. 316

orchidorrhaphy (or″kĭ-dor′ə-fe) orchiopexy or suturing a testicle for fixation purposes. 320

orchiectomy (or″ke-ek′tə-me) excision of one or both testes.

orchiepididymitis (or″ke-ep″ĭ-did″ĭ-mi′tis) inflammation of a testicle and an epididymis. 320

orchiopathy (or″ke-op′ə-the) any disease of the testes. 320

orchiopexy (or″ke-o-pek′se) surgical fixation of an undescended testis in the scrotum. 316

orchioplasty (or′ke-o-plas″te) plastic surgery of a testis.

orchiotomy (or″ke-ot′ə-me) incision and drainage of a testis. 320

orchitis (or-ki′tis) inflammation of a testis. This is not a common disorder, but it can occur in a variety of infectious diseases. 320

orifice (or′ĭ fis) the entrance or outlet of any cavity in the body; any foramen, meatus, or opening. 131

oropharyngeal (or″o-fə-rin′je-əl) pertaining to the mouth and pharynx. 166, 203

    o. mucosa (mu-ko′sə) the lining of the mouth and pharynx. 204

oropharynx (or″o-far′inks) that part of the pharynx between the soft palate and the upper edge of the epiglottis. 166, 167

orotracheal (or″o-tra′ke-əl) pertaining to the mouth and trachea. 170

orthodontics (or″tho-don′tiks) the branch of dentistry concerned with irregularities of teeth and malocclusions and associated facial problems. 22

orthodontist (or″tho-don′tist) a dentist who specializes in orthodontics. 22

orthopedic (or″tho-pe′dik) pertaining to the correction of deformities of the musculoskeletal system. 22

    o. surgeon (sur′jen), a surgeon specialized in orthopedics.

orthopedics (or″tho-pe′diks) that branch of surgery that is specially concerned with the preservation and restoration of the function of the skeletal system, its articulations, and associated structures. 22

orthopedist (or″tho-pe′dist) an orthopedic surgeon. 22

orthopnea (or″thop-ne′ə, or″thop′ne-ə) a condition in which breathing is possible only when the person is in an upright position. 158

ossicle (os′ĭ-kəl) a small bone. 344

    auditory o. (aw′dĭ-tor″e), the malleus, incus, and stapes of the middle ear. 344

ossification (os″ĭ-fĭ-ka′shən) the formation of bone or a bony substance. 341

ostealgia (os″te-al′jə) pain in a bone. 340

ostectomy, osteectomy (os-tek′tə-me, os″te-ek′tə-me) excision of a bone or a portion of a bone. 339

osteitis (os″te-i′tis) inflammation of a bone. 338

    o. deformans (de-for′manz), a disease of bone marked by repeated episodes of increased bone resorption followed by excessive attempts at repair, resulting in weakened deformed bones of increased mass; called also Paget's disease. 374

osteoarthritis (os″te-o-ahr-thri′tis) degenerative joint disease characterized by degeneration of the articular cartilage, hypertrophy of bone at the margins, and changes in the synovial membrane. 356

osteoarthropathy (os″te-o-ahr-throp′ə-the) any disease of the bones and joints. 359

osteoblast (os′te-o-blast″) embryonic form of a bone cell. 339, 368

osteochondritis (os″te-o-kon-dri′tis) inflammation of the bone and cartilage. 361

osteocyte (os′te-o-sīt″) a cell that makes up the bone matrix. 339

osteodynia (os″te-o-din′e-ə) pain in the bone. 340

osteogenesis (os″te-o-jen′ə-sis) the formation of bone. 341

osteoid (os′te-oid) resembling bone. 338

osteolysis (os″te-ol′ĭ-sis) destruction of the bone. 340

osteomalacia (os″te-o-mə-la′shə) a skeletal disorder characterized by a disturbance in bone metabolism. 373

osteometry (os″te-om′ə-tre) measurement of bones. 338

osteomyelitis (os″te-o-mi″ə-li′tis) inflammation of the bone and bone marrow caused by a pyogenic organism. 374

osteopenia (os″te-o-pe′ne-ə) reduced bone mass owing to insufficient bone synthesis to keep pace with normal bone destruction. 371

osteoplasty (os′te-o-plas″te) plastic surgery of the bones. 338

osteoporosis (os″te-o-pə-ro′sis) reduction in the amount of bone mass, leading to fractures after minimal trauma. 373, 374f

osteosarcoma (os″te-o-sahr-ko′mə) a malignant primary neoplasm of bone composed of a malignant connective tissue stroma with evidence of malignant, osteoid, bone, or cartilage formation. 374

osteosclerosis (os″te-o-sklə-ro′sis) the hardening or abnormal density of bone. 340

osteotome (os′te-o-tōm″) an instrument used to cut bone. 338

osteotomy (os″te-ot′ə-me) the surgical cutting of a bone. 375

osteotrophy (os″te-ot′rə-fe) nutrition of bone. 341

ostomy (os′tə-me) a general term for surgery in which an artificial opening is formed. 184

otalgia (o-tal′je-ə) pain in the ear; earache. 415

otic (o′tik) pertaining to the ear. 33

otitis (o-ti′tis) inflammation of the ear. 58

    o. media (me′de-ə), inflammation of the middle ear. 58, 415

otodynia (o″to-din′e-ə) pain in the ear; earache. 59

otolaryngologist (o″to-lar″ing-gol′ə-jist) a physician who specializes in otolaryngology. 24

otolaryngology (o″to-lar″ing-gol′ə-je) that branch of medicine concerned with medical and surgical treatment of the head and neck, including the ears, nose, and throat. 24

otologist (o-tol′ə-jist) a specialist in otology. 24

otology (o-tol′ə-je) the study of the ear. 24

otopathy (o-top′ə-the) any disease of the ear. 59

otorhinolaryngology (o″to-ri″no-lar″in-gol′ə-je) the branch of medicine that deals with diseases of the ear, nose, and throat. It is also called otolaryngology. 24

otorrhea (o″to-re′ə) discharge from the ear. 415

otosclerosis (o″to-sklə-ro′sis) a pathological condition of the ear in which there is formation of spongy bone and that usually results in hearing loss. 418

otoscope (o′to-skōp) an instrument for viewing inside the ear. 415, 417f

otoscopy (o-tos′kə-pe) viewing the inside of the ear using an otoscope. 415, 417f

ovarian (o-var′e-ən) pertaining to an ovary or ovaries. 282

ovary (o′və-re) the female gonad; either of the paired female organs in which eggs are formed. 282, 468f

ovulation (ov″u-la′shən) the discharge of an egg from a vesicular follicle of the ovary. 287

ovum (o′vəm) an egg; the female reproductive germ cell. 287

oximeter (ok-sim′ə-tər) a photoelectric device for determining the oxygen saturation of the blood. 182

oximetry (ok-sim′ə-tre) determination of the oxygen saturation of arterial blood using an oximeter. 182, 183f

oxytocin (ok″sĭ-to′sin) a pituitary hormone that stimulates uterine contractions and milk ejection. 471, 472

pacemaker (pās′ma-kər) the natural cardiac pacemaker or an artificial cardiac pacemaker. 128

Paget's disease (pă-jəts dĭ-zēz) a skeletal disease of the elderly with chronic inflammation of bones, resulting in thickening and softening of bones. 374

palate (pal′ət) the roof of the mouth, which separates the nasal and oral cavities. 164

    hard p., the anterior portion of the palate. 164

    soft p., the posterior portion of the palate. 164

palatine (pal′ə-tīn) pertaining to the palate. 141, 164

palatitis (pal″ə-ti′tis) inflammation of the palate. 164

palatoplasty (pal′ə-to-plas″te) plastic reconstruction of the palate. 164

pallor (pal′or) paleness or absence of skin coloration. 79

palmar (pahl′mər) pertaining to the palm. 48

palpation (pal-pa′shən) the act of feeling with the hand; the application of the fingers with light pressure to the surface of the body for the purpose of determining the consistency of the parts beneath in physical diagnosis. 444

palsy (pawl′ze) paralysis. 407

    Bell's p. (belz), unilateral facial paralysis of sudden onset, due to lesion of the facial nerve and resulting in characteristic distortion of the face. 418

pancreas (pan′kre-əs) a large, elongated gland situated transversely behind the stomach, between the spleen and the duodenum. The external secretion of the pancreas contains a variety of digestive enzymes. An internal secretion, insulin, is concerned with the regulation of carbohydrate metabolism. Glucagon is also produced by the pancreas. 232, 468f, 484

pancreatectomy (pan″kre-ə-tek′tə-me) excision of the pancreas. 233

pancreatic (pan″kre-at′ik) pertaining to the pancreas. 232

pancreatitis (pan″kre-ə-ti′tis) inflammation of the pancreas. 232

pancreatography (pan″kre-ə-tog′rə-fe) X-ray examination of the pancreas, performed during surgery by injecting contrast medium into the pancreatic duct. 233

pancreatolith (pan″kre-at′o-lith) a pancreatic stone. 232

pancreatolithectomy (pan″kre-ə-to-lĭ-thek′tə-me) the removal of a stone from the pancreas. 232

pancreatolysis (pan″kre-ə-tol′ĭ-sis) destruction of pancreatic tissue. 233

pancreatopathy (pan″kre-ə-top′ə-the) any disease of the pancreas. 233

pancreatotomy (pan″kre-ə-tot′ə-me) incision of the pancreas. 233

Papanicolaou's smear (pă″pə-nĭ″ko-la′ōoz smēr) collection of material from areas of the body that shed cells, especially the cervix and the vagina, followed by microscopic study of the cells for diagnosing cancer. This is also called the Pap test or smear. 302

papule (pap′ūl) a red elevated, solid, and circumscribed area of the skin. 444

paraappendicitis (par″ə-ə-pen″dĭ-si′tis) inflammation of the tissues adjacent to the appendix. 235

paracentesis (par″ə-sən-te′sis) surgical puncture of a cavity for aspiration of fluid. 52

    thoracic p. (thə-ras′ik), thoracentesis. 174

paracolitis (par″ə-ko″li′tis) inflammation of the outer coat of the colon. 235

paralysis (pə-ral′ĭ-sis) loss or impairment of motor function owing to neural or muscular lesions. 407

paranasal (par″ə-na′zəl) situated near or alongside the nasal cavities. 165

paranoia (par″ə-noi′ah) a term used to describe behavior characterized by well-systematized delusions of persecution, delusions of grandeur, or a combination of the two. 422

paraplegia (par″ə-ple′jə) paralysis of the legs and lower part of the body, often caused by disease or injury to the spine. 407

parasite (par′ə-sīt) a plant or animal that lives upon or within another living organism at whose expense it obtains some advantage. 176t

parasplenic (par″ə-sple′nik) beside the spleen. 235

parasympathetic (par″ə-sim″pə-thet′ik) referring to the nerves that are part of the autonomic system and work against the sympathetic nerves. 410

parathyroid (par″ə-thi′roid) situated beside the thyroid gland; any one of the four glands that lie beside the thyroid gland and are responsible for secreting a hormone that regulates calcium and phosphorus in the body. 475, 485

paraurethral (par″ə-u-re′thrəl) near the urethra. 284

parenteral (pə-ren′tər-əl) injection into the body, not through the alimentary canal. 200, 456

parietal (pə-ri′ə-təl) pertaining to the walls of a cavity; pertaining to or located near the parietal bone. 52, 172, 397

Parkinson's disease (pahr′kin-sənz dĭ-zēz′) a chronic nervous disease characterized by a fine, slowly spreading tremor; muscular weakness and rigidity; and a peculiar gait. 403

paronychia (par″o-nik′e-ə) inflammation involving the folds of tissue surrounding the fingernail. 451t

parotid (pə-rot′id) situated or occurring near the ear. 226

parotitis (par″o-ti′tis) inflammation of the parotid gland. 226
    epidemic p. (ep″ĭ-dem′ik), mumps. 226

parous (par′əs) having borne one or more offspring. 298

paroxysmal (par″ok-siz′məl) occurring in sudden, periodic attacks or recurrence of symptoms of a disease. 178t

parturition (pahr″tu-ri′shən) childbirth. 299

patella (pə-tel′ə) the kneecap, a lens-shaped bone situated in front of the knee. 343, 352

patellectomy (pat″ə-lek′tə-me) excision of the kneecap. 352

patellofemoral (pə-tel″o-fem′ə-rəl) pertaining to the kneecap and the femur. 352

patent (pa′tənt) open, unobstructed, or not closed. 170

pathogen (path′o-jən) any disease-producing agent or microorganism. 34

pathogenic (path-o-jen′ik) disease-causing. 34

pathologic, pathological (path-o-loj′ik, path″o-loj′ĭ-kəl) indicating or caused by some morbid process. 34

pathologist (pə-thol′ə-jist) a physician who is specialized in the study of the essential nature of disease. 18
    clinical p. (klin′ĭ-kəl) a physician specialized in the branch of pathology that is applied to the solution of clinical problems, especially the use of laboratory methods in clinical diagnosis. 18
    surgical p. (sur′jĭ-kəl) a physician specialized in the study of disease processes that are surgically accessible for diagnosis or treatment. 18

pathology (pə-thol′ə-je) the study of the changes caused by disease in the structure or functions of the body. 17-18

pathophysiology (path″o-fiz″e-ol′ə-je) the study of causes of disordered function. 17

pediatrician (pe″de-ə-trĭ′shən) physician who specializes in the treatment of children's diseases. 27

pediatrics (pe″de-at′riks) the branch of medicine that is devoted to the study of children's diseases. 27

pediculicide (pə-dik′u-lĭ-sīd) destroying lice; an agent that destroys lice. 461

pediculosis (pə-dik″u-lo′sis) infestation with lice of the family *Pediculidae*. 455

pedodontics (pe-do-don′tiks) the branch of dentistry that deals with the teeth and mouth conditions of children. 22, 27

pedodontist (pe-do-don′tist) a dentist who specializes in the teeth and mouth conditions of children. 22, 27

pelvic (pel′vik) pertaining to the pelvis. 51
    p. inflammatory disease (in-flam′ə-tor″e dĭ-zēz′), an ascending pelvic infection involving the genital tract beyond the cervix uteri. 308

pelvis (pel′vis) the lower portion of the trunk. The word also means any basinlike structure. 52
    renal p. (re′nəl), in the kidney, the funnel-shaped structure at the upper end of the ureter. 252

penile (pe′nīl) pertaining to or affecting the penis. 312

penis (pe′nis) the male organ of urination and copulation. 312

peptic (pep′tik) pertaining to pepsin or digestion; related to action of gastric juices. 215

percussion (pər-kŭ′shən) the act of striking a part with short, sharp blows as an aid in diagnosing the condition of the underlying parts by the sound obtained. 182

percutaneous (per″ku-ta′ne-əs) performed through the skin. 132

periappendicitis (per″e-ə-pen″dĭ-si′tis) inflammation of the tissues around the vermiform appendix. 236

pericardial (per″ĭ-kahr′de-əl) around the heart. 113

pericarditis (per″ĭ-kahr-di′tis) inflammation of the pericardium. 113

pericardium (per″ĭ-kahr′de-əm) the sac enclosing the heart and the roots of the great vessels. 112f, 113
    parietal p. (pə-ri′ə-təl), the outer layer of the double membrane that surrounds the heart. 112f, 113
    visceral p. (vis′ər-əl), the innermost of the double membrane that surrounds the heart. 112f, 113

perichondrial (per″ĭ-kon′dre-əl) pertaining to or composed of perichondrium. 361

perichondrium (per″ĭ-kon′dre-əm) the layer of fibrous connective tissue that invests all cartilage except the articular cartilage of synovial joints. 361

pericolic (per′ĭ-ko′lik) around the colon. 236

pericolitis (per″ĭ-ko-li′tis) inflammation of the tissue surrounding the colon. 236

peridental (per″ĭ-den′təl) surrounding a tooth.

perihepatitis (per″e-hep′ə-ti′tis) inflammation surrounding the liver. 236

perimetrium (per″ĭ-me′tre-əm) the serous coat of the uterus. 286

perinatologist (per″ĭ-na-tol′ə-jist) a specialist in perinatology. 33

perinatology (per″ĭ-na′tol′ə-je) the branch of medicine (obstetrics and pediatrics) dealing with the fetus and infant during the perinatal period. 33

perineal (per″ĭ-ne′əl) pertaining to the perineum. 284

perineum (per″ĭ-ne′əm) the pelvic floor and the associated structures occupying the pelvic outlet; it is bounded anteriorly by the pubic symphysis, laterally by the ischial tuberosities, and posteriorly by the coccyx; the region between the thighs, bounded in the male by the scrotum and anus and in the female by the vulva and anus. 284

periodontal (per″e-o-don′təl) around a tooth; pertaining to the periodontium. 206

periodontics (per″e-o-don′tiks) the branch of dentistry that deals with the study and treatment of the periodontium. 207

periodontist (per″e-o-don′tist) a dentist who specializes in periodontics. 207

periodontitis (per″e-o-don′ti′tis) inflammation of the periodontium, caused by residual food, bacteria, and tartar that collect in the spaces between the gum and the lower part of the tooth crown. 206

periodontium (per″e-o-don′she-əm) the tissues investing and supporting the teeth. 206

periosteum (per″e-os′te-əm) a tough fibrous membrane that surrounds a bone. 338

peripancreatitis (per″ĭ-pan″kre-ə-ti′tis) inflammation around the pancreas. 236

peripheral nervous system (pə-rif′ər-əl ner′vəs sis′təm) the various nerve processes that connect the brain and the spinal cord with receptors, muscles, and glands. 391, 409

peristalsis (per″ĭ-stal′sis) movement by which the alimentary canal propels its contents. It consists of a wave of contraction passing along the tube for variable distances. 201

peritoneal (per″ĭ-to-ne′əl) pertaining to the peritoneum. 52
    p. cavity (kav′ĭ-te), the potential space between the parietal and visceral layers of the peritoneum. 52

peritoneum (per″ĭ-to-ne′əm) the serous membrane that lines the walls of the abdominal and pelvic cavities and invests the internal organs in those cavities. 52, 213
    parietal p. (pə-ri′ə-təl), the peritoneum that lines the abdominal and pelvic walls and the undersurface of the diaphragm. 52, 213
    visceral p. (vis′ər-əl), a continuation of the parietal peritoneum reflected at various places over the viscera. 52, 213

peritonitis (per″ĭ-to-ni′tis) inflammation of the peritoneum. 213

peritonsillar (per″ĭ-ton′sĭ-lər) around a tonsil. 236

perspiration (per″spĭ-ra′shən) sweating; sweat. 442

pertussis (pər-tus′is) an acute, highly contagious infection of the respiratory tract, most frequently affecting young children, usually caused by *Bordetella pertussis*. 178t

petechia (pə-te′ke-ə) a pinpoint, nonraised, perfectly round, purplish red spot caused by intradermal or submucous hemorrhage. 445, 446f, 448f

phagocyte (fag′o-sīt) any cell that ingests something else. The term usually refers to polymorphonuclear leukocytes, macrophages, and monocytes. 89, 138, 197

phagocytic (fag″o-sit′ik) exhibiting phagocytosis; pertaining to phagocytosis or phagocytes. 89, 197

phagocytize (fag′o-sīt″īz) to eat or ingest by phagocytosis.

phagocytosis (fag″o-si-to′sis) the engulfing of microorganisms, other cells, and foreign particles by phagocytes. 89

phagomania (fag″o-ma′ne-ə) an abnormal craving for food; obsessive preoccupation with eating. 421

phagomaniac (fag″o-ma′ne-ak) one who suffers obsessive preoccupation with eating. 421

phalangectomy (fal″ən-jek′tə-me) excision of a finger or toe. 352

phalanges (fə-lan′jēz) bones of the fingers or toes. 343, 351f, 352

phalangitis (fal″ən-ji′tis) inflammation of one or more bones of the fingers or toes. 352

pharmaceutics (fahr″mə-soo′tiks) pharmacy (the science); pharmaceutical preparations. 30

pharmacist (fahr″mə-sist) one who is licensed to prepare, sell, or dispense drugs and compounds and to make up prescriptions. 30

pharmacologist (fahr″mə-kol′ə-jist) a specialist in pharmacology. 30

pharmacology (fahr″mə-kol′ə-je) the study of drugs and their origin, properties, and effects on living systems. 30

pharmacotherapy (fahr″mə-ko-ther′ə-pe) treatment of disease with medicines. 30

pharmacy (fahr′mə-se) the science of preparing, compounding, and dispensing medicines; a place where drugs and medicinal supplies are prepared, compounded, and dispensed. 30

pharyngalgia (far″in-gal′jə) pain in the pharynx. 166

pharyngeal (fə-rin′je-əl) pertaining to the throat. 166

pharyngitis (far″in-ji′tis) inflammation of the throat. 166

pharyngodynia (fə-ring″go-din′e-ə) pain in the throat; sore throat. 166

pharyngomycosis (fə-ring″go-mi-ko′sis) any fungal infection of the pharynx. 184

pharyngopathy (far″ing-gop′ə-the) any disease of the pharynx. 166

pharyngoplasty (fə-ring′go-plas″te) plastic repair of the pharynx. 166

pharyngoscope (fə-ring′go-skōp) an instrument for examining the throat. 166

pharynx (far′inks) the throat; the cavity behind the nasal cavities, mouth, and larynx, communicating with them and with the esophagus. 24, 161

phimosis (fi-mo′sis) constriction of the preputial orifice so that the prepuce cannot be retracted back over the glans. 325

phlebectomy (flə-bek′to-me) removal of a vein or a segment of a vein. 124

phlebitis (flə-bi′tis) inflammation of a vein. 122

phleboplasty (fleb′o-plas″te) plastic repair of a vein. 122

phlebosclerosis (fleb″o-sklə-ro′sis) fibrous thickening of the walls of veins. 122

phlebostasis (flə-bos′tə-sis) controlling the flow of blood in a vein. 143

phlebotomist (flə-bot′ə-mist) one who practices phlebotomy. 108

phlebotomy (flə-bot′ə-me) incision of a vein, as for the letting of blood; needle puncture of a vein for the drawing of blood; venesection. 108

phobia (fo′be-ə) any persistent abnormal dread or fear. 421

phobophobia (fo″bo-fo′be-ə) irrational fear of one's own fears or of acquiring a phobia. 421

phonic (fon′ik, fo′nik) pertaining to the voice. 182

photodermatitis (fo″to-der″mə-ti′tis) an abnormal skin reaction produced by light. 458

photofluorogram (fo″to-floor′o-gram) the film produced in photofluorography. 210

photophobia (fo″to-fo′be-ə) abnormal intolerance of light. 402

photoreceptor (fo″to-re-sep′tor) a nerve ending that detects light, found in the human eye. 411

phrenic (fren′ik) pertaining to the diaphragm; pertaining to the mind. 162

phrenitis (frə-ni′tis) inflammation of the diaphragm. 162

phrenodynia (fren″o-din′e-ə) pain in the diaphragm. 162

phrenogastric (fren″o-gas′trik) pertaining to the diaphragm and the stomach. 210

phrenoplegia (fren″o-ple′jə) paralysis of the diaphragm. 163

phrenoptosis (fren″op-to-sis) downward displacement of the diaphragm. 163

physician (fĭ-zish′ən) an authorized practitioner of medicine, as one graduated from a college of medicine or osteopathy and licensed by the appropriate board; one who practices medicine as distinct from surgery. 16, 17

    p. assistant (ə-sis′tənt), one who has been trained in an accredited program and certified by an appropriate board to perform certain physician's duties, including history taking, physical examination, diagnostic tests, treatment, certain minor surgical procedures, all under the responsible supervision of a licensed physician. 29

physiologist (fiz″e-ol′ə-jist) a specialist in physiology. 19

physiology (fiz″e-ol′ə-je) the science that deals with the function of living organisms and their parts. 17

pia mater (pi′ə ma′tər, pe′ə mah′tər) the innermost of the three meninges covering the brain and the spinal cord. 395

pituitary (pĭ-too′ĭ-tār″e) the hypophysis, a small oval two-lobed body at the base of the brain. It regulates other glands by secretions of hormones. 469-471

    p. cachexia (kə-kək′se-ə), a profound and marked state of constitutional disorder with general ill health caused by hypopituitarism. 475

placenta (plə-sen′tə) an organ characteristic of true mammals during pregnancy, joining mother and offspring. 291

    p. previa (pre′ve-ə), a placenta that develops in the lower uterine segment, in the zone of dilatation, so that it covers or adjoins the internal os. 297t, 298f

plane (plān) a flat surface determined by the position of three points in space; a specified level; to rub away or abrade; a superficial incision in the wall of a cavity or between layers of tissue. 44, 48

plantar (plan′tər) pertaining to the sole of the foot. 48

plaque (plak) any patch or flat area; a superficial, solid, elevated skin lesion equal to or greater than 1.0 cm (0.5 cm according to some authorities) in diameter. 125

    dental p. (den′təl), a soft, thin film of food debris, mucin, and so forth, deposited on the teeth, providing the medium for the growth of various bacteria.

plastic surgery (plas′tik sur′jər-ə) the branch of surgery that deals with the repair or reconstruction of tissue or organs. 21

pleura (ploor′ə) serous membrane investing the lungs and lining the walls of the thoracic cavity. 172

    parietal p. (pə-ri′ə-təl), pleura that lines the walls of the thoracic cavity. 172

    visceral p. (vis′ər-əl), pleura that surrounds the lungs. 172

pleural (ploor′əl) pertaining to the pleura. 172

    p. cavity (kav′ĭ-te), the space between the parietal and visceral pleurae. 172

    p. effusion (ə-fu′zhən), the presence of liquid in the pleural space. 172

pleurisy (ploor′ĭ-se) inflammation of the pleura. 173

pleuritis (ploo-ri′tis) inflammation of the pleura, or pleurisy. 173

pleurocentesis (ploor″o-sen-te′sis) thoracentesis; puncture of the chest wall for aspiration of fluid. 174

pleurodynia (ploor″o-din′e-ə) pain of the pleura; pleurisy. 176

pleuropneumonia (ploor″o-noo-mo′ne-ə) pain of the pleura complicated by pneumonia. 176

pneumectomy (noo-mek′tə-me) removal of lung tissue. 176

pneumocardial (noo″mo kahr′de-əl) pertaining to the lungs and the heart. 176

pneumocentesis (noo″mo-sən-te′sis) surgical puncture of a lung. 177

pneumoconiosis (noo″mo-ko-ne-o′sis) any lung condition caused by permanent deposition of substantial amounts of dust particles in the lungs. 176, 177

pneumoencephalography (noo″mo-ən-sef′ə-log′rə-fe) radiographic visualization of the fluid-containing structures of the brain using air to more clearly define the structures. 401

pneumohemothorax (noo″mo-he″mo-thor′aks) gas or air and blood in the pleural cavity. 176

pneumomalacia (noo″mo-mə-la′shə) softening of lung tissue. 177

pneumomelanosis (noo″mo-mel″ə-no′sis) black condition of the lung caused by inhaled coal dust, soot, etc. This is generally called pneumoconiosis. 176

pneumomyelography (noo″mo-mi″ə-log′rə-fe) roentgenographic examination of the spinal canal, using air to define the structure. 407

pneumonectomy (noo″mo-nek′tə-me) surgical removal of all or part of a lung. 176

pneumonia (noo-mo′ne-ə) inflammation of the lung with consolidation; pneumonitis. 171

pneumonic (noo-mon′ik) pertaining to the lung or to pneumonia.

pneumonitis (noo″mo-ni′tis) inflammation of the lung; pneumonia. 171

pneumoperitoneum (noo″mo-per″ĭ-to-ne′əm) the presence of air or gas in the peritoneal cavity. 307f

pneumothorax (noo″mo-thor′aks) air or gas in the pleural space, which may occur spontaneously (spontaneous p.) or as a result of trauma or disease process or which may be introduced deliberately (artificial p.) 176, 177f

podiatrist (po-di′ə-trist) one who specializes in the care of the human foot. 54

podiatry (po-di′ə-tre) the specialized field dealing with the study and care of the foot, including its anatomy, pathology, and medical and surgical treatment. 54

podogram (pod′o-gram) a print of the foot. 54

poikilocyte (poi′kĭ-lo-sīt) an abnormally shaped red blood cell. 84, 85f

poikilocytosis (poi′kĭ-lo-si′to′sis) the presence of abnormally shaped red blood cells. 84

poliomyelitis (po″le-o-mi″ə-li′tis) an acute viral disease characterized clinically by fever, sore throat, headache, and vomiting, often with stiffness of the neck and back. In its more severe form, the central nervous system is involved and paralysis can result. 408

polyarthritis (pol″e-ahr-thri′tis) inflammation of several joints. 359

polycystic (pol″e-sis′tik) containing many cysts. 252

    p. kidney (kid′ne), a condition in which multiple cysts occur in both kidneys. 252, 253f

polycythemia (pol″e-si-the′me-ə) an increase in the total red cell mass of the blood. 81

polydactylism, polydactyly (pol″e-dak′təl-iz-əm, pol″e-dak′tə-le) the presence of supernumerary digits on the hands and feet. 354

polydipsia (pol″e-dip′se-ə) excessive thirst. 198, 484

polymorph (pol′e-morf) a term for polymorphonuclear leukocyte. 82

polymorphonuclear (pol″e-mor″fo-noo′kle-ər) having a nucleus that is so divided that it appears to be multiple; a polymorphonuclear leukocyte. 82

polymyalgia (pol″e-mi-al′jə) pain affecting more than one muscle. 358

    polymyalgia rheumatica (pol″e-mi-al′jə roo-mat′ik-ə) a syndrome in the elderly characterized by proximal joint and muscle pain and a self-limiting course. 359t

polymyositis (pol″e-mi″o-si′tis) a chronic, progressive inflammatory disease of skeletal muscle, characterized by symmetrical weakness of the limb girdles, neck, and pharynx, usually associated with pain and tenderness. 358, 359t

polyneuralgia (pol″e-noo-ral′jə) pain of several nerves. 407

polyneuritis (pol″e-noo-ri′tis) inflammation of many nerves simultaneously. 407, 418

polyneuropathy (pol″e-noo-rop′ə-the) a disease involving several nerves. 407, 418

polyp (pol′ip) any growth or mass protruding from a mucous membrane. 165

polyphagia (pol″e-fa′jə) excessive eating; craving for all kinds of food. 197, 484

polyuria (pol″e-u′re-ə) excessive urination. 97, 484

pons (ponz) the part of the central nervous system that lies between the medulla oblongata and the mesencephalon and ventral to the cerebellum; called also pons varolii. 398f

postanesthetic (pōst″an-əs-thet′ik) after anesthesia is administered. 34

posterior (pos-tēr′e-or) situated behind. 44

posteroanterior (pos″tər-o-an-tēr′e-or) from back to front. 44

posteroexternal (pos″tər-o-ek-ster′nəl) situated on the outside of a posterior part. 44

posterointernal (pos″tər-o-in-tər′nəl) situated within and to the rear. 44

posterolateral (pos″tər-o-lat′ər-əl) situated on the side and toward the posterior aspect. 44

posteromedial (pos″tər-o-me′de-əl) situated in the middle of the back side. 46

posterosuperior (pos″tər-o-soo-pēr′e-or) situated behind and above. 46

postesophageal (pōst″ə-sof″ə-je′əl) behind the esophagus. 235

postmortem (pōst-mor′təm) occurring or performed after death. 34

postnatal (pōst-na′təl) occurring after birth. 301

postpartum (pōst-pahr′təm) after childbirth. 299

postuterine (pōst-u′tər-in) behind the uterus. 301

precancerous (pre-kan′sər-əs) used to describe an abnormal growth that is likely to become cancerous. 235

preeclampsia (pre″e-klamp′se-ə) a complication of pregnancy characterized by hypertension, edema, and/or proteinuria; when convulsions and coma are associated, it is called eclampsia. 297t

premenstrual (pre-men′stroo-əl) occurring before menstruation. 307

> *p. syndrome* (sin′drōm), a condition that occurs several days before the onset of menstruation, characterized by one or more of the following: irritability, emotional tension, anxiety, depression, headache, breast tenderness, and water retention. 307

premolar (pre-mo′lər) one of the eight permanent teeth (two on either side of each jaw) anterior to the molars and posterior to the canine teeth. 207

prenatal (pre-na′təl) referring to the time period before birth. 293

prepuce (pre′pūs) a foreskin; a fold over the glans penis. 284, 312

presentation (pre″zən-ta′shən) in obstetrics that portion of the fetus that is touched by the examining finger through the cervix, or during labor, is bounded by the girdle of resistance. 300

> *breech p.* (brēch), presentation of the buttocks or feet of the fetus in labor. 300, 301f
> *cephalic p.* (sə-fal′ik), presentation of any part of the fetal head in labor, including occiput, brow, or face. 300, 301f
> *shoulder p.* (shōl′dər), presentation of the fetal shoulder in labor. 300, 301f

primigravida (pri″mĭ-grav′ĭ-də) a woman who is pregnant for the first time. 298

primipara (pri-mip′ə-rə) a female who is bearing or has borne her first child. 299

proctalgia (prok-tal′jə) pain of the lower rectum. 223

proctoclysis (prok-tok′lĭ-sis) slow introduction of large quantities of liquid into the rectum. 245

proctodynia (prok″to-din′e-ə) pain of the rectum. 223

proctologist (prok-tol′ə-jist) a physician who specializes in diseases of the rectum. 223

proctopexy (prok′to-pek″se) the surgical fixation of the rectum to some other part. 223

proctoplasty (prok′to-plas″te) plastic surgery of the rectum. 223

proctoplegia (prok″to-ple′jə) paralysis of the rectum. 223

proctoptosis (prok″top-to′sis) sagging of the rectum. 223

proctorrhagia (prok″to-ra′jə) hemorrhage from the rectum. 234

proctorrhaphy (prok-tor′ə-fe) suture of the rectum for the purpose of repair. 223

proctoscope (prok′to-skōp) the instrument used to examine the rectum. 223

proctoscopy (prok-tos′kə-pe) examination of the rectum. 223

progesterone (pro-jes′tə-rōn) the hormone produced by corpus luteum in the ovaries, adrenal cortex, and placenta. It prepares and maintains the uterus during pregnancy. 289, 291

progestin (pro-jes′tin) the name originally given to the hormone of the corpora lutea. The term is now used for synthetic and naturally occurring progestational agents. 327

prognosis (prog-no′sis) prediction of the probable outcome of a disease. 303

prolactin (pro-lak′tin) one of the hormones of the anterior pituitary gland that stimulates lactation in postpartum mammals. 472, 476

prolapse (pro-laps′) dropping or sagging of a body part. 135

pronation (pro-na′shən) assuming the prone position, or being prone (lying face downward). Applied to the hand, the act of turning the palm backward or downward. 60, 366f, 367

prone (prōn) lying face downward. 60

prophylaxis (pro″fə-lak′sis) protection against disease. 91

prostaglandin (pros″tə-glan′din) any of a group of components derived from unsaturated 20-carbon fatty acids. They are extremely potent mediators of a diverse group of physiologic processes. 487

prostate (pros′tāt) a gland that surrounds the neck of the bladder and the urethra in the male. 312, 313

prostatectomy (pros″tə-tek′tə-me) surgical removal of the prostate or part of it. 319

prostatic (pros-tat′ik) pertaining to the prostate. 313

prostatitis (pros″tə-ti′tis) inflammation of the prostate. 318

prosthesis (pros-the′sis) an artificial substitute for a missing body part, such as an arm or leg, eye or tooth, used for functional or cosmetic reasons, or both. 317

protease (pro′te-ās) a proteolytic enzyme. 199

proteinase (pro′tēn-ās) an enzyme that breaks down proteins. 199

proteinuria (pro″te-nu′re-ə) the presence of protein in urine. 199, 269

proteolysis (pro″te-ol′ĭ-sis) the breaking down of proteins into simpler components by means of enzymes. 199

proteuria (pro″te-u′re-ə) protein in the urine; proteinuria. 199

protozoon (pro″to-zo′on) a primitive animal organism consisting of a single cell. 323

proximal (prok′sĭ-məl) nearest the origin or point of attachment. 46

pruritus (proo-ri′təs) itching; an unpleasant skin sensation that provokes the desire to scratch to obtain relief. 451

pseudesthesia (soo″dəs-the′zhə) a sensation occurring in the absence of the appropriate stimuli; an imaginary sensation. 418, 423

pseudocyesis (soo″do-si-e′sis) false pregnancy. 296

pseudogout (soo″do-gout) an arthritic condition marked by attacks of goutlike symptoms, usually affecting a single joint. 358, 359t

pseudomania (soo″do-ma′ne-ə) false or pretended mental disorder; a mental disorder in which the patient admits to crimes of which he is innocent. 421

pseudoplegia (soo″do-ple′jə) hysterical paralysis; apparent loss of muscle power without real paralysis. 421

psoriasis (sə-ri′ə-sis) a common chronic dermatosis, marked by exacerbations and remissions and having a polygenic inheritance pattern. 445, 446f, 448f

psychiatric (si″ke-at′rik) pertaining to or within the purview of psychiatry. 26, 420

psychiatrist (si-ki′ə-trist) a physician who specializes in psychiatry. 26

psychiatry (si-ki′ə-tre) the branch of medicine that deals with the recognition and treatment of mental disorders. 26, 420

psychoanalysis (si″ko-ə-nal′ĭ-sis) a method of diagnosing and treating mental and emotional disorders by ascertaining and studying the facts of the patient's mental life. 420

psychobiologic (si″ko-bi″o-loj′ik) pertaining to the study of the biological aspects of mental processes. 421

psychologist (si-kol′ə-jist) one who specializes in the science that deals with the mind and mental processes. 420

> *clinical p.* (klin′ĭ-kəl), a psychologist who uses psychological knowledge and techniques in the treatment of people who have emotional difficulties. 26

psychology (si-kol′ə-je) the branch of science that deals with the mind and mental operations, especially as they are shown in behavior. 26

> *clinical p.* (klin′ĭ-kəl), the use of psychological knowledge and techniques in the treatment of emotional difficulties. 26

psychopharmacology (si″ko-fahr″mə-kol′ə-je) the study of drugs that affect the mind. 420

psychophysiologic (si″ko-fiz″e-o-loj′ik) pertaining to physiologic psychology. 57

psychosis (si-ko′sis) any major mental disorder of organic or emotional origin characterized by derangement of the personality and loss of contact with reality. 53

psychosomatic (si″ko-so-mat′ik) pertaining to the mind-body relationship; having body symptoms of emotional origin. 57

psychotherapy (si″ko-ther′ə-pe) treatment of functional nervous disorders that uses psychological methods. 420

ptosis (to′sis) prolapse of an organ or part; drooping of the upper eyelid from paralysis of the third nerve or from sympathetic innervation. 163

puberty (pu′bər-te) the period during which the secondary sex characteristics begin to develop and the capability for sexual reproduction is attained. 287

pubes (pu′bēz) the hairs growing over the pubic region; the pubic region. 349

pubic (pu′bik) pertaining to the pubis, a bone of the pelvis. 349

pubis (pu′bis) the anterior portion of the hip bone. 284

pubofemoral (pu″bo-fem″ə-rəl) pertaining to the pubis and the femur. 352

pulmonary (pool′mo-nar″e) pertaining to the lungs. 108, 116

> *p. edema* (ə-de′mə), effusion of fluid into the air spaces and tissues spaces of the lungs. 175

pulmonic (pəl-mon′ik) pertaining to the lungs. 174

pulse (puls) the rhythmic expansion of an artery that may be felt with a finger. 128

> *p. rate* (rāt), the number of pulsations of an artery per minute. 128

Purkinje's fibers (pər-kin′jēz fi′bərz) modified cardiac fibers that constitute the terminal ramifications of the conducting system of the heart. 171

purulence (pu′roo-ləns) condition consisting of pus or containing pus. 450

pus (pus) a product of inflammation, composed of leukocytes, cellular debris, and fluid. 94

pustule (pus′tūl) a visible collection of pus within or beneath the epidermis, often in a hair follicle or sweat pore. 444

pyelitis (pi″ə-li′tis) inflammation of the renal pelvis. 255

pyelogram (pi′ə-lo-gram) the record produced after the kidney and the ureter have been rendered opaque in pyelography. 257

> *intravenous p.* (in″trə-ve′nəs), a pyelogram after intravenous injection of a radiopaque material. 257

pyelography (pi″ə-log′rə-fe) radiography of the renal pelvis and ureter after injection of a contrast medium. 257

pyelolithotomy (pi″ə-lo-lĭ thot′ə-me) excision of a renal calculus from the pelvis of the kidney. 257

pyelonephritis (pi″ə-lo-nə-fri′tis) inflammation of the kidney and its accompanying renal pelvis. 252

pyeloplasty (pi′ə-lo-plas″te) plastic repair of the renal pelvis. 257

pyelostomy (pi′ə-los′tə-me) formation of an opening into the renal pelvis for diversion of urine from the ureter. 257

pyloric (pi-lor′ik) pertaining to the pylorus or the pyloric part of the stomach. 210
 p. sphincter (sfingk′tər) the thickened muscle at the lower end of the stomach that regulates flow of food into the duodenum. 215
pyloromyotomy (pi-lor″o-mi-ot′ə-me) incision of the muscles of the pylorus. 215
pyloroplasty (pi-lor′o-plas″te) plastic surgery to relieve pyloric obstruction or to accelerate gastric emptying. 215
pyloroscopy (pi″lor-os′kə-pe) endoscopic inspection of the pylorus. 215
pylorostenosis (pi-lor″o-stə-no′sis) a narrowing of the caliber of the pylorus. 215
pylorotomy (pi″lor-ot′o me) surgical incision of the pylorus. 215
pylorus (pi-lor′əs) the opening betwen the stomach and the duodenum. 210
pyodermatitis (pi″o-der″mə-ti′tis) a skin infection in which pus is produced. 462
pyogenesis (pi″o-jen′ə-sis) formation of pus. 450
pyogenic (pi″o-jen′ik) producing pus. 450
pyonephrosis (pi″o-nə-fro′sis) purulent inflammation of the kidney. 252
pyorrhea (pi″o-re′ə) a discharge of pus. 207
pyothorax (pi″o-tho′raks) accumulation of pus in the chest cavity. 184
pyrexia (pi-rek′se-ə) a fever or febrile condition. 61, 442
pyrogen (pi′ro-jən) a fever-producing substance. 61
pyromania (pi″ro-ma′ne-ə) an abnormal preoccupation concerning fire.
pyromaniac (pi″ro-ma′ne-ak) one affected with a compulsion to set fires. 421
pyrophobia (pi″ro-fo′be-ə) an abnormal fear of fire. 421
pyuria (pi-u′re-ə) the presence of pus in the urine. 269

quadrant (kwod′rənt) any one of four corresponding parts or quarters, as of the abdominal surface. 49, 50f
quadripara (kwod-rip′ə-re) a woman who has had four pregnancies that resulted in viable offspring. 299
quadriplegia (kwod″rĭ-ple′jə) paralysis of all four extremities. 407

rabies (ra′bēz) hydrophobia, an acute viral disease of the central nervous system, usually spread by contamination with virus-laden saliva of bites inflicted by rabid animals. 423
rachialgia (ra″ke-al′jə) pain in the spine. 346
rachiodynia (ra″ke-o-din′e-ə) pain of the vertebral column. 346
rachischisis (ra′kis′kĭ-sis) split spine; spina bifida. 371
rachitis (ra-ki′tis) rickets; inflammatory disease of the vertebral column.
radiogram (ra′de-o-gram″) a radiograph; film produced in radiography. 458
radiograph (ra′de-o-graf″) a film produced by radiography. 458
radioisotope (ra″de-o-i′sə-tōp) a radioactive isotope; an isotope that has an unstable nucleus and emits characteristic radiation during decay to a stable form. 479
radiologic (ra″de-o-loj′ik) having to do with radiology; having to do with radiant energy. 31
 r. technologist (tek-nol′ə-jist), one who specializes in the use of x-rays and radioactive isotopes in the diagnosis and treatment of disease and who works under the supervision of a radiologist. 31
radiological (ra″de-o-loj′ĭ-kəl) pertaining to radiology. 31, 104
radiologist (ra″de-ol′ə-jist) a physician who uses roentgen rays, radium, and other forms of radiant energy in the diagnosis and treatment of disease. 25, 31
radiology (ra″de-ol′ə-je) the science concerned with the use of various forms of radiant energy in the diagnosis and treatment of disease. 25, 31
radiopaque (ra″de-o-pāk′) impervious to x-ray or other forms of radiation. 25, 339
radiopharmaceutical (ra″de-o-fahr″mə-soo′tĭ-kəl) a radioactive pharmaceutical or chemical used for diagnostic or therapeutic purposes. 36
radius (ra′de-əs) in anatomy the bone of the thumb side of the forearm. 343
rale (rahl) an abnormal nonmusical respiratory sound heard in some pathological conditions. 171
reabsorption (re″əb-sorp′shən) the act or process of absorbing again, as the selective absorption by the kidneys of substances (glucose, proteins, sodium, etc.) already secreted into the renal tubules, and their return to the circulating blood. 255
receptor (re-sep′tər) a sensory nerve ending that responds to various stimuli. 409
rectocele (rek′to-sēl) hernia of the rectum, with protrusion of part of the rectum into the vagina. 223, 261f
rectoclysis (rek-tok′lĭ-sis) proctoclysis; slow introduction of large quantities of liquid into the rectum.
rectoplasty (rek′to-plas″te) surgical repair of the rectum. 234
rectorrhaphy (rek′tor-ə-fe) suture of the rectum for the purpose of repair. 223, 234
rectoscope (rek′to-skōp) proctoscope; a tubular instrument with illumination for inspecting the rectum. 223
rectoscopy (rek-tos′kə-pe) inspection of the lower part of the intestine with a proctoscope; proctoscopy. 223
rectourethral (rek″to-u-re′thrəl) pertaining to the rectum and urethra. 262
rectovaginal (rek″to vaj′ĭ nal) pertaining to the rectum and vagina. 311
rectum (rek′təm) the distal portion of the large intestine. 203

reduction (re-duk′shən) pulling the broken ends of a fractured bone into alignment. 371
 closed r., restoring a fractured bone to its normal position by manipulation without surgery. 371
 open r., exposing a fractured bone by surgery to realign it. 371
rejection (re-jek′shən) an immune reaction against transplanted tissue. 92
renal (re′nəl) pertaining to the kidney. 249
 r. dialysis (di-al′ə-sis), diffusion of blood across a semipermeable membrane to remove materials that would normally by removed by the kidneys if they were present or were functioning properly. 250
 r. failure (fal′yər), inadequate functioning of the kidneys, which leads to uremia. 252, 254
 r. pelvis (pel′vis), a funnel-shaped cavity in the kidney that collects urine from many nephrons. 252
 r. transplant (trans′plant), replacement of a diseased kidney with a healthy one from a donor. 249
 r. tubule (too′būl), the part of a nephron in which urine forms. 254
renovascular (re″no-vas′ku-lər) pertaining to or affecting the blood vessels of the kidney. 252
resection (re-sek′shən) removal of a portion of an organ or other structure.
respiration (res″pī-ra′shən) the exchange of oxygen and carbon dioxide between the atmosphere and the cells of the body; the metabolic processes in living cells by which molecular oxygen is taken in, organic substances are oxidized, free energy is released, and carbon dioxide, water, and other oxidized products are given off by the cell. 155, 163f
respiratory (res″pī-rə-tor″e) pertaining to respiration. 155
 r. distress syndrome (dis-tres′ sin′drōm), a condition of newborns formerly known as hyaline membrane disease, marked by dyspnea and cyanosis. 177, 178t
resuscitation (re-sus″-ĭ-ta′shən) restoration of life to one who is apparently dead or whose respiration has ceased. 129
 cardiopulmonary r. (kahr″de-o-pul′mə-nar-e), an emergency first aid procedure to reestablish heart and lung action, consisting of external heart massage and artificial respiration. 129
retention (re-ten′shən) the process of keeping in position, as the persistent keeping within the body of matters normally excreted or the maintaining of a dental prosthesis in proper position in the mouth. 270
retinoid (ret′ĭ-noid) resembling the retina; retinol, retinal, or any structurally similar natural derivative or synthetic compound. 441
retinopathy (ret″ĭ-nop′ə-the) any disease of the retina. 412
retrocecal (ret″ro-se′kəl) behind the cecum. 235
retrocolic (ret″ro-kol′ik) behind the large intestine. 235
retroflexion (ret″ro-flek′shən) the bending of an organ so that its top is turned backward; the bending of the body of the uterus toward the cervix. 310f
retromammary (ret″ro mam′ər-e) behind the breast. 474
retronasal (ret″ro-na′zəl) behind the nose. 185
retroperitoneal (ret″ro-per″ĭ-to-ne′əl) behind the peritoneum. 235
retrosternal (ret″ro-ster′nəl) situated or occurring behind the breastbone. 376
retroversion (ret″ro-ver′zhən) the tipping of an entire organ backward. 310f
rheumatism (roo′mə-tiz-əm) any of a variety of disorders marked by inflammation, degeneration, or metabolic derangement of the connective tissue structures of the body, especially the joints and related structures. 28
rheumatoid arthritis (roo′mə-toid ahr-thri′tis) a chronic systemic disease characterized by inflamed joints and related structures that often results in crippling deformities. 357, 359t
rheumatologist (roo″mə-tol′ə-jist) a specialist in rheumatic conditions. 27
rheumatology (roo″mə-tol′ə-je) the branch of medicine dealing with rheumatic disorders. 22, 28
rhinitis (ri-ni′tis) inflammation of the mucous membranes of the nose. 165
rhinodacryolith (ri″no-dak′re-o-lith″) a tear stone in the nasal duct. 414
rhinolith (ri′no-lith) a calculus or stone in the nose. 165, 166
rhinolithiasis (ri″no-lĭ-thi′ə-sis) a condition marked by the presence of nasal calculi or stones. 165
rhinoplasty (ri′no-plas″te) plastic surgery of the nose. 165
rhinorrhagia (ri″no-ra′je-ə) nosebleed. 184
rhinorrhea (ri″no-re′ə) a discharge from the nose; a runny nose. 165
rhytidoplasty (rit′ĭ-do-plas″te) plastic surgery to eliminate wrinkles from the facial skin by excising loose or redundant tissue. 438
rib (rib) any one of the paired bones, 12 on either side, forming the major part of the thoracic skeleton. 347f
 false r., one of the five ribs on each side of the body that is not attached to the sternum. 347f
 floating r., one of the last two pairs of false ribs, so called because it is attached only on the posterior side. 347f
 true r., the upper seven ribs on each side, which directly join the sternum. 347f
rickets (rik′əts) a condition caused by a deficiency of vitamin D, especially in infancy and childhood, with disturbance of normal ossification. 373
roentgen (rent′gen) the international unit of x-ray. 25
roentgenology (rent″gən-ol′ə-je) the branch of radiology that deals with x-rays. 25

rubella (roo-bel′ə) an acute but usually benign infectious viral infection usually affecting children and nonimmune young adults; also called German measles and three-day measles. 451t

rubeola (roo-be′o-lə, roo-be-o′lə) the measles; a highly contagious viral disease, common among children who have not been immunized. 451t

rugae (roo′je) ridges, wrinkles, or folds, as of mucous membranes. 210

sacral (sa′krəl) pertaining to the sacrum, the triangular bone below the lumbar vertebrae. 346

sacrodynia (sa″kro-din′e-ə) pain in the sacrum, the triangular bone below the lumbar vertebrae. 346

sacrum (sa′krəm) the triangular bone at the base of the spine. 346

sagittal (saj′ĭ-təl) shaped like an arrow; denotes a plane that is parallel to the midsagittal line vertically dividing the body into right and left portions. 48

saliva (sə-li′və) the clear, alkaline, somewhat viscid secretion from the salivary glands of the mouth. 227

salivary (sal′ĭ-var-e) pertaining to saliva. 227
  s. gland (gland), any of several glands of the oral cavity that produce saliva. 227

salpingectomy (sal″pin-jek′tə-me) excision of a uterine tube. 282, 308

salpingitis (sal″pin-ji′tis) inflammation of a uterine tube. 308

salpingocele (sal-ping′go-sēl) hernial protrusion of a uterine tube. 308

salpingo-oophorectomy (sal-ping″go-o″of-ə-rek′tə-me) surgical removal of a uterine tube and an ovary. 305

salpingopexy (sal-ping′go-pek″se) surgical fixation of a uterine tube. 308

salpingorrhaphy (sal″ping-gor′ə-fe) suture of the uterine tube. 308

salpingostomy (sal″ping gos′tə-me) formation of an opening into a uterine tube for the purpose of drainage; surgical restoration of the patency of a uterine tube. 308

sarcoma (sahr-ko′mə) any of a group of tumors usually arising from connective tissue, although the term now includes some of epithelial origin; most are malignant. 142

scabicide (ska′bĭ-sīd) used in the treatment of scabies; an agent for destroying the itch mite. 461

scabies (ska′bēz) a contagious dermatitis of humans and various wild and domestic animals caused by the itch mite. 455

scan (skan) shortened form of *scintiscan,* as brain scan, thyroid scan, etc; a visual display of ultrasonographic echoes. 347, 400f, 479

scapula (skap′u-lə) the shoulder blade, the flat triangular bone in the back of the shoulder. 343, 349

scapular (skap′u-lər) of or pertaining to the scapula. 349

scapuloclavicular (skap″u-lo-klə-vik′u-lər) pertaining to the scapula and the clavicle. 350

scarlet fever (skahr′lət fe′vər) infection with group A streptococci that varies in intensity and is characterized by pharyngitis, tonsillitis, increased body temperature, and a rash that eventually disappears, followed by shedding of dead skin cells. 451t

schizophrenia (skiz″o-fre′ne-ə, skit″so-fre′ne-ə) a mental disorder or group of disorders comprising most major psychotic disorders and characterized by disturbances in form and content of thought, mood, and sense of self and relationship to the external world and behavior. 422

sciatic nerve (si-at′ik nerv) the largest nerve in the body, arising in the pelvis and passing down the back of the leg. 398

sciatica (si-at′ĭ-kə) a syndrome characterized by pain radiating from the back into the buttock and into the lower extremity along its posterior or lateral aspect; pain anywhere along the course of the sciatic nerve. 398

scleroderma (sklēr″o-der′mə) chronic hardening and thickening of the skin. 358, 455

scleroprotein (sklēr″o-pro′tēn) a protein that is characterized by its insolubility and fibrous structure. 435

sclerosis (sklə-ro′sis) hardening, chiefly applied to hardening of the nervous system or to hardening of the blood vessels. 119
  multiple s. (mul′tĭ-pəl), a chronic disease of the central nervous system in which there is development of disseminated glial patches called plaques. 408
  progressive systemic s. (pro-gres′iv sis-tem′ik), a systemic disorder of the connective tissue characterized by induration and thickening of the skin, by abnormalities involving both the microvasculature (telangiectasia) and larger vessels (Raynaud's phenomenon), and by fibrotic degenerative changes in various body organs, including the heart, lungs, kidneys, and gastrointestinal tract. 359t

sclerotic (sklə-rot′ik) hard or hardening; affected with sclerosis. 408

scoliosis (sko″le-o′sis) lateral curvature of the vertebral column. 371

scrotal (skro′təl) pertaining to the scrotum. 312

scrotum (skro′təm) the pouch that contains the testes and their accessory organs. 312

sebaceous (sə-ba′shəs) pertaining to sebum or secreting sebum. 440
  s. gland (gland), oil-secreting gland of the skin. 440-441

seborrhea (seb″o-re′ə) excessive secretion of sebum; seborrheic dermatitis. 436

seborrheic (seb″o-re′ik) affected with seborrhea. 436
  s. dermatitis (der″mə-ti′tis), an inflammatory condition of the skin caused by overactive sebaceous glands. 436, 437f

sebum (se′bəm) the oily material secreted by a sebaceous gland. 436

secundipara (se″kən-dip′ə-rə) a woman who has had two pregnancies that resulted in viable offspring. 299

sedative (sed′ə-tiv) allaying activity and excitement; an agent that allays excitement. 425

semen (se′mən) fluid consisting of gland secretions and sperm, discharged at ejaculation. 313

semicoma (sem″ĭ-ko′mə) a mild coma from which the patient can be aroused. 405

semiconscious (sem″ĭ-kon′shəs) only partially aware of one's surroundings. 405

semilunar (sem″ĭ-loo′nər) resembling a half-moon. 116

seminal (sem′ĭ nəl) pertaining to semen. 315
  s. fluid (floo′id), semen; the fluid discharged from the penis at the height of sexual excitement. 315

seminiferous tubules (sem″ĭ-nif′ər-əs too′būlz) channels in the testis in which the spermatozoa develop. 314

semipermeable (sem″ĭ-per′me-ə-bəl) permitting passage of only certain molecules. 405

sensory (sen′sə-re) pertaining to sensation. 390, 394f
  s. nerve cells (nerv selz), cells of the afferent nervous system that pick up stimuli. 390, 394f

sepsis (sep′sis) a poisoned state caused by bacteria. 453

septal (sep′təl) pertaining to a septum. 113

septemia (sep-te′me-ə) septicemia. 86t, 453

septicemia (sep″tĭ-se′me-ə) a morbid condition caused by the presence of bacteria or their toxins in the blood. 86t, 453

septum (sep′təm) a dividing wall or partition. 113
  cardiac s. (kahr′de-ak), the membranous partition that divides the left and the right side of the heart. 113
  nasal s. (na′zəl), the partition between the two nasal cavities. 164

serosa (sēr-o′sə, sēr-o′zə) any serous membrane; the chorion. 210, 217

serotonin (ser″o-to′nin) a vasoconstrictor, found in various animals, in bacteria, and in many plants. It has many physiologic properties. 393

shock (shok) a sudden disturbance of mental equilibrium; a condition of profound hemodynamic and metabolic disturbance characterized by failure of the circulatory system to maintain adequate perfusion of vital organs. 135

shunt (shunt) to turn to one side, divert, or bypass; a passage or anastomosis between two natural channels, especially between blood vessels. 93

sialadenitis (si″əl-ad″ə-ni′tis) inflammation of a salivary gland. 227

sialitis (si″ə-li′tis) inflammation of a salivary gland or duct. 227

sialography (si″ə-log′rə-fe) radiographic demonstration of the salivary glands after injection of radiopaque substances. 227

sialolith (si-al′o-lith) a chalky concretion or calculus in the salivary ducts or glands. 227

sickle cell (sik″əl sel) abnormal red blood cell that has a crescent shape. 84

sigmoid (sig′moid) having the shape of the letter *S* or *C;* the sigmoid colon. 222

sigmoidoscope (sig′moi′do-skōp) a rigid or flexible endoscope with appropriate illumination for examining the sigmoid colon. 222

sigmoidoscopy (sig″moi-dos′kə-pe) inspection of the sigmoid colon through a sigmoidoscope. 222

sign (sīn) an indication of the existence of something as opposed to the subjective sensations (symptoms) of the patient. 28

silicosis (sil″ĭ-ko′sis) pneumoconiosis caused by inhalation of the dust of stone, sand, or flint containing silicon dioxide, with formation of generalized nodular fibrotic changes in both lungs. 177

sinoatrial (si″no-a′tre-əl) pertaining to the sinus venosus and the atrium of the heart. 116
  s. node (nōd), a node in the wall of the right atrium that is the source of impulses that initiate the heartbeat. 116, 128

sinus (si′nəs) a recess, cavity, or channel. 165
  paranasal s. (par-e″nā′zəl), one of several cavities that communicate with the nasal cavity and are lined with a mucous membrane. 165

sinusitis (si″nə si′tis) inflammation of a sinus. 165

Sjögren's syndrome (shər′grenz sin′drōm) a symptom complex of unknown etiology, usually occurring in middle-aged or older women, marked by keratoconjunctivitis, xerostomia, and the presence of a connective tissue disease, usually rheumatoid arthritis but sometimes systemic lupus erythematosus, scleroderma, or polymyositis. 359t

skin cancer (skin kan′sər) cancer that arises on the surface of the body and manifests as a small ulcer, pimple, or mole. 179, 449, 450f

somatic (so-mat′ik) pertaining to the body. 56

somatogenic (so″mə-to-jen′ik) originating in the cells of the body. 56

somatomegaly (so″mə-to-meg′ə-le) increased size of the body; gigantism. 57

somatopsychic (so″mə-to-si′kik) pertaining to both body and mind, denoting a physical disorder that produces mental symptoms. 57

somatotropic (so″mə-to-trop′ik) having an affinity for or stimulating the body or the body cells; having a stimulating effect on body nutrition and growth; having the properties of somatotropin. 475

superior (soo-pe′re-or) situated above, or directed upward. 46

supination (soo″pĭ-na′shən) the act of assuming the supine position, or the state of being supine. Applied to the hand, the act of turning the palm forward or upward. 60, 366f, 367

supine (soo′pīn) lying with the face upward. 60

supracostal (soo″prə-kos′təl) above or outside the ribs. 376

suprahepatic (soo″prə-hə-pat′ik) above the liver. 235

supranasal (soo″prə-na′səl) above the nose. 185

suprapelvic (soo″prə-pel′vik) above the pelvis. 376

suprapubic (soo″prə-pu′bik) above the pubes. 271, 376

suprarenal (soo″prə-re′nəl) above the kidney. 271, 480

suprasternal (soo″prə-ster′nəl) above the breastbone. 345, 376

suprathoracic (soo″prə-thor-as′ik) above the chest. 62

supratonsillar (soo″prə-ton′sĭ-lər) above the tonsil. 143

suppuration (sup″u-ra′shən) forming pus; the act of discharging pus. 450

surgery (sur′jər-e) the branch of medicine that treats diseases, injuries, and deformities by manual or operative methods; the place in a hospital where surgery is performed. 21

  general s. (jen′ər-əl), surgery that deals with operations of all kinds. 21

  oral s. (or′əl), the branch of medicine that deals with surgical treatment of diseases, injuries, and defects of the mouth, jaws, and associated structures. 21, 22

  plastic s. (plas′tik), surgery that is concerned with restoration, reconstruction, correction, or improvement in the shape and appearance of body structures. 21

  reconstructive s. (re″kən-struk′tiv), plastic surgery. 21

surgical (sur′jĭ-kəl) of, pertaining to, or correctable by surgery. 21

  s. pathology (pə-thol′ə-je), the pathology of disease processes that are surgically accessible for diagnosis or treatment. 18

susceptibility (sə-sep″tĭ-bil′ĭ-te) a state of vulnerability, readily affected or acted upon, such as a diminished immunity to infection. 89

suture (soo′chər) the act of uniting a wound by stitches; a type of joint in which the opposed surfaces are closely united, as in the skull; material used in closing a surgical or traumatic wound with stitches; a stitch or stitches made to secure the edges of a wound. 212, 213

sympathectomy (sim″pə-thek′tə-me) transection, resection, or other interruption of some portion of the sympathetic nervous pathways. 410

sympathetic (sim″pə-thet′ik) a sympathetic nerve or the sympathetic nervous system; pertaining to sympathy. 410

symphysis pubis (sim′fĭ-sis pu′bis) the joint formed by union of the bodies of the pubic bones. 284

symptom (simp′təm) any subjective evidence of disease or of a patient's condition. 28

symptomatic (simp″to-mat′ik) pertaining to or of the nature of a symptom. 34

symptothermal (simp″to-thər′məl) pertaining to symptoms and change in body temperature. 293

  s. contraceptive method (kon″trə-sep′tiv meth′əd), a natural method of family planning that incorporates ovulation and basal body temperature. 293

synapse (sin′aps) the junction between two neurons. 392

syncope (sing′kə-pe) a temporary loss of consciousness owing to generalized cerebral ischemia; a faint. 79

syndactylism, syndactyly (sin-dak′tə-liz-əm, sin-dak′tə-le) a congenital anomaly characterized by the fusion of the fingers or toes. 377

syndrome (sin′drōm) a set of symptoms that occur together and collectively characterize or indicate a particular disease or abnormal condition. 177

  adrenogenital s. (ə-dre″no-jen′ĭ-təl), a general term for the group of syndromes in which inappropriate virilism or feminization results from disorders of adrenal function that also affect gonadal steroidogenesis. 482

  carpal tunnel s. (kahr′pəl tun′əl), a complex of symptoms resulting from compression of the median nerve in the carpal tunnel. 375

  Down s. (doun), a chromosome disorder characterized by a small, anteroposteriorly flattened skull; short, flat-bridge nose; epicanthal fold; short phalanges; widened spaces between the first and second digits of hands and feet; and moderate to severe mental retardation; called also trisomy 21 (formerly called mongolism). 296

  irritable bowel s. (ir′ĭ-tə-bəl bou′əl), a chronic, noninflammatory disease characterized by abdominal pain, altered bowel habits consisting of diarrhea or constipation or both, and no detectable pathological change; also called irritable colon syndrome. 225

  malabsorption s. (mal″əb-sorp′shən), a group of disorders in which there is decreased absorption of dietary constituents and thus excessive loss of non-absorbed substances in the stool. 225

  Meniere's s. (men″e-ārz′), a recurrent and usually progressive group of symptoms including progressive deafness, ringing in the ears, dizziness, and a sensation of fullness or pressure in the ears. 418

  Sjögren's s. (shər′grenz) a symptom complex, usually occurring in middle-aged or older women, marked by keratoconjunctivitis sicca, xerostomia, and the presence of a connective tissue disease, usually rheumatoid arthritis. 359t

  sudden infant death s. (sə-dən in′fənt deth), sudden and unexpected death of an apparently healthy infant that is not explained by careful postmortem studies. 178

  tarsal tunnel s. (tahr′səl tun′əl), a complex of symptoms resulting from compression of a nerve in the tarsal tunnel, with pain, numbness, and a tingling sensation of the sole of the foot. 375

synovial (sĭ-no′ve-əl) pertaining to, consisting of, or secreting synovia, the lubricating fluid of the joints, bursae, and tendon sheaths. 355

synovitis (sin″o-vi′tis) inflammation of a synovial membrane. 357

syphilis (sif′ĭ-lis) a sexually transmitted disease caused by *Treponema pallidum*, which is characterized by lesions that may involve any organ or tissue. 268f, 321

  congenital s. (kən-jen′ĭ-təl), syphilis acquired in utero and manifested by any of several characteristic malformations and by neurologic changes and active mucocutaneous syphilis at the time of birth or shortly afterward. 321

systemic (sis-tem′ik) pertaining to or affecting the body as a whole. 107

systole (sis′to-le) the contraction or period of contraction of the heart, especially of the ventricles. 126

systolic (sis′tol′ik) pertaining to or produced by the systole. 126

tachycardia (tak″ĭ-kahr′de-ə) fast heartbeat; fast pulse. 79, 128

tachyphasia (tak″ĭ-fa′zhə) fast speech. 183

tachypnea (tak″ip-ne′ə, tak″e-ne′ə) rapid breathing. 59

target organ the organ or structure toward which the effects of a drug or hormone are primarily directed. 468

tarsal (tahr′səl) pertaining to the tarsus of an eyelid or to the instep; any of the bones of the tarsus. 343, 375

tarsoptosis (tahr″sop-to′sis) falling of the tarsals; fallfoot; fallen arch. 353

tarsus (tahr′səs) the seven bones composing the articulation between the foot and the leg; also the cartilaginous plates of the eyelids. 353

telecardiogram (tel″ə-kahr′de-o-gram) a heart tracing that registers distant from the patient by means of electrical sending of the signal. 47

temporal (tem′pə-rəl) pertaining to the lateral region of the head. 397

temporomandibular (tem″pə-ro-mən-dib′u-lər) pertaining to the temporal bone and the mandible. 209, 378

tenalgia (te-nal′jə) pain in a tendon. 359

tendinitis (ten″dĭ-ni′tis) inflammation of tendons and tendon-muscle attachments. 358

tendon (ten′dən) a fibrous cord by which a muscle is attached. 355

tendonitis (ten″də-ni′tis) tendinitis; inflammation of a tendon. 358

tendoplasty (ten′do-plas″te) surgical repair of a tendon. 359

tenodynia (ten″o-din′e-ə) pain of a tendon. 359

tenomyoplasty (ten″o-mi′o-plas″te) surgical repair of a tendon and muscle. 368

tenorrhaphy (tə-nor′ə-fe) union of a divided tendon by a suture. 359

tenotomy (tə-not′ə-me) cutting of a tendon. 359

testalgia (tes-tal′jə) testicular pain.

testectomy (təs-tek′tə-me) surgical removal of a testicle.

testicular (tes tik′u lər) pertaining to a testicle. 312

testis (tes′tis) the male gonad; either of the egg-shaped glands located in the scrotum, in which sperm are formed. 312, 314, 468f

testosterone (təs-tos′tə-rōn) a hormone secreted by the testes that brings about induction and maintenance of male secondary sex characteristics. 314, 315

tetanus (tet′ə-nəs) an acute, often fatal, infectious disease caused by the anaerobic bacillus *Clostridium tetani*. The bacteria usually enter the body through a contaminated puncture wound. 408

tetany (tet′ə-ne) a nervous condition characterized by intermittent or continuous tonic muscle contractions involving the extremities. 367

tetraiodothyronine (tet″rə-i″o-do-thi′ro-nēn) thyroxine, a thyroid hormone. 478

thalamus (thal′ə-məs) the largest subdivision of the diencephalon. 397, 398f

therapeutic (ther″ə-pu′tik) pertaining to therapeutics or to therapy; curative. 30

therapist (ther′ə-pist) a person skilled in the treatment of disease or other disorder. 31

  physical t. (fiz′ĭ-kəl), one skilled in the techniques of physical therapy and qualified to administer treatments prescribed by a physician. 31

  respiratory t. (res′pĭ-rə-tor″e), one skilled in the techniques of respiratory therapy. 32

therapy (ther′ə-pe) treatment of disease. 31

  physical t. (fiz′ĭ-kəl), the use of physical agents and methods in rehabilitation and restoration of normal bodily function after illness or injury. 31

  respiratory t. (res′pĭ-rə-tor″e), the technical specialty concerned with the treatment of cardiopulmonary disorders. 32

thermolysis (thər-mol′ĭ-sis) destruction by heat.

thermoplegia (thər″mo-ple′jə) heatstroke or sunstroke. 442

thermoreceptor (thər″mo-re-sep′tor) a nerve ending, usually in the skin, that is sensitive to a change in temperature. 411